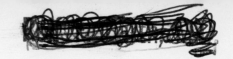

Nuclear Medicine
In Vitro

NUCLEAR MEDICINE
In Vitro

Edited by

Benjamin Rothfeld, M.D.

*Chief, Nuclear Medicine; Associate Chief of
Staff for Research and Education; Assistant
Chief, Medical Service, Veterans Administration
Hospital, Perry Point, Maryland
Assistant Professor of Medicine, The Johns Hopkins
University School of Medicine, Baltimore, Maryland*

J.B. Lippincott Company
Philadelphia and Toronto

ISBN 0-397-50320-2

Library of Congress Catalog Card Number 74-14921

Printed in the United States of America

1   3   5   4   2

Library of Congress Cataloging in Publication Data

Rothfeld, Benjamin
    Nuclear medicine—in vitro.
    Includes bibliographical references.
    1. Radioisotopes in medicine. I. Title.
[DNLM: 1. Nuclear medicine. WN440 R846n]
RM858.R67   616.07′575   74-14921
ISBN 0-397-50320-2

To Fil, Alan, Barbara and Debbie

Contributors

SOLOMON N. ALBERT, M.D.
Director, Anesthesiology Research Laboratory
Washington Hospital Center, Washington, D.C.

KITTI ANGSUSINGHA, M.D.
Fellow in Pediatric Endocrinology
The Children's Hospital of Pittsburgh
Pittsburgh, Pa.

GEORGE A. BELLER, M.D.
Cardiac Unit, Massachusetts General Hospital
Instructor in Medicine, Department of
Medicine, Harvard Medical School
Boston, Mass.

KEVIN CATT, M.D., PH.D.
Chief, Section on Hormonal Regulation
Reproduction Research Branch
National Institute of Child Health and
Human Development, National Institutes of
Health, Bethesda, Md.

GERARD CERNIAK, M.D.
Senior Resident in Medicine (Gastroenterology)
Veterans Administration Hospital, Hines, Ill.
Clinical Instructor in Medicine
Stritch School of Medicine, Loyola
University, Maywood, Ill.

FRANK H. DeLAND, M.D.
Chief of Nuclear Medicine
University of Kentucky Medical Center
Lexington, Ky.

JANICE DOUGLAS, M.D.
Senior Staff Fellow, Section on Hormonal
Regulation, Reproduction Research Branch
National Institute of Child Health and
Human Development, National Institutes of
Health, Bethesda, Md.

BEN I. FRIEDMAN, M.D.
Professor and Chairman, Department of
Nuclear Medicine, University of Tennessee
College of Medicine, Memphis, Tenn.

STANLEY J. GOLDSMITH, M.D.
Director, Andre Meyer Department of Physics
(Nuclear Medicine), Mount Sinai Hospital
Assistant Professor of Medicine, Mount
Sinai School of Medicine of the City
University of New York

CARLOS R. HAMILTON, JR., M.D.
Clinical Assistant Professor
Endocrine Division, Department of Internal
Medicine, Baylor College of Medicine
Houston, Tex.

VICTOR HERBERT, M.D., J.D.
Clinical Professor of Pathology and Medicine
College of Physicians and Surgeons
Columbia University, Chief, Hematology
and Nutrition Laboratory
Bronx Veterans Administration Hospital
New York, N.Y.

CHARLES S. HOLLANDER, M.D.
Chief, Endocrine Division,
Department of Medicine and
Director, Special Clinical Unit,
School of Medicine, New York University
Medical Center

T. H. HSU, M.D.
Assistant Professor of Medicine, The Johns
Hopkins University School of Medicine
Baltimore, Md.

ARTHUR KARMEN, M.D.
Chairman, Department of Laboratory Medicine
Albert Einstein College of Medicine
Bronx, N.Y.

FREDERIC M. KENNY, M.D.
Professor of Pediatrics
University of Pittsburgh School of Medicine
and The Children's Hospital of Pittsburgh
Pittsburgh, Pa.

MARVIN A. KIRSCHNER, M.D.
Director of Medicine and Professor
of Medicine, Newark Beth Israel
Medical Center, New Jersey Medical School
Newark, N.J.

ARTHUR KLEIN, M.D.
Director, Departments of Nuclear Medicine
Norwood Hospital, Norwood, Mass. and Glover
Memorial Hospital, Needham, Mass.

IONE A. KOURIDES, M.D.
Thyroid Unit, Assistant in Medicine
Massachusetts General Hospital
Instructor in Medicine, Harvard Medical School
Boston, Mass.

HENRY KRAMER, PH.D.
Senior Group Leader, Clinical Diagnostics
Union Carbide Corporation, Tarrytown
Technical Center, Tarrytown, N.Y.

STEVEN V. LARSON, M.D.
Assistant Professor of Radiology
Instructor in Medicine and Assistant
Professor of Environmental Health,
The Johns Hopkins University School of
Medicine, Baltimore, Md.

A. M. LAWRENCE, M.D.
Associate Chief of Staff/Education
Veterans Administration Hospital, Hines, Ill.
Professor of Medicine
Stritch School of Medicine
Loyola University, Maywood, Ill.

FARAHE MALOOF, M.D.
Chief, Thyroid Unit
Massachusetts General Hospital
Associate Professor of Medicine, Harvard
Medical School, Boston, Mass.

J. M. MENEFEE, M.A.
President, Bicron Corporation,
Newbury, Ohio

THOMAS J. MERIMEE, M.D.
Head, Division of Endocrinology
University of Florida School of Medicine
Gainesville, Fla.

JONATHAN P. MILLER, PH.D.
Director, Scientific Affairs, Abbott
Diagnostics Division, Abbott Laboratories
North Chicago, Ill.

RALPH M. MYERSON, M.D.
Veterans Administration Hospital
Philadelphia, Pa.

LACY R. OVERBY, PH.D.
Director, Division of Experimental Biology
Abbott Laboratories, North Chicago, Ill.

THADDEUS PROUT, M.D.
Associate Professor of Medicine
The Johns Hopkins University School
of Medicine, Baltimore, Md.

DAVID RABINOWITZ, M.D.
Head of Department of Chemical Endocrinology
Hadassah University Hospital and Hebrew
University Medical School, Jerusalem, Israel
Currently Visiting Scientist, Diabetes Branch
National Institutes of Arthritis, Metabolism,
and Digestive Diseases, National Institutes of
Health, Bethesda, Md.

JOSEPH L. RABINOWITZ, PH.D.
Chief, Radioisotope Research
Veterans Administration Hospital
Philadelphia, Pa.

E. CHESTER RIDGWAY, M.D.
Thyroid Unit
Assistant in Medicine, Massachusetts
General Hospital; Instructor in Medicine
Harvard Medical School, Boston, Mass.

BENJAMIN ROTHFELD, M.D.
Chief, Nuclear Medicine, Veterans
Administration Hospital, Perry Point, Md.
Assistant Professor of Medicine,
The Johns Hopkins University School of
Medicine, Baltimore, Md.

LOUIS SHENKMAN, M.D.
Endocrine Division, Department of Medicine
School of Medicine, New York University
Medical Center, New York, N.Y.

THOMAS W. SMITH, M.D.
Cardiac Unit, Massachusetts General Hospital
Associate Professor of Medicine, Department
of Medicine, Harvard Medical School
Boston, Mass.

MALCOLM M. STANLEY, M.D.
Section Chief, Gastroenterology
Veterans Administration Hospital, Hines, Ill.
Professor of Medicine, Abraham Lincoln
School of Medicine, University of Illinois,
Chicago, Ill.

RONALD STEELE, PH.D.
Assistant Professor of Pediatrics, The Johns
Hopkins University School of Medicine
Baltimore, Md.

JOHN H. WALSH, M.D.
Associate Professor of Medicine
School of Medicine, The Center for the
Health Sciences, University of California
Los Angeles, Cal.

Preface

The purpose of this book is to disseminate more widely knowledge of isotopic techniques which are of value in clinical medicine. These methods offer to physicians highly specific and sensitive techniques that can be of immeasurable help with difficult diagnostic and therapeutic problems.

In Vitro Nuclear Medicine may be defined as that area of nuclear medicine in which the results may be expressed in a quantitative fashion. This is in contrast to the field in which cameras and scanners are used to make interpretations on a qualitative (subjective) basis. In this latter field interpretations are made for the most part by examining an image. It may be argued that even in this field results are expressed in quantitative terms at times because of the increasing use of computers and on-line data. However, in the vast majority of cases these additional tools are not used. By contrast, *in vitro* nuclear medicine expresses the results almost invariably in numerical terms.

Qualitative and quantitative nuclear medicine have both had rapid growth in the last twenty years. At first nuclear medicine was almost entirely quantitative with blood volumes, Schilling tests and iodine uptakes predominating. Then in the mid-1950's there was a rapid growth in imaging techniques, first with the scanner and then with the gamma camera. At the present time in most nuclear medicine laboratories, the bulk of the work is done by means of imaging techniques. More recently, with the development of immunoassay and protein-binding techniques, quantitative nuclear medicine has begun to catch up.

While the qualitative area is becoming a more and more expensive field in which to keep up-to-date, with the increasing complexity of the imaging devices and the introduction of computer techniques, the quantitative area has remained a relatively less expensive area in which to participate.

As previously mentioned, *in vitro* nuclear medicine continues to be a rapidly growing field with its quantitative techniques presenting useful tools for clinical situations. For instance, the ability to do assays for digitalis fairly rapidly by isotopic techniques has facilitated greatly the handling of persons suspected of being either over- or under-digitalized. Instead of proceeding as previously in a cautious manner with a therapeutic trial, it is now possible to get helpful therapeutic guidance from the serum digitalis level. Another example is the test for Australia antigen, a test of prognostic value in serum hepatitis. Additionally, the value of isotopic techniques for detecting Australia antigen in prospective blood donors is becoming increasingly recognized. Also, the entity of T-3 toxicosis is being diagnosed with increased frequency by means of these isotopic techniques. There are numerous other examples of valuable clinical applications of these techniques throughout this book. It was for this reason that it was felt appropriate to prepare a book covering these techniques employed at the present time.

It is impossible, of course, to be all-inclusive in this field, discussing every possible technique used in *in vitro* nuclear medicine. It has been the effort of the editor, therefore, to cover those areas of greatest interest to internists, clinical pathologists and nuclear medicine specialists.

The book is appropriately arranged by subject matter in five parts with related chapters being grouped together as follows: Methods—Chapters 1 through 4; Blood: Volume and Production—Chapters 5 through 7; Radioassays of Compounds Having Naturally Occurring Binding Substances —Chapters 8 through 12; Radioassays of Compounds Without Naturally Occurring Binding Substances—Chapter 13 through 22; Gastrointestinal Diagnostic Tests— Chapters 23 and 24; Infection—Chapters 25 and 26; and Chapter 27 suggesting and predicting Future Directions of this highly important field of *in vitro* nuclear medicine.

BENJAMIN ROTHFELD, M.D.

Acknowledgment

I wish to acknowledge with gratitude the help, encouragement and advice of Arthur Karmen, M.D., Henry Wagner, M.D., Turner Bledsoe, M.D., Theodore Bayless, M.D., and Moses Paulson, M.D. which made this book possible. I would also like to acknowledge the patience and skill of Miss Ruth Reynolds who helped me with the stenographic work. Also, the patience and good humor of Mrs. Winifred Wheeler made a real contribution to this work.

Contents

Nuclear Medicine
In Vitro

1 *Crystal Scintillation Counting*

J. M. MENEFEE, M.A.

INTRODUCTION

When the need arises to measure the amount or type of gamma-emitting isotope within a sample, the most efficient and economical method to date is with a crystal scintillation detector system. Within this chapter we shall describe the components of this system, briefly look at the detection mechanism, discuss its operation and performance, quality control and commonly encountered problems. Because we are seeking a broad understanding of the subject matter, some of the topics are of necessity treated superficially. Excellent references are available on detector design,[1] interaction of radiation with matter[2] and scintillator theory.[3]

Crystal scintillation counting is today a well-developed technology. While its origin dates back to Rutherford's spinthrascope in the 1890's, its development as a practical tool began with the electron multiplier tube developed during World War II and the discovery of NaI(Tl) (thallium-activated sodium iodide) as a scintillator by Hofstadter in 1948. The first photomultipliers had to be emersed in liquid nitrogen to separate signal from noise and before NaI(Tl) the next best material was naphthalene or anthracene. It was from this somewhat shaky foundation of mothball detectors and noisy electron tubes that scintillation counting was launched. Extensive commercial development was carried on in the 1950's and the last major innovation was accomplished in the 1960's

with the application of solid state components to counting circuitry. Today's scintillation counting systems, although somewhat complex, are quite accurate, reliable, and simple to operate.

COMPONENTS OF THE SYSTEM

To obtain maximal utilization from one's counter system, a general knowledge of its operation is essential. Therefore we shall look at the separate components of the counter and discuss briefly their individual contributions to the overall system operation.

Principle of Operation. Any crystal scintillation counter, whether desk-top or large multisample console may be schematically visualized (Fig. 1-1). In one form or another it will always include a detector, high voltage (H.V.) power supply, amplifier, analyzer, and readout.

Detector. The first and possibly most important element of the system is the detector. It consists of a scintillation crystal optically coupled to an electron multiplier tube (usually referred to as a photomultiplier tube or PMT). Figure 1-2 is a diagram of a typical well detector.

Almost without exception, the crystal will be NaI(Tl). Many other crystals are available including CsI(Tl), CsI(Na), and $CaF_2(Eu)$,

---

Credit is given to Mr. H. Suscheck of Bicron Corporation for the original artwork on the many line drawings and to Miss D. Apanovitch for typing the manuscript.

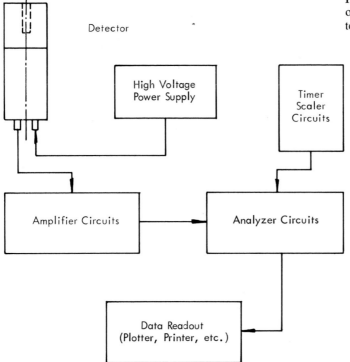

Detector

High Voltage
Power Supply

Timer
Scaler
Circuits

Amplifier Circuits

Analyzer Circuits

Data Readout
(Plotter, Printer, etc.)

Fig. 1-1. Functional diagram of a crystal scintillation counter system.

but are rarely used due to cost factors.* Properties and a discussion of their application may be found in papers by Schmidt and Menefee and an excellent survey of these and other scintillation crystals is available in Birks, and Kaiser.[3-7] Although our considerations are limited in this chapter to NaI(Tl), in most cases, the comments generally apply to any crystal that is used. For references, some basic properties of NaI(Tl) are given in Table 1-1.

DETECTION PROCESS

Crystal and PMT. Before proceeding further, we must examine the detection process within the crystal and PMT. Gamma rays entering a NaI crystal may be absorbed by one or more of 3 mechanisms—photoelectric effect, Compton scatter, or pair production. Each of the absorption processes has an in-

---

* Plastic or anthracene crystals have also been used but with these materials gamma rays with energies between 100 to 300 kev usually interact to produce scatter, rather than the more desirable photoelectric collisions.

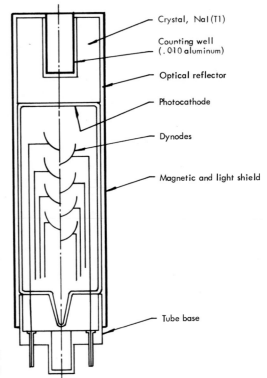

Crystal, NaI(Tl)

Counting well
(.010 aluminum)

Optical reflector

Photocathode

Dynodes

Magnetic and light shield

Tube base

Fig. 1-2. Cross-section of a typical well detector.

Table 1-1. Properties of Sodium Iodide (Thallium) Crystals.

Density	Emission Wave Length	Refraction Index	Conversion Efficiency	Decay Constant
Gm/cc 3.67	4,200 Å	1.77	Approximately 9 cathode photoelectrons per kev	250 Nanoseconds

dependent statistical probability of occurring and each changes in probability as a function of energy. At low energies, a few kev up to 200 to 300 kev the most probable interaction is photoelectric, in which the gamma ray gives up its entire energy to a sodium or more likely an iodine* atom's orbital electron. This electron is then brought to rest in the crystal through many thousands of ionizing collisions. The many secondary electrons which are generated by the photoelectron finally interact with the scintillating centers† to produce light photons in the crystal. Going back to the original photoelectron, we note that even though the gamma ray gives up its entire energy, the photoelectron produced is always lacking the binding energy used up in removing or knocking it out of its atomic shell. The majority of photoelectrons are produced from iodine K shell electrons and consequently the photoelectron's energy is low, approximately 32 kev. At gamma energies above approximately 100 kev, there is no need to be concerned at this apparent energy loss because coincidentally a free electron drops in to fill the K shell hole, and in so doing radiates a 32 kev x-ray, which finally, in all but the smallest crystals, is totally absorbed giving them a "full energy" absorption pulse equivalent to the energy of the initial gamma ray. Below approximately 100 kev, however, gamma ray absorption can take place near the crystal surface and a significant number of these x-rays may escape without detection. The following section, "Gamma Ray Spectrums" p. 5, discusses the effect of this energy loss in more detail.

Near 300 kev the photoelectric cross-section rapidly decreases and Compton scatter becomes the most probable absorption mechanism. Compton scatter has its best analogy in billard-ball behavior. If the incoming gamma ray strikes an electron in the crystal head-on, it gives up the maximal energy it is capable of giving and is scattered 180° back on its own path. The energetic electron produced by the scattered gamma is brought to rest in the crystal through many thousands of collisions in a manner similar to that of the photoelectron in our first consideration. Again, each of the ionizing collisions produces secondary electrons which in turn recombine with the scintillation centers to eventuate in light photons. When the Compton scatter occurs at angles less than 180°, the resultant electron energy is necessarily smaller. Pair production, because it has a threshold of occurrence near one Mev, does not become significant until gamma rays of several Mev energy are encountered.

When a gamma ray is totally absorbed in the crystal through one or a combination of the above processes, the number of secondary electrons produced in the process is always directly proportional to the energy of the gamma ray absorbed. Each secondary ionization electron which combines with a scintillation center produces a light photon. These photons are then (sometimes after multiple reflections) directed out of the crystal to impinge upon the cathode of a photomultiplier. They are here converted back to electrons, and through multiple collisions down the dynodes, they are amplified into a usable charge pulse. In summary then, the detection process is nothing more than a

---

* Iodine is the principal absorber by several orders of magnitude, since it has a much higher atomic number.

† Scintillation center refers to an electron-trapping lattice defect produced by the thallium activator.

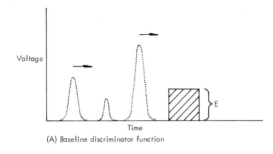

(A) Baseline discriminator function

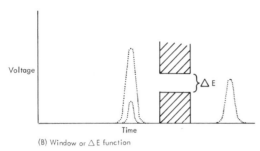

(B) Window or △ E function

Fig. 1-3. Signal analysis in the single channel analyzer.

series of conversions—the gamma ray is first converted to electrons, the electrons to photons, and the photons back again to electrons at the photocathode.

As previously stated, these cathode electrons are accelerated through the tube's dynode structure, knocking off additional electrons as they proceed. This amplification process is very large and one electron at the cathode results in 10^7 electrons being collected at the anode of a typical photomultiplier. The conversion processes, on the other hand, are relatively inefficient. One kev of gamma ray energy typically produces about 10 photoelectrons at the photocathode of a high-efficiency bi-alkali tube.

Although the detection process is reasonably fast, it is somewhat slower than detection in a liquid scintillation system. The time required for the gamma ray to be converted to electrons in the crystal is negligible, but the time required for these electrons to recombine with scintillation centers and eventuate in light photons is substantial. The recombination and subsequent photon production occurs logarithmically with time, and

in NaI(Tl) crystals 250 nsec are required for the light intensity to decay to 1/e (approximately 37%) of its initial value.* This time, incidentally, is defined as the decay constant of the crystal and is a characteristic of the material. CsI(Tl) has a decay constant of approximately 1 microsecond. Electron multiplication and collection in the phototube is a bit faster. While there can be a considerable variation from one type to another the typical time required for the electrons to transit the dynodes and be collected at the anode is 80 to 100 nsec.

All of these detection, conversion, and amplification processes are practically linear and as a result the electronic charge at the anode is directly proportional to the energy of the detected gamma ray. The charge pulse at the anode is coupled into the counter circuitry by allowing a load capacitor to become charged by the anode and then discharging across a load resistor. Because of the times involved, this period is normally adjusted to approximately 1 μ sec (microsecond) and ultimately determines the maximal counting rate that may be accommodated.

Amplifiers. Signal pulses at the detector anode vary from a few millivolts to over 100 and thus require considerable additional amplification before analysis. Most counters have several circuits which amplify the pulses to a level of several volts. An acceptable circuit outputs a clean noise-free pulse at 1 volt and does not saturate below 10 volts, yielding a dynamic range for a particular setting of about 10 to 1.

Analyzers. The function of the analyzer, regardless of type, is to measure the voltage height of each pulse presented to it by the amplifier. This voltage height is, of course, still proportional to the energy of the original gamma ray. The two basic types of analyzers available are single channel and multichannel. Single-channel analyzers usually output to scalers and printers and multichannels output into a memory bank which displays into a cathode ray tube. The multichannel

---

* e = 2.718, the base of the natural logarithm system

memory bank can, of course, be read out to a printer or plotter.

Figure 1-3 shows how the single-channel analyzer measures a pulse.

Consider a series of various voltage height pulses proceeding into the analyzer as (A). Through a transistor trigger circuit an electronic barrier is provided with a voltage height (E). Close examination shows that while the first and last pulse satisfy the voltage requirements the center pulse is too small and is blocked by the *Baseline discriminator* (E function). Thus, one can sort out all pulses above a particular E setting. Through a similar circuit an upper discriminator function is provided (B). The combined functions then are capable of blocking the first and center pulse while allowing the last pulse to pass through. The "window" or ΔE function also may be varied and thus at a particular setting the analyzer passes only those voltage pulses between E and E+ ΔE.

By setting ΔE at say 0.1 volt and varying E from 0 to 10 volts in steps of 0.1 volt and using equal counting times at each interval, a 100-channel histogram or spectrum may be plotted.

Timer/Scaler. Integral to the analysis circuitry is a timer which is normally settable from 0.1 minutes to several hours. A scaler circuit is also included to count the pulses emanating from the analyzer. In some cases the scaler may be "blind" or without display and automatically prints its contents on a paper tape at the termination of the counting interval. In most systems, the counting interval may also be determined by a preset count in which the time is recorded to obtain a predetermined number of counts.

Multichannel analyzers are functionally identical to the single-channel type described, but through a complex ramp circuit and ferrite core memory they are able to produce a 100-channel or more, spectrum in one simultaneous counting interval.

High Voltage Power Supply. Incorporated in all scintillation counting systems is a high-voltage power supply. Its sole function is to supply acceleration voltage to the photomul-

tiplier dynodes. A typical tube contains 10 dynodes and requires a total voltage of approximately 1,000 volts positive DC. The gain or amplification factor of the PMT (photomultiplier tube) is linearly proportional to the high voltage applied. However, nonlinearity results if the voltage is too low (typically below 800 volts) and too high a voltage (usually above 1,200 volts) produces excessive low-energy noise. A rule of thumb states that for each 100 volts increase, the detector gain is approximately doubled.

Gamma Ray Spectrums. If the counting systems which we have discussed were free of statistical variation, interpretation of our data would be greatly simplified. Ideally, monoenergetic gamma rays absorbed in the crystal by photoelectric effect would produce a narrow line (Fig. 1-4).

Those gamma rays which were Compton scattered would produce a band of events starting below the full energy line and ending at the zero energy point. The high-energy side of this band would represent those gamma rays scattered 180° back on their own path (giving up the maximal energy allowable) and the zero energy would represent those gamma rays which escaped the crystal after a very small angle of scatter.

While the statistical variations in the counter circuits are negligible, those in the photomultiplier and crystal are not. Variations in the number of light photons produced in the crystal, the uniformity of light collection as a function of position within the crystal and variations in the number of electrons produced in the PMT all contribute to widen the line in Figure 1-4 to a "peak"

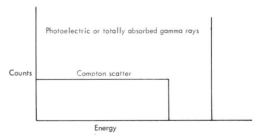

Fig. 1-4. Ideal monoenergetic gamma spectrum with no statistical variations.

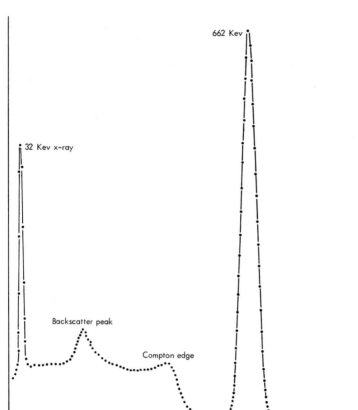

Fig. 1-5. Gamma ray spectrum of cesium-137.

662 Kev

32 Kev x-ray

Backscatter peak

Compton edge

(Fig. 1-5). These variations also smear the edges of the Compton continuum. Figure 1-5 is an actual gamma spectrum of cesium-137. The single gamma ray has a monochromatic energy of 662 kev. The width of the peak is, of course, representative of the resolving power of the system, that is, its ability to distinguish between adjacent gamma lines (see p. 11). Sample containers and crystal shape or "geometry" also contribute to spectrum appearance. Sample containers with any substantial mass result in gamma rays being "backscattered" in the container material. These scattered gammas which are detected by the crystal produce a broad peak with an energy equal to the difference between full energy and Compton edge energy. A backscatter peak may be seen in the cesium spectrum of Figure 1-5.

When a sample is placed inside the crystal,

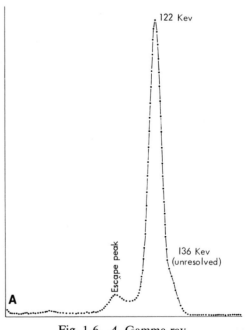

122 Kev

Escape peak

136 Kev
(unresolved)

A

Fig. 1-6. *A*, Gamma ray spectrum of cobalt-57.

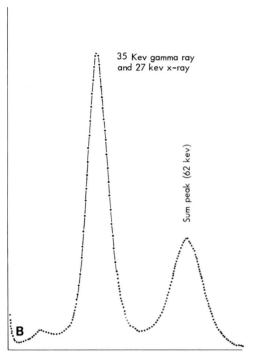

Fig. 1-6. *B*, Gamma ray spectrum of iodine-125.

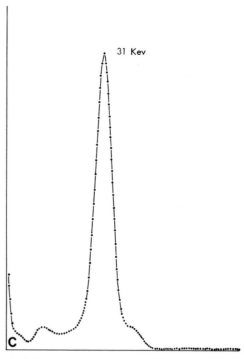

C, Gamma ray spectrum of iodine-129.

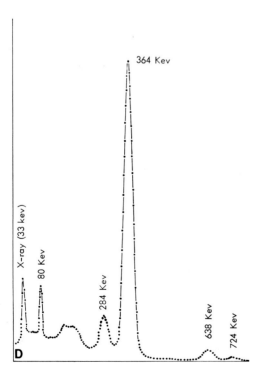

D, Gamma ray spectrum of iodine-131.

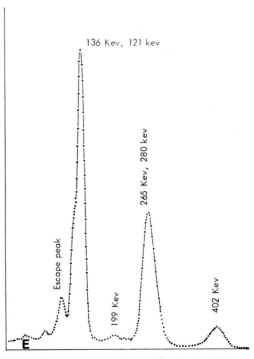

E, Gamma ray spectrum of selenium-75.

such as with the conventional well-type geometry, many gamma rays which are scattered inside the crystal traverse the well and are subsequently absorbed by the other side of the crystal. As a result, the Compton edge is often absent or poorly defined.

At this point, it should be apparent that isotopes producing several gamma lines, or mixtures of isotopes, yield spectra which are exceedingly complex and difficult to analyze accurately. This can be especially true when using a single channel analyzer where the spectra cannot be readily visualized. Figures 1-6, *A* through *E* help visualize how the spectra from some of the more commonly used isotopes may appear.

At gamma ray energies near 100 kev and below, some events are detected with less than "full energy." The Cobalt-57 spectrum (Fig. 1-6*A*) is a good example of this effect. Most of the 122 kev (or 136 kev) gamma rays are absorbed by photoelectric effect near the surface of the crystal. The so-called "escape peak" seen below the 122 kev line is the result of the x-ray, produced during the absorption process, escaping the crystal without being detected. Since the energy of the x-ray, in NaI(Tl), is approximately 32 kev, the escape peak always appears 32 kev below the full energy peak.

Figure 1-6*B* is the spectrum of Iodine-125 taken with a well-type detector. The "sum peak" represents the 27 kev Iodine-125 x-ray and 35 kev gamma ray being detected coincidentally by the crystal. When a solid crystal is used, these coincidental absorptions are infrequent and the sum peak all but disappears.

Because Iodine-125 has a relatively short half-life, Iodine-129 is frequently used as a substitute standard for calibration. Its spectrum is illustrated in Figure 1-6*C*. Iodine-131 and Selenium-75 spectra are depicted in Figures 1-6*D* and *E*. A compilation of most of the commonly used isotope spectra is available in Heath.[8]

OPERATION AND PERFORMANCE

Specifying a System. The choices available in types of scintillation counting systems are unlimited and include a small, single sample, desk-top counter with preset counting windows, a large automatic sample changer type console with several adjustable channels, or a counting system of separate modules, multichannel analyzer, and computer interface. The usual parameters of work load, economics, and flexibility must be applied. The minimal requirements should include a variable H.V. supply, and at least one counting channel with settable baseline (E) and window (ΔE) discriminators. Fixed H.V. supplies unnecessarily limit the dynamic energy range and a manually settable counting window allows one to count the occasional complex or unusual sample.

Performance criteria to consider include gain stability (as a function of time and count-rate change), resolution, minimal detectable energy, background levels and efficiency. (These are discussed and operationally defined in the following paragraphs.) A system, regardless of quality, should exhibit a stability of better than ±2 percent. That is, if a calibration is made so that a particular peak is centered at channel 100, it should not change more than 2 channels up or down during the day or with normal changes in counting rate. The resolution one should expect, of course, depends on the crystal geometry. Resolutions at 662 kev for most standard well crystals vary from 7.5 to 10 percent, solid crystals are rarely worse than 8.5 percent, and crystals with side wells are poorest with a range of 10 to 15 percent. In applications where they are needed, crystals with selected resolutions are available from most manufacturers at a reasonable extra charge.

Minimal detectable energy depends on both the thickness or mass of material between source and crystal and the signal to noise capabilities of the system. Present-day detectors are usually equipped with 0.010-inch aluminum well liners and readily transmit gamma or x-rays down to about 20 kev. If a system has a good signal to noise capability, it easily resolves the 22 kev peak of Cadmium 109 from the system noise.

Background varies with the amount of

shielding provided; 1 or 2 inches of lead is typical in most systems. The only sure way to specify a suitable value for background, or for that matter efficiency, is by trial and error (see p. 11).

Mechanical and electric reliability are of primary importance although difficult to specify. An interesting situation would derive if purchasers insisted on being given values for "mean time between failure" and "failure modes" before buying a particular counter. This would certainly put equipment reliability on a quantitative basis.

Counter Evaluation and Operation. Before using a scintillation counting system for routine procedures, become acquainted with its capabilities and be assured that it is accurately calibrated and operating properly. Accomplishing this goal requires not only an initial evaluation, but a follow-up program of quality control. Items to initially evaluate include an energy calibration procedure, plots of spectra and resolution measurement, background and gain stability check, and an evaluation of count-rate limitations. After this initial evaluation, make a daily check of energy calibration, count rate for a standard sample and background.

On a weekly basis, or at least once a month, plot a spectrum for a standard sample, measure the resolution, and if desirable perform a χ^2 test. Assign a notebook to each counter to include the evaluation data, notes on special procedures required, and a log of the daily and weekly system checks.

In the following discussion, each of the above procedures will be treated in detail. In performing the initial evaluation, a consultant versed in experimental nuclear physics can be an immense help; especially if the user is generally unfamiliar with counting procedures.

Energy Calibration. All of the detection and amplification processes are linear. Thus, the voltage height of the signal pulse is directly proportional to the gamma ray that produced it. For example, if a 300 kev gamma ray gave rise to a 1-volt pulse, then a gamma ray with twice that energy, or 600 kev, would produce a signal of twice that

voltage—in this case, 2 volts. These signal voltages may also be changed by varying H.V. or amplifier settings. If for the case at hand, the amplification were doubled, then the 300 kev gamma ray would give rise to a 2-volt signal and the 600 kev gamma ray to a 4-volt signal. Since the typical analyzer measures pulses over a range of 0 to 10 volts, it is apparent that while 0 volts always corresponds to 0 energy, 10 volts may be caused to correspond to any energy that is convenient. Calibration then, is simply adjusting the H.V. and amplifier so that the 0- to 10-volt analyzer range corresponds to the desired energy range. Good practice dictates that a calibration be chosen that allows the counting window, or E function, to fall in the mid- to upper range of the analyzer. Avoid counting in the lower 5 or 10 percent of the analyzer's range. In addition to encountering electronic noise in this region, the normal errors in instrument settings are usually magnified.

If a calibration procedure is provided by the instrument manufacturer, follow it. Lacking that, most analyzers may be calibrated as follows: if you wish to count ^{125}I, you might arbitrarily choose a counting range of 0 to 100 kev. For a reference energy, you could use an ^{125}I source or any other isotope with a gamma peak in this range. The 60 kev gamma from [241]Am would do very well.

If the 60 kev [241]Am is used, set the baseline discriminator or E dial to 5.5 volts and the window or ΔE dial to 1.0 volt. This establishes a counting window from 5.5 volts to 6.5 volts with a midpoint of 6.0 volts. The objective is to have 10 volts correspond to 100 kev or 0.1 volt/kev. With the amplifier set at approximately half total gain, and the instrument in the "count" mode, slowly increase the H.V. while watching the scaler or ratemeter. As the voltage increases there is a point at which the count rate begins to rise. At this point, adjust the "fine" H.V. control or the "fine" gain control until a maximal counting rate is observed. To visualize what is happening, imagine that at low H.V. settings the entire spectrum is "compressed" into the lower portion of the analyz-

even adjoining floors, or a nearby x-ray or radiation therapy unit. This type of background, as well as the build-up from occasional spills may distort a laboratory's results. It can best be evaluated and monitored by setting the E dial at 0.1 volts, ΔE at 10 volts, and taking a 5-minute count over the entire calibration range which is normally used for counting. The energy calibration must be the same, of course, in each measurement.

Gain Stability. Any shift in a systems gain directly and proportionally changes the energy calibration. Where narrow ΔE windows are used, a change in calibration as small as 3 to 4 percent can create substantial counting errors. To accurately interpret data, be aware of the degree of gain shift present in the system being used.

Contributions from the counter circuitry are usually negligible in even the poorest quality systems. In fact, almost every case of gain shift can be pinned down to the photomultiplier tube. PMT's characteristically drift with both time and count rate change. In a good tube it can amount to about one percent; in a poor tube, however, it may reach a level of 5 or 6 percent. The variations are random above and below some mean value. Gain shifts in any system may be minimized by leaving the power on at all times and this practice also helps prolong the life of the components within a system.

Testing the gain stability of a counter system requires an entire day and is accomplished as follows:

1. Allow the equipment at least an hour to stabilize after the power is turned on.

2. Perform an energy calibration with any convenient source and place tape across the gain and H.V. controls to assure that they are not changed.

3. Using a ΔE of 0.2 volts, scan across the gamma peak being utilized and record the E value corresponding to maximum counting rate (i.e., the peak channel or voltage).

4. Introduce into the detector chamber a second source which has approximately 10 times the activity. It need not be the same isotope.

5. Repeat the peak scanning operation and record the peak channel or voltage.

6. Wait 15 minutes and again measure the peak channel.

7. Remove the second source, wait 15 minutes, and once more measure the peak channel.

8. Divide the mean of the 4 values of E into the maximal deviation between them. A good system has drift versus count rate change of 1 or 2 percent.

Leaving the original source in the detector, repeat the peak channel or voltage measurement and record the value approximately once each hour for the remainder of the workday and again the following morning. A similar computation as before indicates the percentage drift as a function of time. Again a good system will exhibit a value of 1 or 2 percent. This effect on counting rate in any particular situation may, of course, be evaluated by manually changing the calibration by an equivalent percentage and observing the resultant difference in count rate.

Count Rate Limitations. Where it is not necessary to count sources in excess of 50,000 cps with a single channel analyzer or 50,000 cpm with a multichannel analyzer this evaluation consideration may be omitted.

However, if high activity sources must be counted, be aware that at these high counting rates a significant number of events will fail to be counted per unit time. The unresolved pulses will exhibit a partially summed voltage height and as a result be analyzed as having higher than actual energy. To evaluate properly the systems capabilities, seek a consultant or advice from the manufacturer.

QUALITY CONTROL PROGRAM

The quality of the data is no better than the condition of the counting system. The quality assurance program described here is easy to institute, requires very little extra time, and ensures that a system is always in proper operating condition.

Procure a notebook and standard source for each machine. Choose an isotope for the standard which has (a) a long half-life,

Month of: _____ 19 _____

Laboratory: _____ Instrument ID _____

Day	Calibration Check	Standard Count (S)	Background Count	$S_n - \bar{S}$ (Absolute value)	$(\bar{S}_n - S)^2$
1					
2					
3					
4					
5					
6					
7					
8					
9					
10					
Column Totals					
Average (÷10)					
11				QC summary:	
12				Calibration = v /kev	
13				Standard count E = v	
14				ΔE = v	
15				Background E = v	
16				ΔE = 10.0v	
17				Resolution = %	
18				x^2 test:	
19					
20				$x^2 = \dfrac{\text{Total of } (S_n - \bar{S})^2*}{\text{Average stand count, } \bar{S}}$ _____	
21					
22					
23				$4.17 \leq$ _____ ≤ 14.68	
24				(limits of x^2 using 10	
25				measurements	
26					
27				Notes:	
28					
29					
30					
31					

*This is the sum of the squares of the differences between individual counts and the mean of all the counts.

Fig. 1-8. Monthly quality control form.

Table 1-2. Properties of Commonly Used Radioisotopes.

SHORT-LIVED GAMMA EMITTERS (Medical Life Science Applications)

	Mass Symbol At. No.	Half-Life	Peaks of Interest—Gamma Energy in Mev (X-ray energy in kev)
Technetium—99m	$^{99m}Tc_{43}$	6.0 hr	0.141
Iodine—125	$^{125}I_{53}$	60.2 d	0.035 (27 kev)*
Iodine—131	$^{131}I_{53}$	8.1 d	0.365, 0.638 (Others) (33 kev)
Xenon—133	$^{133}Xe_{54}$	5.3 d	0.083 (30 kev)
Chromium—51	$^{51}Cr_{24}$	27.8 d	0.322
Indium—113m	$^{113m}In_{49}$	1.7 hr	0.393 (24 kev)
Selenium—75	$^{75}Se_{34}$	120 d	0.136, 0.121, 0.265, 0.280*
Sodium—24	$^{24}Na_{11}$	15 hr	1.368, 2.750
Iron—59	$^{59}Fe_{26}$	45 d	0.145, 0.191, 1.097, 1.289
Mercury—197	$^{197}Hg_{80}$	65 hr	0.0778

LONG-LIVED GAMMA EMITTERS (Calibration Sources)

	Mass Symbol At. No.	Half-Life	Peaks of Interest—Gamma Energy in Mev (X-ray energy in kev)
Thorium (Oxide)	$^{232}Th\ O_2$	1.4x10^10 yr	2.615 [from T1-208], Others
Cobalt—60	$^{60}Co_{27}$	5.62 yr	<u>1.173</u>, <u>1.332</u>† [2.505 Sum]
Sodium—22	$^{22}Na_{11}$	2.62 yr	<u>0.511</u> [B⁺ annihilation] <u>1.275</u> (1.786 Sum)
Zinc—65	$^{65}Zn_{30}$	245 d	0.511 [B⁺ annihilation] 1.115 (8.2 kev)
Manganese—54	$^{54}Mn_{25}$	303 d	0.835 (5.5 kev)
Cesium—137	$^{137}Cs_{55}$	30.0 yr	0.662 (33.0 kev)
Krypton—85	$^{85}Kr_{19}$	10.6 yr	0.670 Beta, [Bremsstrahlung, 0.515 Gamma Ray]
Barium—133	$^{133}Ba_{56}$	7.2 yr	0.080, 0.276, <u>0.302</u>, <u>0.356</u>, 0.382* (32.0 kev)
Cobalt—57	$^{57}Co_{27}$	270 d	<u>0.014</u>, <u>0.122</u>, 0.136* (6.5 kev)
Cadmium—109	$^{109}Cd_{48}$	453 d	0.088 (23.0 kev)
Americium—241	$^{241}Am_{95}$	458 yr	0.060
Iron—55	$^{55}Fe_{26}$	2.6 yr	(5.7 kev)

* Adjacent peaks are unresolved using scintillation detectors.
† Peaks underlined are coincident with one another.

(b) at least one easily resolved peak, and (c) if possible, a spectral range similar to the samples being counted. Iodine-129 with a half-life of 16,000,000 years and essentially the same photon energy as Iodine-125 is an ideal standard. A list of other long half-lived sources is given in Table 1-2. Make up a form to record the data as shown in Figure 1-8.

At the start of each day make a calibration check, count the standard, and take a background. Of course, use the same calibration value, and window settings from day to day for this data to be accurate and meaningful. Record these values for reference in the space provided in the Quality Control summary block.

At the end of the tenth day, make a χ^2 test. This calculation is a statistical test to determine the probability that a series of measurements are derived from a Poisson distribution.* From the statistical nature of radioactive decay, if you use the same sample for all of the measurements, the Poisson distribution will be satisfied. Therefore, if the test is not within proper limits, you can conclude that the counting system is working improperly and take necessary corrective action. Chi square is given by

$$\chi^2 = \sum_{n=1}^{N} \frac{(S_n - \overline{S})^2}{\overline{S}}^\dagger$$

Where N measurements have been made having values of S_n and the average of all N measurements is $\overline{S}$.

Using the form

1. Find the total of the standard counts in column 2.

2. Divide by 10 to get the average, $\overline{S}$.

3. Compute the absolute difference between S_n and $\overline{S}$ for each measurement and record in column 4.

4. Square each of these and record in column 5.

5. Divide the total of column 5 by $\overline{S}$, to obtain χ^2.

Where 10 measurements are used in the calculation, χ^2 should be equal or greater than 4.17 and less than or equal to 14.68. A detailed discussion of χ^2 tests and a table of limits for other than 10 measurements is given in Hoel.[9]

At the end of the month plot a full spectrum of the standard source and compare closely with the previous spectrum taken during the evaluation tests. Compute the reso-

lution and record in the Quality Control summary section (see p. 11 for details on computing resolution). If this is done carefully, any change greater than ±15% of the resolution value obtained during the evaluation indicates malfunction.

Data Reduction. Fortunately, most clinical counting procedures involve samples with single isotopes. In these situations count either at a particular peak in the spectrum or over the entire spectrum. Quite often, when backgrounds are not a problem, the counting times for lower activity samples may be shortened by counting over the entire spectrum. This procedure also tends to minimize any errors introduced by gain drift and calibration accuracy. Under any circumstance, try to avoid using narrow counting windows which include only a portion of a peak. Small changes in gain can produce substantial errors in count rate, under these conditions.

When a standard solution is not included in the clinical procedure being used, it is suggested that no attempt be made to compute the microcuries of activity from any formula involving detector efficiency, geometry, and so on. These variables are extremely difficult to determine accurately and the resulting computation rarely is more than a crude estimate. In this situation, fabricate a standard using a calibrated activity solution diluted to the desired level. These solutions are available from both radioisotope suppliers and the National Bureau of Standards, Gaithersburg, Maryland. Comparing an unknown with a fabricated standard of this type yields errors of less than 5 percent in terms of microcurie estimations.

COMMONLY ENCOUNTERED PROBLEMS

Equipment Problems. While most repairs are beyond the capability of the normal laboratory, it is very often helpful to identify a problem. A reasonably accurate diagnosis of a particular problem can be made by comparing the findings with those described below. No attempt is made here to discuss the

---

* Since radioactive decay follows a Poisson distribution, this is essential.

$\dagger$ $\overline{S}$ is the mean of all the counts.

$(S_n - \overline{S})^2$ is the sum of the squares of the differences between individual counts and the mean of all the counts.

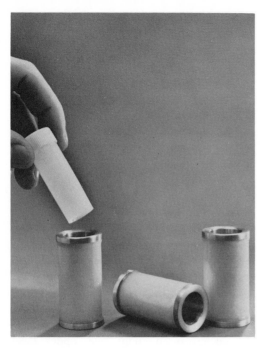

Fig. 1-9. LSC—Gamma vials.

procedures for signal tracing and analysis using an oscilloscope.

Extraneous Peaks in the Spectrum. If unidentified peaks appear in the spectrum in counting times of under 60 minutes it is unlikely that they are produced by the detector. If the width of a peak is narrower than a gamma peak of equal energy, it is almost certain to be a result of the electronic system. If the peak is the same width as a gamma line it is likely due to unshielded sources near the detector.

Background. Background from the detector is usually not significant unless one hour or more counting time is taken in heavily shielded (4 to 6 inches of lead) chambers. Background spectra are complex and are the result of many sources, including cosmic rays and natural radioactivity. Where low-level samples must be counted, a specially designed detector and massive shield may be obtained from detector manufacturers.

Noise. Noise in a spectrum is generally defined as the extraneous events counted near the zero energy end of the spectrum. It is nearly always a product of the photomultiplier due to spontaneous emission from the photocathode and other phenomena within the tube. It appears as a near exponentially decreasing curve extending into the spectrum and often obscuring low energy peaks. Acceptable noise level varies with the type of phototube used but probably would be considered excessive if it extended far enough into the spectrum to obscure 15 to 20 kev x-ray peaks.

Distorted Spectra and Poor Resolution. Scintillation detector crystals, especially NaI(Tl), are highly sensitive to both moisture and thermal shocks or thermal gradients. Therefore, care must be taken not to puncture or break the hermetically sealed container or expose a detector to extreme temperature changes—transfer from a heated to an unheated room, being placed in front of an airconditioner, or on a sun-warmed surface. Where the detector is mounted in an equipment cabinet or counter console it will be adequately protected against a normal laboratory environment.

Any unexplained changes in the gamma-ray spectrum or a deteriorating resolution can normally be traced to a fractured or leaky detector. If a detector becomes fractured but the crack is not excessive and if it has proper orientation it will not impair performance. Usually, however, fractured crystals produce asymetrical peaks and may exhibit multiple peaks for a single gamma line. Once a fracture has occurred, it is usually stable and will not extend.

Moisture leaks always produce hydration on the crystal surface and without exception degrade resolution. It has an effect on performance similar to that of fractures. It can be distinguished from fracturing, however, because here performance degrades over an extended period of time. Hydrate appears as a spotty, yellowish tint on the crystal surface.

RECENT DEVELOPMENTS

Through a new product recently available, crystal scintillation counting capabilities have been added to liquid scintillation counting machines. The devices are called LSC-Gamma vials and provide comparable counting efficiencies with conventional gamma counters for most isotopes. Figure 1-9 illustrates these vials which have approximately the same outside dimensions as the standard liquid vials. The counting well is 17 mm in diameter and accommodates samples up to 2⅛ in. long. Sample bottles are inserted directly into the gamma vials, which, in turn, are placed directly into a liquid scintillation counter machine. While gamma counting has previously been accomplished with lead loaded cocktails, these units eliminate volume dependence and quench corrections, since no cocktail is used. Prokop has described these gamma vials and evaluates their performance in counting T-3, T-4, and other radioimmunoassay samples.[10]

References

1. Adams, F., and Dams, R.: Applied Gamma-Ray Spectrometry. ed 2. Oxford, Pergamon Press Ltd., New York, 1970.

2. Evans, R. D.: The Atomic Nucleus, pp. 672-745. New York, McGraw-Hill, 1955.

3. Birks, J. B.: The Theory and Practice of Scintillation Counting. Oxford, Pergamon Press, 1967.

4. Schmidt, C. T.: Cesium Iodide as a Gamma-Ray Spectrometer. IRE Tran. Nucl. Sci., NS7, p. 25, June-Sept., 1960.

5. Menefee, J.: Nuclear Science. vol. NS14-1, p. 464. Institute of Electrical and Electronics Engineers, Inc., Oct., 1966.

6. Menefee, J., Swinehart, C. F., and O'Dell, E. W.: IEEE Tran. Nucl. Sci., NS-13, (1), 720, Feb., 1966.

7. Kaiser, W. C.: Scintillation spectrometry. Anal. Chem. 38:(11), 1964.

8. Heath, R. L.: Scintillation Spectrometry Gamma-Ray Spectrum Catalogue. vol. 1 and 2. Phillips Petroleum Company—Idaho Operations Office, Aug., 1964.

9. Hoel, P. G.: Introduction to Mathematical Statistics. ed. 2. New York, John Wiley & Sons, 1954.

10. Prokop, E. K.: Personal communication. Baltimore. Johns Hopkins University Hospital.

2 *Liquid Scintillation Counting*

ARTHUR KARMEN, M.D.

When ionizing radiation deposits energy in solutions of certain fluorescent compounds, the solutions emit bursts of light or scintillations. Under ideal conditions, the number of bursts of light in a given time period is a function of the rate of disintegration of the radioisotope present. The number of photons emitted in each burst is related to the energy deposited. The liquid scintillation counter detects, measures and determines the rate of emission of the scintillations.

The radioactive sample can usually be incorporated directly into the solution of the scintillator. Losses of energy from absorption in a counter window, the covering of a crystal or from self-absorption in the sample itself are thus minimized. As a result, even beta particles of very low energy, such as those from tritium, can be counted with high efficiency and often with a minimum of sample preparation. Larger quantities of sample can generally be counted than with gas counting methods and preparation of the sample for counting is simpler. Several isotopes which emit particles of different energies can be counted simultaneously through the use of scintillation spectrometry and pulse-height analysis.

Liquid scintillation counting can be used to analyze many types of ionizing radiation. It is particularly useful for assaying emitters of alpha and low-energy beta particles and is often the method of choice for assaying ^{14}C and ^{3}H.

Generation of the Scintillations

The liquid scintillator consists of a dilute solution of one or more fluorescent compounds dissolved in a solvent. The radioactive particle deposits energy in the solvent causing excitation. This excitation energy is transferred to the fluorescent solutes which release the energy as a burst of light. This light is detected by a photomultiplier tube giving rise to an electric pulse which is amplified, analyzed, sorted according to size, and counted.

The solvent serves 2 functions: it dissolves the sample and the fluorescent solutes, and it absorbs and transfers the energy of the radioactive particle to the fluorescent solute. Not all liquids transfer electronic excitation with equal efficiency. Those that are most effective are the aromatic liquids, such as toluene, xylene, dioxane and several other alkyl benzenes. Many organic compounds are soluble in these solvents. Others can be solubilized by the addition of small quantities of other solvents provided that these do not interfere markedly with either the transfer of the energy or the emission of the scintillations.

The Primary Solute. PPO (2,5 diphenyloxazole), PPD (phenyldiphenyloxadiazole) and p-terphenyl are examples of primary solutes. Their function is to receive excitation energy from the solvent and to emit it as a burst of light. The most important criterion for choice of a primary solute is the number of photons emitted per unit of energy deposited in the solvent. Since concentrations of 5 to 10 Gm per 1 of these compounds are generally required for maximal light output, the usefulness of a fluorescent compound as a primary solute may be limited by its solubility in toluene. p-Terphenyl, for example, was one of the first compounds used, and is still one of the least expensive, but because of its low solubility in cold toluene, it has been replaced by PPO in most applications. A second criterion is that the light be emitted at a wavelength to which the photomultiplier tube is most sensitive. Emission of light at close to 400 nm is therefore desirable.

The Secondary Solute. Since the wavelength of the light emitted by most useful primary solutes is shorter than 400 nm, a secondary fluorescent solute, such as POPOP (1, 4-bis-2[5-phenyloxazolyl]-benzene) is frequently added. This solute absorbs the photons emitted by the primary solute and re-emits fluorescent light at a longer wavelength. A compound may be an effective secondary solute or wavelength shifter at concentrations one-tenth that of the primary solute, or at approximately 0.5 Gm per liter of toluene. In general, low solubility in toluene prevents these compounds from being used as primary solute.

Detecting the Scintillations

Since the small quantities of energy deposited by disintegrations of radioisotopes such as ^{14}C and ^{3}H give rise to bursts of small numbers of photons, sensitive photomultiplier tubes are required. The photocathodes of sensitive tubes tend to emit electrons in the absence of light which are not distinguishable from those emitted when light photons interact. To reduce the resulting noise or background counting rate, several measures may be employed.

1. The photomultiplier tubes may be refrigerated to reduce thermionic emission. Advances in photomultiplier tube technology, which resulted in the development of tubes with a smaller tendency toward thermionic emission, reduced the compelling need for refrigeration. However, to maintain the sensitivity of the photocathode and the dynodes so that equal size electrical pulses are generated for equal numbers of photons emitted by the scintillator, thus simplifying scintillation spectrometry, the maintenance of the photomultiplier tube at a constant temperature is desirable. Refrigeration is now used primarily to provide that constancy.

2. A second measure to reduce noise is to use pulse-height analysis. The interaction of a burst-of-light photons with the photocathode generally gives rise to a number of electrons simultaneously. The electrical pulses that result are thus generally larger than those resulting from the emission of individual thermionic electrons. Pulse-height analysis is therefore helpful in distinguishing signal from noise pulses.

3. The most effective measure is coincidence counting. When a scintillator absorbs a beta particle it emits a number of light photons simultaneously. If 2 photomultiplier tubes view the scintillator, and their outputs are arranged so that only pulses appearing in both tubes simultaneously are counted, pulses in each tube from thermionic electrons may be disregarded. This is effective in reducing background because of the low probability of thermionic emission of electrons from both photocathodes simultaneously. As a result of these measures background counting rates can be reduced to less than 10 counts per minute under conditions suitable for ^{14}C assay at 80 percent efficiency and ^{3}H assay at 60 percent efficiency or better.

Samples are generally counted in 10 to 15 ml of scintillator solution in 20 ml glass or polyethylene counting vials which are coupled to the photosensitive surfaces of the 2 photomultiplier tubes by a light guide. The electrical pulses in the outputs of the photomultiplier tubes are fed to the coincidence network where they are electrically summed so as to reflect more closely the total number of photons detected. The sum-pulse is amplified, subjected to pulse-height analysis, and sorted into one or more scalers according to size.

The factors determining the size of the electrical pulse, in addition to the energy deposited by the radioactive event, include the chemistry of the scintillator, the voltage on the photomultiplier tube, and the gain of the amplifiers. To achieve comparable efficiencies of counting for each sample in a series, the chemistry of the scintillator is kept as constant as possible. Small changes such as might arise from the presence of materials that interfere with the generation of the scintillation can be compensated for by suitable adjustments in electrical settings. In selecting these settings we generally choose those conditions for counting that permit the detection and accurate measurement of the smallest quantity of each isotope. Because of statistical considerations this may best be indicated by the efficiency squared to background ratios (E^2/B). An example of selection of these settings follows.

A sample of liquid scintillator containing tritium is placed in the sample well. The lower discriminator of a channel of the scaler is set high enough to exclude most amplifier noise. The upper discriminator is set at its maximum, thus defining a "wide window."

With amplifier gain set at mid-scale, the high voltage on the photomultiplier tube is adjusted until the counting rate in the window is maximal. In an unquenched sample, most of the tritium pulses are counted under these conditions and most of the larger pulses originating from background radiation are excluded. Following this procedure a known quantity of tritium dissolved in the same scintillation solution as the unknown sample is placed in the well and the amplifier gain is increased until the counting rate in the window is again maximal. These settings may be close to optimal for tritium in the samples to be assayed.

Amplifier gain settings may be adjusted for each isotope in the same way. Since the beta particle of ^{14}C is more energetic than that of ^3H, it gives rise to larger pulses. At settings optimized for tritium, many of these pulses exceed the level of the upper discriminator. To adjust the instrument for optimal counting of ^{14}C, a solution of scintilla-

tor containing ^{14}C is counted, and the amplifier gain is decreased until the maximal number of ^{14}C counts appear in the window.

To facilitate counting many samples, liquid scintillation spectrometers which employ completely automated sample changers and turntables with capacities as high as 400 samples are available. The spectrometer can sort pulses into several different scalers. Several different approaches to radioassay are made possible. A series of samples each containing different isotopes can be counted together.

By proper choice of amplier gain and window settings, each channel of the spectrometer can be set to count only one isotope. An automatic counter can thus be set up to assay the results of several experiments or determinations during the same time period. A single automated scintillation spectrometer set to count overnight can thus supply the needs of several different studies in the same laboratory.

Monitoring for Counting Efficiency

Certain samples contain compounds that interfere with the generation or the emission of light pulses. Compounds such as carbon tetrachloride interfere with the transfer of energy from solvent to solute or with the emission of light by the solute. Other compounds, particularly those that are yellow, interfere by absorbing the light that is emitted. The effect of these interferences is to change the number of photons detected per radioactive event. The change in the height of the pulse that results may cause the pulse to be sorted out of the channel set to count that isotope and thus cause the loss of that count. This tends to decrease the efficiency of counting. Since most samples cause some degree of quenching, particularly when the sample is in high concentration in the scintillation solute, the efficiency of counting in each sample is estimated. There are several methods for doing this.

Channels-ratio Method. This method of determining counting efficiency is based mainly on pulse-height analysis. The window and gain settings in one channel are optimized for an unquenched sample of the isotope to be assayed. A second channel is set to record only a fraction of those pulses, generally those above the average pulse height. The division of counts between the 2 channels remains constant if the ratio of counts remains the same. If a quenching agent changes the number of photons emitted, the distribution of pulses between the 2 channels changes. Once the relationship between the ratio and efficiency of counting has been determined, the ratio can be used to monitor the efficiency in unknown samples.

The channels-ratio method is somewhat difficult to apply to samples containing more than one isotope. In these instances, the more energetic isotope gives rise to counts that may be displaced to a greater or lesser degree into the channel of the less energetic isotope. When a more accurate estimate of efficiency is required, it is generally useful to determine the efficiency for each isotope in each sample in each channel. This can be done by first counting the sample and then repeating the count after addition of known quantities of ^{14}C and then of ^{3}H (the "internal standard" method). When this method is used it is important that the ^{3}H or ^{14}C standard that is added be similar in solubility and chemical form to the labeled material to be assayed. For samples which are counted in toluene solution, ^{14}C or ^{3}H labeled toluene, which do not themselves quench, are useful. When the sample to be counted distributes between 2 phases, the choice of standard may be somewhat more difficult.

Determination of Efficiency with External Standards. Another approach for monitoring efficiency is to expose the sample to a high-energy gamma source and to measure the spectrum of pulses that results. The discriminator and amplifiers are set to record portions of the spectrum of pulse heights that are generally larger than those resulting from any of the radioactivity contained in the sample. Samples with quenching agents present generally show a shift in the spectrum that can be related to the efficiency of

counting. A series of samples containing known quantities of either ^{14}C or ^{3}H and graded quantities of quenching agents are generally counted first to determine the relationship between the efficiency of counting the isotopes in their respective channels and the counting rates of the external standards in its channels. Once this relationship is known the efficiency of unknown samples can be estimated directly from the counting rate and spectrum of the external standard.

There have been several instruments introduced in which the efficiency of counting, determined by the external standard method, is used as the basis for correcting for changes in efficiency. Several instruments employ built-in computers to read out the quantities of radioisotope present from the counting rates and the measured efficiency. In other devices, the data is used to modify the gain of the amplifier in an attempt to restore the efficiency to a preselected, constant value. One of the more imaginative devices changes the electron multiplication factor of the photomultiplier tube for each sample so as more nearly to approximate the efficiency of a reference sample.

The objective in most analyses is to insure that each of the samples is counted with approximately equal efficiency. One instrumental approach is to optimize the amplifier setting and then reduce the setting of the upper discriminator so that a small fraction of the larger pulses is excluded from the window. If a quenching agent is present the amplitude of all pulses is reduced. The amplitude of larger pulses is reduced sufficiently to fall within the counting window. At the same time, the amplitude of some of the small pulses is reduced so that they are too small to be counted. If the number of counts in the window is increased and decreased equally the counting rate is scarcely changed. The addition or removal of small quantities of quenching agents thus has no effect on efficiency. The overall efficiency is decreased only slightly. This approach is termed "balance point" counting.

Simultaneous Counting of Two Isotopes

Two isotopes emitting beta particles of different energies such as ^{14}C and ^{3}H can often be assayed simultaneously in the same sample through the use of pulse-height analysis. However, since the energy of the beta particles of each isotope extends over a spectrum from very low levels up to the maximal energy characteristic of the isotope, the beta spectra of different isotopes all overlap at low levels. Some of the pulses arising from the more energetic isotope always appear in the channel optimized for the isotope with the lower energy. In order to perform a simultaneous assay one channel is generally optimized for each isotope. The efficiency of counting of each isotope in each channel is then determined by counting known samples. In a mixture containing both, the quantity of each can be calculated from the counting rates in each window through the use of simultaneous equations.

In simultaneous ^{14}C and ^{3}H counting, the lower level discriminator of the ^{14}C channel is generally raised somewhat above the optimal level to exclude most or all of the ^{3}H pulses. The counting rate in this channel is then due only to ^{14}C. The quantity of ^{3}H present is calculated from the counting rate in the lower channel minus the contribution of ^{14}C to that channel. Automatic equipment is now available which offers automatic background subtraction, automatic external standardization, and built-in special purpose computers for calculating and printing out the number of disintegrations per minute of each isotope in each sample.

Sample Preparation. A sample can be counted dissolved in a scintillator, suspended in a scintillator, coated on the surface of a scintillator, or, alternatively the scintillator can be dissolved or suspended in the sample. The chemical state of radioisotope can also be changed when necessary by convenient automated methods in order to achieve uniform efficiency for all samples in a series.

Solution Counting. The simplest method is to dissolve the sample in a scintillation solution. Toluene, one of the best scintillation solvents, is good for lipids, hydrocarbons and other such relatively nonpolar compounds. Some of these compounds cause quenching and are counted efficiently only in dilute solution. The efficiency can be monitored and corrected for by the electronic methods described above.

Polar compounds that are not very soluble in toluene can often be counted in toluene solution containing small quantities of solvents such as ethanol. The counting efficiency is usually appreciably less than that of toluene solutions alone. Small changes in electronic settings can usually compensate for these difficulties. It is rather important, however, to take care that the labeled compounds remain in solution. Proteins, for example, may tend to precipitate out and be counted with less efficiency than substances which are completely dissolved.

Counting of Suspensions. Many samples are most effectively assayed for radioactivity by suspending them in liquid scintillator. Carbon dioxide can be precipitated as barium carbonate and then suspended with the help of a thixotropic gelling agent. Other beta emitters such as strontium-90 can often be prepared as water and toluene-insoluble precipitates and counted effectively the same way. Silica gel from thin-layer chromatography plates can also be assayed this way. Samples deposited on filter paper such as sections of paper chromatograms are counted by depositing the entire strip of paper in the liquid scintillator.

The material to be assayed by this approach should be in the same chemical form in each sample. When the chemical forms are different, the distribution between solution and precipitate may vary somewhat and with this variation may come differences in counting efficiency. In general, the efficiency with which suspended materials are counted is surprisingly good. Light scattering is not as great a problem in liquid scintillation counting as it is in spectrophotometry or other similar optical systems in which the light must be transmitted to the phototube along a defined axis. Many samples that appear quite opaque can be counted with high efficiency.

The counting of suspensions has provided one of the most effective tools for the assay of radioactivity in aqueous solution. There are several detergents available that facilitate the preparation of colloidal suspensions of aqueous droplets in toluene. These emulsions can contain as much as 40 percent of water in toluene with acceptable counting efficiencies. One peculiarity of the mixtures of toluene, water and surfactant is that as the percentage of water is increased there is a sudden diminution in counting efficiency when the suspension separates into 2 phases; however, as the percentage of water is increased further a semi-opaque gel results and the counting efficiency increases to levels close to that obtained previously. Large or small concentrations of water are thus incorporated with good counting efficiency but not intermediate. The usual explanation given for this phenomenon is that at low concentrations the water acts as a quenching agent. At higher concentrations 2 phases are formed, and the radioactive material soluble in the water is effectively separated from the scintillator. The efficiency is decreased further and rather sharply when separation occurs. At still higher water concentrations an emulsion forms and the 2 phases are intimately associated with each other. The counting efficiency then is restored. Only at very high concentrations of water do the individual water droplets increase to a size sufficient to cause self-absorption. The occurrence of large droplets thus forms the upper limit of the volume of water that can be tolerated.

A distinct advantage offered by this approach is that potential quenching materials which may be present in aqueous solutions do not come in contact with, and therefore do not interfere with, the action of the scintillator.

Calibrating the efficiency of emulsion counting is somewhat difficult. Internal standards are useful only if the standard particions between the water and organic phases in the same way as the substance being counted. The use of external standardization requires very careful attention to the composition of the mixture. The channels-ratio method is helpful, particularly if the isotope to be counted is in only one chemical form so that its distribution between phases can be defined.

A number of prepared counting mixtures utilizing the emulsion counting approach are available from the major manufacturers of scintillation counters and scintillation counting reagents.

Counting of Aqueous Solutions by Placing them in Contact with Finely Divided Crystal Insulators

Another method for counting liquid solutions is to suspend finely divided crystals of organic scintillator in them. Steinberg, et al poured the solution to be counted over a weighed quantity of crystalline anthracene in a conventional counting vial.[1] The efficiency of ^{14}C was quite high but the efficiency for tritium was low. This system has formed the basis of the use of finely divided anthracene crystals for detecting the radioactivity in flowing liquid effluents of ion exchange and other columns such as are used for amino acid analysis. Similar instrumentation can be used for assaying radioactivity in flowing gas streams. Successful application of this approach requires that the materials to be assayed not precipitate upon or become adsorbed to the crystalline scintillator. Adsorption on the organic scintillator may constitute a severe limitation in some assays, since materials that are retained on the scintillator provide more counts in a flowing system than materials remaining in contact with the scintillator for a shorter time.

An advantage of the use of a flow-through detector is that the same scintillator can be used for the assay of an entire group of samples. This can result in a considerable saving of reagent expense when a large volume of solution is to be assayed, as in the assay of compounds separated by chromatography.

Automatic Conversion of ^{14}C and [3]H Labeled Compounds to [14]CO₂ and [3]H₂O by Combustion

A straightforward approach to counting complicated organic compounds, such as proteins or sections of acrylamide gel columns with uniform efficiency is to combust the samples. Automatic equipment is now available from several manufacturers for handling individual samples with a minimum of difficulty. Collection of $^{14}CO_2$ and ^3H_2O in scintillator solution is quantitative and convenient.

A second, and in time, an earlier approach to the assay of colored solutions was to subject the sample to bleaching with hydrogen peroxide. This method requires that care be taken to avoid chemiluminescence by gradually heating and then allowing the sample to stand prior to counting. The use of automatic combustion is probably preferable in most situations.

Interpretation of Results

In all metabolic studies we cannot assume that the radioactivity in a particular tissue or body fluid is in the same chemical form as the original compound administered. This is particularly true for ^{14}C and ^{3}H labeled compounds, most of which are readily metabolized. Correct interpretation of results frequently hinges on the accuracy with which the radioactive compounds are identified prior to an assay, which depends directly on the adequacy of the chemical methods used to isolate and purify the sample.

In the use of ^{3}H and ^{14}C labeled materials as chemical or biological reagents, such as in radioimmunoassays, the problems are similar. Most samples can generally be assayed effectively by emulsion counting. After they are separated by appropriate chemical techniques the compound bound to protein and that free in aqueous solution can be counted with equal efficiency, and a true bound-to-free ratio can be determined. It is generally important to maintain the same ratio of sample-to-scintillation-fluid volume for all samples in a group. With this minor caution the use of liquid scintillation counting is often comparable in convenience with the use of the gamma counter.

In many radioimmunoassay procedures iodine-125 can be effectively used to label the compound of interest. Iodine-125 can be assayed conveniently by liquid scintillation counting with generally superior sensitivity than that obtainable by crystal counting. The procedures used are similar to those used in counting [14]C.[2]

References

1. Steinberg, D.: Radioassay of aqueous solutions mixed with solid crystalline fluors. Nature, *183*:1253, 1959.
2. Rhodes, B.: Liquid scintillation counting of radio iodine. Anal. Chem., *37*:955, 1965.

Suggested Additional Reading

Price, L. W.: Practical Course in Liquid Scintillation Counting. Laboratory Practice. pp. 27-31, 110-114, 181-194, 277-283, 352-358, 417-422, 480-484, 571-574 (January through September 1973).

3 *Activation Analysis*

Benjamin Rothfeld, M.D.
Henry Kramer, Ph.D.

HISTORICAL BACKGROUND

Neutron activation analysis is used to determine the *elemental* concentrations in a sample material by measuring the radioactivity induced in specific isotopes of the elements after bombarding them with neutrons. This technique has been used to analyze liquid, solid and gaseous samples for about 70 elements, some with sensitivities as low as 10^{-12} Gm (0.000 000 000 001 Gm).

In this chapter the historical background of activation analysis, its basic principles and applications are presented.

The phenomenon of radioactivity was first identified in 1898. In 1934 Joliot and Curie demonstrated the phenomenon of induced radioactivity. Two years later, in 1936, Hevesy and Levi[1] suggested the application of the principle of induced radioactivity. However, years elapsed before there was any systematic application of this process. There were several reasons for this time lag including the scarcity of neutron sources and the fact that they were not readily available for biological experimentation. After World War II this became less of a problem. Furthermore, sophisticated instrumentation, specifically multichannel gamma-ray spectrometry, the most commonly used counting method in neutron activation analysis, only became available about 1957. Activation analysis without this is possible but is quite tedious.

PRINCIPLES OF NEUTRON ACTIVATION ANALYSIS

There are 3 basic steps involved in neutron activation analysis (NAA)[2]: activation, isolation and counting. These steps are dealt with in more detail below. Although the great majority of studies involving neutron activation analysis deals with elements, in the material to be studied there is a variation in which enriched stable isotopes are used. Here the stable isotope is utilized as a tracer and subsequent quantitation is done by neutron activation of the enriched isotope. This means tracer studies can be performed in biologic systems in human beings without radiation exposure.

Activation

Although the terms activation analysis and neutron activation analysis are often used synonymously this is, strictly speaking, not correct. Actually, any type of nuclear particle or radiation may be used to alter an atomic nucleus. Protons, deuterons and high-energy electromagnetic radiation, as well as neutrons, may be used. However, neutrons have certain definite advantages over these alternative sources. Since they have no charge and therefore are neither attracted nor repelled by nuclei, the probability of an interaction is more likely. Additionally, the charged particles are more likely to raise the target material to a high temperature than are neutrons, thus limiting practical applications. Also, the technology involved with charged particles is more complex than with neutrons. The use of high-energy photons requires very intense generating sources. Therefore, all in all, neutrons are the most practical material for these reactions.

In NAA, the sample to be analyzed is exposed to a high-neutron flux, so that radioactivity is induced and the radioisotopes thereby formed may be analyzed.

There are several possible neutron sources available to generate this flux—nuclear reactors, neutron generators and isotopic sources.[3] For practical purposes, the reactor is the only source which permits analyses in the range of importance for trace element work, because its flux of 10^{11} to 10^{14} neutrons per cm^2 per second permits analyses in the 10^{-12} to 10^{-6} Gm range, which is the range of importance for trace element analysis. Neutron generators such as the Cockcroft-Walton generator and the VandeGraff generator produce fluxes in the range of 10^7 to 10^{10} neutrons per cm^2 per second ($n/cm^2 \cdot sec$) and the accompanying reduction in sensitivity makes these devices unsuitable for most trace element applications. The yield of isotopic sources is, in general, still lower and their main function is in teaching. However, recent innovations[4] using the radionuclide Californium-252 have produced usable fluxes of 10^8-10^9 $n/cm^2 \cdot sec$, approaching that of neutron generators.

On the whole, thermal neutrons are much preferable to fast neutrons in activation analysis, because the probability of their interaction with nuclei is usually greater than that with fast neutrons, thereby yielding a more sensitive analysis. However, for lower atomic weight elements (lower than sodium) fast neutrons are the only practical source for activation analysis. This is discussed further below.

In neutron activation analysis, once a nucleus captures a neutron a compound nuclide is formed. The compound nuclide is highly unstable and immediately releases excess energy by emitting "prompt radiation."

In the process, the compound nuclide is transformed to an isotope that may be either stable or radioactive. Studies of "prompt radiation" are of value in providing information about the particular reaction and are of interest primarily to physicists; but recently, prompt radiation analysis is being studied for elemental analyses.[4] It is the nucleus formed after the prompt radiation is given off which is of prime interest for trace element analysis. If it is radioactive, it is its radiation which is detected and measured in neutron activation analysis.

The amount of radioactivity created by an isotope capturing a neutron may be expressed by the 2 following formulas:[5]

$$(1) \quad A_t = A_\infty \left(1 - e^{\frac{-.693t}{T\frac{1}{2}}}\right)$$

$$(2) \quad A_\infty = N \phi \sigma$$

$t =$ neutron exposure time

$T\frac{1}{2} =$ half-life of isotope produced

$N =$ number of atoms present of isotope being activated

$\phi =$ neutron flux in neutrons/cm^2 per second

$\sigma =$ neutron activation cross-section of target nuclei in $10^{-24} cm^2$ per nucleus

A_∞ is the radioactivity at saturation after neutron exposure of infinite time in disintegrations/unit of time. A cross-section or σ of a stable isotope for neutrons represents the probability of a neutron being captured by a nucleus of that isotope. This probability is a specific characteristic of the isotope and also a function of the energy of the bombarding neutron. This cross-section is usually expressed as barns. The greater the number of barns involved in a reaction the greater is the probability of capture.

Separation

In studying various biological tissues and fluids, sodium and chloride are so common that when they are activated they often swamp out all other elements. Therefore, it is often necessary to have a preliminary step in order to separate these elements from those which are of interest. These separations are made only after the radioactivity is induced (after neutron bombardment) in the sample. Preirradiation separations are virtually never done because of possible sample contamination.

All methods of separation may be listed under the following categories: time, pulse height analysis, computer and chemical. Three of these separation methods are unique to neutron activation analysis and are used routinely to permit direct analysis of the sample without any postirradiation chemical processing. They give the NAA a flexibility no other analytical method has.

Time. By varying the amount of radiation time and the decay time periods before counting, one is able to take advantage of the differences between the half-lives of the various nuclides being studied. By these means it is possible to increase or decrease the yield of a given isotope compared to other isotopes.

Instrumental. One of the reasons that beta emitters are not used often in activation analysis is because their spectrum is a continuum extending over a wide range of energies. Unlike gamma rays which have discrete energies, beta energies cannot be resolved by pulse height analysis. Instrumental technique uses pulse height analysis to separate the radiations produced by one gamma emitter from those produced by others. This permits simultaneous analysis of a number of radionuclides in the same sample.[6] However, if the gamma energies of several of the elements being studied are close together, pulse height analysis becomes impractical and it becomes necessary to use computer or chemical methods.

Computer Methods. These involve least squares, multiple regression, linear programming, machine stripping and stepwise fitting. These methods are mentioned for completeness and will not be gone into in any detail here.

Chemical Methods. In these methods a known amount of the stable element of interest is added as a carrier. The chemical separations need not be quantitative, because the radioactivity measurements can be corrected by the known efficiency of the chemical processing. A procedure following standard quantitative analysis is followed to separate out the element of interest, which is then counted using standard radionuclide measurement techniques.

Counting

The basic tool here is the gamma-ray pulse height analyzer. From this, both quantitative and qualitative information can be obtained. The gamma-ray energy provides the qualitative determination of the radionuclides in the sample while the total counts collected for a given energy provide the quantitative determination.

For quantitation, a small sample of the stable element of known weight is irradiated. The expected number of radioactive atoms can be calculated and the radioactivity per unit weight of stable element determined. The same degree of activity is expected in the unknown, and hence the initial weight of the stable element in the unknown may be calculated. Although quantitative measurements can be made from calculations using basic nuclear information, the use of the standard cancels out various inaccuracies which may develop during the procedure and is inevitably more accurate than calculations based on theoretical computations.

The radiations emitted from a neutron activated sample are measured using either a NaI(Tl) or a Ge(Li) detector. The latter provides much better energy resolution and makes possible the analysis of many samples which must be radiochemically separated before they can be analyzed using the former. NaI(Tl) detectors are useful for the analysis of a small number of elements in a sample; however, it has the advantage of having a greater efficiency relative to a Ge(Li) detector. Both these detectors are used with multichannel pulse height analyzers, although a more sophisticated system is required for optimal utilization of a Ge(Li) detector. More recently Ge(Li) detectors have increased in sensitivity, and this combined with their higher resolution has led to their in-

Table 3-1. Typical Uses of Neutron Activation Analysis.

Element Determined	Material Analyzed	Concentration Found (µg/g)
IN BIOCHEMISTRY		
Antimony	Blood	0.1-1.
Arsenic	Blood, Hair, Urine	0.1-0.0005
Vanadium	Hair, Tissue	1-0.0005
Iodine	Blood proteins	0.0001-1.
Cobalt	Plant ash	0.001
Iron	Grasses and Grains	100-1000
Molybdenum	Sugar cane	.01-0.1
Selenium	Fish meal, Crab meal	1.0-0.01
IN METALLURGY		
Oxygen	Steel, Tantalum, Aluminum	10-100
Gold	Silicon	0.1-1.0
Chromium	Aluminum, Silicon, Arsenic	1.
Manganese	Beryllium	10-100
Potassium	Silicon, Tungsten	0.1
Tantalum	Silicon	1.
IN SEMICONDUCTOR MATERIALS		
Gold	Arsenic	0.0001
Sodium	Gallium	100
Oxygen	Silicon	10
IN GEOCHEMISTRY		
Thorium	Ores, Water, Soils	0.01-1.
	Minerals	0.001
Uranium	Various ores	0.1-0.001
IN PLASTICS		
Chromium, Aluminum	Polyethylene	0.01-10.0
Sodium, Rubidium, Copper	Fluorocarbons	1.0-0.001
Iron, Cesium, Zinc, Sodium	Epoxies	1.0-0.0001

creasing use recently. If there are only a few elements being analyzed in the sample, the calculations are relatively simple. However, if there are a large number of elements in the sample, computer data reduction is necessary. This is especially true if a crystal containing Ge(Li) is used, since here a large number of peaks are resolved in the spectrum (there are often over 100 such peaks).[7]

TYPES OF ELEMENTS TO WHICH NAA IS APPLICABLE

The elements which can be assayed for by neutron activation analysis vary depending on whether thermal or fast neutrons are used. In using thermal neutrons, only elements from sodium on up in the periodic table can be readily measured. If it is desired to assay for elements of lower atomic number, it is

Table 3-2. Elemental Sensitivities—Neutron Activation Analysis.

SENSITIVITIES:

■ Representative of the sensitivities possible for short irradiations are the values shown below for some of the elements:

Element	Micrograms
Oxygen	100.
Fluorine	1.
Sodium	.02
Magnesium	.06
Aluminum	.0009
Silicon	.5
Sulfur	20.
Chlorine	.004
Potassium	.2
Calcium	.2
Scandium	.0003
Titanium	.005
Vanadium	.0001
Chromium	0.1
Manganese	.0002
Cobalt	.001
Nickel	.2
Copper	.005
Zinc	.05
Gallium	.01
Arsenic	.0001
Selenium	.01
Bromine	.001
Rubidium	.1
Strontium	.08
Yttrium	1.0
Columbium	.01
Molybdenum	.04
Ruthenium	.08
Rhodium	.0001
Palladium	.01
Silver	.001
Cadmium	1.0
Indium	.00002
Tin	.07
Antimony	.007
Tellurium	.02
Iodine	.001
Cesium	.001
Barium	.1
Lanthanum	.002
Cerium	.9
Praseodymium	.005
Neodymium	.03
Samarium	.004
Europium	.00004
Gadolinium	.006
Terbium	.01
Dysprosium	.0001
Holmium	.002
Erbium	.003
Thulium	.08
Ytterbium	.01
Lutetium	.0004
Hafnium	.005
Tantalum	.005
Tungsten	.009
Rhenium	.002
Osmium	.2
Iridium	.00001
Platinum	.05
Gold	.0001
Mercury	.05
Thorium	.001
Uranium	.0001

necessary to use fast neutrons. This has an advantage in that in organic tissues the predominant elements are carbon, hydrogen, oxygen and nitrogen, and they will not become activated and interfere with tests for other elements when using thermal neutrons.

Isotopes which give off beta particles after activation present many problems in the analysis. It is only practical to use beta particles for analysis if they are the sole analytic indicators of the isotope of interest or if the element under study can be conveniently isolated in pure form. On the whole, elements which yield gamma-ray emitters when neutron activated are much preferable for this type of work.

Another factor to be taken into consideration in deciding whether to assay an element using neutron activation analysis is whether a radiochemistry step is necessary. In a biological sample, elements such as bromine, iron, potassium, sodium, phosphorus, rubidium and zinc may be analyzed without chemical separations. Also toxicologic investigations[8] for elements present in abnormally high concentrations are sometimes possible without a chemical separation. Under some conditions the following elements may also be analyzed for without such separations: silver, calcium, cadmium, cobalt, chromium, cesium, mercury, magnanese, antimony, and selenium.[9] The previous statement is applicable only when using Ge(Li) detectors. In general, neutron activation analysis is used to analyze for trace, as well as macro, amounts of elements in all types of materials.[10] Its sensitivity, specificity, and versatility, have led to its use in all areas of science. Typical uses are shown in Table 3-1; typical elemental sensitivities are shown in Table 3-2.

SOURCES OF ERROR IN HANDLING OF SAMPLES

Needless to say, as in all analytic methods, pains should be taken to obtain a representative sample. The sample should reflect accurately the characteristics of the material being analyzed.

Sources of contamination must be excluded with great care. Since this method is so sensitive, constant awareness must be maintained to eliminate possible sources of contamination.[11] Thus, use ethyl alcohol instead of antiseptics containing iodine and mercury for cleansing skin prior to venipuncture. Be careful in using stainless steel needles, since their hubs are often plated with nickel or chromium. It is preferable to use needles without hubs. Avoid using syringes (plastic syringes are preferable), metal plated knives and scissors and also metal storage vessels, since many trace elements may be found in them. Avoid using autoclaves, since trace amounts of elements are distilled from the soldered joints and from the water used to produce the steam. Preferably sterilize by ethylene oxide or by ionizing radiation. Avoid the use of drying ovens, also for the same reason, using infrared lamps in their place. Of course, once the material has been neutron activated there is no need for these precautions in terms of the various tools used in handling the material. Contamination with nonradioactive trace elements at this point will not affect the final result. In addition, since no chemistry is performed on the sample until after activation, one does not have to be concerned with reagent blanks (the inherent trace elements contamination in reagents that are virtually impossible to remove). This is one of the great advantages of neutron activation analysis over other techniques for trace metal studies: contamination with trace amounts of any element after activation does not interfere with the analysis.

ADVANTAGES AND DISADVANTAGES OF NEUTRON ACTIVATION ANALYSIS

Advantages. The great advantage of neutron activation analysis is its great sensitivity. Using this method it is possible to detect most of the elements in any matrix at a concentration of less than 0.1 parts per billion. Additionally, the element in question can be determined no matter what its chemical form or oxidation state, that is, there is essentially no matrix effect, nor is there a blank effect. After irradiation the careful technique needed in other analytic chemical techniques is not necessary since contamination of the sample is unimportant. This method is usually nondestructive especially when no radiochemical separations are necessary.[12] Because of its nondestructive character many elements can be determined in a single sample. It is in this area of application that activation analysis is most cost effective.[7]

Other advantages are its high accuracy and precision and its high specificity. In addition, activation analysis can be used to measure the concentration of a specific isotope of an element, since the bombarding neutrons interact with the isotope of an element to give rise to a unique product for each isotope.

Disadvantages. The primary disadvantage of this method is usually its cost. Construction and operation of a nuclear reactor is extremely expensive. Although it is possible to do neutron activation using the less expensive neutron generators and isotopic neutron sources, the relatively low neutron flux available here limits the sensitivity that can be obtained. Furthermore, sophisticated nuclear instrumentation is required to take full advantage of this method. It has been recommended that for the investigator who needs an in-house capability for analysis at low cost, atomic absorption and flame emission are preferable.[7]

Another limitation of this method is that its practical application is limited to about 65 elements. Additionally, no information can be obtained regarding the matrix of the material, and it cannot be used for quantitation of organic compounds.

Thus, unless there is some definite advantage to be gained from the increased sensitivity available from neutron activation analysis, its application is often limited because of cost factors. Currently there are several highly sensitive techniques for trace metal analysis.[7] These are spark's source mass spectroscopy, atomic absorption, flame emission spectroscopy, anodic stripping voltametry, and x-ray fluorescence.[13-16] If the cost is left out of account, activation analysis provides a great advantage in that it has the greatest freedom from reagent and laboratory contamination and, in general, the greatest elemental sensitivity.

What then are the indications for neutron activation analysis? They may be summarized as follows:

1. *Repetitive analyses for a few elements which can be done instrumentally.* In this case large numbers may be done automatically. It is in this area that NAA is most cost effective and based on cost per element per sample it can compete effectively with atomic absorption.[7]

2. *Special analyses requiring high sensitivity:* for example, the rare earths, manganese and arsenic.

3. *Analyses of enriched stable isotopic tracers.*[17] This is especially important where radiation exposure should be minimized.[12]

4. *General exploration.* Since NAA has an extremely good sensitivity for virtually all the heavy elements (elements of atomic number greater than sodium), it can be used to seek out those elements that show the greatest correlation with what one is looking for. Then one can often develop a cheaper methodology to assay a large number of samples for the few elements of interest.

5. *Assay for a large number of elements in a single, small (<10 mg) sample.* Because of the sensitivity and time manipulation characteristics of the NAA technique, it is readily possible to assay for many (>20) elements in a single needle biopsy sample. This is a unique ability of NAA.

As was pointed out above, to do NAA for trace assays, one really needs a nuclear reactor and expensive counting equipment. This is an expensive "set-up." However, there are a number of commercially available NAA services. The most current listing is given in Nuclear News Buyers Guide *17*: (No. 3), 1974. Many of those on the list do not do their own NAA but subcontract out the assay to another on this same listing. In addition, costs per assay are not standardized and can vary significantly from outfit to outfit depending on the element, sample matrix and

number of samples. It is best to shop around for costs, reliability, and accuracy.

MEDICAL APPLICATIONS

The main use of NAA in the medical area is in analyzing for trace elements.[18] Using this technique a large number of studies have been done on trace elements in various tissues. Thus elements such as antimony, arsenic, molybdenum, nickel, selenium, zinc, etc. have been studied using this technique. The hope was that changes in these elements could be related to various disease processes.[19,20,21] Additionally this technique has been used, as described above, for the study of enriched stable isotopic tracers.[17] In the latter application its advantage is that radiation exposure to human subjects is minimized.[22]

A large number of studies have been done seeking for changes in trace elements in various diseases. These may be divided into skin diseases and systemic disorders. In the former certain workers[23] found that patients with scleroderma, basal cell carcinoma, and psoriasis erythroderma all had zinc levels below normal in their skin biopsies. Other authors state that previous investigators found zinc levels in psoriatic skin ranged from below to above normal.[24] In their work they found zinc levels to be higher than normal. Copper levels were normal in skin. Serum copper levels in psoriatic patients were elevated but not serum zinc levels. Also, studies in skin reveal that in malignant melanoma selenium, scandium and copper are elevated.

A fair amount of work has been done on changes in trace metals in systemic disorders using NAA. Thus it was found that serum cadmium was increased in hypertension.[25] Others have found that NAA applied to nail clippings[26] and sweat[17] revealed higher than normal levels of sodium in patients with cystic fibrosis. They felt that this was a reliable screening technique for this disorder.[27] Other workers[28] applied this technique for determining the stable iodine uptake of the thyroid. Additionally it has been found that

Table 3-3. Concentrations of Elements in Biological Substances in Various Diseases.

Condition	Matrix Analyzed	Element*
Myocardial infarction	Serum	Mn ↑[30], Zn ↓, Mg ↓, Cu ↑, Na ↑[31]
	Urine	Mn ↑, Cu ↑[32]
	Tissue	As ↑, Mo ↓, Cu ↓, Ce ↑[33]
Uremia	Blood	As ↑, Mo'↑[34]
Chronic myelogenous leukemia	Leukocytes	Cu ↓, Mn ↓[35]
Rheumatoid arthritis	Blood	Cu ↑[36], Zn ↓, Na ↓[31]
Cancer	Tissues	↓ (many)[37,38]
Muscular dystrophy	Skeletal muscle	K ↓, Na ↑[39]
Melanoma	Tissue	Se ↑, Sc ↑, Cu ↑[40]
Wilson's disease	Serum	Cu ↓[41]
Hyperphagia and obesity	Tissue	Au ↑[42]
Fatty cirrhosis	Tissue	Mn ↓[43]
Trauma	Hair	Zn ↓[44]
Atherosclerosis	Hair	Zn ↓[44]
	Blood	Zn ↓[44]

* Arrows pointing up indicate an elevated concentration; arrows pointing down, a decreased concentration. (Adapted from Kramer, H.: Wagner Nuclear Medicine. chap. 20. W. B. Saunders, 1968)

in white muscle disease in cattle tissue selenium is depressed, and this disease may be prevented by supplementing the animals' feed with selenium. Much other work has been done in associating disease states to trace metal content and some is summarized in Table 3-3. Much of the work done in this field has been conflicting, possibly because of the problems with sample collection and preservation as discussed above.

Although this book is devoted to in vitro techniques, mention is made of in vivo techniques at this point. This involves whole body radiation to produce neutron activation analysis.[45] By this means the calcium status of subjects has been evaluated, as well as that of body nitrogen.[46,47] Needless to say, this is currently a research technique.

All in all, a large amount of data has been accumulated with regard to trace element composition in various disorders. So far the practical applications have been disappointing with regard to human disease states. A number of tantalizing results have been obtained but no breakthroughs have occurred. Currently one has to wonder whether breakthroughs in various disorders will be made which will render these results somewhat irrelevant. Situations which come to mind

are those with regard to the painstaking studies of the biology of the pneumococcus which were rendered moot when penicillin came along, and the detailed studies done on the tubercle bacillus which, although interesting, became more or less irrelevant when INH was developed. Or contrariwise will we have a situation as with polio vaccine in which a large number of very carefully applied facts were synthesized into the production of a vaccine which brought a dreaded disease under control? Only time will tell.

References

1. Hevesy, G. von, and Levi, H.: Actions of neutrons on the rare earth elements, Kgl. Danske Vivensk. Selsk. Math-Fys. Medc., *14*:5, 1936.
2. Wahl, W. H., and Kramer, H. H.: Neutron activation analysis. Sci. Amer., *216*:68, 1967.
3. Kramer, H., and Wahl, W.: Chapter 20, Wagner, H. N.: Principles of Nuclear Medicine. Philadelphia, W. B. Saunders, 1968.
4. Californium-252 Progress. vol. 16, December, 1973.
5. Taylor, T. I., and Havens, W. W., Jr.: Neutron spectroscopy and neutron interactions chemical analysis. *In* Berl, W. G. (ed.): Physical Methods of Chemical Analysis. vol. 3. New York, Academic Press, 1956.

6. Nadkarni, R. A., and Morrison, G. H.: Multielement instrumental neutron activation analysis of biological materials. Anal. Chem., 45:1957, 1973.

7. Vogt, J. R.: Methodology and problems in analysis of trace elements activation analysis. Ann. N.Y. Acad. Sci., 199:237, 1972.

8. Smith, H.: Neutron Activation Analysis and Toxicology. J. Radioanal. Chem., 15: 71, 1973.

9. Parr, R. M.: Applications of Ge (Li) detectors in medical activation analysis. Br. J. Radiol., 45:797, 1972.

10. Lutz, G. L., et al.: Activation Amelysis: A Bibliography Through 1971. National Bureau of Standards Technical Note 467.

11. Versieck, J. M. J., and Speecke, A. B. H.: Contaminations Induced by Collection of Liver Biopsies and Human Blood in Nuclear Activation Techniques in the Life Sciences, pp. 39-49. Yugoslavia Conference, April, 1972; IAEA Proceedings (Vienna), 1972.

12. Bethard, W. F., and Blahd, W.: Nuclear Medicine. New York, McGraw-Hill, 1965.

13. Hopps, H. C., and Cannon, H. L.: Geochemical environment in relation to health and disease. Ann. N.Y. Acad. Sci., 199: 137, 1972.

14. Sunderman, F. W., Jr.: Atomic absorption spectrometry of trace metals in clinical pathology. Human Path., 4:549, 1973.

15. Puumalainen, P., et al.: A selective microscale x-ray fluorescence analyzing method for determination of trace elements. Int. J. Appl. Rad. Isot., 24:617, 1973.

16. Baglin, R. J., et al.: Application of nondispersive x-ray fluorescence techniques for in vitro studies. IEEE Trans. Nucl. Sci., NS20, 1:379, 1973.

17. Wahl, W. H., Nass, H. W., and Kramer, H. H.: Use of stable isotopes and activation analysis for in vivo diagnostic studies, pp. 191-204. Radioactive Pharmaceuticals CONF-651111, U. S. Department of Commerce, Washington, D. C., 1965.

18. Nuclear Activation Techniques in the Life Sciences. Yugoslavia Conference, April 10-14, 1972, IAEA Proceedings (Vienna), 1972.

19. Schroeder, H. A., and Nason, A. P.: Trace element analysis in clinical chemistry. Clin. Chem., 17:461, 1971.

20. Nielsen, F. H.: Newer Trace Elements in Human Nutrition. Food Technology, 38, January, 1971.

21. Lisk, D. J.: Ecological aspects of metals. N.Y. State J. M., 71:2541, 1971.

22. Glomski, C. A., et al.: Survival of [50]Cr-labeled erythrocytes as studied by instrumental activation analysis. J. Nud. Med., 12:31, 1971.

23. Gooden, D. S.: Nondestructive neutron activation analyses for the determination of manganese and zinc in human skin biopsies. Phys. Med. Biol. 17:26, 1972.

24. Mohamed, M., Molokhia, and Portnoy, B.: Neutron activation analysis of trace elements in skin. Br. J. Dermatol., 83:376, 1970.

25. Schroeder, H.: Journal of Chronic Diseases, 18:217, 1965.

26. Kopito, L., and Shwachman, H.: Spectroscopic analysis of tissues from patients with cystic fibrosis and controls. Nature, 202: 501, 1964.

27. Johnson, C. F., et al.: Neutron activation analysis technique for nail sodium concentration in cystic fibrosis patients. Pediatrics, 47:88, 1971.

28. Wagner, H. N., Nelp, W. B., and Dowling, J. H.: Use of neutron activation analysis for studying stable iodine uptake by the thyroid. J. Clin. Invest., 40:1984, 1961.

29. Kramer, H.: Personal communication.

30. Kanabrocki, E. L., et al.: Neutron activation studies of biological fluids: Manganese and copper. Int. J. Appl. Radiat., 15:175, 1964.

31. Danis, J., and Kusleikaiti. Quantitative changes of trace elements in some internal diseases. Ter. Arkh., 44:9, 1972.

32. Kanabrocki, E. L.: Manganese and copper levels in human urine. J. Nucl. Med., 6: 780, 1965.

33. Wester, P. O.: Trace elements in human myocardial infarction determined by neutron activation analysis. Acta Med. Scand., 178:765, 1965.

34. Brune, D., Samsahl, K., and Wester, P. O.: A comparison between the amount of As, Au, Br, Cu, Fe, Mo, Se, and Zn in normal and uraemic human whole blood by means of neutron activation analysis. Clin. Chim. Acta, 13:285, 1966.

35. Frischauf, H.: Studies on the content of trace elements in leukocytes with neutron activation analysis. Folia Haematol. (Leipzig) 7:291, 1963.

36. Plantin, L. O., and Strandberg, P. O.: Whole blood concentrations of copper and zinc in rheumatoid arthritis studied by activation analysis. Acta Rheumatol. Scand., 11:30, 1965.

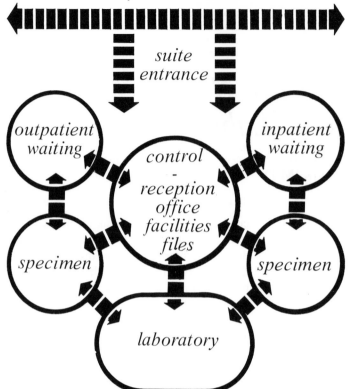

Fig. 4-1. The relationship to one another of the various divisions of an RIA unit.

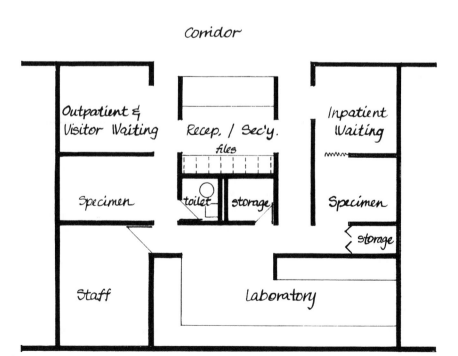

Fig. 4-2A.

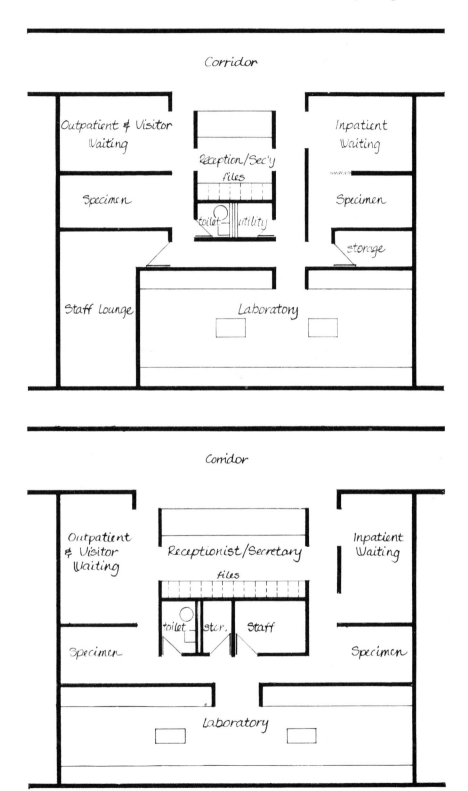

Fig. 4-2. *A, B,* and *C.* Model **RIA** units based on space availability.

a practical standpoint it is an advantage to have the unit in conjunction with a nuclear medicine department so that waiting rooms, record keeping, staff facilities and equipment may be shared, and there is more room for actual bench operations.

Figure 4-1 shows how each area of an in vitro nuclear medicine unit relates to the other. Figures 4-2*A, B* and *C* are model layouts which may be considered based on space availability. These layouts can, of course, be built in stages if there are insufficient funds, but actually they represent an essential minimum. They incorporate several concepts which are vital to success and which are discussed below.

Separate Waiting Rooms for Inpatients and Outpatients. It is essential to keep inpatients separate from outpatients because of the possibility of nosocomial infections. Studies have stressed the risks involved in taking inpatients to x-ray departments[1] as well as to nuclear medicine departments. The outpatient and his accompanying family significantly increase the risks of nosocomial infections to the inpatient. There is also a loss of privacy and dignity for the inpatient involved in exposing him to outpatients and their accompanying families.

Reception Area. It is important to have a member of the unit available to greet the patient as he comes to the unit. Being placed at ease in a comfortable area promptly facilitates patient control and increases accuracy in many determinations in which the patient's position and anxiety are capable of altering test results. Also, if the reception area is situated in such a way as to provide visibility into both waiting rooms the staff can better control the area.

Record Area. Placing records adjacent to the reception area permits ready identification and processing of requisitions and data. Use of this space adds to the sense of privacy without blocking patient and staff movement.

Separate Areas for Drawing Specimens. Having such a separate area has two advantages. First, there is the opportunity to cut down on cross-infection. Second, patients have privacy while specimens are being obtained. They are not isolated from others but neither are they the objects of stares and comments.

Laboratory Area. The layout of this area presents the greatest complexity. It is difficult to be specific, because the design of this area depends on the type of equipment to be used. For instance, is equipment to be located on the floor or on workbenches? For equipment on the floor it is necessary to allow access to all parts of it for servicing. For bench equipment it is essential that it not be situated against the back of the bench because access and air flow are essential. Because benches come in various depths, order the most practical depth suitable for the size of your equipment.

One potential layout for a workbench equipment unit which may be employed with the overall unit layout (Fig. 4-2*A*) is Figure 4-3. With this scheme the technologist at one bench may use one of the detectors; another

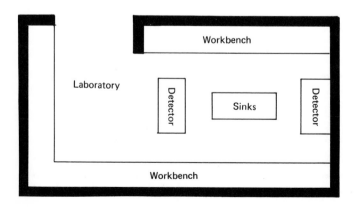

Fig. 4-3. A potential laboratory layout.

technologist can use the opposite bench and detector. Sufficient distance between the two detectors eliminates significant background interference. While two detector systems constitute an extra expense this cost is justified, since there is an increase in efficiency and the laboratory is not crippled if one of the detectors malfunctions.

Plan protected facilities for storage of fresh materials and temporary disposal of waste material. It is advisable to have a "permanent" disposal area for waste decay at a safe place outside the laboratory unit. Choose surfaces—floors, walls, bench—that are nonabsorbent and smooth so that spills can be properly taken care of and make sure they are strong enough to hold heavy equipment and lead bricks. There is no need for lead lining of walls unless x-ray units are nearby and constitute a source of altered background. This may be determined by monitoring equipment.

General Considerations. *Size.* The size of each area has not been specified because it may be quite variable. With careful planning, waiting rooms of 175 to 200 square feet are sufficient to handle a large amount of activity and specimen drawing areas of 100 square feet may suffice. The laboratory itself should, if possible, be at least 400 square feet. Thus, an overall area of 1,500 square feet allows operation, although with time it will undoubtedly require expansion. If possible in the initial planning, obtain an additional 500 square feet. Think in terms of the anticipated work load which will have to be managed several years from the inception of the laboratory. Experience has shown that utilizing every inch of space does not increase efficiency; the contrary is usually the result. If it is impossible to allow for this growth at the beginning, locate the unit in a place which does not preclude later expansion. Consult the plant engineer from the start, so that he can point out where walls may or may not be removed and where other obstacles to expansion exist which cannot be overcome.

Location. The location of the unit in terms of its interrelationship with the other facilities of the hospital is vital. With proper location and careful organization of the work of the laboratory, it is possible to cut down on the number of inpatients in the department at any one time.

Decoration. The decor of the unit reflects the attitude of the hospital and the staff and indicates the type of unit one has, just as one's house reflects the personality of its occupants. Since walls are often confining, do not use full walls where partial walls are possible, or omit walls entirely. Choose furniture that is stylish as well as utilitarian. Mirrors can often add to the general appearance of the laboratory. An FM radio playing soft, pleasant music can help relax anxious patients in the waiting areas.

Lighting. For areas in which people are sitting or standing use fluorescent or regular, ceiling, wall-mounted or free-standing lighting. In areas where patients are on beds or stretchers eliminate ceiling lights which may glare in the patient's eyes; rather use recessed, or corner, or wall lighting. There is a disadvantage to using floor lamps in these areas because they may be struck by moving stretchers.

The question has been raised whether fluorescent lighting is satisfactory for the bench area of the laboratory. It probably has little if any effect on gamma-detector units, since the background for these instruments appears to be caused chiefly by external radiation, including cosmic rays and radiation from radionuclides in shielding and other construction materials. In most instances, this amount of external radiation provides a relatively constant background level. However, with liquid scintillation counting (LSC) there does seem to be an effect.[2] Laboratory fluorescent lighting has been shown to increase background counts here; for example, it has been shown that white screw caps on the LSC vials give a higher background than black screw caps because of the greater effect of fluorescent lighting on the white caps.[3] Therefore, it is suggested that fluorescent lighting not be used in the area where liquid scintillation counting is done.

RECORDS

Requisition Slip. You will have to determine how many copies of the requisition slip are necessary. At least 4 copies are essential:

1. One copy slip to remain at the initiating source (to allow the ward clerk to check that the result has gone back to the floor, whereupon she can destroy her copy as she enters the complete report on the patient's chart).

2. One copy for the accounting office, so that the proper charge may be made (forwarded to accounting from the laboratory after completion of the test).

3. If your laboratory does not have a computer print-out, one copy for the ward to serve as the result slip.

4. One copy to the laboratory for a permanent record.

You may need more copies if the situation requires it (e.g., if separate professional component billing is to be done).

Allow room on the requisition slip for a short history. In the past more often than not, no history was forwarded to the laboratory. However, with the Joint Commission on Accreditation of Hospitals insisting on a history, the chances are that compliance will improve. The available assays may be pre-printed on the requisition slip if so desired. If the accounting department is computerized, preprinting with the assignment of a computer number is essential.

Several methods are used to identify the requisition. These may include name, hospital number, social security number and assigned unit number. One problem with using the social security number as identification is that children may not have them. Furthermore, while inpatients and many outpatients have hospital numbers and identification cards, some of the work is done on samples sent in without the patient's number attached.

The use of an assigned number by the nuclear medicine department requires a second system, a name system, in order to reclaim the permanent record for follow-up studies and comparison. Thus, it seems most practical to use the name system from the outset.

EQUIPMENT

The Scintillation Counter. Before deciding which scintillation counter to purchase—beta or gamma—it is important to consider the physics involved in radioimmunoassay.

One of the characteristics of radioactive disintegration is the *constancy* of the rate of disintegration. In any radioisotope a specific percentage of all of the atoms of the element disintegrate per unit of time. The actual rates vary tremendously with the varying radionuclides, in some cases a very small percentage, in others a very high percentage. That is, the half-life of ^{125}I is 60 days, of ^{131}I is 8 days, of ^3H is 12.26 years and of ^{14}C is 5,730 years. It is apparent that for a given number of atoms there are many more disintegrations of ^{131}I available for detection than of ^3H per unit of time. Similarly, more disintegrations of ^{125}I are available than of ^3H and ^{14}C.

A second factor to be considered is the *energy* of the disintegration and its effect on the efficiency of counting. ^{131}I can be counted with greater efficiency than ^3H. ^3H and ^{14}C (beta emitters) are isotopes which require liquid scintillation counters. ^{131}I and ^{125}I (gamma emitters) may be counted in a well-type scintillation counter. Thus, there seems to be definite advantages to counting gamma-emitters. From the above facts, however, it appears that ^{131}I has advantages over ^{125}I. From a theoretical point of view this is true, although ^{131}I has a lower specific activity (commercially available preparations of ^{131}I contain up to 80 to 85 percent ^{127}I, while ^{125}I contamination is much less).[4] When this factor is taken into account the difference between ^{131}I and ^{125}I is relatively small. Therefore, the longer half-life of ^{125}I becomes the determining factor. A kit labeled with ^{125}I has a longer shelf-life than one labeled with ^{131}I.

A third factor to consider is that more and more manufacturers are using the ^{125}I label rather than ^{3}H label. Therefore, a gamma counter is more practical than a beta counter. However, one must remember that not having a beta counter precludes the possibility of performing certain radioimmunoassays, and it is possible that some of them will never be feasible with gamma emitters.

The size of the crystal used in the gamma well detector must also be considered. A 3-inch crystal gives a higher sensitivity than a 2-inch crystal for ^{125}I and it also gives a higher background. At low energies practically all pulses fall within the photo-peak and the 2-inch crystal will be very efficient.[6] All in all, the 2-inch crystal seems quite practical for this type of counting and saves money.

A fourth factor concerns *automation*. Should the automatic counting equipment have a 100-, a 300- or a 500-sample capacity? It is the author's opinion that a 100-sample capacity (whether for gamma or beta) is sufficient. The limiting factor in handling samples is not in the counting but in the preparation. The money saved here can be put into sample and data handling rather than in counting capacity. A very practical use for the money saved involves refrigeration and temperature regulation.

Because some of the tests done in a nuclear medicine laboratory require centrifuging in the cold, it is wise to purchase a refrigerated centrifuge (approximately $3,500). Efforts to avoid this by placing the centrifuge tube into a second tube which has ice and/or dry ice at the bottom, or placing an ordinary centrifuge inside a refrigerator are unsatisfactory. Performing centrifugation in a cold room may have possibilities but it does not totally prevent the temperature rise involved in the centrifugation process.

Additional Equipment. Other essential equipment include: a water bath, timer, test tubes and test tube racks, glass and plastic pipets with rubber bulbs, air compressor, vortex-type mixer, automatic dispenser, vacuum aspirator, automatic pipetes with disposable tips, micropipets, and radiation safety equipment and materials. These are discussed below.

ATOMIC ENERGY COMMISSION (AEC) REGULATIONS

The AEC regulations are embodied in the Code of Federal Regulations, Title 10—Atomic Energy.[7] The authorization to use radioisotopes must come from the United States Atomic Energy Commission or from one's state if it is an "Agreement State." Part 30.3 specifies activities requiring a license and states that "except for persons exempt as provided . . . no person shall . . . receive, acquire, own, possess, use . . . by-product material except as authorized in a specific or general license issued pursuant to the regulations . . .". The exemptions refer to agreement states (states with which the AEC has entered into an effective agreement—where there are equivalent regulations—under subsection 274b. of the Act) and "when it makes a finding that the exemption . . . will not constitute an unreasonable risk . . . to the health and safety of the public." A person is exempt from the requirements for a license when the concentrations possessed do not exceed those in a specific schedule (Part 30.70). With regard to a radioimmunoassay unit (RIA) one cannot, from a practical standpoint, function without a license because the quantities involved exceed the maximal exempt amounts. These are:

$$^{125}\text{I}—1 \ \mu\text{Ci}$$
$$^{131}\text{I}—1 \ \mu\text{Ci}$$
$$^{3}\text{H}—1 \ \text{mCi}$$
$$^{14}\text{C}—100 \ \mu\text{Ci}$$

Institutions and physicians using more than one isotope must have a license, even if the amount involved for each isotope is an exempt quantity. Licenses for by-product material are of two types: *specific* and *general*. A specific license is necessary if any isotope is to be administered to a person internally or externally.

Specific License. The specific license requires AEC approval of an applicant's Form AEC-313 in which he verifies that:

1. His equipment and facilities are adequate to protect health.

2. He is qualified to use safely the materials for the purpose requested.

3. The maximal quantities he will possess at a time are appropriate.

4. He has satisfactory radiation detection and monitoring equipment.

5. He has adequate waste disposal facilities.

6. There is proper supervision in terms of record keeping and radiation protection, including a radioisotope committee.

General License. A general license may be obtained for limited diagnostic use—for thyroid uptakes with ^{131}I, for blood plasma volume determinations with ^{131}I and ^{125}I human serum albumin and for the use of Cobalt^{58} and Cobalt^{60} and Chromium^{51} for intestinal absorption of cyanocobalamin and red blood cell volumes and survival. This requires the filing of Form AEC-482 "Registration Certificate—Medical Use of By-product Material Under General License." It is possible also to obtain a general license for the use of ^{125}I and for ^{131}I for in vitro testing, but there are severe limitations on this general license: (a) It may not be used in units exceeding 10 μc each for in vitro tests; (b) the general licensee may not possess at any one time a total amount of ^{125}I and/or ^{131}I in excess of 200 μc and (c) the material must be in labeled prepackaged units. To obtain this permission, form AEC-483, "Registration Certificate—In Vitro Testing with By-product Material Under General License" must be filed with the Director, Division of Materials Licensing, U.S. Atomic Energy Commission, Washington, D.C. 20545, and one must receive back a validated copy of Form AEC-483 with a registration number assigned. The application form requires that one specify that he has the appropriate radiation measuring instruments to perform the in vitro tests with

the ^{125}I and ^{131}I (as noted above) and that these tests be performed only by personnel competent in the use of such instruments and in the handling of by-product materials.

Agreement States. At the present time the states which have signed agreement certificates with the AEC include: Alabama, Arizona, Arkansas, California, Colorado, Florida, Georgia, Idaho, Kansas, Kentucky, Louisiana, Maryland, Mississippi, Nebraska, New Hampshire, New York, North Carolina, North Dakota, Oregon, South Carolina, Tennessee, Texas and Washington. If you are starting your facility in one of these states, consult the State Health Department for advice.

RECORD KEEPING

It is necessary to account completely for all isotopes received, their use and the amount and type of disposition. Keep additional records with regard to radiation exposure of personnel, the monitoring of the facility and also data on instrumentation calibration and service.

It is also essential to comply with the requirement that any area in which radioactive material is stored or used (over the exempt quantities) must have a sign stating CAUTION—Radioactive Material or CAUTION—Radiation Area if the amount of radiation is 5 mr/hour or in excess of 100 mr in 5 consecutive days.

In complying with AEC requirements:

1. Check all deliveries of isotopes when they are received to be sure that there has been no breakage or contamination.

2. Keep down the level of exposure of personnel to radiation by proper storage of isotopes with proper shielding.

3. Dispose of liquid waste into the sanitary sewerage system, but be sure that it does not exceed the authorized limit. The material must be readily soluble or dispersible in water. The quantity of radioactive material added, diluted by the average daily quantity of sewage released into the sewerage system must result in an average concentration not

exceeding in any one day or any one month:

^{14}Carbon $2 \times 10^{-2}\ \mu Ci/ml$
^{3}Hydrogen $1 \times 10^{-1}\ \mu Ci/ml$
^{125}Iodine $4 \times 10^{-5}\ \mu Ci/ml$
^{131}Iodine $6 \times 10^{-5}\ \mu Ci/ml$

or 10 times the quantity of material specified in Appendix C of Title 10, Chapter 20:

^{14}Carbon $50\ \mu Ci$
^{3}Hydrogen $250\ \mu Ci$
^{131}Iodine $10\ \mu Ci$
^{125}Iodine   (not specifically noted but accepted at $6\ \mu Ci$)

The gross quantity of radioactive material released into the sewerage system by the licensee must not exceed 1 curie per year. The amount of flow into the sewerage system may be obtained from the hospital engineer or obtain from the local water department the specifics of the hospital water consumption.

4. Store solid wastes in shielded containers with plastic linings. Seal off the linings when filled, identify them with a date and place in an appropriate shielded area for decay, away from ready contact by personnel, patients, visitors and employees. Be sure to post the proper sign for this area.

5. Specify on company data sheets for the RIA kits that no AEC license is required for purchase or use of their materials. This statement is valid if you use only the one isotope in an amount not exceeding the exempt quantity.

If you already possess a specific license for the administration of radioactive material to humans it is sufficient for in vitro tests.

A new law, No. 30.41 has been added to 10 CFR Part 30. This was implemented in March 1974 and requires each manufacturer to verify that the user's license authorizes the receipt of the type, form and quantity of by-product material before it may be shipped to him.

In addition to the Atomic Energy Commission, the Department of Labor has a certain jurisdiction over Nuclear Medicine Laboratories. The appropriate rules are outlined in the Occupational Safety and Health Act.[8] Careful examination of the current standards indicates that there is no conflict between AEC and Occupational Safety and Health Administration regulations and that compliance with the AEC regulations as detailed above, places one in compliance with OSHA regulations.

FACTORS RELATING TO TECHNIQUE AND EQUIPMENT

Deciding whether to purchase prepackaged RIA kits or bulk supplies in setting up an assay requires an analysis of the relative costs of the reagents as against the number of assays to be performed. All things considered it is wiser to use a prepared kit at the outset, no matter what the volume, until experience has been developed with the test. Thereafter, when the number of tests to be performed (including controls) require more than one large prepackaged kit per week, you may consider buying bulk supplies because there is a considerable price saving. Take into consideration the capabilities of the personnel in the laboratory and be sure that you have facilities available for, and personnel experienced in, producing antisera and in labeling material with a radioactive tag. In most situations it is not practical to prepare your own antibodies and tag your antigens.

When the shipment of radioactive material arrives, note the label on the outside of the box. If the background color of the label is *all white,* the radiation level is so low that no special handling is required. If the background of the upper half of the label is *yellow,* the radiation level at the outside of the package must be considered. When the package has an *all yellow* label with 3 stripes, the vehicle in which it is carried must have a placard. All packages having a diameter of less than 21 inches have a surface radiation limitation of 200 mr/hr. The handler's hands are the main problem for this type of container. For packages larger than 21 inches in diameter, the surface radiation limitation is 10 mr/hr at 3 feet from the surface of the package, because the exposure is more likely to be to the whole body of the worker and because of the need to control the exposure to anyone near the package by chance. (The general population may not be exposed to more than 0.5 r/yr whole body dose and should not receive more than 0.17 r/yr whole body dose from all sources of radiation other than natural background and medical exposure.) Radiation must be controlled to avoid having a large number of packages producing cumulatively a much higher radiation level than desirable.

The package label, therefore, must specify the name of the isotope, the number of curies, millicuries or microcuries, vertical red lines and a "transport index" (number assigned to the package which relates directly to the radiation level so that there is no absolute need to determine the radiation level at a specified distance). The transport index is related to the radiation level in millirem per hour at 3 feet from the nearest accessible surface of the package. A number equivalent to the number of mr/hr, rounded to the nearest one-tenth of a unit, is assigned to the package as it is to be transported, and this number is called the "transport index." If the transport index exceeds zero a white

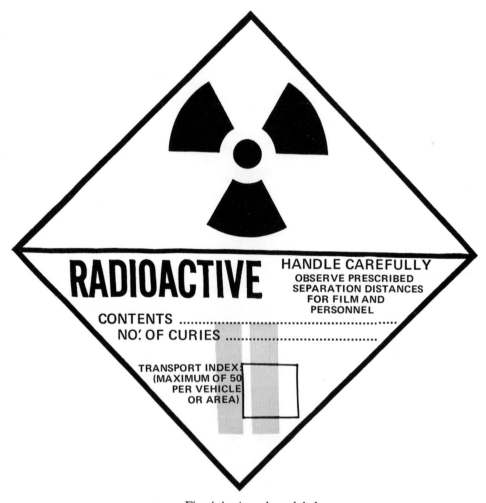

Fig. 4-4. A package label.

label may not be used; a yellow label is required and the transport index is then recorded on this yellow label. When shipping, the sum of the transport indices (TI) of all the yellow labeled packages present in one specific area may not exceed 50 at any time. The smallest outside dimension of any radioactive materials package must be 4 inches or greater. Liquid radioactive material requires packaging in a leakproof and corrosion resistant inner container which must be able to withstand a 30-foot drop-test without loss of liquid contents, and there must be enough absorbent material to absorb twice the volume of the radioactive liquid contents. If absorbent material is not used there must be an equally effective method of containment.

The vertical red lines on the label refer to the Fissile Classification, that is classification according to the controls needed to provide safety during transportation. The fissile classes are:

1. Fissile Class I—packages which may be transported in unlimited numbers and require no nuclear criticality safety controls during transportation. The external radiation level may or may not require a transport index number.

2. Fissile Class II—packages which may be transported together in any arrangement but in numbers which do not exceed an aggregate transport index of 50 without requiring a nuclear criticality safety control by the shipper.

3. Fissile Class III—shipments controlled in transportation to provide nuclear criticality safety. Reproduced in Figure 4-4 is a sample label. Your laboratory staff must be familiar with this label and what it means.

While wipe tests of the container are not required by law, it is a good practice to perform such a maneuver as soon as possible after receiving the shipment and to record the result on the inventory page. Surveying for contamination outside and inside as well as correlation with the amount of shielding, relate to the class of the shipment.

MONITORING

It is essential to have adequate monitoring equipment to obtain a specific AEC license. In addition to having a survey meter ($350-$500) laboratory personnel should have monitoring devices such as inexpensive film badges and finger ring badges. The film badge is not adequate for monitoring low-energy beta-radiation such as ^{14}C. It is possible to arrange contracts with firms which provide a monthly analysis of exposures and a cumulative print-out of exposures to date. It is necessary to keep records showing radiation exposures of all personnel on Form AEC-5; these company forms meet this requirement. Pocket dosimeters are suitable for daily use; they check exposure between badge and ring reports, and while not essential they are worthwhile. These types of personnel monitoring equipment are essential for each person who enters a restricted area. The maximal permissible exposures in rems per calendar quarter are:

1. Whole body; head and trunk; active blood-forming organs; lens of eyes; or gonads—1¼.

2. Hands and forearms; feet and ankles—18¾.

3. Skin of whole body—7½.

The forms must be kept for 5 years after termination of the individual's employment. Microfilm records are acceptable and each employee, former or present, has a right to a copy of this information. Each licensee must also maintain records of the results of surveys of his department and of his disposal area. Always remember that radiation areas must have conspicuously posted the required sign—CAUTION (or DANGER)—Radiation Area—with the conventional 3-bladed radiation design with the crosshatched area in magenta or purple on a yellow background. Each area or room in which licensed material is used or stored, and which contains any radioactive material in an amount exceeding 10 times the exempt amount, must also be conspicuously posted with a sign bearing the radiation caution symbol and the words CAUTION (or DANGER)—Radioactive Materials.

Form AEC-3 "Notice to Employees" must be conspicuously posted where employees are involved in activities licensed by the AEC. This form may be obtained by writing to the nearest AEC Regional Compliance Office or to AEC Division of Materials Licensing, Washington, D.C.

QUALITY CONTROL

Quality control starts with an attitude. Are you willing to pay for doing the work to the very best of your ability? Quality control costs money, time, and a great deal of effort. It is initiated with a thorough knowledge of the test itself, information such as is available in this volume. Know the correlations between the test results and the course of the disease state. If the test is to have any value, know the parameters that affect the results. For example, in CPB tests for T3 and T4, is the patient on oral contraceptive medication? In the digoxin assay is the patient on spironolactone? Use a special request blank for the ordering of a test which obtains such pertinent information before the test is started.

Then look at the labels on the materials you will use. Be sure to evaluate specific activity, expiration date and recommendations for storage. Also become familiar with the normal appearance of the material.

Patient and Laboratory Control. Consider quality control in terms of (a) the overall population making up your potential patient load, (b) the individual patient, and (c) the laboratory.

Potential Patient Load. The category of population means that it is necessary to develop a set of normal values for your own unit by constant attention to the possibility that the local normal is not identical to a textbook normal, or, to be more specific, to the limits of normal given with the kit. A recent (1972) survey of the College of American Pathologists in consultation with the American College of Radiology and the Society of Nuclear Medicine[9] comparing results showed that there existed with various methods considerable differences between laboratories and duplicates, and in clinical interpretation. As an example, in the survey the serum digoxin assays emphasized the need for defining an individual laboratory's own therapeutic range. Measured amounts of digoxin were added to serum samples (not containing digoxin at the start) to achieve concentrations of 2, 3, and 4 ng/ml. Participants in the survey, using 4 different assays, registered varying results. The digoxin assay method using ^{125}I digoxin consistently gave higher results than the method using the ^3H label. The clinical interpretation applied was based on the numerical values obtained in the assay. When the actual concentration of the digoxin was 2 ng/ml, the results reported by 83 percent of the RIA units using the iodinated antigen considered it to be in the toxic range. Almost half of the units reported digoxin levels within the therapeutic range when there was no digoxin present. The conclusion of the survey was that the lack of accuracy was in part due to the reliance for therapeutic and toxic ranges on the values supplied by the manufacturer with the kit. It urged that the determination of normals for each test be established by each RIA unit for itself.

Individual Patient. Be aware of the potential for change in "normals." For example, radioactive iodine uptake results were listed with a normal range of 15 percent to 45 percent in standard textbooks for years. More recently many laboratories have been lowering their "normals" to roughly 8 percent to 33 percent. This drop is felt to be due to an increased dietary iodine intake by the general population. It is necessary to do many controls and keep on doing spot-checks. The individual patient's variation is another factor. Not only do patients differ from one another but they differ from themselves over a period of time. Such things as circadian rhythms of hormone secretion reflect the stimuli acting on the body; in specific instances the RIA data reported have value only in the context of time, which must be specified in a report if it is to have meaning.

The Laboratory. Here you have the greatest opportunity to enforce control. In its simplest form laboratory control may be divided into (a) the difference obtained on duplicate or triplicate tests in any one run-through of an assay at one time, and (b) the difference obtained in the same RIA on today's test as compared to yesterday's or last month's.

The Number of Samples per Patient. A question frequently raised is the necessity for performing each unknown patient's sample in duplicate or triplicate. Although it is more expensive, studies should be done at least in duplicate. As a corollary to this it is quite apparent that emergency studies are especially expensive. Therefore, as much as possible, avoid stat requests. Careful scheduling and staff education help here. If grossly abnormal results are obtained it is prudent to do another sample from the patient on the next assay run (again in duplicate) to verify the data. The patient charge for the first run should be high enough to cover reruns on an all-inclusive basis. If the overall economics of a test preclude its being done in the best possible manner, consider not doing the test at all.

RIA Kits Versus Preparing Your Own Materials. Obviously, kits present fewer problems than preparation of your own materials or bulk purchase of materials. The problems of ordering, receipt, storage, dating, and so on are still present but to a much lesser degree. As the use of RIA kits increase throughout the country and as new manufacturers enter the field, the cost of kits should drop steadily. The cost of ^{3}H labeled kits is generally less than the ^{125}I gamma kits but the cost of the ancillary supplies for the former is higher so that the liquid scintillation approach may be a bit more expensive.

The quality of an antiserum tends to deteriorate with time. Although this is not a practical consideration in general for kits, it can be with bulk materials. With the kit,

the specific activity of the labeled antigen is appropriate; with bulk and individual laboratory preparations it is necessary to check the specific activity and keep it within a suitable range. In time you may want to start making periodic checks for the degrading of the label (free iodine) by passing the labeled compound through a Sephadex column, or by dialysis or electrophoresis. The iodine may be attached to nonspecific proteins.

Precision of Pipetting. Another important factor is the precision of the pipetting. Here small changes may have great significance in the final results. It is almost impossible to detect a small error in the volume delivered visually. Therefore, other approches must be used to evaluate this, that should be done at the start and finish of every assay run.

One means of checking an automatic pipet is to take ink or colored water and draw up the particular amount, such as 5 μl or 10 μl as the case may be, into a fine glass pipet (where one may see the exact level). Deposit this on a fine quality, uniform diffusion-type filter paper. Measure the diameter of the spot several times. Then with the plastic-tipped automatic pipetter duplicate the same procedure several times. The diameter of the 2 dots should be the same. Once you have determined the diameter of the fine glass pipet spot a sufficient number of times to be certain of its value, do only the automatic pipetter to check its accuracy. Use slow, "ashless" filter paper such as Whatman No. 42 or its

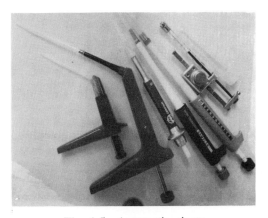

Fig. 4-5. Automatic pipets.

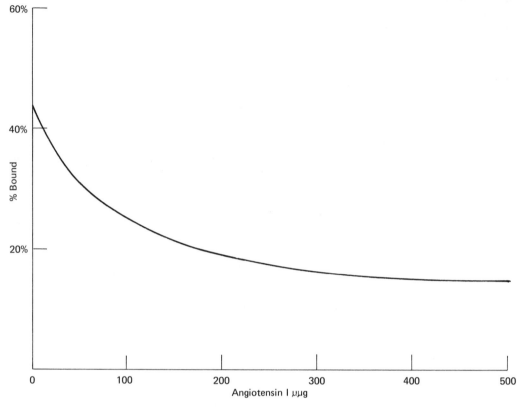

Fig. 4-6. Sample assay curve.

equivalent. It will not provide 100 percent accuracy but will give a good approximation of the accuracy of the automatic pipetter.

Standard Curve. The next phase is a careful analysis of the standard curve. Though the curve changes somewhat with each assay run, it should be similar to the preceding assay. The typical curve (Fig. 4-6) shows that there may be difficulty in obtaining accurate results from it. One of the mathematical techniques for handling this type of exponential curve is to use loga-

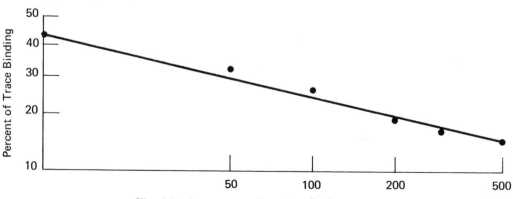

Fig. 4-7. Assay curve plotted on log-log paper.

rithms. Another approach is to plot the data on log-log paper to convert the curvilinear function to a straight-line function. The slope of the line is related to the sensitivity of the assay and it varies with the value of the exponent. This gives a curve which is related to the formula $y = kx^n$ (Fig. 4-7).

To develop an appreciation of the statistics involved in these techniques it is necessary to study the literature.[10,11,12] One of Rodbard's suggestions should be followed carefully. To maintain a grasp on "between assay" precision, graph the data. One method of doing this is to graph 3 (or more) known standards as they are determined for each assay run. They should be low, middle and high values. Plot duplicate values for each and draw a line representing the mean from assay to assay (Fig. 4-8). Such a curve suggests that unknown patient samples done in assays 5 and 6 might well have low values

but really not be in the abnormally low range. This type of chart can point out focal or generalized defects. Assay No. 9 reads lower in the high range and higher in the mid-range and assay No. 10 reads lower in the low range. When you have accumulated enough experience you will be able to calculate significant standard deviations and confidence limits.

Establishing Norms. Establishing one's own normals[9] involves instrumentation (dose calibrators in this case). With one make of dose calibrator, all determinations were found to be above the National Bureau of Standards value. A few laboratories reporting values very close to the National Bureau of Standards value were calibrating their own equipment rather than using the manufacturer's calibration. The conclusion was that the data provided by the manufacturer is not dependable and you must establish your

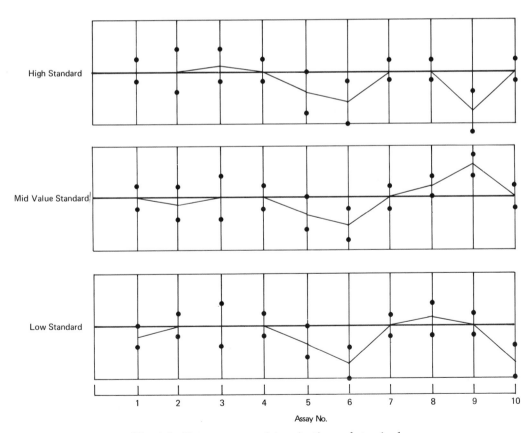

Fig. 4-8. Between assay determinations of standards.

own controls on the equipment. However, this paints a somewhat unfair picture in that most manufacturers sell at a fair price a service policy which provides for periodic field-checking of their equipment. Give careful consideration to purchase of a service policy.

Instrument Testing. In May 1970 the New England Chapter of the Society of Nuclear Medicine and the New England Radiological Physics Organization formed a Standards Committee. This Committee has been developing protocols for testing the performance of instruments. It has prepared a protocol for testing source calibrators and has established a Quality-Control Center for analyzing data. The performance of each instrument at different times may be reviewed and each laboratory may obtain analysis of instrument performance and pertinent intercomparisons. This may alert laboratories to possible variances in their equipment relative to the best possible performance of such equipment. The Committee believes that the best type of quality control may be obtained through regional cooperation. As further protocols become available, this approach will become even more valuable. The address of the New England Center is: Nuclear Medicine Quality-Control Center, Houseman Bldg.–Room 13, 80 East Concord Street, Boston, Mass. 02118.

Two other methods of checking a laboratory's work are readily available. This first is by subscription to the quality control program of the American College of Clinical Pathologists. This organization sends out unknowns and reports individual laboratory results back to them as well as the results obtained by other units. The second is to use other laboratories directly. This may involve other laboratories in one's area with whom one may be able to collaborate for this purpose or some of the excellent commercial laboratories throughout the country.

Acquiring the Equipment. In determining the necessary equipment to provide for your laboratory, consider the possibility of leasing it. Consult the hospital comptroller about the relative advantages of leasing versus outright purchase. The major advantage of leasing as it relates to quality control is that it is easier to upgrade equipment as improvements reach the market without suffering severe financial embarrassment. Under current regulations, ownership of equipment allows only a depreciation deduction (perhaps, the life of the equipment must be considered to be 5 or more years), whereas the cost of leasing is fully deductible as an expense each year and is fully reimbursable through Blue Cross and Medicare. Under some circumstances this can result in a substantial saving to the hospital.

References

1. Haskin, M. E., Bondi, A., Holmes, R., *et al.*: Possible role of radiology depts in cross infection and resistant bacterial mutagenesis. Surg. Clin. N. Amer., *50*:945, 1970.
2. Moghissi, A. A.: Low-level liquid scintillation counting of α and β-emitting nuclides. *In* Bransome, E. D., Jr.: The Current Status of Liquid Scintillation Counting. New York, Grune & Stratton, 1970.
3. Garfinkel, S. B., Mann, W. B., Medlock, R. W., and Yura, O.: Calibration of N.B.S. tritiated toluene standard of radioactivity. Int. J. Appl. Radiat. Isotop., *16*:27, 1965.
4. Parker, C. W.: Radioimmunoassays. *In* Stefanini, M.: Progress in Clinical Pathology. vol. IV, chap. 2, pp. 110-111. New York, Grune & Stratton, 1972.
5. Davidson, J. D.: Continuing Education Lectures of Southeastern Chapter of the Society of Nuclear Medicine. vol. 11, chap. 18, p. 18, 1971.
6. Hine, G. R.: X-ray sample counting. *In* Hine, G. R.: Instrumentation in Nuclear Medicine. Chap. 12, p. 285. New York, Academic Press, 1967.
7. Code of Federal Regulations. Title 10. Atomic Energy. U.S. Government Printing Office, Washington, D.C.
8. Federal Register. vol. 37, no. 202, part II. Department of Labor, Title 29. Occupational Safety and Health Administration. Occupational Safety and Health Standards Rules and Regulations, Paragraph 1910.96. Ionizing Radiation. pp. 22158-22162.
9. Hansell, J. R., Hauser, W., and Herrera, N. E.: Analysis of the Data from a Quality

Evaluation Program for Nuclear Medicine. Presented at Society of Nuclear Medicine, Miami Beach, June 1973.

10. Feldman, H., and Rodbard, D.: Mathematical theory of radioimmunoassay. *In* Odell, W. D., and Daughaday, W. H.: Principles of Competitive Protein-Binding Assays. chap. 7, p. 163. Philadelphia, J. B. Lippincott, 1971.

11. Rodbard, D.: Statistical aspects of radioimmunoassays. *In* Odell, W. D., and Daughaday, W. H.: Principles of Competitive Protein-Binding Assays. chap. 8. Philadelphia, J. B. Lippincott, 1971.

12. Rodbard, D., Rayford, P. L., Cooper, J. A., and Ross, G. T.: Statistical quality control of radioimmunoassays. J. Clin. Endocrinol. Metab., *28*:1412, 1968.

5 Blood Volume in Clinical Practice

Solomon N. Albert, M.D.

BLOOD VOLUME

Measuring circulating blood has been the physiologist's dream ever since circulation of the blood was discovered. A cursory review of the physiological basis of such a measurement certainly stimulates the curiosity of clinicians and researchers as to the importance of knowing the actual amount of the vehicle (blood) that fills the vascular system.

Circulation is basically a conveyor system that serves to maintain the cells constituting the body in contact with the outside world. Regardless of the route by which food, gases, drugs, and so forth are administered into the system, they have to enter the blood stream, be carried to the distal parts of the microcirculation, and be transferred to the interstitial fluid space to finally reach the cellular level. End products of metabolism follow the reverse route. In order to maintain tissue function, an adequate perfusion system and volume of blood must be maintained.

Perfusion depends on the adequacy of the cardiac pump system and the vasculature. Physical, mechanical and physiological responses govern the ultimate rate of tissue perfusion. The efficacy of the pump system, the heart, depends on the filling pressure and volume of blood that distends the cardiac chambers during diastole and regulates the stroke volume. The contraction of the muscle fiber and force of ejection of blood follows Starling's law of the heart. Cardiac output and stroke volume are directly related, from a mechanical point of view, to vascular tonicity and the amount of blood that fills the intravascular bed.

From a physiological point of view cardiac function is responsive to tissue requirements, need for oxygen, elimination of end products of metabolism, delivery of basic metabolic nutrients and distribution of synthetic end products (hormones, amino acids, the building blocks of cellular regeneration).

The Carrier Medium–Blood. This non-Newtonian fluid is composed of a liquid vehicle and a cellular suspension. Each element of blood has its specific function. The cellular element, the red cell, is responsible for carrying oxygen and for elimination of carbon dioxide. The quality, in terms of concentration, is just as important as the total quantity available to maintain an adequate and efficient rate of delivery through the microvasculature. Perfusion rate at the capillary level, the area of the circulatory vasculature where transfer actually occurs, is the basis of maintaining effective delivery and transfer of the various elements necessary for life. When the quality and/or quantity are deficient, self-regulatory systems come into effect that increase perfusion rate. Cardiac output is increased, resulting in an overburden on myocardial activity, in order to maintain oxygen delivery and sustain vital functions.

Clinical Considerations. Whenever a patient is in circulatory distress, one is concerned with the adequacy of the cardiac pump and the balance between vascular tonicity and blood volume. One of the many mechanisms that regulate tissue perfusion with blood is the amount of blood in the vascular tree. With improved technology, we have learned to measure blood volume and the 2 compartments which constitute blood, plasma and red cell volume. As we progressed, we found that the accepted tests, such as hemoglobin in Gm percent and hematocrit percent, are essentially measurements of concentration and do not indicate volume or mass.

Numerous reports have appeared on humans who survived operative procedures with 3 to 4 Gm percent hemoglobin or a 10 percent hematocrit. In animal experiments, blood was replaced by fluids of various compositions and the subjects survived temporarily. These heroic measures are only possible at the expense of an increase in cardiac output to compensate for a deficit in the oxygen-carrying capacity of the blood.[1] The average hospital patient should not be called on to compensate for the effects of diminished blood volume in addition to the stress of surgery and the depressant effects of anesthetic agents on the central nervous system and myocardium. If this necessitates an increased cardiac output for a prolonged period of time, there is a definite increase in the possibility of an unfortunate result. Hardaway and associates[2] in their studies on shock recommend that the red cell mass be maintained within normal limits at all times while trying to reestablish venous return and circulatory dynamics.

Blood Volume Regulation. Several mechanisms are in effect to maintain an adequate blood volume. Acute mechanisms are responsible for rapid shifts in the fluid component of blood and tend to maintain the physiomechanical system effectively. This entails the rapid transfer of fluid from the interstitial space into the intravascular compartment and vice versa. There are baroreceptors located about the base of large vessels, surrounding their portal of entry into the heart, which operate by reflex systems and control vascular tone. Also renal intra-arteriolar pressure changes may result in activation of the angiotensin and aldosterone systems, which have to do with fluid balance and vascular tone.[3] Additionally, there are osmoreceptors in the central nervous system activating mechanisms that compensate for fluid loss. In contrast to the above rapid–acting mechanisms for increaseing intravascular blood volume, there is a slower process that is activated by the need of oxygen—the acceleration of erythropoiesis by the erythropoietin liberated by the kidneys. Bone marrow responds to this stimulus but is limited by the responsiveness of the erythropoietic system.

Replacement Therapy. The need of replacing or supplementing blood elements by blood transfusion has reached a critical stage. One must justify the necessity of replacement of the specific component of blood to restore physiological function: red cells for oxygen-carrying capacity, fluids and colloids for plasma deficit, immunological factors in cer-

Table 5-1. Indications for Blood Volume.

Preoperative Evaluation	In Obstetrics	Postoperative Evaluation	Medicine
Geriatric patient	Anemia	Proper replacement	Possible anemia
Chronic disease	Hypotension	Persistent hypotension	Possible high output failure
Anemia	Blood loss	Evaluate blood loss	Renal disease
Chronic or acute blood loss		Oliguria	Hypertension
Cardiovascular surgery			Cardiovascular disorders
Pulmonary surgery			Polycythemia
Trauma			
Burns			
GI bleeding			

Central venous pressure. This procedure is attractive because of its simplicity. Some claim that this method can detect a 10 percent change in blood volume.[6-10] In our experience and the experience of others, it does not accurately reflect changes in volume.[11-15] Active venomotor tone tends to restore venous pressure in the presence of hypovolemia in an effort to maintain venous return.[16] The following 2 cases demonstrate the poor correlation of central venous pressure and blood volume.

For practical purposes, central venous pressure is considered to be the resultant of many factors. It reflects essentially the efficacy of the pumping action of the right side of the heart. Figure 5-1 shows the various forces involved in registering a manometric reading from the superior vena cava or right auricle, central venous pressure. In simple terms, the relationship of blood volume, vascular tonicity and cardiac competence to central venous pressure is expressed in the following equation.[17]

Case 3. Hip Fracture: 92 F, 5'4", 121 lbs.

Compart-ment	Normal Values	Measured Values	Ml Diff.	% Diff.
RCV	1,460 ml	1,000 ml	−460	−31.5
PV	2,015	1,900	−115	− 5.7
TBV	3,475	2,900	−575	−13.6
LVH-corr.		38.4%		
CVP		11cm H_2O		
BP		160/110		
Pulse		92		

Case 4. Hip Fracture: 84 F, 5'4", 124 lbs.

Compart-ment	Normal Values	Measured Values	Ml Diff.	% Diff.
RCV	1,465 ml	1,750 ml	+285	+19.4
PV	2,020	2,600	+580	+28.7
TBV	3,485	4,350	+865	+24.7
LVH-corr.		44.2%		
CVP		9cm H_2O		
BP		190/100		
Pulse		70		

to develop with a low central venous pressure.[18,19] It is felt that pulmonary artery pressure is more indicative of blood volume changes than is central venous pressure.[20,21]

$$\text{Central Venous Pressure} = \frac{\text{Effective Blood Volume}}{\text{Cardiac Function} + \text{Vascular Capacity}}$$

An increase in CVP can result from an increase in effective blood volume, a decrease in cardiac function, or a decrease in vascular capacity. Pulmonary edema has been seen

Complications reported with insertion of catheters for monitoring CVP are vein trauma, pneumothorax, hemothorax, rupture of the right auricle, sepsis and air embo-

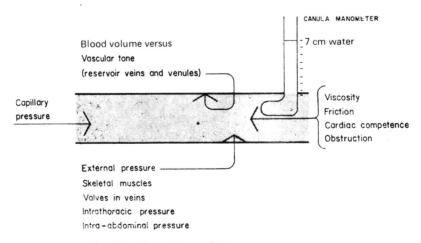

Fig. 5-1. These factors influence venous pressure.

lism.[22] The combined determination of CVP and blood volume measured by isotopic methods give the best information on the hemodynamic status.[23] Thus both techniques give useful information and supplement each other.

Vital Signs. Blood pressure and pulse rate vary with compensatory mechanisms that come into effect provided the autonomic nervous system is responsive and the cardiac pump has the capacity to maintain adequate perfusion. In the early stages, prior to the point of decompensation and especially when the patient is under the influence of narcotics or in metabolic deficit, blood pressure and pulse rate may vary in a paradoxical manner to normal physiological principles as described in the textbooks.

Urine Output. Urine output varies between 40 to 60 ml per hour with an osmolality ordinarily higher than plasma osmolality. Urine output depends on the state of hydration, renal blood flow, pressure gradients in the glomeruli and tubular function. Once hemostasis is established and baseline measurements determined, urinary output can serve as an index of blood volume only as it reflects perfusion of glomeruli, and thereby determines the efficacy of fluid replacement. Here again, we are referring only to the problem of hydration and not to the oxygen and carbon dioxide transport.

MEASURING BLOOD VOLUME

Progress has been made from the time that blood volume measurements were performed by direct methods with total body washout, a very impractical method. Later techniques were indirect methods that involved dilution of blood with known volumes of fluid and determining changes in concentration of blood elements, the tracers in this instance being the elements of blood. This method was very unreliable since large volumes of fluid had to be administered in order to obtain a measurable difference in the elements of blood. The first reliable indirect methods were developed at the turn of the century when dyes were utilized. The most popular dye was Evan's blue (T-1824). Dyes were used essentially as plasma tracers; technically the photometric measurements of the concentration of the dyes is fraught with errors. Moreover, with repeated determinations the tissues absorbed the dye, resulting in skin discoloration. Radioactive nuclides gained prominence as tracers for blood volume measurement, since small doses can be administered and radioanalysis is specific and practical.

Measuring fluid volumes by the indirect dilution technique with radioactive tracers has been subjected to both criticism and praise.[24,25] Also, one can note in the literature changes in methodology from oversimplified single tracer techniques to more sophisticated multiple tracer techniques.[26,27] The logical conclusion at this time is that in vivo volume measurements are reliable and meaningful provided the basic principles governing the dilution technique are understood.

PRINCIPLES OF MEASUREMENT

The fundamentals of the dilution principle are based on the following equation:

$$V = \frac{Q}{C}$$

Volume = Volume of diluent
Q = Amount of tracer
C = Concentration in the diluent

Prerequisites for tracer

1. The tracer material should mix evenly with the volume of the diluent.
2. Reach equilibration.
3. During the period of mixing and equilibration be sure there is no loss of the tracer from the compartment.

Tracers for measuring blood volume fall into two groups.

1. Tracers Bound to the Red Cell. The component that is most accurately measured is the red cell volume—the oxygen- and carbon dioxide-carrying element. The labeled cells are distributed in the red cell mass. The extent to which blood and plasma volume are underestimated depends on the ratio be-

Table 5-3. Variations in F_{cell} Ratio.

Low F_{cell} Ratio (Below 0.91)	High F_{cell} Ratio (Above 0.91)
Apprehension	Anesthesia
Vasopressors	Sedation
Hypertension	Sympatholytic and ganglionic blocking agents
Hypovolemia	High spinal
Pheochromocytoma	Hypervolemia
Shivering	Neurogenic shock
Chronic diseases	Cardiac decompensation
Dehydration	Overcompensation
Intestinal obstruction	Pediatric patients
Geriatric patients	Late pregnancy
Hypothermia	Splenomegaly
	Diseases of the bone marrow

tween WBH/LVH, the F_{cell} ratio. The hematocrit of blood obtained from a large vessel (LVH) is higher than the average whole body hematocrit (WBH), on the average by a factor of 1.1, equal to the reciprocal of the ratio of WBH/LVH (0.915), termed F_{cell} ratio. Under normal conditions this ratio is fairly constant, but it varies in different pathologic conditions.

2. Tracers Bound to Plasma Proteins. Tracers bound to plasma proteins tend to cross the capillary membrane and equilibrate with the body albumin pool. Correction for the rate of elimination of the protein-bound tracers from the intravascular pool must be taken into consideration. The blood and red cell volume are overestimated on the average by a factor of 1.1, equivalent to the reciprocal of the F_{cell} ratio.

Table 5-4. Labeled Albumin and Labeled Red Cells Versus True Values.

Compartment	Labeled Protein	Labeled Cells	True Values
RCV	2,113	[1,830]	1,830
PV	[3,170]	2,745	3,170
TBV	5,283	4,575	[5,000]
LVH-corr.	40.0%	40.0%	
WBH			36.6%

Under labeled protein, the only correct measurement is the plasma volume. Under labeled red cells, the only correct measurement is the red cell volume.*

---

* Correct by definition.

Table 5-4 is an example of over- and underestimates of blood compartments by the 2 methods.

Equilibration of Tracer in Circulating Blood. The basic principle of measuring volume by the dilution principle involves complete mixing of the tracer administered in the intravascular compartment. To determine the value of C, the concentration of the tracer in the diluent, establish that mixing is complete, equilibration has been reached, and if there is any loss of tracer from the intravascular space, establish the rate and amount of loss during this period of time. The latter is essential with plasma labels but less so with red cell labels. This can only be determined by multiple postinjection sampling, samples drawn at different time intervals. Examples of equilibrating problems are presented in the following 2 cases.

^{51}Cr Labeled Red Cells. Red cells are labeled with radioactive chromium by mixing blood with hexavalent $Na_2^{51}CrO_4$. The chromate penetrates the red cell membrane

Case 5. Blood Volume Measured with Radioactive Iodinated Albumin.

Time (min)	Volume (ml)
5	3,300
10	3,600
20	4,350

Extrapolated volume to zero-time = 2,950 ml. Note steadily increasing blood volume with time; true value is extrapolated zero-time value.

Case 6. Blood Volume Measured with ^{51}Cr Labeled Red Cells.

(Colon Resection Under Hypothermia at 32°C)

Time (min)	Volume (ml)
5	3,650
10	3,800
20	3,950
30	4,200
40	4,520
50	4,500

Equilibrated volume = 4,500 ml
Note prolonged time to obtain equilibration with labeled cells when patient is in marked vasoconstriction.

and is attached to the hemoglobin molecule. Tagging is rapid and the free hexavalent chromium is reduced to trivalent chromium with ascorbic acid. The cells are washed with normal saline solution. ^{51}Cr is a gamma-emitting nuclide and the concentration of the tracer is determined by placing an aliquot in a gamma-counting device. ^{51}Cr lends itself especially well to measuring blood volume with the dual tracer technique (vide infra). The International Committee for Standardization in Hematology has approved methods for labeling red cells with ^{51}Cr.[28]

^{99m}**Tc-Technetium Labeled Red Cells.** Red blood cells can be labeled with technetium. The radiation dose to the patient with ^{99m}Tc red cells is about one-tenth of that with ^{51}Cr, an important consideration when measuring red cell volume in children.[29,30,31] Since this nuclide has a short half-life, counting statistics and uniform dosage can be maintained when repeated studies are necessary. The pertechnetate is fixed in the cell with stannous chloride solution. The stannous chloride is prepared in a nitrogen-purged commercial glove box by adding 50 mg $SnCl_2 \cdot 2H_2O$ to 0.43 ml of 11.4 N HCl and diluting to 5 ml with sterile water. This solution is stable for 2 weeks. One-tenth ml of the stannous solution is added to 5 ml citrate solution (3% sodium citrate, 1% citric acid), resulting in a dilution containing 200 Ug $SnCl_2 \cdot 2H_2O$ per ml which is stable for 8 hours.

Procedure for Labeling Red Cells

1. Add 2 ml $T_cO_4^-$ to 3 ml of citrate anticoagulant solution.
2. Add TcO_4^- citrate solution (step 1) to 5 ml of heparinized whole blood.
3. Mix for 5 minutes.
4. Add 1 ml of tin citrate solution.
5. Mix for 1 minute.
6. Add 30 ml saline and centrifuge.
7. Repeat saline wash and resuspend cells for injection.

Two saline washes are sufficient to decrease the unbound technetium to less than 1 percent.

The reducing agent is critical. It may be ineffective if an excessive amount of tin is added and may result in deterioration of the red cell which is sequestered by the spleen. Nouel and Brunelle[32] developed a technique whereby O-Rh-negative red cells are pretreated with stannous chloride washed with EDTA (5%) and the pertechnetate solution obtained from the generator is added. They claim a 95 to 99 percent tag.

Labeled Plasma Protein. Human serum albumin labeled with radioactive iodine is

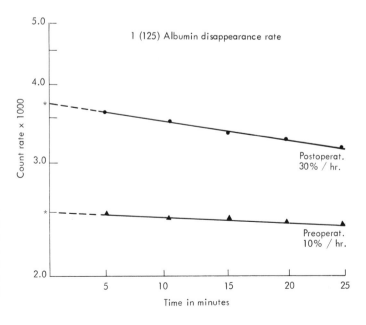

Fig. 5-2. Rate of disappearance of ^{125}I albumin. Note the change in rate of disappearance of radioiodinated albumin from the preoperative to postoperative period—an increase from 10 percent to 30 percent per hour loss.

1 (125) Albumin disappearance rate

Postoperat.
30% / hr.

Preoperat.
10% / hr.

Count rate x 1000

Time in minutes

commercially available in two forms: [131]I and [125]I. The difference between these 2 nuclides is their energy and half-life. [131]I has a half-life of 8 days and has a number of different gamma and beta emissions. [125]I has a half-life of 60 days and is a pure gamma emitter.

Procedure. Draw a sample of blood prior to administration of the tracer to determine the radiation background of the recipient (preinjection sample). Accurately determine the tracer quantity and administer intravenously. Make injection directly into a vein and not through existing intravenous tubing. Draw two or three samples of blood 10-, 20-, or 30-minute intervals in order to obtain proper mixing of the tracer and to establish the rate of loss of albumin from the intravascular system. Plot the counts in the various samples against time on semilogarithm paper. Extrapolate back to zero to obtain the true count (Fig. 5-2).

Protein Labeled With Short-lived Radionuclides—[99m]Tc Labeled Albumin. Efforts are in progress to prepare a usable ^{99m}Tc albumin. These preparations must be made at the time of use, since the tracer has a relatively short half-life.

[113]In[m] Labeled Proteins. Hosain, et al.,[33] have prepared plasma protein labeled with [113]In[m]. The half-life of this tracer is 1.66 hours and the parent [113]Sn-generator 115 days. [113]In[m]-chloride in gelatin solution at acid pH, when injected intravenously binds with plasma transferrin to form a stable compound. Several methods of administering the [113]In[m]-chloride have been utilized. One of the methods consists in directly injecting [113]In[m]-chloride (10-50 μCi). It is desirable to keep the pH of the solution between 2 and 3. A rise in pH favors the formation of colloidal hydroxide that is rapidly removed from the blood. Results compare favorably to ^{99m}Tc-labeled protein and iodinated albumin. However, both the technetium and indium methods give plasma volumes about 5 percent higher than R[131]ISA.

The advantages of utilizing short-lived nuclides are numerous and include:

1. A smaller radiation dose.

2. Tests can be repeated with negligible background build-up and increase in radiation dosage.

3. They can be utilized in infants, in pregnancy and experimentally in small animals.

4. They produce higher count rates with more reliable statistics.

CALCULATIONS

Blood Volume Measured with a Single Tracer.

Labeled Red Cells

$$\text{Dilution Volume} = \frac{\text{Labeled Red Cell Count (tracer administered)} - \text{Residue}}{\text{Count of labeled red cells in blood} - \text{Bkg}}$$

Red Cell Volume = Dilution Volume $\times$ LVH (LVH is corrected for trapped plasma)

Blood Volume   = Dilution Volume $\times$ 1.1 (reciprocal of F_{cell} Ratio 0.915)

Plasma Volume = Blood Volume—Red Cell Volume

Labeled Albumin

$$\text{Dilution Volume} = \frac{\text{Labeled Albumin Count (tracer administered)} - \text{Residue}}{\text{Count of labeled albumin in blood} - \text{Bkg}}$$

Plasma Volume = Dilution Volume $\times$ (1-LVH)

Blood Volume   = Dilution Volume $\times \left[\dfrac{1-\text{LVH}}{1-(0.915 \text{ LVH})} \right]$ or D_f Factor*

* See Table 5-2.

Technical developments depend on the ingenuity of the user; the reliability of the test depends on methodology, accuracy of aliquot measurements and reproducibility of results. The automatic pipets (Clay-Adams) with disposable tips have proven to be valuable additions to our armamentarium, adding simplicity to accuracy, and avoiding contamination as well as being economical.

The advantages of labeled albumin with radioactive iodine is that the preparation is readily available and can be used without the necessity of preparing the standard dose to be administered for each determination. Iodine-125 has longer shelf-life, and lends itself for dual tracer techniques with ^{51}Cr-labeled cells—simultaneous measurement of red cell and plasma volume.

The major drawback in measuring blood volume with plasma protein-bound tracers is that the primary compartment measured is plasma volume. Red cell and blood volume are calculated values and depend on hematocrit. By taking into account the rate at which albumin disappears from the intravascular compartment, and correcting for the F_{cell} ratio, the results obtained are reasonably accurate.

Table 5-5 presents the distribution of the F_{cell} ratio in 200 patients. Some received multiple transfusions. The error in volume was established by comparing results with the true volume measured with 2 tracers compared to values obtained with ^{125}IHSA alone, as seen in the equations on page 60 using labeled albumin.

Simultaneous Measurement of Red Cell and Plasma Volume. To achieve greater accuracy the two compartments of blood, red cell and plasma volume, should be measured separately and simultaneously with appropriate tracers.

A two-position well-type scintillation counter was developed which simplifies the procedure. The concentration of two gamma-emitting nuclides, ^{51}Cr and ^{125}I, are measured simultaneously on all samples, ^{51}Cr-labeled cells for red cell volume (RCV) and ^{125}I

Table 5-5. 200 Blood Volume Determinations with Dual Tracers Compared to Results. With Single Tracer—^{125}I

No. of Cases	Percentage of Cases		F_{cell} Range	Error
165	82.5		0.85 to 1.00	±2.5
18	9.0	98%	0.80 to 0.84	+4.5
13	6.5		1.01 to 1.05	−5.0
1	0.5		0.75 to 0.79	+7.0
3	1.5		1.06 to 1.15	−6.5

40 cases = Preoperative elective surgery
60 cases = Postoperative with no blood replacement
100 cases = Postoperative patients who received from 2 to 10 units of banked blood
In 98 percent of instances the error varied ±5 percent.

albumin for plasma volume (PV). Both tracers are mixed in a single syringe and counted simultaneously in a dual-channel scaler analyzer.

Counting ^{51}Cr and ^{125}I (Tracer Dose). ^{51}Cr and ^{125}I are analyzed simultaneously in a dual-scaler analyzer. The well-type scintillation detector has 2 counting positions, a front and a rear well. The front well facing the 2-inch NaI (thallium-activated) crystal is used for measuring the concentrated tracer dose syringe. About 7 to 8 ml of the tracer dose is administered to the patient. The residue (the amount of tracer remaining in the dose syringe) is also measured in the front position.

Counting Samples. The rear well is an opening through the crystal and is used for counting samples of low concentration (the preinjection and postinjection blood samples). Blood is drawn in heparinized syringes and 2 ml aliquots in plastic tubes are prepared with an automatic pipet. The 2 tracers utilized in this technique have distinct energy peaks that are easily separated and identified, with minimal spillover. One channel of the two-channel analyzer (scaler A with analyzer A) is pulse-heighted for the energy of [51]Cr (320 kev); the second channel (scaler B with analyzer B) for [125]I (35.4 kev). Since ^{51}Cr has an energy approximately 10 times higher than ^{125}I, there is some spillover of ^{51}Cr onto the ^{125}I band, but none of the ^{125}I appears on the ^{51}Cr band. The extent of ^{51}Cr activity appearing on the B scaler can be adjusted to less than a 3 percent spillover. Since both tracers are diluted by approximately the same volume, the error introduced by such a low spillover is negligible.

Standardization of the Two-position Modified Well Counter (Omniwell). When the 2 tracers, ^{51}Cr and ^{125}I, are counted in the presence of each other, certain problems arise as to coincidence, summation effect, and spectral changes when the geometrical exposure to the detector is altered (i.e., when samples are moved from the front to the rear position). In an attempt to correct these variables, the geometric ratio equivalent between the front and rear positions of samples for each of the tracers is established by in vitro volumetric measurements, utilizing approximately the same proportion of ^{125}I to ^{51}Cr normally administered as the standard dose in vivo. A tracer dose of 7 to 8 ml (standard) containing both tracers is drawn into a 10 ml plastic syringe which is placed in the front position of the well counter to determine the total dose of the tracers. The dose is introduced into a glass flask containing an accurately measured volume of water (4,000 ml). The empty syringe is filled with water to the 7 to 8 ml mark and measured in the same position as the standard, the front well, establishing the amount of the 2 tracers remaining (residue) in the syringe (Fig. 5-3).

A dilution sample from the 4,000 ml flask is drawn and the concentration of the 2 tracers in the known dilution is established. The front-to-rear ratio (F/R) is calculated for each tracer (scaler A set for ^{51}Cr to determine the ^{51}Cr count rate, and scaler B set for ^{125}I to determine the ^{125}I count rate). Three or four in vitro experiments are performed and the average ratio is established. Although

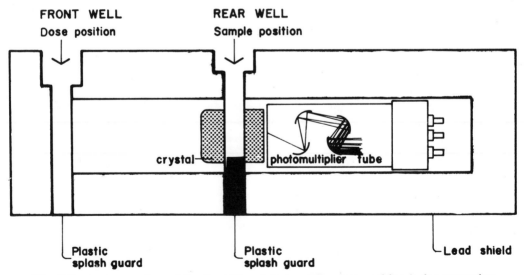

Fig. 5-3. A cross-section of the 2-position detector. The dose position is for measuring standard in plastic syringes—total volume exposed to sensing crystal is 7 to 8 ml. The well position (sample position) through the crystal opening accommodates disposable plastic test tubes. The patient background and a sample analysis are performed in this position.

the F/R ratio for each tracer is stable, it is advisable to recheck these constants once a week by repeating and performing a spot-check in vitro determination.

$$\text{Ratio (F/R)} = \frac{\overset{(^{51}\text{Cr or }^{125}\text{I})}{4,000 \times (\text{count of dilution sample} - \text{atmospheric background})}}{\underset{(^{51}\text{Cr or }^{125}\text{I})\qquad(^{51}\text{Cr of }^{125}\text{I})}{\text{Count of standard} - \text{residue in syringe}}} \qquad (2)$$

Calculating Red Cell and Plasma Volume (Dual-Tracer Technique). The equations to calculate RCV and PV are based on the dilution of each of the tracers in blood.

$$\text{RCV (scaler A set for }^{51}\text{Cr)} = \frac{(\text{Ct of standard} - \text{residue}) \times \text{F/R}^* \times \text{LVH}}{\text{Equilibrated}\dagger \text{ net ct of sample}} \qquad (3)$$

$$\text{PV (scaler B set for }^{125}\text{I)} = \frac{(\text{Ct of standard} - \text{residue}) \times \text{F/R}\ddagger \times (1\text{-LVH})}{\text{Zero-time extrapolated net ct determined on 2 samples}\S} \qquad (4)$$

$$\text{TBV (total blood volume)} = \text{RCV} + \text{PV} \qquad (5)$$

$$\text{WBH (whole body hematocrit)} = \frac{\text{RCV}}{\text{TBV}} \qquad (6)$$

$$F_{\text{cell}} \text{ Ratio} = \frac{\text{WBH}}{\text{LVH}}$$

---

* F/R for ^{51}Cr.
† When 2 samples of blood at different time intervals have the same count.
‡ F/R for ^{125}I.
§ 10- and 20-minute sample counts extrapolated to zero-time.

Predicted Values

Blood volume varies with metabolic needs and tissue requirements. Normal values established according to body weight do not accurately fit expected values for a particular individual. Norms calculated according to body surface are more realistic and adaptable to most clinical conditions. For this purpose the values established by Hidalgo, Nadler and Bloch[34] for blood volume have been utilized as a basis for norms.

$$\text{BV} = 0.0236 \, H^{0.725} \, M^{0.423} - 1.229 \text{ (Males)}$$

$$\text{BV} = 0.0248 \, H^{0.725} \, M^{0.425} - 1.954 \text{ (Females)}$$

Normal blood volume values are based on 2 body parameters—height in centimeters, weight in kilograms—as well as sex of the individual.

The red cell volume is calculated as 40 percent of the total volume.

$$\text{Predicted Red Cell volume} = \text{Predicted BV} \times 0.40$$

$$\text{Predicted Plasma Volume} = \text{Predicted BV} \times 0.60$$

We feel that a patient can tolerate a 20 percent deficit in red cell volume if no further blood loss is contemplated. On the other hand, a 10 percent overload cannot be tolerated for any length of time.

SHORTCOMINGS OF AVAILABLE COMPUTERS UTILIZING SINGLE TRACERS

No computer can detect technical errors such as those resulting from contamination of the well counter. Nor is the computer capable of interpreting results.

Automated blood volume measuring devices, to be of value, should be flexible and adaptable for measuring blood volume, taking into account the complexities of the various calculations involved. Recorded data for each step in the procedure is necessary. A method to feedback data when needed should be available. With all of the sophistication of electronics, we still find that a simple slide rule is just as good as the most expensive equipment available on the market. A circular slide rule was adapted for blood volume computations and to measure hematocrit percent on microhematocrit capillary tubes.[35,36]

Volumĕtron. Volumĕtron* is capable of computing blood volume by utilizing 2 balanced detector systems on the basis of preset count or time. The detectors are geometrically adjusted 2 positions for counting "hot" standard and dilute samples. The total volume of tracer is counted by the sensing crystal and the standard and residue are counted in one position. The steps of the procedure follow the standard procedure for measuring dilution volume. The standard, in prepackaged syringets, is analyzed. The residue in the syringet is counted and is then subtracted from the standard count. Patient background and sample count are counted simultaneously in preset volume aliquots.

Initially, the Volumĕtron was developed for $R^{131}ISA$ single sample determinations. Due to errors that single sample blood volume determinations carry, the machine was

modified and a manually set memory system was incorporated in the circuit so that the net standard count ($Q - Bkg_1$) could be reinserted for determining dilution volume on subsequent sampling. The machine was further modified to enable the utilization of different energy tracers, ^{51}Cr, ^{125}I and ^{131}I.[37]

Hemolitre.† This single detector system has a memory system to retain the count of the standard administered. This enables dilution volume to be determined on subsequent samples. The detector system consists of a single photomultiplier tube to which is adapted a 2-inch crystal with a through-and-through opening that permits insertion of aliquots into the center of the crystal. The "hot" sample, standard, is placed in a geometrically fixed position distal to the sensing crystal and the total volume administered is counted by the detector. One can utilize prepackaged syringets of prepared standards in volumes from 6 to 8 ml. The residue is measured in the same position.

Blood Volume Computer.‡ This lightweight portable unit was developed for counting $^{125}IHSA$. It works on the general principle of the Volumĕtron. Patient background and blood samples are counted in constant volume containers placed in the well counter in the opening through the crystal.[38,39]

BLOOD VOLUME MEASUREMENTS

Contraindications to Blood Volume Measurements

Inaccessible vessels for injecting or withdrawing blood, poor methodology, and shortcuts in methodology and calculations can render this valuable measurement an unreliable laboratory determination. There is no substitute for good technique. A poor measurement can make the best postoperative care look inferior. It is advisable not to measure blood volume if there are questions about the technique of performance.

---

* Trademark, Ames Company.

† Trademark, Picker-Nuclear Corp.

‡ Trademark, D. A. Pitman, Ltd.

COMMON PITFALLS IN MEASURING BLOOD VOLUME

1. Errors Due to Contamination

(a) Contamination of syringes and counting equipment.

(b) Injecting tracer through plastic tubing.

(c) Sampling blood in a contaminated syringe (results abnormally low).

(d) Blood removed from the same site used for injecting standard (gives low measurements).

(e) Removal of sample from infusion tubing or vein used to administer blood or fluids. The sample of blood is not a representative sample of circulating blood in which the tracer was distributed (gives high measurement values).

2. Patient Background Not Taken

With the increased use of radioactive isotopes for diagnostic procedures, it is erroneous to assume that the patient has no radioactive background level. Therefore, take a patient control sample at all times before administering a dose of radioactive tracer. Otherwise, abnormally low blood volume determinations result.

3. Dose of Standard

(a) Measuring blood volume, in a patient actively bleeding from a vessel near a main arterial trunk, results in substantial loss of the tracer dose; the calculated blood volume determinations are abnormally high.

(b) Extravascular administration of standard.

(c) Inaccurate measurement of volume of standard injected gives normally high volume measurements unless the total dose is measured and the residue accounted for.

(d) Counting of a poorly mixed standard preparation gives inaccurate results.

(e) Excessive amounts of free tracer element in the preparation.

4. Blood Sampling

(a) Inadequate mixing time allowed. Normally with slow injection, mixing is complete within 2 minutes. With vascular stasis, poor circulation, shunts in the vascular system, intestinal obstruction and pressure on large vessels, allow more time for proper distribution—15 to 30 minutes.

(b) Clotted blood in syringe. Clots, agglutination, aggregation of cells, may offset uniformity of cell distribution in the sample to be analyzed and lead to an erroneous count. Most difficulties encountered with tagging red cells (clots and aggregation of labeled cells) are obviated when stock-O-Rh-Kell-negative cells labeled with ^{51}Cr are utilized. Syringes containing blood samples are shaken well before counting.

(c) Injection of tracer dose through a minute vein, veins in spasm, thrombosed veins, into infusion tubing or extravascular injection result in loss of tracer and exaggerated large dilution volume.

Technical Difficulties Encountered with RISA. Iodinated preparations may have substantial quantities of free tracer element. Part of the tracer can be lost since RISA adheres to glass, metal, plastic tubing and the vascular wall at the site of injection. Rinse the syringe gently with blood before withdrawing the needle from the vein. Obtain dilution samples in heparinized syringes from a site other than the site of injection, preferably from the opposite arm. It is desirable to withdraw blood samples without a tourniquet so that stagnation of blood does not alter the red cell/plasma ratio.

Points to Remember

1. Injection of iodinated labeled protein may lead rarely to anaphylactic reaction.

2. It is advisable to block the thyroid with Lugol's solution in order to eliminate thyroid uptake of radioiodine.

3. There is the danger in pregnancy that part of the free iodine may cross the placental barrier.

Problems Encountered in Labeling Red Cells with ^{51}Cr

1. Chromium-51 will not label red cells if blood drawn from the patient contains a con-

siderable amount of reducing agents, vitamins or antibiotics, that reduce hexavalent chromium into nontagging trivalent chromium. Under these conditions, it is advisable to utilize banked O-Rh-Kell-negative blood labeled with ^{51}Cr. Hexavalent chromate salt, when allowed to remain in contact for a long period of time with the ACD solution, may be reduced to nontagging trivalent chromic salt; ACD acts as a reducing agent.

2. Rouleau formation and blood clots in the standard result in uneven distribution of the tracer in circulating blood. This is prevented by using O-Rh-Kell-negative labeled red cells filtered through a microfilter.

3. Hemolysis of labeled cells may occur during manipulation of samples.

4. Intravascular hemolysis may occur because of increased fragility of washed labeled cells resulting from manipulation and changes in temperature during the washing procedure.

Conclusions

One facet of tissue perfusion depends on the quality and quantity of blood that fills the vascular bed. Many other factors come into play and contribute to our prime concern—tissue perfusion.

Proper hydration and blood replacement are important in the management of problem medical and surgical patients. Volume disorders are best monitored by actual measurements. This is more reliable than depending on the concentration of the various elements that constitute blood or indirect indices such as blood pressure, heart rate, oxygen tension, and pH and urine output that are frequently misleading.

Measuring blood volume is important in determining the quantity and nature of replacement necessary in the management of the individual surgical and medical patient.

The techniques for measuring plasma and red cell volume simultaneously, by the dilution method utilizing 2 tracers, are practical and applicable in clinical practice. These measurements when performed on the seriously ill, chronically ill, geriatric or complicated surgical patient reduce morbidity and mortality. They are well worth the additional trouble involved.

A major area of concern is the interpretation of results. The physician's estimate of what is and what is not a deviation from normal[40] in a particular individual, who may be in physiologic imbalance, is open to all the vagaries of individual judgments. Blood volume must be measured, not estimated. But if blood volume is to be meaningful, the measurement and calculations must be reliable.

Blood volume measurements to be meaningful must be performed with painstaking attention to detail. There are no shortcuts and the problems encountered are many. Gregersen and Rawson[41] clearly bring into focus many problems and stress the fact that methodology plays an important role in evaluating results. It is wiser not to perform blood volume measurements if the technique is poor.

Regardless of the tracers utilized, two important facts must be taken into account: (a) equilibration of the tracer with the component of blood being measured; (b) with plasma tracers, the extent of loss of tracer from the intravascular system must be considered and values corrected for this.

On repeated measurements, the count rate of samples should be adjusted for the differences in hematocrit between samples.

References

1. Takaori, M., and Safar, P.: Treatment of massive hemorrhage with colloid and crystalloid solutions. J.A.M.A., *199*:297, 1967.
2. Hardaway, R. M., James, P. M., Anderson, R. W., Bredenberg, C. E., and West, R. L.: Intensive study and treatment of shock in man. J.A.M.A., *199*:779, 1967.
3. Davis, J. O.: The control of aldosterone secretion. Physiologist, *5*:65, 1962.
4. Strumia, M. M., and Strumia, P. V.: Blood substitutes. Hosp. Med., *7*:36, 1967.
5. Hoye, R. C.: Simultaneous measurement of red cell, plasma and extracellular fluid volume in the surgical patient. J. Lab. Clin. Med., *69*:683, 1967.
6. Borow, M., Aquilizan, L., Krausz, A., and Stefanides, A.: The use of central venous pressure as an accurate guide for body fluid

replacement. Surg. Gynecol. Obstet., *120*: 545, 1965.

7. Jenkins, L. C., and Screech, G.: Central venous pressure monitoring in anaesthesia. Can. Anaesth. Soc. J., *13*:513, 1966.

8. Danes invent device to record venous pressure. Med. World News, *7*:45, December 9, 1966.

9. Sykes, M. K.: Venous pressure as a clinical indication of adequacy of transfusion. Ann. R. Coll. Surg. Eng., *33*:185, 1963.

10. Wilson, J. N., Grow, J. B., Demong, C. V., *et al.*: Central venous pressure in optimal blood volume maintenance. Arch. Surg. (Chicago), *85*:563, 1962.

11. Askrog, V.: The cardiovascular response of normal anaesthetized man to rapid infusions of saline. Br. J. Anaesth., *38*:455, 1966.

12. Beard, J.: Venous pressure and other thoughts. Proc. R. Soc. Med., *62*:635, 1969.

13. Friedman, E., Grable, E., and Fine, J.: Central venous pressure and direct serial measurements as guides in blood-volume replacement. Lancet, *2*:609, 1966.

14. Keddie, N. C., Provan, J. L., and Austen, W. G.: Central venous pressure, blood volume determinations, and the effects of vasoactive drugs in hypovolemic shock. Surgery, *60*:427, 1966.

15. Ryan, G. M., and Howland, W. S.: An evaluation of central venous pressure monitoring. Anesth. Analg., *45*:754, 1966.

16. Landis, E. M., and Hortenstine, J. C.: Functional significance of venous blood pressure. Physiol. Rev., *30*:1, 1950.

17. Turndorf, H.: Central venous pressure, Anesth. Rounds. vol. 1, no. 6, New York, Ayerst Labs., 1967.

18. Buchman, R. J.: Subclavian venipuncture. Milit. Med., *34*:451, 1969.

19. Hallin, R. W.: Continuous venous pressure monitoring as a guide to fluid administration in the hypotensive patient. Amer. J. Surg., *106*:164, 1963.

20. Prout, W. G.: Relative values of central-venous-pressure monitoring and blood-volume measurement in the management of shock. Lancet, *1*:1108, 1968.

21. Waltz, C. A., and Shumacker, H. B., Jr.: Further studies on vascular pressure and of graded exercise on stroke volume in man. J. Clin. Invest., *39*:1051, 1960.

22. Levinsky, W. J.: Fatal air embolism during insertion of CVP monitoring apparatus. (Letter to editor.) J.A.M.A., *209*:1721, 1969.

23. Editorial. J.A.M.A., *202*:1099, 1967.

24. Cartmill, T. B., Ricks, R. K., Garrett, H. W., Williams, J. A., and DeBakey, M. E.: Blood volume measurements in cardiovascular surgical patients. Surg. Gynec. Obstet., *121*:1269, 1965.

25. McMurrey, J. D., Garrett, H. E., and DeBakey, M. E.: Blood volume measurements in patients receiving cardiovascular surgical treatment. Cardiovasc. Res. Cent. Bull., *1*:51 (Winter) 1962-63.

26. Albert, S. N.: Plasma-volume and red-cell mass determinations. (Letter to editor.) J. Nucl. Med., *9*:504, 1968.

27. Grable, E., and Williams, J. A.: Simplified method for simultaneous determinations of plasma volume and red-cell mass with ^{125}I-labeled albumin and ^{51}Cr-tagged red cells. J. Nucl. Med., *9*:219, 1968.

28. International Committee for Standardization in Hematology (Panel on Diagnostic Applications of Radioisotopes in Haematology): Recommended methods for radioisotope red-cell survival studies. Br. J. Haematol., *21*:241, 1971.

29. Dillman, L. T.: Radionuclide decay schemes and nuclear parameters for use in radiation-dose estimation. J. Nucl. Med., *10*:(suppl. 2) 1, 1969.

30. Loevinger, R., and Berman, M.: A scheme for adsorbed-dose calculations for biologically distributed radionuclides. J. Nucl. Med., *9*:(suppl. 1), 1968.

31. Sayder, W. S., Ford, M. R., Warner, G. G., and Fisher, H. L., Jr.: Estimates of adsorbed fractions for manoenergetic photon sources uniformly distributed in various organs of a heterogeneous phantom. J. Nucl. Med., *10*:(suppl. 3), 1969.

32. Nouel, J. P., and Brunelle, P.: Le marquage des hematies par le technetium 99m. La Presse Medicale, *78*:73, 1970.

33. Hosain, P., Hosain, F., Iqbal, Q. M., Carulli, N., and Wagner, H. N., Jr.: Measurement of plasma volume using ^{99}Tc^m and ^{113}In^m labeled proteins. Br. J. Radiol., *42*:627, 1969.

34. Hidalgo, J. U., Nadler, S. B., and Bloch, T.: The use of electronic digital computer to determine best fit of blood volume formulas. J. Nucl. Med., *3*:94, 1962.

35. Albert, S. N., and Zekas, E.: Modifications of technique for blood volume measurements. Anesthesiology, *21*:564, 1960.

36. Albert, S. N., and Zekas, E.: Technical improvements in diagnostic techniques. Amer. J. Med. Techn., *22*:24, 1960.

37. Williams, J. A., and Fine, J.: Measurement of blood volume with a new apparatus. N. Eng. J. Med., *264*:842, 1961.
38. Albert, S. N.: Letter to editor. Anaesthesia, *24*:288, 1969.
39. Heath, M. L., and Vickers, M. D.: An examination of single-tracer, semi-automated blood volume methodology. Anaesthesia, *23*:659, 1968.
40. Brucer, M.: St. Thomas and the cannibals. The blood volume problem, (Vignettes in Nuclear Medicine). vol. 44. St. Louis, Mallinckrodt Chemical Works, 1970.
41. Gregersen, M. I., and Rawson, R. A.: Blood volume. Physiol. Rev., *39*:307, 1959.
42. Albert, S. N.: Blood Volume and Extracellular Fluid Volume. ed. 2. Springfield, (Ill.), Charles C Thomas, 1971.

6 B_{12} and Folate Deficiency

VICTOR HERBERT, M.D., J.D.

In 1953, Schilling described the first simple method for measuring vitamin B_{12} absorption in man.[1] The "Schilling test," along with blood volume determinations and radioiodine uptakes, became one of the staple diagnostic tests used to justify the creation of nuclear medicine units, and has since expanded from that base through a large range of diagnostic procedures. In the fields of hematology, gastroenterology, and nutrition, tests of radioactive-vitamin B_{12} absorption continue to play a primary role in the differential diagnosis of vitamin B_{12} deficiency states.[2]

Rapidly following on the report in 1958 of the use of radioactive vitamin B_{12} to determine the quantity of the vitamin in an unknown solution by competitive inhibition radioassay,[3] a number of radioassays for B_{12} capitalizing on this principle appeared in rapid succession.[3-7] In 1971, radioassay for serum folate level was described by the techniques of both competitive and sequential inhibition.[8] Subsequent reports indicate that radioassay for serum folate will eventually replace microbiologic assay for this vitamin, just as radioassay for B_{12} has substantially replaced microbiologic assay for that vitamin.

Nuclear medicine has also contributed to the diagnostic armamentarium related to the field of vitamin B_{12} deficiency three in vitro tests which so far can be done in no way other than by using radioactive vitamin B_{12} —in vitro assay: (1) for intrinsic factor in human gastric juice, (2) for antibody to intrinsic factor in human serum and other body fluids, and (3) for measurement of the unsaturated vitamin B_{12}-binding capacity of human serum and other body fluids.[9]

Another nuclear medicine technique that has proven of value in differential diagnosis of megaloblastic anemias is the dU-suppression test, which has also recently been explored for its possible value for in vitro prediction of therapeutic response of various human malignancies to various chemotherapeutic drugs, as well as for predicting selective suppression of just one of the two main cell lines of lymphocytes.[10,11,12]

Radiofolate absorption tests have been of some research value, but because of difficulties in specificity and sensitivity, as well as lack of methodologic simplicity, these tests remain primarily research tools, having proved of considerable value in conjunction with use of the triple-lumen tube.[13-19] The triple-lumen nasogastric tube is used by infusing the substance, whose absorbability is to be measured through the proximal port, and collecting infusion fluid mixed with intestinal juices at the second port (proximal collecting site) 15 cm distal to the perfusion port, and also collecting fluid from the third port (distal collecting site) 30 cm distal to port No. 2. The difference between the

This work of the author was supported primarily by United States Public Health Service grant, AM-15163, by a Veterans Administration Medical Investigatorship, and by Career Scientist Award I-683 of the Health Research Council of the City of New York.

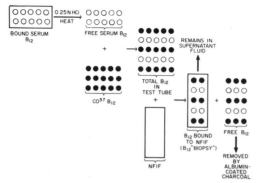

Fig. 6-1. The concept of competitive inhibition assay is applied to the assay of serum vitamin B_{12} levels.

quantity of nutrient removed from port No. 2 and port No. 3 quantitates the amount of nutrient which was absorbed.

Diagnosis of Vitamin B_{12} Deficiency (Serum Vitamin B_{12} Level)

The basic physiology of vitamin B_{12} is delineated elsewhere.[20,21] Briefly, the vitamin is found only in animal protein, and therefore all individuals on strict vegetarian diets eventually develop vitamin B_{12} deficiency. For normal vitamin B_{12} absorption, gastric intrinsic factor must combine with food B_{12}, and the complex must be "plastered" onto specific receptors on the brush border of the ileal mucosa cell in the presence of ionic calcium and an adequate alkaline pH. Therefore, vitamin B_{12} deficiency may result from any structural or functional damage to stomach, ileum, or pancreas. The diagnosis of malabsorption of vitamin B_{12} due to gastric or intestinal dysfunction is discussed below.

The sole definitive diagnostic test for vitamin B_{12} deficiency in man is the demonstration of a serum vitamin B_{12} level below 100 pg/ml. Microbiologic assay of serum B_{12} levels has defects—at least an overnight period must be allowed for the organism to grow before the assay can be "read," and various drugs (e.g., antibiotics, antimetabolites, and tranquilizers) inhibit bacterial growth and produce false low results.[22,23]

Radioassay of vitamin B_{12}, on the other hand, may be completed in less than an hour, and is unaffected by any of the abovementioned drugs. However, recent evidence shows that large doses (such as 2 Gm daily) of oral ascorbic acid may produce artifactually low serum vitamin B_{12} levels by radioassay. We have not yet determined whether such doses also produce low microbiologic assay results for vitamin B_{12}. However, if a patient is taking such doses of ascorbate to keep his urine acid, as is true of many paraplegics, the possibility of a false low serum B_{12} level should be kept in mind.[24] Furthermore, large amounts of fluoride are added in vitro to blood samples for certain procedures; such blood samples should not be used for B_{12} assay, since large fluoride doses also appear to produce artifactually low serum B_{12} levels by radioassay.[25]

The principle of radioassay of vitamin B_{12} in any fluid (Fig. 6-1), popularly known as "competitive inhibition," is a subcategory of isotope dilution assay.[26,27] Because vitamin B_{12} in serum is attached to a binding protein (Fig. 6-1), the first step in assay of the vitamin is to free it from its binder. To do so heat it in 0.25NHCl for 15 minutes at 100°C. Add to the free vitamin B_{12} in the test tube a known amount of radioactive vitamin B_{12}. Briefly shake it thoroughly so that it mixes the nonradioactive vitamin with the radioactive; add to the mixture a binder (or "carrier") of a known fixed maximal capacity to bind approximately two-thirds of the amount of radioactive B_{12} previously added to the unknown sample. In Figure 6-1, National Formulary Intrinsic Factor (NFIF) is used. The carrier will "biopsy" the pool of mixed radioactive and nonradioactive B_{12} (Fig. 6-1) by taking out a piece of that pool equal to the binding capacity of the carrier. For simplicity, Figure 6-1 shows the competition between labeled and unlabeled B_{12} for the carrier to be in a 1:1 ratio, although this is not necessary; all that is necessary is that the competition ratio be reproducible from test tube to test tube. The test tube now contains some B_{12} attached to the carrier, yielding a com-

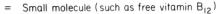 = Large molecule (such as intrinsic factor, alone or complexed with vitamin B₁₂)

○ = Small molecule (such as free vitamin B₁₂)

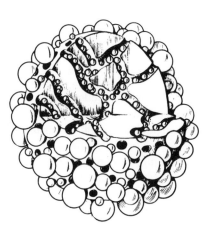
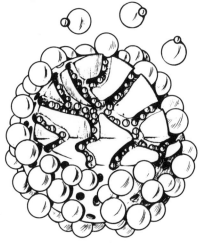

Uncoated-charcoal particle absorbs large and small molecules on its surface. Molecules small enough to get through its pores are absorbed on the walls of its channels.

Charcoal particle presaturated with large molecules can only absorb small molecules. (They go through its pores and are absorbed on the walls of its channels.)

Charcoal nonspecifically absorbs many large and small molecules. Large molecules (such as intrinsic factor and serum proteins) cannot get into charcoal particle channels through small pores? and thus are absorbed only on outer surface and walls of larger channels.

Fig. 6-2. The "coated-charcoal" concept. A number of workers allege that "uncoated charcoal" separates small molecules from large, but only when a very small amount of charcoal is used in comparison to a large amount of plasma. These workers fail to realize that the relatively large amount of plasma protein coats the relatively small amount of charcoal, thereby creating "coated charcoal." As a rule of thumb, charcoal is fully coated when the weight of the serum protein exceeds about 10 percent of the weight of the charcoal. (Gottlieb, C., *et al.*: Blood, *25*:875, 1965)[9]

plex with a molecular weight greatly in excess of B₁₂ alone (i.e.: 1,355) and some free B₁₂. Then separate the free and bound B₁₂ by any modality capable of separating large molecules from small.

Separation can be carried out by any of many different modalities, ranging from dialysis,[28] through DEAE,[29] to separating columns.[30] We have found batch separation with coated charcoal the simplest and most rapidly reproducible method (Fig. 6-2).[9,26] The preferred coating for vitamin B₁₂ assay is hemoglobin, although dextran or albumin will also serve. The coating insures that only small molecules are adsorbed. To pre-

pare hemoglobin-coated charcoal, add to a flask containing 100 ml of distilled water, 5 Gm of Norit A pharmaceutical-grade neutral charcoal. To another flask, add 0.25 Gm hemoglobin solution and make up to 100 ml with distilled water. Pour the content of the latter flask into the former, swirl for 10 seconds—the result is hemoglobin-coated charcoal. Prepare hemoglobin by washing discarded human red cells twice with 0.9 percent saline, then hemolyzing them with an equal volume of distilled water, followed by adding one-half volume of toluene. Shake the mixture vigorously for 5 minutes, then centrifuge it for 15 minutes at 3,000 rpm.

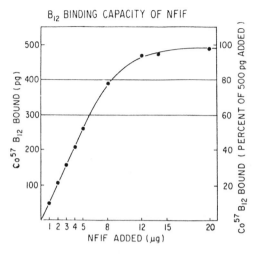

Fig. 6-3. Percentage of Co^{57} B_{12} bound by increasing quantities of a particular lot of National Formulary Intrinsic Factor Concentrate (NFIF). The results of this study demonstrate that this particular lot of NFIF has a maximal capacity to bind approximately 400 pg of $B_{12}/8$ μg of NFIF, and that therefore the amount of this lot of NFIF to add to each unknown as "standard amount of binder" is 5.5 μg.

Discard the top two layers, consisting of toluene and cell debris, and pass the bottom layer consisting of hemoglobin, through Whatman No. 1 filter paper to yield a clear red filtrate. Determine the hemoglobin content of the filtrate in the conventional manner, and adjust the hemoglobin concentration with distilled water to 10 Gm/100 ml.[26]

After the content of the test tube (an unknown amount of nonradioactive B_{12}, a known amount of radioactive B_{12}, and a known amount of binder) has been allowed to incubate for half an hour at room temperature, add 2 ml of the coated-charcoal suspension; mix the sample by inverting thrice, centrifuge for 10 minutes, and determine the supernatant radioactivity using the formula.[26]

pg B_{12} per ml serum =

$$\frac{1}{n} \times pg\ Co^{57}B_{12}\left(\frac{B}{B'} - 1\right)$$

n = ml of serum assayed

B = net cpm of intrinsic factor concentrate control tube

B′ = net cpm of tube with unknown serum

For B_{12} radioassay work with any reproducible binder ("carrier") of B_{12}. We have been using the "intrinsic factor, 10X NF without B_{12}."* Others have successfully used saliva, serum from patients with chronic myelogenous leukemia, and chicken serum.[31-35] Regardless of what binder is used, prior to its use, determine the capacity to bind B_{12} (Fig. 6-3).

As Figure 6-3 illustrates, set up a series of test tubes; put no binder in the first; put one unit of binder in the second; put 2 units of binder in the third, and so on until there is a series of 10 or 15 test tubes with sequentially increasing amounts of binder. Then, to each test tube add an identical amount of radioactive vitamin B_{12}. Since one wants to assay normal serum B_{12} levels, select the amount of radioactive vitamin B_{12} in the middle of the normal serum B_{12} range, namely 500 pg of radioactive B_{12}. Then briefly agitate the test tubes and allow them to incubate for one-half hour at room temperature (or 37°C), so that association of B_{12} and intrinsic factor concentrate goes essentially to completion. (Our original report did not mention this important half-hour incubation period, but we subsequently pointed out its importance.)[26,31] Then separate the free vitamin from the bound using coated charcoal, and count the radioactivity in the supernatant or in the precipitate, from which data construct a curve similar to that in Figure 6-3. On the curve seek the point at which it begins to "break," represented by the upper horizontal line (Fig. 6-3). Move downward from that "break" point approximately one-quarter (represented by the lower horizontal line in Fig. 6-3) to one-third of the way down toward the baseline. This point (i.e., one-quarter to one-third of the way back down toward the baseline from the point where the curve ceases to be an ascending straight line) represents the standard amount of that particular batch of that particular binder which

---

* Nutritional Biochemicals Corporation, Cleveland, Ohio.

may be used in all subsequent B_{12} assays until the batch is exhausted. Immediately after that quantity of binder is determined, divide the entire stock solution of binder among a large number of test tubes, so that each test tube contains an adequate quantity of binder for whatever number of vitamin B_{12} assays will be run in an average day. Then store these individual test tubes frozen at −20 degrees C. When a vitamin B_{12} assay is to be done, thaw and use one tube; discard any remaining binder in the thawed tube after the assay of the day.

The ability of intrinsic factor concentrate to bind B_{12} does not decrease with time when the concentrate is continuously frozen. However, it is altered by repeated thawing and refreezing.

Although we have not found it necessary to use either cyanide or albumin to stabilize our assays, others have found these additions desirable.[36,37] As a general rule, the best way to set up a radioassay for vitamin B_{12} is to send the person who is actually going to do the assay to spend the day in the laboratory of someone who is successfully doing radioassays for vitamin B_{12}. Workers who have attempted to set up radioassay for vitamin B_{12} from the literature alone have often experienced difficulty; such difficulty usually is overcome after a visit to any laboratory successfully doing these assays by any of the many modifications of the basic methodology. Commercial kits are now available for determination of serum B_{12} by radioassay.

Anomalous values of serum vitamin B_{12}—in the presence of liver disease, or myeloproliferative disorders, B_{12} binding proteins may be released into the serum. These proteins may bind vitamin B_{12} irreversibly, resulting in a normal (or elevated) serum vitamin B_{12} level, despite tissue depletion and biochemical deficiency of the vitamin.[82]

During the progress of pregnancy, the serum vitamin B_{12} level tends to fall, and serum vitamin B_{12} binding capacity tends to rise. This phenomenon appears to be physiologically analogous to the fall in serum iron and rise in iron-binding capacity.

Red Cell Vitamin B_{12} Levels

As vitamin B_{12} deficiency develops, the serum vitamin B_{12} level falls first and is only slowly followed by the red cell vitamin B_{12} level.[38] For this reason, measurement of the red cell vitamin B_{12} level is of much less value in the diagnosis of vitamin B_{12} deficiency than 'are measurements of the serum vitamin B_{12} level. However, red cell vitamin B_{12} level is of clinical value when the serum vitamin level is artificially elevated due to chronic myelogenous leukemia, liver disease, or an injection of vitamin B_{12} within the previous 48 hours.[38] Since vitamin B_{12} enters mainly reticulocytes[39,40,41] and not mature erythrocytes, the erythrocyte vitamin B_{12} level may be a more valid measure of tissue B_{12} stores when the serum vitamin level is artificially elevated. Radioassay for red cell vitamin B_{12} level is carried out in much the same manner as radioassay for serum vitamin B_{12} level.[38]

Diagnosis of Pernicious Anemia (Assay of Intrinsic Factor in Gastric Juice and Antibody to Intrinsic Factor in Serum)

Pernicious anemia is that form of vitamin B_{12} deficiency due to inadequate or absent gastric parietal cell secretion of the intrinsic factor of Castle. It is of unknown cause.[42] Thus, the sine qua non for the diagnosis is inadequate or absent gastric intrinsic factor secretion. The only in vitro procedures for assay of intrinsic factor require the use of radioactive vitamin B_{12}. The simplest, and therefore the most popular, assay is the one using coated charcoal;[9] but the guinea pig intestinal mucosa homogenate assay, although not as popular, has the advantage of measuring not only the capacity of intrinsic factor to bind B_{12} (which the coated-charcoal test measures) but also transfer of the vitamin to specific intestinal receptors.[43,44]

The methodology is identical for coated-charcoal assay of intrinsic factor and antibody to intrinsic factor.[9] For assay of the quantity of intrinsic factor in an unknown sample of gastric juice, use a serum known

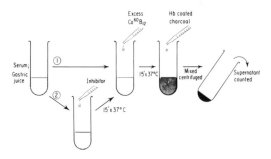

Fig. 6-4. The above steps are used in measuring the unsaturated B_{12} binding capacity of serum or gastric juice (pathway 1) and in measuring inhibitor (antibody to intrinsic factor, pathway 2) using coated charcoal.

to contain antibody to intrinsic factor. To determine whether a given sample of serum contains antibody to intrinsic factor, use a normal juice known to contain intrinsic factor. The measurement of gastric intrinsic factor is depicted in Figure 6-4.[27] To determine the total vitamin B_{12} binding capacity of the gastric juice specimen add an excess of radioactive B_{12}, remove the free B_{12} with coated charcoal, and count the radioactivity of the supernatant. That portion of this total B_{12} binding capacity which is due to intrinsic factor is determined by following pathway 2 in Figure 6-4 (i.e., to another aliquot of gastric juice add "inhibitor"—serum containing antibody to intrinsic factor). Incubate this mixture for 15 minutes at 37°C, during which time the antibody to intrinsic factor combines with the intrinsic factor in such a manner as to make the intrinsic factor no longer able to bind vitamin B_{12}. After this 15-minute incubation period, add an excess of radioactive vitamin B_{12} and incubate for another 15-minute period. During this period, the radioactive B_{12} will bind to that portion of the total binding capacity of the gastric juice which is "nonintrinsic factor B_{12} binder." Separate the excess free radioactive B_{12} from the bound B_{12} by the coated charcoal and count the supernatant radioactivity. It represents that portion of the total B_{12} binding capacity of the gastric juice specimen which is not due to intrinsic factor; by

simple subtraction, the fraction due to intrinsic factor is determined.[9,45] Chanarin has compiled data on intrinsic factor content of gastric juice in a wide range of situations including pernicious anemia.[46]

Antibody to intrinsic factor is discovered in serum by the same method as intrinsic factor is measured. For this purpose start with a normal gastric juice known to contain intrinsic factor as a standard (Fig. 6-4). To this add (pathway 2) the sample of unknown serum (inhibitor, Fig. 6-4). The rest of the procedure is identical to that for assay of intrinsic factor. If the normal gastric juice binds the same amount of radioactive B_{12} in the presence of the serum as it does in its absence, the serum contains no antibody to intrinsic factor. (Actually, the amounts of radioactive B_{12} bound by normal gastric juice in the presence of added serum are actually a little greater than in the absence of serum, because the serum contributes its own B_{12} binding capacity as an addition to the B_{12} binding capacity of the gastric juice.) If the serum contains antibody to intrinsic factor, then the normal gastric juice, in the presence of that serum, binds substantially less (20% less or an even more substantial decrement) radioactive vitamin B_{12} in the presence of the serum-containing antibody than in its absence.

Results of in vitro assay for intrinsic factor are generally expressed as "the unsaturated vitamin B_{12} binding capacity of this gastric juice is X pg of vitamin B_{12} per ml, of which Y pg are due to intrinsic factor."[45] Results of assays for antibody to intrinsic factor are expressed either qualitatively (antibody absent; antibody present) or quantitatively (by serial dilution of the serum and reporting that "maximal dilution is still able to inhibit radioactive vitamin B_{12} uptake by the intrinsic factor contained in normal gastric juice").

Diagnosing Malabsorption of Vitamin B_{12} Due to Gastric or Intestinal Dysfunction

Once the diagnosis of vitamin B_{12} deficiency has been made by demonstrating a low-serum vitamin B_{12} level, the question

Table 6-1. The Amount of Vitamin B_{12} Normally Absorbed from a Single Oral Dose of Vitamin B_{12}.

Oral Dose of Vitamin B_{12} (μg)	Approximate Amount Absorbed			Percentage in Urine in 24 hr*	
	μg	Percentage Mean	Range	Mean	Range
0.1	0.08	77	52–92	26	13–48
0.25	0.19	75	32–92		
0.5	0.35	71	33–97	23	8–46
0.6	0.38	63	20–92		
1.0	0.56	56	26–87	17	6–35
2.0	0.92	46	4–83	11	4–29
5.0	1.4	28	2–50		
10.0	1.6	16	0–34		
20.0	1.2	6			
50.0	1.5	3			

* The percentage normally found in the urine in 24 hr after Schilling-type tests is approximately one-third of the amount absorbed; a second 24-hr urine collection following a second flushing dose raises percentage normally in urine to approximately half the amount absorbed.

(From Chanarin as modified by Herbert)[2,46]

arises as to whether the B_{12} deficiency is due to inadequate gastric secretion of intrinsic factor or to ileal dysfunction. These questions are answered by determining the absorbability of an orally fed dose of radioactive vitamin B_{12} under various conditions described as Stage 1, Stage 2, and, if necessary, Stage 3.[2]

The radioactive vitamin B_{12} used is labeled with [56]Co (half-life, 77 days), [57]Co (half-life, 270 days), [58]Co (half-life, 71 days), or [60]Co (half-life, 5.26 years). The amount absorbed is determined by measuring the amount of radioactivity in urine (the Schilling test[1]), stool,[47] liver (Glass test),[48] plasma,[49] or whole body.[50,51]

It is important that the test record state the quantity of vitamin B_{12} fed by mouth, because the mean and range for the percentage of vitamin B_{12} normally absorbed from a single oral dose is inversely proportional to the weight of the vitamin B_{12} fed to the patient. The dose should not exceed 2 μg, since that dose approximates the maximal functional capacity of the intrinsic factor mechanism and the ileal intrinsic factor receptors.[52] A significant percentage of doses in excess of 2 μg is absorbed by diffusion; therefore such doses are useless in assessing the absorbability of the small amounts of B_{12} normally made available for absorption

from food.[52] It is important to remember that postgastrectomy and achlorhydric patients have less than normal ability to release vitamin B_{12} from food and to thereby make it available for absorption. For this reason, such patients may have normal absorption of B_{12} from a radioactive dose of the vitamin (because the radioactive dose is crystalline vitamin and does not have to be freed from anything prior to being absorbed), and yet may subnormally absorb vitamin B_{12} from food.[53]

Table 6-1 lists the amount of vitamin B_{12} absorbed from a single oral dose of radioactive vitamin.[2,46]

The most popular method for measuring vitamin B_{12} absorption is the urinary excretion test originally devised by Schilling.[1] The patient is fed a dose of 2 μg of radioactive vitamin B_{12} and given an injection of 1 mg of nonradioactive vitamin B_{12} to block all potential tissue sites of vitamin B_{12} binding, thus causing the subsequently absorbed radioactive vitamin B_{12} to be flushed out into the urine which is collected for 24 hours. The modification of the Schilling test we use extends the test period by giving a second 1 mg injection of nonradioactive vitamin B_{12} at the end of the first 24-hr period, and then collecting a second 24-hr urine.[54] The second 24-hr urine collection is of value

Table 6-2. Average Urinary Excretion of an Oral Dose of 2 μg of Radioactive Vitamin B$_{12}$, Measured as Percent of the Oral Dose.

Day	Oral Treatment	Normals	Pernicious Anemia	Sprue
1	Vitamin B$_{12}$ alone	10.5 (64)	0.7 (124)	0.7 (7)
2		4.4 (45)	0.3 (100)	0.3 (6)
3	B$_{12}$ + Intrinsic factor	12.1 (23)	7.2 (128)	0.8 (8)
4		5.3 (20)	3.3 (117).	0.4 (8)

Figures in parentheses represent the number of patients.
(Data provided by Ellenbogen, L., et al.: Proc. Soc. Exp. Biol. Med., *99*:257, 1958)[54]

Table 6-3. Range of Urinary Excretion of an Oral Dose of 2 μg of Radioactive Vitamin B$_{12}$, Measured as Percent of the Oral Dose.

Day	Oral Treatment	Normals	Pernicious Anemia	Sprue
1	Vitamin B$_{12}$ alone	4.1–29.2	0.0– 2.7	0.1–2.2
2		0.7–20.0	0.0– 1.5	0.1–0.6
3	B$_{12}$ + Intrinsic Factor	3.6–22.4	2.0–16.4	0.2–1.5
4		1.4–12.8	0.1–10.3	0.1–1.1

(Data provided by Ellenbogen and Williams)[54]

Table 6-4. Results of the 24-Hour Urinary Radioactivities in 206 Control Subjects, with Varying Time Intervals Between Oral Dose of 0.56 μg B$_{12}$ Containing 0.39 or 0.5 μc ^{60}Co and Single Flushing Injection of 1 mg Cold B$_{12}$.

No. of Urinary Tests	Time Between Oral Dose and Intramuscular Injection (hr.)	8-hr Plasma Absorption pg/ml Plasma			Urinary Radioactivity Percent of Oral Dose		
		No. of Tests	Average	Range	Average	SD	Range
10	0	0			17.3	±7.1	10.6–31.0
28	2	0			22.4	±8.0	6.5–44.7
11	4	3	6.8	5.6– 8.6	23.5	±6.2	11.2–33.1
42	6	42	8.0	3.2–15.1	28.9	±8.5	13.2–48.2
10	8	10	4.6	3.1– 6.0	26.6	±7.4	16.8–39.7
10	10	10	4.8	2.5– 9.9	23.6	±5.1	16.5–31.7
10	12	10	4.2	3.1– 6.4	21.4	±6.5	12.3–30.8
10	24	10	3.9	2.1– 7.3	12.8	±4.8	5.6–21.6
10	48	5	5.5	3.3– 7.0	7.8	±3.0	3.6–11.4
12	72	7	3.8	2.8– 5.6	3.6	±1.8	0.6– 6.8
12	96	8	5.6	2.9–11.4	2.9	±1.5	0.7– 6.2
10	120	7	4.3	3.7– 5.3	1.6	±0.6	0.9– 3.1
10	144	10	5.2	3.3– 7.5	1.5	±0.7	0.7– 2.8
10	168	10	5.2	3.1– 8.1	1.3	±0.4	0.8– 2.0
11	336	11	5.7	2.9–10.3	0.5	±0.2	0.2– 0.7

Urine radioactivity may be sharply increased by a 50 μg injection of cold B$_{12}$ 24 hr before starting this test.
(From Doscherholmen, A.: Studies in the Metabolism of Vitamin B$_{12}$. Univ. of Minn. Press, Minn., 1965)[56]

since it picks up radioactive vitamin B_{12} excreted in delayed fashion because of renal damage, intestinal edema, or unknown factors. Tables 6-2 and 6-3 present the average and range of urinary excretion, over 48 hours, of radioactive vitamin B_{12} in this modification of the Schilling test.[55] The absorption of radioactive B_{12} is recorded as the percent of the oral dose excreted in the urine. This measurement may be made on the entire 24-hr urine collection, on an aliquot thereof, or on the entire urine concentrated by evaporation, or by boiling (0.4 ml of Tween 80 added to 500 ml of urine allows the urine to be boiled down to 50 ml without foaming), or the vitamin B_{12} may be removed by shaking the urine with 1 Gm of Norit A charcoal per 100 ml of urine, and then counting the radioactivity in the charcoal.

To prevent food interference in absorption of radioactive vitamin B_{12}, the patient is given no food for 2 hours before the feeding of the material to 2 hours afterward.

We find it convenient to give the non-radioactive flushing injection of vitamin B_{12} at the same time the oral dose of radioactive B_{12} is fed; there is good separation of normal results from subnormal, and there is economy of time for both physician and patient. Others give the injection at different times in relation to the oral dose; Doscherholmen found the highest urine (and plasma) radioactivity when the injection was given 6 hours after the oral dose; his study of the relationship of varying time intervals to quantity of radioactivity found in the urine and the plasma is summarized in Table 6-4.[56]

The "first-stage" test consists in feeding the patient a dose of radioactive vitamin B_{12} and determining whether its absorption is normal or subnormal. The "second-stage" test consists in feeding the radioactive B_{12} with intrinsic factor concentrate, and determining the degree of radioactive B_{12} absorption as influenced by intrinsic factor. If the second-stage test is subnormal, it means that

the cause of the subnormal vitamin B_{12} absorption will be found in the intestine or the pancreas. Since approximately half the patients with vitamin B_{12} deficiency due to inadequate gastric secretion of intrinsic factor have secondary intestinal mucosal cell damage,[57,58] the "third-stage" test may simply be a repeat of the second-stage test after 2 months of vitamin B_{12} therapy in order to allow return to normal of the intestinal mucosa damaged by lack of vitamin B_{12}. If this repeat test then becomes normal, and the patient still lacks intrinsic factor by in vitro assay, the diagnosis of pure pernicious anemia is made, and the ileal dysfunction is diagnosed as simply secondary to vitamin B_{12} deficiency.

Also perform a third-stage test whenever a patient is suspected of having pancreatic disease, fish tapeworm, blind-loop syndrome, or a drug-induced vitamin B_{12} malabsorption (which may be produced by para-aminosalicylic acid, colchichine, neomycin, ethanol, oral contraceptives, or metformin).[2] For the third-stage test, if pancreatic disease is suspected, repeat the first-stage protocol but feed pancreatin or bicarbonate with the radioactive B_{12}.[59,60,61] Either of these agents corrects the subnormal B_{12} absorption associated with pancreatic disease.

If the subnormal intestinal absorption of vitamin B_{12} is believed due to blind-loop syndrome or fish tapeworm, treat the patient with antibiotics or anthelmintics for an appropriate period of time; then measure the ability to absorb radioactive vitamin B_{12}. If drug-induced vitamin B_{12} malabsorption is suspected, the third-stage test is the test of ability to absorb radioactive B_{12} after withdrawal of the offending drug.

The first- and second-stage tests may be carried out simultaneously using 2 different radioisotopes of vitamin B_{12}.[62,63] The simultaneous feeding of both free and intrinsic factor-bound vitamin B_{12} has the advantages that inadequate urine collection and variability in intestinal absorption are eliminated as problems, since the ratio of free to bound vitamin B_{12} absorbed is not affected when both reach the sites of absorption and excretion at the same time.

Reporting on the relationship between the Schilling test, the 8-hour plasma radioactivity test, and the 9-day whole-body retention test, Cottrall, et al.[64] confirmed that approximately one-third of the activity absorbed from a 1 μg oral radioactive vitamin B_{12} dose is excreted in the urine following a single intramuscular injection of 1 mg of nonradioactive vitamin B_{12}. They further confirmed that the administration of the flushing dose did not significantly reduce the amount of radioactive B_{12} absorbed and that the flushing dose approximately doubled the plasma radioactivity at 8 hours after ingestion of the oral dose. The authors pointed out that among these 3 methods of measuring radioactive B_{12} absorption, "the method of choice will be dependent on the facilities available and the cooperation that may be expected from the patient." While the plasma radioactivity test has the assets of convenience and rapidity, it suffers from some overlap between normal and subnormal values, and from being the poorest quantitative measure of ability to absorb vitamin B_{12}. If the patient is to have a therapeutic trial with one μg of vitamin B_{12} daily[65] as part of his evaluation, do not perform the Schilling test, which requires injection of a massive dose of the vitamin, until the therapeutic trial has been completed. In this situation, either delay the Schilling test or carry out a hepatic uptake test or plasma radioactivity test. These tests are not mutually exclusive, and 2 or more may be carried out after the same single oral radioactive vitamin B_{12} dose has been administered.

Diagnosis of Folate Deficiency
(the Serum and Red Cell Folate levels)

The basic physiology of folate is delineated elsewhere.[20,21] Although folate is present in nearly all natural foods, much of it is destroyed by cooking and other processing. Therefore, folate deficiency is common whenever the diet does not contain at least fresh uncooked fruit or vegetables (or fruit juice) daily. Since folate is absorbed from the upper third of the small bowel, any structural or functional derangement involving that section of the intestine may result in folate deficiency. Radiofolate absorption tests are discussed below.

Measurement of the serum and red cell folate levels together constitute the best diagnostic test for folate deficiency in man.[42,66] Serum folate falls rapidly after cessation of ingestion or absorption of the vitamin, and is low (i.e., below 3 ng/ml) after only 3 weeks of dietary deprivation or poor absorption; this is well before tissue folate stores are exhausted, and therefore the serum folate measure alone is too sensitive. The serum folate is *too* sensitive, because a patient with tissue folate depletion may have transiently normal serum folate level after a single meal of adequate folate content.[67] A low red cell folate is diagnostic for tissue folate depletion,[42,66,68] but such depletion occurs not only because of folate lack but because of lack of vitamin B_{12}, since vitamin B_{12} is required for folate to be incorporated into red cells.[69] Thus, determination of both serum and red cell folate together overcomes the objection to measurement of either one alone as the sole index for diagnosing folate deficiency.

The microbiologic assay for serum folate with *Lactobacillus casei*[70] has been the standard folate assay for almost 15 years. However, radioassays of improving quality are now coming on the horizon and should eventually replace microbiologic assay.

The first radioassay for measurement of serum folate levels mixed tritiated methyltetrahydrofolate with unknown serum, "biopsied" this pool with a measured aliquot of powdered milk as folate binder, and separated free from bound using hemoglobin-coated charcoal.[8] In an addendum to their original report, the same workers reported a sequential rather than simultaneous radioassay for serum folate.[8] In this modification, the serum to be assayed was incubated with the milk binder and, after 30 minutes, tritiated PGA (pteroylglutamic acid) was added. Separation was by coated charcoal. The method was subsequently reported in more detailed form, and applied to red cell folate assay, using commercially available lacto-globulin instead of powdered milk, since Salter, et al. have demonstrated that lacto-globulin was the major folate binder in milk.[71,72,73]

Rothenberg and his associates used a purified milk binder in their radioassay for folate, and felt it necessary to stabilize the reaction by carrying out their incubation in the cold. They have extended their method to red cell folate assays.[74,75]

Kamen and Caston used a partially purified folate binder extracted from hog kidney, which may well prove to be hog kidney conjugase.[76] Hog kidney conjugase is a peptidase for folate polyglutamates, and therefore binds folate tightly. Mincey, et al. were the first to report on radioassay for red cell folate, but of course any methodology applicable to serum folate is also applicable to red cell folate, since what is applicable to serum is applicable to any aqueous extract.[77]

Which, if any, of the above methodologic modifications of the basic radiofolate assay protocol proves most generally applicable for routine use awaits determination. Various modifications continue to appear.[78]

Anomalous values of serum folate—in liver and kidney disorders, folate binding proteins may be released into the serum. These binding proteins prevent measurement by radioassay of the folate attached to them, but this problem may be solved by freeing the folate by acid or other means.

During the progress of pregnancy, the serum folate level falls and folate-binding capacity rises. This is similar to the fall in serum iron and the rise in serum iron-binding capacity.

Studies of Folate Absorption Using Radioactive Folate

Unlike studies of absorption of radioactive vitamin B_{12}, which are of great importance in clinical differential diagnosis of vitamin

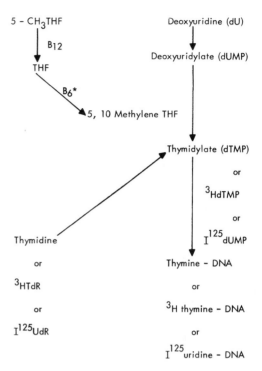

* Only one of several possible THF → 5,10 methylene THF pathways is B_6 - dependent

Fig. 6-5. The dU suppression test. Normally preincubation with dU suppresses the incorporation of subsequently added DNA precursor, so that the resultant DNA has low radioactivity relative to a no-dU control. If there is deficiency of vitamin B_{12} or folate, dU suppression will be subnormal, and the resulting DNA will have high radioactivity relative to the no-dU control.

B_{12} deficiency states (see above), tests of radiofolate absorption have been confined largely to research studies, in which they have had great value.[13-19] There is a lack of clinical application because the radioisotope used is not a gamma emitter. Counting beta emissions in urine and stool is cumbersome and it is impossible to count beta emissions from the whole body. To overcome this problem, Dr. Scott in our laboratory prepared ^{125}I-labeled PGA. This did not work out, because when folate was labeled with radioactive iodine it no longer acted like folate, its size having become so much

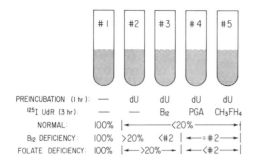

	#1	#2	#3	#4	#5
PREINCUBATION (1 hr):	—	dU	dU	dU	dU
^{125}I UdR (3 hr):	—	—	B12	PGA	CH3FH4
NORMAL:	100%	|←————<20%————→|
B12 DEFICIENCY:	100%	>20%	<#2 | ←—=#2—→|
FOLATE DEFICIENCY:	100%	|←—>20%—→ | ←<#2—→|

Fig. 6-6. Therapeutic trial in the test tube. (See below for detailed explanation.) (Gen. Med. Res. NF# 24422 A, VAH Bronx, New York)

greater. Therefore, studying its absorption was not equivalent to studying the absorption of folic acid. Others may wish to study this possibility further (see addendum).

Therapeutic Trial in the Test Tube (The dU Suppression Test Using ^{125}IUdR)

Prior to the age of radioisotopes, the classic means of demonstrating that a given anemia was due to lack of a given nutrient was by therapeutic trial. Here the patient was given the nutrient parenterally or orally daily, and his reticulocyte response was followed.[65,79] Therapeutic trial is time-consuming, and generally requires an initial control period of 7 to 10 days followed by equivalent test periods for vitamin B_{12} and separately for folate.

"Therapeutic trial in the test tube" accomplishes the same result as in vivo therapeutic trial but does so in a few hours. The concept (Fig. 6-5)[10,80] is as follows: Obtain a bone marrow aspirate from the patient and divide it into 5 aliquots of bone marrow cells suspended in Hanks' medium.[80] Add nonradioactive deoxyuridine (dU) to test tubes No. 2 through 5 (Fig. 6-6); in addition add 1 μg of B_{12} to test tube No. 3, 5 μg of PGA to test tube No. 4, and 5 μg of methyltetrahydrofolic acid to test tube No. 5. Incubate the tubes at 37°C for 1 hour with gentle shaking and in a slanted position to prevent the bone marrow cells from settling at the bottom. After this 1 hour of preincubation,

add ^{125}I deoxyuridine (1 μc, of specific activity 2-5 c per mM) to each of the 5 tubes and continue the incubation for another 2 to 3 hours. At the end of the incubation period, place the tubes in ice water to terminate the reaction and add 5 ml of cold saline containing 50 μl of 0.1 percent nonradioactive iododeoxyuridine to each tube to dilute out the radioactive iododeoxyuridine. Mix the tubes and centrifuge at 1500 G for 20 minutes; decant the supernatants and lyse the red cells (by adding 4.5 ml of distilled water, mixing and then reconstituting tonicity by adding 1.5 ml of 3.5 percent NaCl). Mix the remaining white cell suspension and centrifuge; and again wash the cells with 5 ml of saline, centrifuge, and decant the supernatant. Add 4 drops of 25 percent albumin solution, followed by 4 ml of 10 percent trichloroacetic acid. After mixing and centrifugation, remove the supernatant and determine the radioactivity of the precipitated DNA. The amount of radioactivity in test tube No. 1 is by definition the 100 percent value.

If the patient's bone marrow cells are not deficient in either B_{12} or folate (Fig. 6-6), test tubes Nos. 2 to 5 will have less than 20 percent of the radioactivity in test tube No. 1. If the patient is deficient in B_{12}, test tube No. 3 will have the lowest amount of radioactivity by comparison to test tube No. 1. If the patient is deficient in folate, then test tubes No. 4 and No. 5 will have the lowest amounts of radioactivity by comparison with test tube No. 1.

The sensitivity of the dU-suppression test is such that it can demonstrate biochemical deficiency of vitamin B_{12} or folate in the absence of morphological changes, and in the presence of misleading serum levels of vitamin B_{12} or folate. It does not require an extra bone marrow aspiration, since the test can be carried out using bone marrow cells obtained in the original bone marrow aspiration used to determine morphologic diagnosis of megaloblastic anemia.

Serum (or Plasma) Unsaturated Vitamin B_{12} Binding Capacity

This measurement is made very simply. Add an aliquot of radioactive vitamin B_{12} to a sample of serum (or plasma), shake briefly with coated charcoal, centrifuge, and count the radioactivity in the supernatant, which directly quantitates the unsaturated B_{12} binding capacity of the sample. Normally, the total B_{12} binding capacity of serum is approximately 33 percent saturated.[25,82] In vitamin B_{12} deficiency it is less than 10 percent saturated (unpublished data of VH).[25] Since the unsaturated B_{12} binding capacity of serum consists of 1 component which is "liver-related" TCII (transcobalamin II), and 2 other components which are "granulocyte-related" (TCI and TCIII), the separation of unsaturated vitamin B_{12} binding capacity into its 2 major components is of value in the study of liver disease and of myeloproliferative disorders.[25,82,83]

Summary

Radioassay for serum levels of vitamin B_{12} and folate, and radioassay of red cell folate, constitute the 3 most useful tests in diagnosing deficiency of vitamin B_{12} and/or folic acid. The most specific test for diagnosis of pernicious anemia (which is that vitamin B_{12} deficiency due to inadequate or absent gastric secretion of intrinsic factor of unknown or uncertain cause) is radioassay for quantitation of intrinsic factor in gastric juice. Of value also is radioassay for the presence of antibody to intrinsic factor in serum; such antibody is present in two-thirds of patients with pernicious anemia.

Diagnosis of subnormal absorption of vitamin B_{12} is made by determining the absorbability of a small amount of radioactive B_{12} given orally. Differential diagnosis as to whether the subnormal absorption of B_{12} is due to gastric damage, intestinal damage, pancreatic dysfunction, or some other cause is made by Stage-2 and Stage-3 tests of absorbability of an oral dose of radioactive B_{12} under circumstances altered as indicated in the text.

References

1. Schilling, R. F.: Intrinsic factor studies. II. The effect of gastric juice on the urinary excretion of radioactivity after the oral administration of radioactive vitamin B_{12}. J. Lab. Clin. Med., *42*:860, 1953.
2. Herbert, V.: Detection of malabsorption of vitamin B_{12} due to gastric or intestinal dysfunction. Sem. in Nucl. Med., *2*:220, 1972. Also published in Freeman, L. M., Blaufox, M. D. (eds.): Radionuclide Studies of the Gastrointestinal System. pp. 122-136. Grune & Stratton, New York, 1973.
3. Herbert, V.: Studies on the role of intrinsic factor in vitamin B_{12} absorption, transport, and storage. Amer. J. Clin. Nutr., *7*:433, 1959.
4. Herbert, V., Castro, Z., and Wasserman, L. R.: Stoichiometric relation between liver-receptor, intrinsic factor and vitamin B_{12}. Proc. Soc. Exp. Biol., *104*:160, 1960.
5. Barakat, R. M., and Ekins, R. P.: Assay of vitamin B_{12} in blood: A simple method. Lancet, *2*:25, 1961.
6. Rothenberg, S. P.: Assay of serum vitamin B_{12} concentration using Co^{57}, B_{12} and intrinsic factor. Proc. Soc. Exp. Biol., *108*:45, 1961.
7. Grossowicz, D., Sulitzeanu, D., and Merzbach, D.: Isotopic determination of vitamin B_{12} binding capacity and concentration. Proc. Soc. Exp. Biol., *109*:604, 1962.
8. Waxman, S., Schreiber, C., and Herbert, V.: Radioisotopic assay for measurement of serum folate levels. Blood, *38*:219, 1971.
9. Gottlieb, C., Lau, K. S., Wasserman, L. R., and Herbert, V.: Rapid charcoal assay for intrinsic factor (IF), gastric juice unsaturated B_{12} binding capacity, antibody to IF, and serum unsaturated B_{12} binding capacity. Blood, *25*:875, 1965.
10. Herbert, V., Tisman, G., Go, L. T., and Brenner, L.: The dU suppression test using I^{125}-UdR to define biochemical megaloblastosis. Br. J. Haematol., *24*:711, 1973.
11. Tisman, G., Herbert, V., and Edlis, H.: Determination of therapeutic index of drugs by in vitro sensitivity tests using human host and tumor cell suspensions. Cancer Chemother. Rep., *57*:11, 1973.
12. Tisman, G., Herbert, V., Go, L. T., and Brenner, L.: Marked immunosuppression

with minimal myelosuppression by bleomycin in vitro. Blood, *41*:721, 1973.

13. Bernstein, L. H., Gutstein, S., Weiner, S., and Efron, G.: The absorption and malabsorption of folic acid and its polyglutamates. Amer. J. Med., *48*:570, 1970.

14. Rosenberg, I. H., and Godwin, H. A.: The digestion and absorption of dietary folate. Gastroenterology, *60*:445, 1971.

15. Gerson, C. D., and Cohen, N.: The absorption of folic acid in man: Recent progress. Mt. Sinai J. Med., *39*:343, 1972.

16. Freedman, D. S., Brown, J. P., Weir, D. G., and Scott, J. M.: The reproducibility and use of the tritiated folic acid urinary excretion test as a measure of folate absorption in clinical practice: Effect of methotrexate on absorption of folic acid. J. Clin. Pathol., *26*:261, 1973.

17. Gerson, C. D., Cohen, N., Hepner, G. W., Brown, N., Herbert, V., and Janowitz, H. D.: Folic acid absorption in man: Enhancing effect of glucose. Gastroenterology, *61*: 224, 1971.

18. Gerson, C. D., Hepner, G. W., Brown, N., Cohen, N., Herbert, V., and Janowitz, H. D.: Inhibition by diphenylhydantoin of folic acid absorption in man. Gastroenterology, *63*:353, 1972.

19. Halsted, C. H., Robles, E. A., and Mezey, E.: Intestinal malabsorption in folate-deficient alcoholics. Gastroenterology, *64*: 526, 1973.

20. Herbert, V.: Drugs effective in megaloblastic anemias. *In* Goodman, L. S., and Gilman, A. (eds.): The Pharmacological Basis of Therapeutics. ed. 4, pp. 1414-1444. New York, Macmillan, 1970.

21. Herbert, V.: Megaloblastic anemias. *In* Beeson, P. B., and McDermott, W. (eds.): The Cecil-Loeb Textbook of Medicine. ed. 14. Philadelphia, W. B. Saunders, 1975.

22. Herbert, V., Gottlieb, C. W., and Altschule, M. D.: Apparent low serum-vitamin B₁₂ levels associated with chlorpromazine. An artefact. Lancet, *2*:1052, 1965.

23. Powell, D. E. B., Thomas, J. H., Mandal, A. R., and Dignam, C. T.: Effect of drugs on vitamin B₁₂ levels obtained using the *Lactobacillus leichmanii* method. J. Clin. Pathol., *22*:672, 1969.

24. Jacob, E., Scott, J., Brenner, L., and Herbert, V.: Apparent low serum vitamin B₁₂ levels in paraplegic veterans taking ascorbic acid. Proc. 16th Ann. Meeting, Am. Soc. Hem., Chicago, December, 1973.

25. Scott, J. M., Bloomfield, F. J., Stebbins, R., and Herbert, V.: Studies on derivation of transcobalamin III from granulocytes: En-hancement by lithium and elimination by fluoride of in vitro increments in vitamin B₁₂ binding capacity. J. Clin. Invest., *53*: January, 1974.

26. Lau, K. S., Gottlieb, C., Wasserman, L. R., and Herbert, V.: Measurement of serum vitamin B₁₂ level using radioisotope dilution and coated charcoal. Blood, *26*:202, 1965.

27. Zalusky, R., and Herbert, V.: Isotope dilution methods using coated charcoal. *In* Hayes, R. L., Goswitz, P. A., and Pearson-Murphy, B. E. (eds.): Radioisotopes in Medicine: In Vitro Studies. pp. 395-412. U.S. Atomic Energy Commission, Division of Technical Information, June, 1968.

28. Friedner, S., Josephson, B., and Levin, K.: Vitamin B₁₂ determination by means of radio-isotope dilution and ultrafiltration. Clin. Chim. Acta, *24*:171, 1969.

29. Frenkel, E. P., Keller, S., and McCall, M. S.: Radioisotopic assay of serum vitamin B₁₂ with the use of DEAE cellulose. J. Lab. Clin. Med., *68*:510, 1966.

30. Wide, L., and Killander, A.: A radiosorbent technique for the assay of serum vitamin B₁₂. Scand. J. Clin. Lab. Invest., *27*:151, 1971.

31. Herbert, V., Gottlieb, C. W., and Lau, K. S.: Hemoglobin-coated charcoal assay for serum vitamin B₁₂. Blood, *28*:130, 1966.

32. Carmel, R., and Coltman, C. A., Jr.: Radio-assay for serum vitamin B₁₂ with the use of saliva as the vitamin B₁₂ binder. J. Lab. Clin. Med., *74*:967, 1969.

33. Rothenberg, S. P.: A radioassay for serum B₁₂ using unsaturated transcobalamin I as the B₁₂ binding protein. Blood, *31*:44, 1968.

34. Lau, K. S.: Radioassay of serum B₁₂ using chicken serum. Manual of Procedures, Nutritional Anaemia Research Laboratory Training Course, March 25-April 5, 1968, Department of Pathology, University of Malaya, Kuala Lumpur. (Financed by USPHS Grant Am 11048 to Dr. V. Herbert).

35. Newmark, P. A., Green, R., Musso, A. M., and Mollin, D. L.: A comparison of the properties of chicken serum with other vitamin B₁₂ binding proteins used in radioisotope dilution methods for measuring serum vitamin B₁₂ concentrations. Br. J. Haemat., *25*:339, 1973.

36. Liu, Y. K., and Sullivan, L. W.: An improved radioisotope dilution assay for serum vitamin B₁₂ using hemoglobin-coated charcoal. Blood, *39*:426, 1972.

37. Hillman, R. S., Oakes, M., and Finholt, C.: Hemoglobin-coated charcoal radioassay for

serum vitamin B_{12}. A simple modification to improve intrinsic factor reliability. Blood, *34*:385, 1969.

38. Kelly, A., and Herbert, V.: Coated charcoal assay of erythrocyte vitamin B_{12} levels. Blood, *29*:139, 1967.

39. Herbert, V., and Zalusky, R.: Interrelations of vitamin B_{12} and folic acid metabolism: folic acid clearance studies. J. Clin. Invest., *41*:1263, 1962.

40. Schilling, R. F.: Incorporation of vitamin B_{12} into immature erythrocytes. Trans. Assoc. Amer. Physicians, *77*:79, 1964.

41. Retief, F. P., Gottlieb, C. W., and Herbert, V.: Mechanism of vitamin B_{12} uptake by erythrocytes. J. Clin. Invest., *45*:1907, 1966.

42. Herbert, V.: Megaloblastic anemias. *In* Beeson, P. B., and McDermott, W. (eds.): The Cecil-Loeb Textbook of Medicine. ed. 14. Philadelphia, W. B. Saunders, 1974.

43. Sullivan, L. W., Herbert, V., and Castle, W. B.: *In vitro* assay for human intrinsic factor. J. Clin. Invest., *42*:1443, 1963.

44. Sullivan, L. W.: Quantitative assay of intrinsic factor secretion in humans. *In* Hayes, R. L., Goswitz, F. A., and Pearson-Murphy, B. E. (eds.): Radioisotopes in Medicine: In Vitro Studies. U.S. Atomic Energy Commission, Division of Technical Information, June, 1968.

45. Herbert, V., and Gottlieb, C. W.: Intrinsic factor assay results. (Letter to the editor.) Lancet, *2*:696, 1965.

46. Chanarin, I.: The Megaloblastic Anaemias. Philadelphia, F. A. Davis, 1969.

47. Heinle, R. W., Welch, A. D., Scharf, G., Meacham, C., and Prusoff, W. H.: Studies of excretion and absorption of Co^{60}-labeled vitamin B_{12} in pernicious anemia. Trans. Assoc. Amer. Phys., *65*:214, 1952.

48. Glass, G. B. J.: Gastric intrinsic factor and its function in the metabolism of vitamin B_{12}. Physiol. Rev., *43*:529, 1963.

49. Booth, C. C., and Mollin, D. L.: Plasma, tissue and urinary radioactivity after oral administration of ^{56}Co-labeled vitamin B_{12}. Br. J. Haemat., *2*:223, 1956.

50. Heinrich, H. C.: Metabolic basis of the diagnosis and therapy of vitamin B_{12} deficiency. Sem. Hematol., *1*:199, 1964.

51. Reizenstein, P. G., Cronkite, E. P., and Cohn, S. H.: Measurement of absorption of vitamin B_{12} by whole-body gamma spectrometry. Blood, *18*:95, 1961.

52. Corcino, J., Waxman, S., and Herbert, V.: Absorption and malabsorption of vitamin B_{12}. Amer. J. Med., *48*:562, 1970.

53. Doscherholmen, A., and Swaim, W. R.: Impaired assimilation of egg ^{57}Co vitamin B_{12} in patients with hypochlorhydria and achlorhydria and after gastric resection. Gastroenterology, *64*:913, 1973.

54. Ellenbogen, L., Herbert, V., and Williams, W. L.: Effect of D-sorbitol on absorption of vitamin B_{12} by pernicious anemia patients. Proc. Soc. Exp. Biol. Med., *99*:257, 1958.

55. Herbert, V.: The Megaloblastic Anemias. New York, Grune & Stratton, 1959.

56. Doscherholmen, A.: Studies in the Metabolism of Vitamin B_{12}. Univ. of Minnesota Press, Minneapolis, 1965.

57. Herbert, V.: Transient (reversible) malabsorption of vitamin B_{12}. Br. J. Haemat., *17*:213, 1969.

58. Herbert, V.: Malabsorption syndrome secondary to B_{12} deficiency. *In* Gilson, A. J., Smoak, W. M., and Weinstein, M. B. (eds.): Hematopoietic and Gastrointestinal Investigations with Radionuclides. Charles C Thomas, Springfield (Ill.), 1972.

59. Veeger, W., Abels, J., Hellemans, N., and Nieweg, H. O.: Effect of sodium bicarbonate and pancreatin on the absorption of vitamin B_{12} and fat in pancreatic insufficiency. N. Eng. J. Med., *267*:1341, 1962.

60. Toskes, P. P., Hansell, J., Cerda, J., and Deren, J. J.: Vitamin B_{12} malabsorption in chronic pancreatic insufficiency. N. Eng. J. Med., *284*:627, 1971.

61. Bernstein, L., and Herbert, V.: The role of pancreatic exocrine secretions in the absorption of vitamin B_{12} and iron. Amer. J. Clin. Nutr., *26*:340, 1973.

62. Katz, J. H., DiMase, J., and Donaldson, R. M., Jr.: Simultaneous administration of gastric juice-bound and free radioactive cyanocobalamin. J. Lab. Clin. Med., *61*:266, 1963.

63. Fish, M. B., Pollycove, M., Wallerstein, R. O., Cheng, K. K-S, and Tono, M.: Simultaneous measurement of free and intrinsic factor (IF) bound vitamin B_{12} (B_{12}) absorption: Absolute quantitation with incomplete stool collection and rapid relative measurement using plasma B_{12} (IF): B_{12} absorption ratio. J. Nucl. Med., *14*:568, 1973.

64. Cottrall, M. F., Wells, D. G., Trott, N. G., and Richardson, N. E. G.: Radioactive vitamin B_{12} absorption studies: Comparison of the whole-body retention, urinary excretion, and eight-hour plasma levels of radioactive vitamin B_{12}. Blood, *38*:604, 1971.

65. Herbert, V.: Current concepts in therapy. Megaloblastic anemia. N. Eng. J. Med., *268*:201, 368, 1963.

66. Herbert, V.: The erythrocyte as a biopsy tissue in the evaluation of nutritional status. *In* Surgenor, D. M. (ed.): The Red Blood Cell. ed. 2. Academic Press, New York, 1974.

67. Herbert, V.: Studies of folate deficiency in man. Proc. Roy. Soc. Med., *57*:377, 1964.

68. Hoffbrand, A. V., Newcombe, B. F. A., and Mollin, D. L.: Method of assay of red cell folate activity and the value of the assay as a test for folate deficiency. J. Clin. Pathol., *19*:17, 1966.

69. Tisman, G., and Herbert, V.: B_{12} dependence of cell uptake of serum folate: An explanation for high serum folate and cell folate depletion in B_{12} deficiency. Blood, *41*:465, 1973.

70. Herbert, V., Wasserman, L. R., Frank, O., Pasher, I., and Baker, H.: Value of fasting serum "folic acid" levels. Fed. Proc., *18*:246, 1959.

71. Waxman, S., and Schreiber, C.: Measurement of serum folate levels and serum folic acid-binding protein by ^{3}H-PGA radioassay. Blood, *42*:281, 1973.

72. Schreiber, C., and Waxman, S.: Personal communication.

73. Salter, D. N., Ford, J. E., Scott, K. J., and Andrews, P.: Isolation of the folate binding protein from cow's milk by the use of affinity chromatography. Fed. Eur. Biochem. Soc. Lett., *20*:302, 1972.

74. Rothenberg, S. P., daCosta, M., and Rosenberg, Z.: A radioassay for serum folate: Use of a two-phase sequential-incubation, ligand-binding system. N. Eng. J. Med., *286*:1335, 1972.

75. Rothenberg, S. P., daCosta, M., and Lawson, J.: The determination of erythrocyte folate concentration using a two-phase ligand-binding radioassay. Blood, *43*:437, 1974.

76. Kamen, B. A., and Caston, J. D.: Direct radiochemical assay for serum folate: Competition between ^{3}H-folic acid and 5-methyltetrahydrofolic acid for a folate-binder. J. Lab. Clin. Med., *83*:164, 1974.

77. Mincey, E., Wilcox, E., and Morrison, R. T.: Determination of serum and red cell folate by a radioactive protein binding method. J. Nucl. Med., *14*:633, 1973.

78. Dunn, R. T., and Foster, L. B.: Radioassay of serum folate. Clin. Chem., *19*:1101, 1973.

79. Minot, G. R., and Castle, W. B.: Interpretation of reticulocyte reactions: Their value in determining potency of therapeutic materials, especially in pernicious anemia. Lancet, *2*:319, 1935.

80. Metz, J., Kelly, A., Swett, V. C., Waxman, S., and Herbert, V.: Deranged DNA synthesis by bone marrow from vitamin B_{12}-deficient humans. Br. J. Haemat., *14*:575, 1968.

81. Loo, T. L., Dion, R. L., and Fu, S.-C. J.: 3′-Iodopteroylglutamic acid (iodofolic acid). J. Org. Chem., *30*:2837, 1965.

82. Herbert, V.: Diagnostic and prognostic values of measurement of serum vitamin B_{12}-binding proteins. Blood, *32*:305, 1968.

83. Jacob, E., Brenner, L., and Herbert, V.: Rapid measurement of "granulocyte related" (TC I and III) and "liver related" (TC II) B_{12} binding proteins by instantly adsorbing TC II on Quso G32. Fed. Proc., *33*:715, 1974.

ADDENDUM

...... A simple radioassay giving results essentially identical to *L. casei* in sera and whole blood has recently been reported which appears to solve the three main difficulties in prior radiofolate assays. This assay makes use of three important facts: (1) at pH 9.3, milk binder is incapable of distinguishing PGA from methylfolate; (2) at adequately high quantity of milk folate binder, interference by endogenous folate binding protein can be ignored; and (3) ^{125}I-folate (the monoiodinated monotyramide of PGA) can substitute for PGA in radioassay.

Ref: Longo, D. L. and Herbert, V.: Simple Radioassay for Serum and Red-cell Folate Based on the New Findings. Program, Am. Soc. Hemat., 17th Ann. Mtg., Atlanta, Ga., Dec. 7-10, 1974.

7 Radionuclide Studies Associated with Abnormalities of Iron

BEN I. FRIEDMAN, M.D.

INTRODUCTION*

The role of nuclear medicine procedures in the study of iron absorption, metabolism, and loss has seemingly reached a plateau if not decreased in importance within the realm of clinical medicine. Though absorption is easily evaluated with radionuclide techniques, the importance of iron absorption in the usual clinical practice of medicine and hematology is very limited. Rather, determination of iron absorption is reserved primarily for clinical research in the study of absorptive mechanisms of disease states (e.g., cirrhosis of the liver, subtotal gastrectomy, extirpation or shunting procedures).

The original work of Huff on ferrokinetics followed by the expanded interpretation and processing of Pollycove and Mortimer, promised considerable elucidation of normal and abnormal physiology.[1,2,3] But, the clinical situations in which these methods are helpful have relegated themselves to a position of little importance except for research. Information regarding ineffective erythropoiesis is found by studying patients with pernicious anemia, or hyperplastic bone marrow associated with anemia, as well as studies of iron distribution in hypoplastic and aplastic anemia, but these have limited import in the medical management of a patient.

There is available a radionuclide competitive-binding assay for the study of the transferrin-iron transport mechanism. Unfortunately, this has involved only an evaluation of the latent iron-binding capacity which only inferentially gives information regarding the serum iron and total iron-binding capacity. Consequently, in clinical use it is necessary to obtain a serum iron. However, meaningful new information, which is not easily available by standard techniques, for determining serum iron and iron-binding capacity has not resulted from radionuclide techniques.

Studies of iron loss are possible. Primarily these involve use of whole-body counters which are of limited availability. At one time it appeared that many of the nuclear medicine laboratories would have such equipment, but in light of their narrow utilization in clinical problems general availability of whole-body counting facilities have not emerged on the nuclear medicine scene. Studies involving iron are of some value in ferrokinetics. These studies may help to elucidate the situation in patients with hyperplastic marrow and severe peripheral anemia or polycythemia (p. 92). Also in the future, studies involving isotopic iron will likely be helpful in further clarification of normal iron metabolism, the anemia of infection, refractory anemia, and the anemia associated with chronic diseases. Such studies may help to put the therapy of these anemias on a more rational basis.

---

* Rather than cite the innumerable references available, only those thought most valuable for the reader are listed. Many of them include extensive bibliographies.

The above uses are admittedly limited. Why then should a text on quantitative and in vitro approaches in nuclear medicine concern itself with abnormalities of iron? Perhaps, it is, as Tevye said in "The Fiddler on the Roof," "Tradition." Tradition or not, I hope this initial overview serves to place in perspective the role of iron in nuclear medicine.

ABSORPTION OF IRON

An evaluation of the methods for determining absorption of iron from the gastrointestinal tract first requires an understanding of the physiology of absorption. Though formerly Granick's elaboration of Hahn's "mucosal block" was accepted as the foundation on which to build concepts, more recently it has been shown that the intestinal mucosa has a major but not exclusive role in the control of iron absorption.[4-8]

In a recent review of the absorption of iron, Bothwell and Charlton first divided the factors to be considered into the luminal environment including gastrointestinal secretions or the form of iron in the food. Second, they looked at the influence of mucosal or internal factors, such as the mucosal mechanism for excluding excess iron and the "signal to the mucosa."[9]

They further cited evidence that ferric iron is absorbed better with gastric acid because it chelates with ascorbate and other complexing agents. These chelates remain more soluble in the alkaline duodenum and jejunum where absorption is thereby increased. The role of gastroferrin, which is thought to inhibit iron absorption, is not clear. In addition, increased absorption in patients with chronic pancreatitis need not be pancreatic in origin. In fact, in all likelihood, the pancreas does not play a significant role in control or regulation of iron absorption.

Iron is generally better absorbed in ionic form than in foods since it must be free of an organic attachment. The percent of absorption varies with the form of food iron, being better absorbed from liver and muscle than from some vegetables; this may be the result of hemoglobin iron being more easily absorbed than ferritin iron. Its absorption is enhanced by a substance in gastric intrinsic factor. Some recent work, however, indicates that there is little difference between iron absorption from food and ionic iron absorption.[10]

Most absorption occurs in the duodenum probably because of its position in relation to gastric; biliary, and pancreatic secretions, since isolated loops from any part of the small bowel absorb iron equally well.[11] However, Wheby showed that absorption may be more efficient in the small intestine proximal to the midjejunum.[12]

Iron stores and erythropoiesis are the major determinants of iron absorption. The site of this control is within the mucosal cell. Apparently, the iron enters the developing cells of the crypts of Lieberkühn, and if it is not needed it is discarded into the gut lumen at the time of physiological desquamation of the intestinal epithelium. It is interesting to learn how the mucosal cell is programmed to accept or hold iron. The amount of iron in the mucosal cells has been thought to influence its absorption. It has been hypothesized that the plasma iron provides the link between iron stores throughout the body and erythroid bone marrow on one hand and the mucosal cell on the other.[9] As more iron moves from plasma into the marrow stores, less is returned to developing mucosal cells, thereby increasing absorption. When iron stores are excessive or marrow function decreased, more returns to the mucous membrane and iron absorption decreases. Since patients with both iron deficiency anemia and hemolytic anemia have increased absorption, perhaps the stimulus to deposition of iron in the mucosa is directly related to the plasma clearance. There is less deposition when the plasma clearance of iron is rapid. Suffice it to say, the final answer to the mechanisms and reasons for variations in iron absorption has not been written.

Methods of Studying Absorption. Three radionuclide methods are available which will be discussed. Noteworthy is that all studies must be performed with an oral dose following at least a 12-hour fast, otherwise, there is too much variability in absorption.

1. The *fecal excretion method* for which various techniques may be used. The essentials of these studies are that a given amount of radioactive iron is administered orally and then feces are collected for a prescribed period of time or until less than a given percentage of the administered radioactivity is found in the last 24-hour stool specimen. When the quantity of administered iron is very small, it is possible to determine only a decreased rate of absorption, since a very high proportion of the oral dose is normally absorbed.[13] In order to have a normal range that allows delineation of increased or decreased absorption, a large amount of iron must be used. Seven hundred (700) μg of ferrous ammonium sulfate have been used for this purpose.[14] A normal absorption range of 50% $\pm$ 18.6 was found.

Two major difficulties are encountered in the fecal excretion method. First is adequacy of collection; second is the physiologic difficulty described earlier, namely, that the iron enters the mucosal cell but is subsequently sloughed off at what may be a variable rate. The period of collection must be at least 7 days in order to provide adequately for this.

2. The *dual isotope technique* involves the use of two radionuclides ^{59}Fe and ^{55}Fe. At the time of oral radionuclide administration (^{59}Fe), an intravenous injection of ^{55}Fe tagged to the patient's plasma is made.[15] Though formerly a single nuclide method using the blood level of radioiron 10 to 14 days after oral ingestion was used, it had the severe defect of not being a reliable index of absorption when the patient had hemochromatosis with dilution of the iron pool. Additionally, it could be misleading in clinical states with decreased utilization such as ineffective erythropoiesis or aplastic anemia. To allow for easy adjustment and interpretation in the presence of decreased utilization, the dual isotope technique was evolved. Ten to fourteen days after oral and intravenous iron administration a blood specimen is obtained and counted by a double-counting procedure. When the count rates in the blood, and the total net counts/min (CPM) (activity) of each radioiron given are known, then the percent absorption is calculated from the formula

$$\% \text{ absorption} = \frac{^{59}\text{Fe activity in the blood*}}{^{59}\text{Fe activity given orally in net CPM}} \times \frac{^{55}\text{Fe activity given IV in net CPM}}{^{55}\text{Fe activity in the blood*}} \times 100$$

The ^{55}Fe fraction is a ratio that compensates for decreased utilization of absorbed iron since it is the reciprocal of percent utilization independent of absorption. The greatest problem with this method is the need for counting the two radioirons, frequently necessitating an electroplating technique. It has been suggested that a liquid scintillation procedure after bleaching might simplify this study and make it more clinically applicable.

3. The *whole-body counting method* is probably the best, but least available, for evaluating iron absorption. Whole-body counters are found in relatively few centers in the United States. Studies with the shielded rooms really evaluate retention of iron within the body after an oral dose rather than absorption from the gastrointestinal tract. Though the specifics in each laboratory vary due to differences in equipment, the essentials are the same. Following an oral dose of ^{59}Fe, the fasting patient is counted at 5 hours and again in 10 to 20 days. Percent absorption is determined by this formula

$$\% \text{ absorption} = \frac{\text{Net CPM @ day 20}}{\text{Net CPM @ 5 hr}}$$

---

* Radioiron activity in the blood may be obtained by multiplying CPM/ml $\times$ estimated blood volume.

Basic assumptions are that there has not been excessive loss of blood through bleeding (gastrointestinal, genitourinary, or other sites) and that the geometry of radioactive distribution is the same on all counting days. In order to use small quantities of radioactivity either 4π liquid scintillation counters or large crystal gamma counters (stationary or scanner) in heavily shielded iron rooms are most efficient. However, it has been pointed out by certain authors that a larger dose of iron with a modified counting system in a nonshielded area is probably adequate for clinical studies.[16] This, however, has not received general acceptance.

It has been shown that with the whole-body counting technique using 0.25 mg ferrous iron as ferrous sulfate orally, absorption at 10 to 14 days is 19.0 ± 2.3% in normal young men, 31.7 ± 2.2% in iron-deficient males and 48.1 ± 4.3% in frequent blood donors.[17] Body and Will found a normal absorption of 9.6 percent in males and 11.4 percent in females after 5 mg of carrier iron.[18] Normal absorption was found in patients with rheumatoid arthritis without anemia and in patients with pernicious anemia.[18,19]

Results of Hausmann, et al. verified that reticuloendothelial stores seemed to regulate the absorption of iron in normals and patients with disease of the blood or liver, malignant diseases and infections using the ^{59}Fe-AWBRT (^{59}Fe absorption whole-body retention test).[20] They determined retained radioactivity in 780 people 14 to 21 days after the administration of 0.558 mg Fe[+++] + 17.6 mg of ascorbic acid. They stressed again the need for the *fasting* state. Normal values in 74 controls under their conditions were 25.4 ± 10.7% for males and 29.6 ± 11.5% for females. The subject of whole-body counting is extensively reviewed by Walker and Williams.[11]

The differences between the values obtained by the various above-cited authors appear to be quite definite. The exact reasons for these differences are not certain. Conceivably they might be related to the

Table 7-1. Diseases or Luminal Materials Associated with Altered Iron Absorption.

Increased	*Decreased*
Anemia	Gastrectomy
Iron deficiency	Total
Hemolytic	Subtotal
Idiopathic	Marrow depression
hemochromatosis	Radiation
Chronic pancreatitis	Hypertransfusion
Cirrhosis[14]	Tropical sprue
Hemorrhage	Gluten-induced
High altitude	enteropathy
Phlebotomy	Phytates[21]
Succinic acid[22]	Phosphates[21]
Ascorbic acid	Cholestyramine[23]
Fructose	Tetracycline*[23]
	Anticholinergics

* Not with usual doses in humans

different quantities of iron administered or to differences in measurement time.

Discrepancies between the fecal excretion method and the dual isotope studies have consistently shown greater absorption with the fecal method. It may be that this is due to submucosal radioiron deposition or simply technical difficulties in the collection of feces with loss of counts from incomplete recovery. It does appear that meticulous care may obviate the discrepancies.

The dual isotope and whole-body counting methods are in satisfactory agreement. At this time they appear to be the best of chemical or radionuclide techniques.

A summary of the absorption of iron under varying conditions appears in Table 7-1. The most common clinical conditions are cited.[20,21,22]

FERROKINETICS

Several excellent reviews of ferrokinetics are available. Pollycove and Finch have a detailed review of the subject.[24,25] A study of ferrokinetics does have a role in clinical nuclear medicine, particularly in evaluating the patient who has a hyperplastic bone marrow but manifests severe peripheral anemia or polycythemia.

Normally, iron absorbed from the gastrointestinal tract attaches to one of the 2 binding sites of transferrin (a β_1 globulin with a molecular weight of 88,000). Plasma transferrin and extravascular transferrin are in equilibrium. Only a part of the iron is lost into the tissues when the transferrin is extravascular. The major component of the transferrin iron is released in the bone marrow and becomes available for erythrocyte production. Within the immature erythroid cell less than 20 percent is nonheme iron and this decreases to 5 percent with maturation.[25] A part of the heme iron is lost to the reticuloendothelial system before maturation.

After maturation of the erythrocyte, the iron within the cell returns to the vascular space as hemoglobin iron and circulates for the life span of the red cell. At the time of red cell destruction, the hemoglobin iron is taken up by the reticuloendothelial system with most being reutilized in subsequent erythrocyte production. A small quantity remains in the ferritin-hemosiderin complex within the reticuloendothelial system. That the RE cell cannot take up transferrin-bound iron has been verified by radioautography. Ferrokinetic studies have been very important in elucidating many aspects of normal and abnormal physiology of iron metabolism.

As discussed here, *ferrokinetics* describes the transportation, utilization, and deposition of iron after the intravenous injection of a quantity of ^{59}Fe, either as ferrous citrate or as that which has been tagged to transferrin in vitro (Fig. 7-1). Absorption is not involved. We are dealing with clearance from the plasma space into the bone marrow or other tissues, followed by reappearance of the radioiron in the erythrocytes. The rate of clearance, either as a simple clearance rate or iron turnover rate, provides meaningful information regarding total erythropoietic activity of the bone marrow. When combined with in vivo studies of distribution, further information is available regarding normal or abnormal deposition of the iron. To determine the effectiveness of marrow activity, it is necessary to know the proportion of iron which has appeared in the red cells either as a percent of administered dose

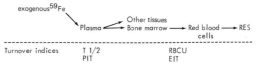

Fig. 7-1. A simplication of the entire ferrokinetic process is above the dotted line. The turnover indices are listed below the process they measure.

or as the quantity of iron turnover per unit of blood per unit of time. These processes are covered by the turnover indices listed in Table 7-2. Abbreviations and terms used vary among different investigators. The most common ones are included in Table 7-2 and may be used interchangeably or noted parenthetically within the text. All of the complex models, terms, and so on, represent explanations of the observations so described.

Methods. The more commonly used indices are the plasma clearance rate, plasma iron turnover rate, % RBC ^{59}Fe uptake, and red cell iron turnover rate. The marrow transit time is used by Finch, et al.[25] Fol-

Table 7-2.

	Normal Values (Approximate)
Plasma iron	50-100 μg/100 ml[a]
Plasma clearance rate (T ½)	90 ± 30 minutes
Plasma iron turnover (PIT) or	0.7 μg/100 ml whole blood per day 37 mg/d
Plasma iron turnover rate (PITR)	0.53 mg/kg/d[b]
Red cell utilization (RBCU) or ^{59}Fe red cell incorporation % RBC ^{59}Fe uptake	80%
Erythrocyte iron turnover (EIT) or	0.56 μg/100 ml whole blood per day 29 mg/d
Red cell iron turnover rate (RCITR)	0.41 mg/kg/d[b]
Marrow transit time (MTT)	3.5 days

[a] Diurnal variation with hypoferremia in evening
[b] Based on 70 kg man

lowing the intravenous injection of a small quantity (approximately 20 μCi of ferrous citrate) plasma is collected at frequent intervals for 3 hours. From data accumulated the plasma clearance rate is calculated and the T 1/2 in minutes obtained.

Some authors have recommended that the radioactive ferrous citrate be attached to either iron-carrying globulin or be incubated in vitro with the patient's plasma so that it would be more representative of transferrin-bound iron. In view of studies which have been performed showing that iron bound to plasma is handled essentially as unbound-ferrous citrate this does not seem necessary.[26]

A plasma iron must be obtained at the time of intravenous injection so that the plasma iron turnover rate can be calculated. It can be calculated from either of these formulas

$$\text{PITR (mg/100 ml whole blood per day)} = \frac{\text{Plasma Iron }(\mu gm/100\ ml)}{\text{T 1/2 (min)}} \times \frac{100 - \text{Hct}}{100}$$

$$\text{PITR (mg per day)} = \frac{0.693^* \times \text{Plasma Iron (mg/ml)} \times \text{Plasma Volume (ml)} \times 24}{\text{T ½ (hr)}}$$

When the clearance rate is rapid (T 1/2 less than 30 minutes), extraction of iron from the plasma by the tissues is maximal; the converse also holds. The PITR allows for recognizing the turnover of large quantities of iron when the plasma clearance rate may be somewhat slow but the plasma iron high. If the level of plasma iron is not taken into account, erroneous interpretation of rapid or slow clearance rates might occur. As stated earlier the PITR has been proposed as an index of "total erythropoiesis." However, this value alone does not differentiate between clearance to erythroid or nonerythroid tissues. Therefore, it can mislead if most of the iron is distributed to nonerythroid tissue.

As has been stressed by Pollycove and Mortimer, a small fraction of the radioiron does return to the plasma after a few hours or days.[3,24] Review the complex model they

proposed to understand this reflux of iron.

Most of the radioiron which cleared to areas of erythroid activity reappeared in the red cells within 10 to 14 days; normally, 80 percent does so. These observations, together with other data, have led to the concept of a rapid turnover of erythropoietic labile iron pool.[27] However, the model for this concept has been challenged by others.[25] Suffice it to say, the rapid appearance of the radioiron in the circulating erythrocytes indicates the presence of both easily utilized and slowly mobilized iron stores with the likelihood of nonhomogenous labeling of an erythroid iron pool in the marrow.

In order to determine the percent appearance (RBCU) (Table 7-2), it is necessary to measure or estimate the red cell mass in addition to determining the CPM/ml of RBC. The red cell iron turnover rate (RCITR) is calculated by the following formula

RCITR = PITR × % RBC ^{59}Fe uptake

It may be expressed as μg/100 ml whole blood/d, mg/d, or as mg/kg/d depending on the value of PITR used.

The importance of the red cell values is that they provide an index of the effectiveness of erythropoiesis, namely, whether the marrow activity results in the delivery of erythrocytes to the circulating red cell mass. This assumption is correct only in the absence of hemolytic anemia. In both hemolytic anemia and in "ineffective erythropoiesis" (see pp. 91-92), the RCITR underestimates effective erythropoiesis. This is also true in patients who have been bleeding.

The marrow transit time (MTT) is that time in days when the RBCU curve reaches 50 percent of its maximal value. It is another index of the rate at which radioiron is

---

* Natural logarithm of 2

being handled after it has been obligated for hemoglobin production.

All of these quantitative determinations utilizing blood obtained from the patient might be construed as "in vitro nuclear medicine." However, in clinical use they are inadequate without in vivo localization studies of the sacral, hepatic, splenic, and precordial radioactivity. The evaluation of these in vivo patterns helps with an understanding of distribution throughout the body. These are the determinations which give the plasma-clearance methods increased meaning regarding the presence of abnormal sites of erythrocyte production and, in some cases, destruction.

The author feels that even the combination of in vitro and in vivo ferrokinetic studies is usually inadequate without ^{51}Cr-tagged red blood cell life and sequestration studies. Only ferrokinetics are considered in this discussion.

Several major patterns of in vivo iron distribution are important. They are presented in the same format as that used by Finch, plus a summary of the relative changes which occur in the ferrokinetic indices (Fig. 7-2).[25] The abscissa is recorded in days after injection and the ordinate in CPM/CPM_0 or the ratio of radioactivity on a given day to that on the day of injection. The blood curve begins at 100 percent after injection only to fall as the radioiron is distributed in erythropoietic tissues and then to rise again as the radioactivity is found in the circulating red blood cells. The normal pattern may be seen in Figure 7-2. As can be seen, there is a rapid rise in radioactivity over the marrow (sacral) area corresponding to the fall in blood (plasma) radioactivity as the radioiron moves into the bone marrow for use in erythrocyte production. The initial drop in splenic and hepatic counts also results from the movement of intravascular radioactivity. This drop is evidence that extramedullary erythropoietic function is absent. As the tagged red cells leave the marrow, with falling marrow (sacral) counts, radioactivity again rises in the blood, spleen, and liver due to the ap-

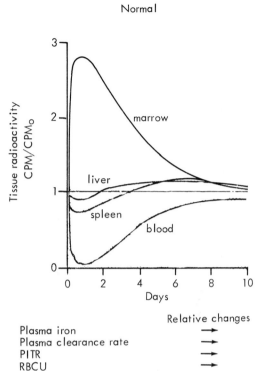

Fig. 7-2. Normal.

pearance of tagged cells in the vascular bed. The half-way point in this movement of red cells, the MTT, is approximately 3.5 days. Normal values appear in Table 7-2.

Interpretation. When dealing with ferrokinetic data it is best to consider the problem under study functionally rather than morphologically. Patterns of hemolytic anemia, ineffective erythropoiesis, reduced erythroid marrow, iron deficiency anemia and polycythemia are considered here.

In the patient with *hemolytic anemia,* marrow function is frequently 3 to 12 times normal (Fig. 7-3). However, in the severe form when many of the red cells are destroyed peripherally, the iron becomes available for red cell production, and, therefore, a low plateau in blood erythrocyte radioactivity is observed. As the cells are hemolyzed, a rise in splenic radioactivity may occur with splenic sequestration (e.g., hereditary spherocytosis, Fig. 7-3). Shifts

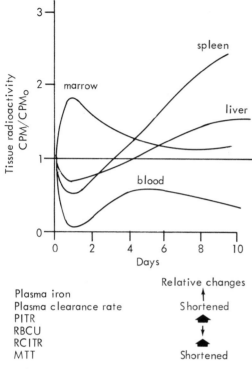

Plasma iron
Plasma clearance rate   Shortened
PITR
RBCU
RCITR
MTT   Shortened

Relative changes

Fig. 7-3. Hemolytic anemia with splenic sequestration.

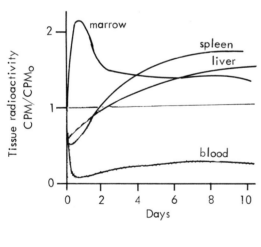

Plasma iron
Plasma clearance rate   Shortened
PITR
RBCU
RCITR
MTT   Shortened but of
         questionable significance

Relative changes

Fig. 7-4. Ineffective erythropoiesis.

occurring in the indices of such a patient are illustrated.

The term *"ineffective erythropoiesis"* refers to the destruction of nucleated red cells which usually occurs in the medullary space but may occur in the liver and spleen. Included in this classification are patients with megaloblastic anemia, sideroblastic anemia, lead poisoning, hyperplastic refractory anemia, and myelofibrosis. In all of these diseases the major feature is a relatively low RCITR when compared with the PITR. Therefore, one must conclude that although total erythropoiesis is normal or considerably increased (as indicated by the PITR), "effective erythropoiesis" is inadequate due to premature red cell destruction (Fig. 7-4). The in vivo studies reveal normal early appearance of radioactivity in the marrow with clearance of the blood, spleen, and liver counts. However, only a small amount of the radioactivity later appears in the blood, since most activity accumulates in the reticuloendothelial cells of the liver, spleen, and bone marrow.

Extramedullary hematopoiesis with myelofibrosis is associated with a change in the in vivo distribution without a corresponding change in the indices. The curve of ineffective erythropoiesis shows the same early uptake and clearance of radioactivity in the involved organ as in the marrow.

Another major group is that in which there is *reduced or absent medullary erythroid marrow* (Fig. 7-5). The ferrokinetic indices are those of decreased red cell production, both "total" and "effective." The in vivo patterns demonstrate a lack of marrow activity. Since much of the iron is rapidly cleared to liver polygonal cells (instead of the erythroid marrow, with subsequent accumulation in the reticuloendothelial cells of the liver), there is an early rise in hepatic radioactivity which persists.

Considerable variation may be noted in the findings with reduced functioning erythroid marrow. Many different disease states demonstrate different degrees of severity. There are the abnormalities of erythropoietic production in renal disease, endocrinopathies, inflammation, and marrow damage associated with drugs, chemicals, malignancies or idiopathic causes.[28]

The abnormality observed in rheumatoid arthritis, inflammation, Hodgkin's disease, and in a case of anemia after a Billroth II gastrectomy, is a problem in reutilization of iron.[29,30,31] Some of the studies of this abnormality in reutilization have been performed with a radioiron dextran complex rather than with radioiron tagged hemoglobin.[32] Dextran is used as a substitute for hemoglobin, since it is a stable compound without the disadvantages or risks associated with transfusions of large quantities of hemoglobin.

In dealing with all of the above-mentioned entities, the concept of relative activity must be kept in mind. A severe hemolytic process to which the patient's erythroid marrow responds, but inadequately, has been described as "relative marrow failure" and leads to a hypoproliferative anemia.

In *iron-deficiency anemia* ferrokinetics are representative of the potential for erythropoiesis if adequate iron is available. The indices are those of increased erythropoietic function (Fig. 7-6). In vivo distribution reveals rapid localization of iron in the erythroid marrow with early appearance in the peripheral blood. There is little localization in the reticuloendothelial cells of the liver and spleen even during the later part of the study (Fig. 7-6). In severe iron-deficiency anemia a hemolytic component appears which may cause some falling of the later portion of the blood radioactivity curve.

A detailed discussion of the findings in *polycythemia* is beyond the scope of this text. A functional classification into 4 groups of polycythemia vera based on ferrokinetics has been reviewed by Pollycove.[24] He describes the normal pattern (class I), a shortened red blood cell life span (class IIa) or intramedullary hemolysis (class IIb) and finally myeloid metaplasia (class III). The pattern of increased erythropoiesis with a normal erythrocyte life span (class I) is that seen in secondary polycythemia.

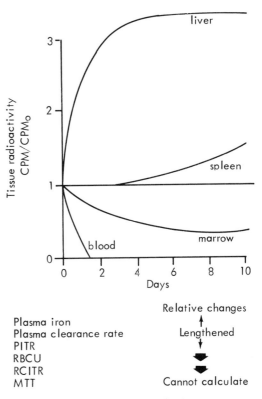

Fig. 7-5.   Reduced erythroid marrow (aplastic anemia).

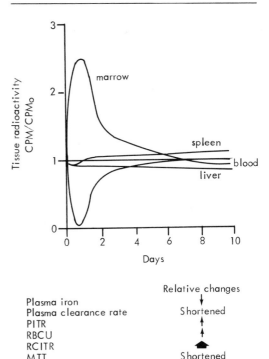

Fig. 7-6. Iron-deficiency anemia.

Ferrokinetics in liver disease are variable with no definitive pattern. According to Finch these techniques do not aid in the differentiation between hemochromatosis and liver disease with iron overload.[25]

RADIOIRON DETERMINATION OF IRON LOSS

In the normal adult male there is effectively no significant loss of iron. Including all avenues of excretion—stool, urine, sweat, and desquamation—less than 1 mg of iron is lost per day.[23] A clinical determination of this minute quantity has not been attempted. Rather the use of radioiron to study excessive loss of blood from the body has been found effective by using the whole-body counter after intravenous injection of ^{59}Fe citrate. In the usual case, the rate of loss of radioactivity is correlated with the quantity of blood lost through the gastrointestinal tract.[33,34,35] However, if whole-body counting alone is used, the exact site of blood loss cannot be determined. This method does allow for long-term studies with periods of observation up to 3 months.[36]

With or without the whole-body counters, if one is attempting to find the site of iron loss it is necessary to perform urinary and fecal iron-excretion studies.[37] This is so since the whole-body counter only determines iron loss inferentially by direct evaluation of iron retention in the entire organism.

MISCELLANEOUS

A radioiron competitive binding assay of the latent iron-binding capacity has been proposed.[38] Commercially available test kits* are available utilizing a resin sponge. These tests have very limited clinical value, since a chemical serum iron and total iron-binding capacity are more important in studying alterations in the iron-carrying capacity of the plasma. Therefore, such a test does not seem to be of clinical or research value.

---

* Irosorb-59, Abbott Laboratories, North Chicago, Ill. 60064.

The use of radioiron for the cohort labeling of red blood cells to determine their life span is not within the purview of this chapter. Cr-51 red cell tagging is usually the method of choice for these studies.

References

1. Huff, R. L., Hennessy, T. G., Austin, R. E., Garcia, J. F., Roberts, B. M., and Lawrence, J. H.: Plasma and red cell iron turnover in normal subjects and in patients having various hematopoietic disorders. J. Clin. Invest., *29*:1041, 1950.
2. Huff, R. L., Elmlinger, P. G., Garcia, J. F., Oda, J. M., Cockrell, M. C., and Lawrence, J. H.: Ferrokinetics in normal persons and in patients having various erythropoietic disorders. J. Clin. Invest., *30*:1512, 1951.
3. Pollycove, M., and Mortimer, R.: The quantitative determination of iron kinetics and hemoglobin synthesis in human subjects. J. Clin. Invest., *40*:753, 1961.
4. Hahn, P. F., Bale, W. F., Lawrence, E. O., and Whipple, G. H.: Radioactive iron and its metabolism in anemia: Its absorption, transportation, and utilization. J. Exp. Med., *69*:739, 1939.
5. Hahn, P. F., Bale, W. F., Ross, J. F., Balfour, W. M., and Whipple, G. H.: Radioactive iron absorption in gastro-intestinal tract: Influence of anemia, anoxia, and antecedent feeding distribution in growing dogs. J. Exp. Med., *78*:169, 1943.
6. Granick, S.: Ferritin: Its properties and significance for iron metabolism. Chem. Rev., *38*:379, 1946.
7. Granick, S.: Ferritin. IX. Increase of the protein apoferritin in the gastro-intestinal mucosa as a direct response to iron feeding: The function of ferritin in the regulation of iron absorption. J. Biol. Chem., *164*:737, 1946.
8. Fairbanks, V. F., Fahey, J. L., and Beutler, E.: Clinical Disorders of Iron Metabolism. pp. 65-87. New York, Grune & Stratton, 1971.
9. Bothwell, T. H., and Charlton, R. W.: Absorption of iron. Ann. Review Med., *21*: 145, 1970.
10. Cook, L. Martinez-Torres, C., *et al.*: Food iron absorption measured by an extrinsic tag. JCI, *51*:805, 1972.
11. Walker, R. J., and Williams, R.: Abnormalities of the gastrointestinal transport of iron. Semin. Nucl. Med., *2*:235, 1972.
12. Wheby, M. S.: Site of iron absorption in man. Scand. J. Haematol., *7*:56, 1970.

13. Lunn, J. A., Richmond, J., Simpson, J. D., Leask, J. D., and Tothill, P.: Comparison between three radioisotope methods for measuring iron absorption. Br. Med. J., 5:331, 1967.

14. Friedman, B. I., Schaefer, J. W., and Schiff, L.: Increased iron-59 absorption in patients with hepatic cirrhosis. J. Nucl. Med., 7:594, 1966.

15. Bothwell, T. H., and Finch, C.: Iron Metabolism. pp. 46-90. Boston, Little, Brown Company, 1962.

16. Brucer, M.: Vignettes in nuclear medicine. No. 62. St. Louis, Mallinckrodt Chemical Works, 1972.

17. Höglund, S., Ehn, L., and Lieden, G.: Studies in iron absorption. VII. Iron deficiency in young men. Acta Haemat., 44: 193, 1970.

18. Boddy, K., and Will, G.: Iron absorption in rheumatoid arthritis. Ann. Rheum. Dis., 28:537, 1969.

19. Boddy, K., and Will, G.: Iron absorption in Addisonian pernicious anemia. Amer. J. Clin. Nutr., 22:1555, 1969.

20. Hausmann, K., Kuse, R., Sonnenberg, O. W., Bartels, H., and Heinrich, H. C.: Interrelations between iron stores, general factors and intestinal iron absorption. Acta Haemat., 42:193, 1969.

21. Dagg, J. H., Cumming, R. L. C., and Goldberg, A.: Disorders of iron metabolism. *In* Recent Advances in Haematology. 77-145. London, Churchill Livingstone, 1971.

22. Hallberg, L., Norrby, A., and Solvell, L.: Oral iron with succinic acid in the treatment of iron deficiency anaemia: An evaluation based on measurements of iron absorption using a whole body counter and a double radioiron technique. Scand. J. Haemat., 8:104, 1971.

23. Greenberger, N. J.: Effects of antibiotics and other agents on the intestinal transport of iron. Amer. J. Clin. Nutr., 26:104, 1973.

24. Pollycove, M.: Iron metabolism and kinetics: The functions, distribution and properties of the iron compounds in the human. Sem. Hemat., 3:235, 1966.

25. Finch, C. A., Deubelbeiss, K., Cook, J. D., Eschbach, J. W., *et al.*: Ferrokinetics in man. Medicine 49:17, 1970.

26. Miller, M., Kereiakes, J. G., and Friedman, B. I.: A simplified method for determination of iron-59 and iron-55 in plasma using liquid scintillation counting. Int. J. Appl. Radiat. Isot., 20:133, 1969.

27. Pollycove, M., and Maqsood, M.: Existence of an erythropoietic labile iron pool in animals. Nature, 194:152, 1962.

28. Peschle, C., Zanjani, E. D., Gidari, A. S., McLaurin, W. D., and Gordon, A. S.: Mechanism of thyroxine action on erythropoiesis. Endocrinology, 89:609, 1971.

29. Haurani, F. I., Burke, W., and Martinez, E. J.: Defective reutilization of iron in the anemia of inflammation. J. Lab. Clin. Med., 65:560, 1965.

30. Beamish, M. R., Jones, P. A., Trevett, D., Evans, I. H., and Jacobs, A.: Iron metabolism in Hodgkin's disease. Br. J. Cancer, 26:444, 1972.

31. Haurani, F. I., and Wirts, C. W.: Unusual type of hyochromic anemia complicating billroth II type gastrectomy. Dig. Dis., 16: 343, 1971.

32. Beamish, M. R., Davies, A. G., Eakins, J. D., Jacobs, A., and Trevett, D.: The measurement of reticuloendothelial iron release using iron-dextran. Br. J. Haemat., 21:617, 1971.

33. Saito, H., Sargent, T. III, Parker, H. G., and Lawrence, J. H.: Whole-body iron loss in normal man measured with a gamma spectrometer. J. Nucl. Med., 5:571, 1964.

34. Leitnaker, F. C.: Research and clinical uses of whole body counters. Med. Bull. U.S. Army, Europe, 24:341, 1967.

35. Stack, B. H., Smith, T., Jones, J. H., and Fletcher, J.: Blood and iron loss in colitis. Proc. Roy. Soc. Med., 62:497, 1969.

36. Holt, J. M., Gear, M. W. L., and Warner, G. T.: The role of chronic blood loss in the pathogenesis of postgastrectomy iron-deficiency anaemia. Gut., 11:847, 1970.

37. Malamos, B., Constantoulakis, M., Gyftaki, E., Kesse-Elias, M., and Augoustaki, O.: Urinary and faecal iron excretion in thalassaemia syndromes. Acta Haemat., 42:321, 1969.

38. Tauxe, W. N.: A rapid radioactive method for the determination of the serum iron-binding capacity. Amer. J. Clin. Path., 35: 403, 1961.

8 Basic Principles of Competitive Radioassay

Stanley J. Goldsmith, M.D.

INTRODUCTION

Competitive radioassay is a generic term used to describe a technique in which small amounts of a radioactive material are displaced from a specific binding substance by small, known or unknown, quantities of a similar nonradioactive substance. The ratio of the bound radioactive material to the displaced radioactive material, estimated by measuring the radioactivity of the bound and unbound fractions after they have been separated, permits an estimate of the concentration of hormones, vitamins, pharmaceuticals and other biological materials in a large number of samples with a specificity, sensitivity, and ease not possible by other means.

The characteristics of radioactive emissions which permit detection and accurate quantitation of small amounts of a material were combined with the specificity of the antigen-antibody interaction by Dr. Rosalyn S. Yalow and the late Dr. Solomon A. Berson in the initial development and refinement of this technique.[1,2,3] The impact on medicine and biology, of the development of this technique of radioassay using immune-binding reagents, is in part expressed by the almost generic use of the term "radio-immunoassay," even when describing non-immune competitive binding radioassay.

Both radioimmunoassay and nonimmune radioassay systems have found a place in many research and clinical laboratories. Opportunities for many workers to contribute to the further development, refinement and application of these techniques are illustrated in the following chapters of this volume. This chapter deals with general principles of the technique and of the laboratory methodology.

Competitive radioassay was developed initially as a method to detect small amounts of a polypeptide, human plasma insulin. One can appreciate the magnitude of this task by comparing the plasma insulin concentration to other plasma concentrations

The author gratefully acknowledges the contribution of Dr. Seymour M. Glick, Dr. Rosalyn S. Yalow and the late Dr. Solomon A. Berson to his training and understanding of radioassay principles and techniques. Gratitude is due to Dr. Avir Kagan for his manuscript review and constructive suggestions. The secretarial assistance of Mrs. Annie Knize, and the photographic and artistic skills of Mr. Nicholas Levycky are acknowledged with thanks.

Table 8-1. Concentration of Commonly Assayed Human Plasma Components.

Substance	Concentration (per 100 ml)
Hemoglobin	10.0-15 Gm
Albumin	3.0-5 Gm
Globulin	1.0-3 Gm
Glucose	50.0-150 mg
Creatinine	1.0-1.5 mg
Calcium	9.0-11 mg
Cortisol	10.0 μg
Thyroxine	30.0-10 μg
Insulin	0.02-0.6 μg
Growth hormone	0.12 μg
Testosterone	0.2 μg
Triiodothyronine	0.1-0.3 μg
Gastrin	0.01-1.0 μg
Vitamin B$_{12}$	0.02-0.1 μg
ACTH	5×10^{-4}-5×10^{-3} μg
Vasopressin	1×10^{-4}-1×10^{-3} μg

Fig. 8-1. Interaction of Binding Reagent and Radioactive Substrate at different concentrations of nonradioactive substrate, demonstrating competition for the fixed limiting concentration of binding sites. *A,* The [binding reagent] = [radioactive substrate]/2, and the radioactivity is partitioned equally between the bound and unbound fractions. In an assay, these fractions would have to be separated prior to counting. In this ideal situation, there is no unlabeled substrate. *B,* Similar condition to *A* with the addition of 4 units of nonradioactive substrate (4 units are arbitrarily selected for illustrative purposes). At [substrate] = 4,

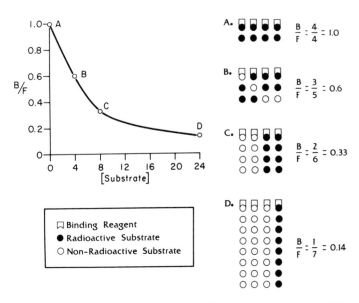

B/F = 0.6 *C,* [substrate] = 8, B/F = 0.33. *D,* [substrate] = 24 B/F = 0.14. A plot of B/F versus [substrate] yields a standard curve which is used to derive [substrate] of unknown samples based upon determining the distribution of radioactivity in the bound and free fractions (B/F).

usually measured by classical chemical spectrophotometric methods (Table 8-1). Following glucose stimulation, plasma insulin in normal subjects may reach a concentration of 0.4 to 0.6 μg/100 ml (100-150 μU/ml). This concentration is at the limit of most classical techniques. By contrast, plasma cortisol in concentrations of 5 to 20 μg/100 ml, with its distinctive cyclopentanophenanthracene structure, is measured with some difficulty by colorimetric assay or by the more sensitive fluorometric assay. Fasting insulin levels of 0.02 to 0.08 μg/100 ml (5-20 μU/ml) are beyond the limit of present spectrophotometric capability, even if a method were available. The problem is compounded as insulin, a polypeptide circulating among other peptides, polypeptides and plasma proteins, is not sufficiently chemically distinct from these compounds to be assayable by colorimetric or chemical analysis in unextracted plasma even if a sufficiently sensitive method were available. It is this ability to detect small concentrations of compounds of biologic interest with great precision, usually in unextracted samples and

in the presence of compounds with similar chemical structures, that characterizes the value of radioassay techniques. In fact, competitive radioassay methods are so sensitive that the sample size frequently may be reduced to 0.1 ml or less. The convenience of handling a large number of samples, and the specificity of the technique has also resulted in its application for assays of compounds such as thyroxine, cortisol, Australia antigen, and others which had previously been determined by other more conventional techniques but with less specificity, convenience and/or economy.

COMPONENTS OF THE RADIOASSAY SYSTEM

There are 3 essential components in a competitive binding radioassay system.

1. A suitable radioactive substrate.
2. A suitable specific binding reagent.
3. A system to separate the free radioactive substrate from the radioactive substrate-binding reagent complex.

A suitable standard is also necessary. It is not obligatory, however, that this standard be available in pure form, or even that the standard be identical to the labeled substrate since relative standards, such as a reference plasma or tissue extract, can be used.

The relationship between these components is described by the now well-known equation

$$\text{Specific Binding Reagent} + \begin{array}{c}\text{Radioactive}\\\text{Substrate}\end{array} \rightleftharpoons \begin{array}{c}\text{Complex of}\\\text{Radioactive}\\\text{Substrate and}\\\text{Binding Reagent}\end{array}$$

$$+ \begin{array}{c}\text{Nonradioactive}\\\text{Substrate}\end{array} \rightleftharpoons \begin{array}{c}\text{Complex of}\\\text{Nonradioactive}\\\text{Substrate and}\\\text{Binding Reagent}\end{array}$$

which describes a radioactive and nonradioactive substrate (hormone, vitamin, enzyme, drug) competitively combining with a specific binding reagent (antibody, naturally occurring circulating binding protein, or cell membrane hormone receptor) to form a complex of substrate and binding reagent. If the concentration of the binding reagent relative to the radioactive substrate (tracer) are small and hence limited in its availability to complex, molecules of the nonradioactive substrate will compete with the radioactive substrate for the available reagent-binding sites, thus altering the distribution of the radioactivity between the complexed or bound components and the noncomplexed or free components. Increasing amounts of substrate will "displace" increasing amounts of labeled substrate (Fig. 8-1). In practice, this relationship of bound versus free radioactive components, determined by counting radioactivity in each fraction following separation of the 2 components, is determined over a range of nonradioactive substrate concentrations. A standard curve is thus constructed comparing substrate concentration with the partition of radioactivity at dif-

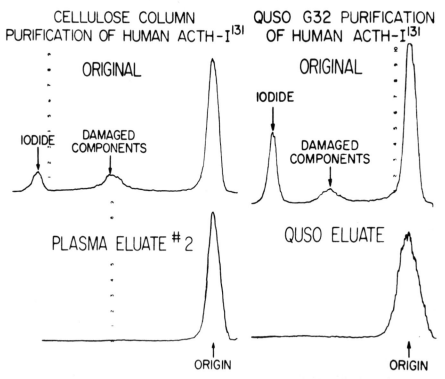

Fig. 8-2. Scans of radioactivity on paper strips following chromato-electrophoresis of ACTH iodination mixture illustrating purification of labeled substrate (ACTH) by 2 different methods: cellulose column separation of original mixture and solid phase adsorption by Quso (silica granules). (Yalow, R. S., and Berson, S. A.: Excerpta Medica, 1968)[7,8]

ferent substrate concentrations. This curve may be constructed to compare the ratio of bound to free radioactivity (B/F) and substrate concentration, or percent (of total radioactivity) bound (%B) and substrate concentration, or any other similar index of the partition of radioactive substrate versus substrate concentration.

Radioactive Substrates (Tracer)

Radioactive substrates may either be purchased or prepared in the laboratory. There is a requirement, however, for purity of the radioactive substrate, and for as high specific activity as possible. The latter requirement determines both the sensitivity of the assay (this concept is developed below) and the counting efficiency.

For nonpeptide tracers, the radionuclide has frequently been incorporated within the structure by biosynthetic production methods (e.g., ^{3}H-cortisol, ^{57}Co-cyanocobalamine, ^{125}I or ^{131}I triiodothyronine and thyroxine). Incorporation of the label directly into the structure of these molecules requires chemical and biosynthetic manipulations beyond the scope of many research and clinical laboratories. The user's laboratory depends upon the commercial developer and supplier. While this source may provide a convenient tracer compound, the user should obtain confirmation of radiochemical integrity. Specifically, one must determine if the tracer compound is contaminated by denatured or altered labeled compounds, or elution of the free radionuclide from the compound. This type of confirmation of purity can be performed readily by a variety of paper, thin layer or column chromatographic techniques within the scope of most laboratories (Fig. 8-2).

In radioassays of polypeptide hormones, the principal use has been made of ^{131}Iodine and ^{125}Iodine. In the initial immunoassay system, insulin was labeled with ^{131}Iodine.[1,2] The method in which elemental iodine was generated from Na^{131}I and dissolved in chloroform prior to combination with the

peptide was cumbersome, requiring prolonged handling of ^{131}Iodine and exposure of personnel to the radioactive material. This inconvenience limited access to labeled substrates. Berson and Yalow, experienced with the labeling of proteins, were able to label insulin and study its biologic survival in normal and diabetic patients.[1] These observations led to the recognition and identification of insulin antibodies in patients receiving insulin. This was followed by the development of techniques for antibody quantitation[4,5] and for the radioimmunoassay of insulin.[2,3] Nevertheless, progress was slow prior to the development of a simple rapid method of iodination by Hunter and Greenwood.[6] This new method afforded laboratories with even modest facilities an opportunity to conveniently and rapidly label insulin, growth hormone, glucagon, parathyroid hormone, adrenocorticotrophin, angiotensin, gastrin and other polypeptide hormones. The iodinated polypeptide must be separated from the unreacted iodine and damaged peptide fragments prior to use in an assay system. This is accomplished by solid-phase tube absorption or column chromatography (see Fig. 8-2), or starch gel electrophoresis.[7] For both peptide and nonpeptide tracers, solvent systems vary with the material being evaluated. While impurities may be determined in thin layer or paper chromatography systems, column chromatography and starch gel electrophoresis, or solid-phase absorption of the tracer offer the additional advantage of preparative fractionation, yielding a purified labeled substrate for use in the assay.

Specific Activity and Assay Sensitivity

Specific activity (radioactivity per unit weight) of the labeled substrate is an important consideration in assay preparation, since the *sensitivity of the assay (smallest assayable amount) depends upon the chemical concentration of the tracer used.*

A brief consideration of the basic principles of the radioassay system should indicate that the theoretical limit of the assay

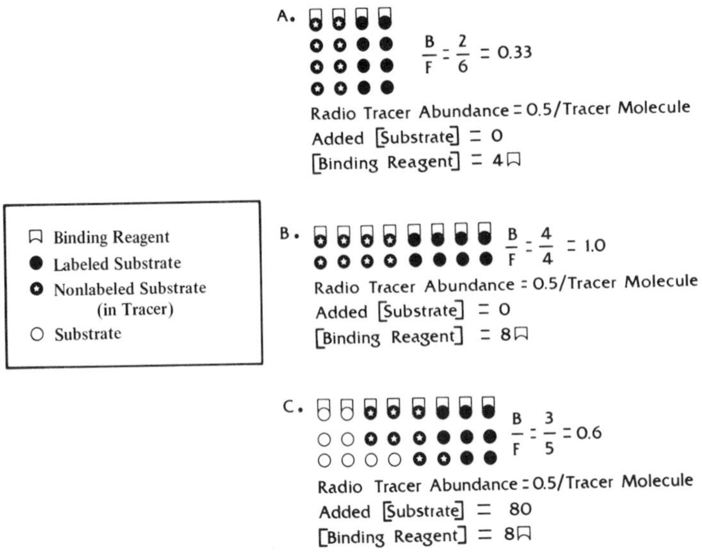

A.

$$\frac{B}{F} = \frac{2}{6} = 0.33$$

Radio Tracer Abundance = 0.5/Tracer Molecule
Added [Substrate] = 0
[Binding Reagent] = 4 ⊓

⊓ Binding Reagent
● Labeled Substrate
◉ Nonlabeled Substrate
    (in Tracer)
○ Substrate

B.

$$\frac{B}{F} = \frac{4}{4} = 1.0$$

Radio Tracer Abundance = 0.5/Tracer Molecule
Added [Substrate] = 0
[Binding Reagent] = 8 ⊓

C.

$$\frac{B}{F} = \frac{3}{5} = 0.6$$

Radio Tracer Abundance = 0.5/Tracer Molecule
Added [Substrate] = 80
[Binding Reagent] = 8 ⊓

Fig. 8-3. *A*, Specific activity of labeled substrate is low, 0.5/molecule (compare with Fig. 8-1). At [substrate] = 0, B/F = 0.33 instead of 1.0 as in Figure 8-1. *B*, If additional binding reagent is added to this poor tracer, the B/F is adjusted to 1.0. However, this is less satisfactory than the alternate adjustment (i.e., use of a higher specific activity tracer; demonstrated in Fig. 8-1). *C*, At [substrate] = 8 molecules, the impact of low specific activity tracer on assay sensitivity is demonstrated. In Figure 8-3 as [substrate] increases from 0 to 8 molecules, B/F decreases from 1.0 to 0.6, for a change of 0.4, in contrast to that

obtained in Figure 8-1 with improved radiotracer abundance (i.e., [substrate] increased to 8 moles), B/F decreases from 1.0 to 0.33, a difference of 0.67. A change of 0.67 in B/F values offers more sensitivity than a change of 0.4 for the same amount of added substrate.

(smallest detectable quantity) is a single molecule of the substance to be assayed. To accomplish this, one ideally needs a single tracer molecule and a single binding-reagent molecule. If the specific activity is lower (e.g., if only 1 of 1,000 molecules is radioactive), the assay system will always contain at least 1,000 molecules of the substrate even at the limit of tracer concentration (i.e., a single radioactive molecule). Therefore, even with a limitingly small amount of tracer (1 radioactive molecule per 1,000 molecules), it is impossible to detect only a few substrate molecules, since only with 1,000 molecules of standard or unknown substrate is the single detectable (radioactive) molecule likely to be displaced (Fig. 8-3A). If the specific activity is even lower (i.e., 1 radioactive molecule per 1 million molecules), the assay will be even less sensitive, detecting no less than 1 million molecules. In practice specific activity is expressed as units of radioactivity (curies or fractional curies) per unit of weight rather than number of radioactive atoms per total number, which is expressed as isotopic abundance.

Selection and Preparation of Tracers

Many organic compounds are composed of carbon, hydrogen, oxygen, nitrogen, and to a very limited extent, sulfur or phosphorus. These elements are not available as gamma-emitting isotopes with suitable half-lives. Since iodine is native to triiodothyronine and thyroxine, and cobalt to cyanocobalamine, [125,131]Iodine and [57,58,60]Cobalt respectively are available as gamma-emitting radionuclides without alteration of the primary molecular structure.

For most organic compounds of biologic interest (polypeptides, steroids, drugs and vitamins), however, there are no naturally occurring atoms for which gamma-emitting radioactive isotopes may be substituted. Liquid scintillation counting equipment can detect and quantitate β-emitting radionuclides of carbon ([14]Carbon) and hydrogen ([3]Hydrogen), but the longer half-lives of these nuclides place limitations on the specific activity* (Table 8-2). This makes them less acceptable for the determination of

---

* There are fewer disintegrations per mole per unit time.

Table 8-2. Commonly Available Radionuclides for Substrate Labeling.

Radionuclide	$T_{1/2}$	Maximal Activity Curies/Grams	Curies/ Gram-atom	Available Isotopic Abundance
^{14}Carbon	5,568 years	4.6	64.8	$\sim$ 20% (as acetic anhydride)
^{3}Hydrogen	12.5 years	9,780	2.96×10^4	$\sim$ 0.1% (acetic anhydride)
^{125}Iodine	60 days	18,000	2.25×10^6	$\sim$ 100% (asNaI)
^{131}Iodine	8.1 days	124,000	1.6×10^7	$\sim$ 30% (as NaI)

physiologic concentrations of many biologic substances, particularly polypeptide hormones, present in low plasma concentrations, despite their potentially longer shelf lives.

Despite the abundance of carbon atoms in organic molecules, ^{14}Carbon is the least desirable tracer because of low specific activity, a consequence of its long half-life of 5,568 years. One μc of ^{14}Carbon weighs 0.215 μg. By contrast, 1 μc of ^{131}Iodine with a half-life of 8.1 days weighs 8.1×10^{-6} μg. Thus, for equivalent counting statistics, if a gram atom of ^{14}Carbon is incorporated into a molecule instead of a gram atom of ^{131}Iodine (and all other considerations such as molecular cross-reactivity are equal), the assay is 4 million times less sensitive. If ^{14}Carbon atoms were incorporated into a molecule at 100 times the frequency of ^{131}Iodine (and again, all other factors are equal) the sensitivity is still 40,000 times less. Moreover, the long half-life results in unacceptably long counting times to ensure acceptable counting statistics. Therefore, despite the potentially greater isotopic abundance of ^{14}Carbon, it is not the tracer of choice even among β-emitting radionuclides.

^{3}Hydrogen is a much better choice for the tracer because of the higher potential specific activity in the carrier-free state as a consequence of its shorter half-life (more disintegrations per mole per unit time). Since 1 μc of ^{3}Hydrogen weighs 1.0×10^{-4} μg, on a gram atomic weight basis, and correcting for counting efficiency, assays using ^{3}Hydrogen are 1/100 as sensitive as the potential sensitivity of assays using ^{131}Iodine as the tracer,

and 2,500 times as sensitive on a similar basis as they are with ^{14}Carbon as the scintillation source.

Despite the supposed structural advantage of substituting a radioactive isotope of the same element for a stable atom naturally occurring in the substrate, the increased tracer specific activity available with the use of higher specific activity/mole radioisotopes of iodine (^{125}Iodine and ^{131}Iodine) yields greater assay sensitivity (Fig. 8-4). In a comparison of the cross-reactivity of digoxin-^{3}H and digoxigenine-^{125}Iodotyrosine (0.02

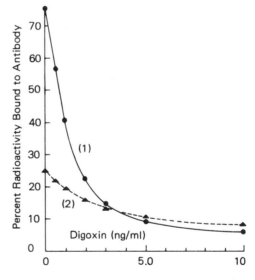

Fig. 8-4. Standard curves from digoxin radioimmunoassay comparing (1) digoxigenin-^{125}iodotyrosine tracer (solid crystal gamma scintillation counting) and (2) digoxin-^{3}H (liquid scintillation beta counting), demonstrating improved sensitivity obtained with gamma-emitting tracers. (Cerceo, E.: Dialogos, *1*:3, 1973)[9]

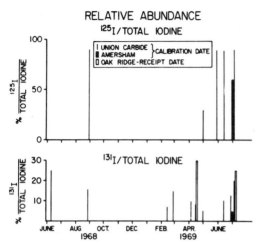

Fig. 8-5. Relative isotopic abundance of [125]iodine and [131]iodine from three different suppliers over a one year period beginning June 1968. Isotopic abundance determined by method described in Berson, and Yalow.[10] Similar values for [131]iodine during 1966 were reported in Yalow, and Berson.[11] Note that the isotopic abundance of [125]iodine frequently approaches 100%. By contrast [131]iodine is rarely supplied with an abundance as high as 30% and sometimes is in the 10% range. (Yalow, R. S., and Berson, S. A.: IAEA, 1970)[12]

Iodine/molecule) to the same antibody under otherwise identical conditions, Cerceo[9] found that use of the iodinated tracer produced a more sensitive curve than the structurally more natural digoxin-^{3}H.

Use of gamma-emitting radionuclides as tracers have the additional advantage of ease of sample counting with none of the problems of quenching and chemoluminescence of liquid scintillation counting techniques.

Since peptides and polypeptides are present in such low concentrations, and usually do not contain potential gamma-emitting atoms in their structure, suitable gamma emitters must be introduced. [131]Iodine and [125]Iodine have proven convenient and satisfactory for this purpose. Iodination, using the Hunter and Greenwood method,[6] is accomplished by reaction of iodine with the tyrosyl moiety within the polypeptide structure. Using a small disposable serology tube as a reaction vessel and a small volume (15

to 20 μl) of a suitable buffer (0.25 M phosphate, pH 7.4) as the reaction medium, add an appropriate concentration of the peptide to be labeled (1-10 μg), then add a small volume of sodium [131]iodide or sodium [125]iodide (50-500 μc). The ratio of iodide to peptide depends upon the desired specific activity of the product based upon some experience with the expected yield (75-90%) and the tyrosyl groups available. Chloramine-T, an oxidizing agent, is added, oxidizing the iodide to I° or I_2, whereupon it reacts with the aromatic ring within the tyrosyl moiety. Sodium metabisulfite is frequently added, reducing excess chloramine-T, and limiting chemical damage. In addition, plasma or albumin may be added to act as a chemical sponge reacting with excess oxidized iodine, oxidizing or reducing agent, and to elute the peptide from the walls of the container. This may result in iodination of albumin and other plasma components. The reaction mixture is assayed by paper or column chromatography to determine efficiency of iodination. Purification by column chromatography, starch gel electrophoresis or differential absorption with solid phase absorbants results in separation of the iodinated peptide from damaged or denatured peptide, other iodinated material, and free iodide. For greatest iodination efficiency, the radioisotopic abundance (hot atoms/total atoms of element) is critical. Although [131]Iodine, even for clinical tracer studies, is purchased as being carrier free, this is an incorrect concept in relation to iodination. Whereas pure [131]Iodine has a theoretical potential specific activity of 124 C/mg, approximately 7 times the specific activity of pure [125]Iodine, the isotopic abundance of [131]Iodine, when examined by a sensitive technique,[10] is frequently only 15 percent and rarely exceeds 30 percent.[11] By contrast [125]Iodine is available in considerably higher isotopic abundance, approaching 100 percent (Fig. 8-5).

Note that for equivalent amounts of radioactivity, the labeled substrate concentration increases with radionuclidic decay, so that 0.1

μCi [131]Iodine labeled insulin/tube in an assay performed 8 days after iodination, contains twice the insulin as 0.1 μCi [131]Iodoinsulin on the day of preparation, as opposed to [125]Iodine-labeled compounds with a 60-day physical half-life, which have 91 percent of their original specific activity after 8 days. These advantages of higher isotopic abundance, longer half-life, and greater sensitivity of NaI (Tl) well counters for the less energetic gamma emission of [125]Iodine has led to [125]Iodine being the radionuclide of choice for substrate labeling.

Maximal specific activity of the labeled substrate is limited by the number of tyrosyl moieties available for iodination, the degree of iodination of the available tyrosyls, and the isotopic abundance of the sodium iodide.[10,11]

Even with the use of [131]Iodine and [125]Iodine, it is sometimes necessary to determine such low concentrations of physiologically active material that tracers of the highest specific activity consistent with maintaining cross-reactivity are required. Ideally, one likes each labeled molecule to be labeled with a single radioactive atom (to offer maximal specific activity and minimal molecular alteration).

One or two iodine atoms may react with each tyrosyl moiety. Although iodine content per mole of peptide is calculated, some tyrosyl groups have no iodine while other groups have one or two iodine atoms. An average number of iodine atoms per molecule, however, can be calculated and prepared. Whereas it is possible to label a molecule with considerably more than an average of 1 iodine atom per insulin molecule thus increasing specific activity, increasing iodine content renders the molecule increasingly different from the native molecule. Although the more highly iodinated compounds may cross-react with antisera to the native compounds, there is usually a measurable (and sometimes, unacceptable) loss of immunologic cross-reactivity (biologic activity likewise decreases progressively with increasing iodine concentration).

Hence, as in other areas of nuclear medicine, the practitioner must accept a compromise. Maximal specific activity and assay sensitivity (smallest assayable quantity) requires as many radioiodine atoms per molecule as possible. Immunologic integrity of the tracer, and therefore immunoreactivity, mandates iodination at lower specific activities than might be otherwise possible.

Binding Reagents

There are two requirements for use of a binding reagent in a competitive binding radioassay—these are *specificity* and *sensitivity*. Several classes of binding reagents are in use in competitive radioassay systems. In the class of assays known as radioimmunoassay, antibodies cross-reacting with the substrate to be measured are used. These assays, based upon antigen-antibody interaction, have the potential of great specificity.[13,14] This specificity, however, is not predictable. Each antiserum must be evaluated, with documentation of the degree of cross-reactivity with substances structurally related to the substrate to be assayed, particularly when these other substrates are apt to be present in the incubation sample (untreated plasma). In nonimmune assay systems, naturally occurring binding reagents are used,[15] i.e., thyroxine-binding globulin for the assay of thyroxine, intrinsic factor in the assay of vitamin B_{12}, and lactoglobulin for the assay of folic acid. Naturally occurring cellular receptor sites from target organs[16,17] and substrate-specific enzymes[18] have also been used as binding reagents in radioassay systems. Since radioimmunoassay was earlier used as a sensitive method to quantitate antigen-antibody interactions, the recognition of specific cellular hormonal binding sites has provided a powerful tool to study the kinetics of hormonal-target cell interaction, and has demonstrated that the effectiveness of internal secretions depends not only upon the plasma concentration but also upon the total number of binding sites on the target cell.

Characteristics of each type of binding reagent should be considered when radioassay techniques are being introduced into a laboratory. First, one should be familiar with the availability, cost, and ease of use. These factors determine the practicality of application of a method. Second, and more significant, is the specificity and sensitivity of the binding reagent, factors which affect the validity of the effort to measure the substrate of interest (hormone, vitamin, etc.).

Availability and Production. Great commercial interest in radioassay components and kits in recent years have made assay systems widely available. Cost per specimen has become acceptable and the cost-to-fee ratio is satisfactory enough to repay over a reasonable period the initial outlay for automatic sample changing counting systems. In this regard, it is well to recall that a wide variety of compounds are all assayed by the same principle using the same equipment, and that the technique lends itself to the processing of hundreds of samples in the same assay almost as conveniently as handling only a few dozen samples.

Human binding proteins. In contrast to the effort involved in preparing antisera, or the dependence upon commercial sources for antisera, some naturally occurring binding globulins are conveniently available to all laboratories. Although there has been some preference for plasma from pregnant women, Murphy[19] does not find this selection advantageous. Outdated blood bank plasma, pooled discarded laboratory samples or donors may be used as sources of binding globulins. Thyroxine-binding globulin, cortisol-binding globulin and testosterone (sex steroid)-binding globulin may be obtained in this manner. These naturally occurring human plasma proteins have been criticized as lacking specificity. While this is generally true, this nonspecificity can be turned to an advantage, since if convenient methods of sample fractionation are available, the single binding globulin can be used to assay a variety of compounds. Murphy reports[19] having measured 8 different corticosteroids with the same cortisol-binding globulin.[18] Despite this cross-reactivity, some quite specific, high-affinity binding is possible with these globulins. Although thyroxine-binding globulin does cross-react with triiodothyronine, the much greater affinity for thyroxine as well as its much higher concentration permits assay of physiologic samples without consideration for the triiodothyronine concentration. In this instance, the reactivity with a seconary ligand can be advantageous. Using thyroxine-binding globulin as the binding reagent, Sterling, et al.[20] measured triiodothyronine by first extracting the T_4 and the T_3 and then separating the T_3 from the T_4 prior to incubation.[19] This astute utilization of the less than totally specific binding properties of thyroxine-binding globulin is not without difficulty. The failure to totally separate thyroxine and other structural analogues by extraction has led to this approach being abandoned for a more specific immunoassay.[21]

Nonhuman binding proteins. Several nonhuman sources of nonimmune-binding proteins are presently available and in use.[19] Dog corticosteroid-binding globulin has a higher affinity for many corticosteroids than does human corticosteroid-binding globulin. Monkey corticosteroid-binding globulin has a higher association constant for corticosterone than for cortisol. Pregnant guinea pig plasma and pregnant rat plasma are sources of relatively specific-binding proteins for progesterone and estrogens, respectively. These binding reagents offer the advantage of greater sensitivity and specificity than is available with human sera. In nonimmune competitive binding radioassays however, it is usually necessary to remove the substrate (ligand) from its parent plasma so that the globulins of the plasma or serum sample do not compete with the added assay binding reagent. Ethanol or other organic solvents are useful for this purpose but also introduce a potential for sample losses. These losses may be corrected by similarly processing known standards in blank plasma. Alternate approaches include the inactivation of the native binding portein by heating, or passage of the sample through small Sephadex columns which retard the lighter molecular weight substrates and permit passage of the heavier plasma proteins.

Enzyme and cellular-binding proteins. The specificity of substrate-enzyme interactions has been employed in the assay of folic acid using the enzyme dihydrofolate reductase.[18] This approach offers considerable potential for further applications. Lefkowitz, et al. isolated adrenal cortex cell membrane-binding sites and used them as the binding agent in a competitive radioassay for ACTH.[22] Subsequently, this approach has been used for insulin, growth hormone, and other peptide hormones.[16] End organ cytosol macromolecules have been used as a binding reagent for the radioassay of estrogens.[17] Since receptor binding as the first step in activating adenyl cyclase is a requisite for biologic activity, this type of binding reagent has the advantage of being more closely correlated with biologic activity than are immune or carrier proteins. Tissue receptors, however, are not always molecular specific. In addition, they are difficult to prepare, and are of limited stability. Receptor-binding observations are of great interest and have been useful in validating physiologic observations which have been obtained with radioimmunoassays. However, widespread application for clinical assays does not appear to be realistic at this time because of the difficulty in preparing and storing the binding macromolecules.

Antisera. The last statement is cautious. Not too long ago, some reviews found the preparation and evaluation of antisera too cumbersome for widespread use. The broad spectrum of reactivity of nonimmune globulins, the necessity for extraction of samples from plasma proteins, and the fractionation of these extracts has instead led to preferential development of radioimmunoassays, even for substances with conveniently available binding reagents. Except for cellular-binding sites, naturally occurring binding proteins for peptide hormones have not been found. By contrast, antisera for many biologically significant compounds are increasingly available. At this time, therefore, despite the effort involved in the preparation and initial evaluation of antisera, it seems likely that the future will see a continued preferential application of this class of binding reagent as opposed to the naturally occurring circulating proteins or the cellular receptors.

The ease of production of insulin antibodies belies the earlier notion that the molecular weight of antigenic material must be 10,000 or greater. Antisera to unconjugated peptide molecules as small as gastrin, M.W. 2,100,[23] ACTH, MW 4,500,[24] and oxytocin, MW 1,000,[25] have been produced and used in assays. Nevertheless, conjugation of other small molecules, such as steroids, thyroid hormones, prostaglandins and some drugs seems to be in order. This is accomplished by coupling to albumin, globulins, polylysine or other larger molecular weight materials by one of several methods.[26]

Production of antisera by a laboratory requires, in addition to animal facilities and the initial expense, foresight and an interest in production. Guinea pigs and rabbits are commonly used as hosts for immunization. Some laboratories favor one or another species. Reiss was more successful in producing parathyroid antisera in chickens,[27] raising speculation by some that there may be some unique species responsiveness to particular antigens. This does not appear to be the case; satisfactory antisera have been produced in many species.

To date, the production of antisera has remained empiric. Immunization is usually carried out with a moderate amount of protein. At moderate protein doses, as opposed to larger doses, only immunocytes with high affinity are thought to be stimulated, hopefully producing higher affinity antibody.[28] Antigens are usually mixed with Freund's adjuvant which delays antigen absorption and retards antigen metabolism providing a prolonged antigenic stimulus as well as nonspecific stimulation of the immune system. Immunization schedules vary without substantial evidence in support of any particular regimen. A frequent pattern is serial immunization every 2 weeks for 3 doses and then booster doses at less frequent intervals. Animals are bled for serum 10 to 14 days after the previous immunization (the classical interval for maximal antibody titers). Several animals are conveniently immunized at a time, increasing the likelihood of obtaining a useful antiserum. Purity of the immunizing dose is not always critical, since specific antibodies may be selected which will react with the highly purified labeled substrate used in the assay.

Summary. Antisera and nonimmune binding reagents may be prepared by laboratories willing to make modest investments of money and time. At the present time, binding reagents in bulk, or as part of kits for competitive binding radioassays, are available commercially. Despite this widespread commercial availability and reasonable cost of many binding reagents, an awareness of the problem of specificity of these binding reagents is essential for regularly meaningful application of competitive binding radioassays. This point seems to be infrequently appreciated or ignored by many distributors of binding reagents (particularly immune sera). Data detailing the cross-reactivity of the binding protein with structurally related substances is generally not provided. The significance of this information is apparently unappreciated by many users also, as indicated by the widespread economic success of these kits and components despite the dearth of this type of information.

Specificity. The question of specificity is one which arises in evaluating a competitive binding radioassay. Relative nonspecificity of nonimmune systems has been reviewed. Immunoassays offer the potential advantage of great specificity. In the early days of radioimmunoassay, this aspect was appropriately crucial in demonstrating the validity of the assay. Despite the present general acceptance of the radioimmunoassay approach, clinicians and investigators must continue to evaluate (or demand evaluation) of each new harvest of antiserum.

Table 8-3. Comparison of Cross-reactivity of Antisera to Triiodothyronine.

Compound	Percent T-3 Immunoreactivity	
	Wien[29]	Gharib, et al.[21]
L-triiodothyronine	100.0	100.0
3,3',5 Triiodo acetic acid	50.0	33.0
L-thyroxine	0.75	0.33
3,5 Diiodothyronine	0.25	1.4
3,3'5-Triiodoproprionic acid	100.0	—
3,5,5'-Triiodoproprionic acid	—	0.01
3,3'5,5'-Tetraiodo proprionic acid	0.90	0.04

The type of data which should be provided is illustrated in Table 8-3. Reactivity with structural analogues is provided for sample antisera from a commercial source[29] and from a research laboratory.[21] Considering the structural similarity between triiodothyronine (T_3) and thyroxine (T_4), it is remarkable that such molecular selectivity is achieved. It should be noted that the degree of thyroxine cross-reaction with the Wien triiodothyronine antisera was 0.75 percent. This contrasts to Gharib's antisera which cross-reacts with thyroxine 0.33 percent as effectively as with triiodothyronine. The practical consequence of this cross-reactivity is that a plasma sample with a thyroxine concentration of 6.0 μg/100 ml overestimates the triiodothyronine concentration by 20 $\mu\mu$g/100 ml with Gharib's antisera, and by 40 $\mu\mu$g/100 ml with Wien's antisera. It is important to recall this antiserum variability when comparing "normal values" from laboratory to laboratory or when looking at small fluctuations in the plasma concentration. As illustrated with this data, the degree of cross-reactivity may be so small as to have little clinical significance. In order to determine if the degree of cross-reactivity is significant, however, it must be known to the laboratory supervisor, either provided by the source of the antisera if

Fig. 8-6. *A,* Plasma parathyroid hormone concentration determined with 2 different antisera, 273 and C329, in 3 patients following removal of parathyroid adenoma (MA), total (PA), and subtotal (FI) parathyroidectomy. Antisera 273 cross-reacts with parathyroid hormone molecules which are not recognized by antisera C329. *B,* Dose response curves comparing inhibition of ^{125}I-b parathyroid hormone binding with 3 antisera by an extract from a normal gland (o) and plasma from a patient with secondary hyperparathyroidism (+). C329 cross-reacts better with glandular extracts than with plasma hormone. (Berson, S. A., and Yalow, R. S.: J. Clin. Endocrinol. Metab., *26*:1037, 1968)[30]

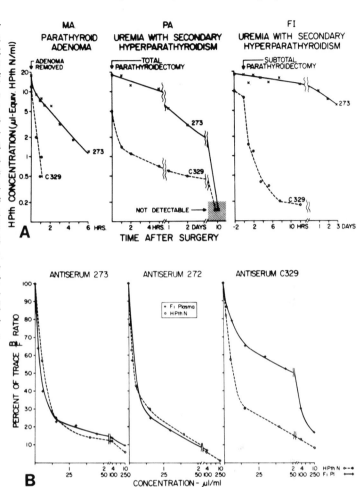

purchased or determined by the laboratory itself, and then evaluated in terms of the application of the assay.

Careful evaluation of antisera has led to an understanding of previously unsuspected aspects of peptide hormone physiology. Based upon thorough evaluation of antisera cross-reactivity with plasma samples and glandular extracts, Berson and Yalow were able to conclude that there was more than one molecular species of human parathyroid hormone.[30] Marked differences in the disappearance rate of endogenous parathyroid hormone following parathyroidectomy were found when assays were performed with different antisera (Fig. 8-6A). Such differences were a consequence of variable recognition by different antisera of an immunoheteroge-neous population of parathyroid hormones (Fig. 8-6B). Subsequently, other investigators have confirmed this observation. Rather than simply invalidating the determination of plasma parathyroid hormone concentrations (although it has slowed the wide availability of this assay), this observation led to the preparation of antisera reactive to different amino acid sequences of the glandular hormone.[31] The recognition and assay of these different immunoreactive parathyroid hormones seems to account for some of the earlier differences in physiologic observations reported by various authors.

Subtle interlaboratory antisera variation accounted also for minor differences among laboratories in the estimation of proinsulin concentration in human plasma samples.

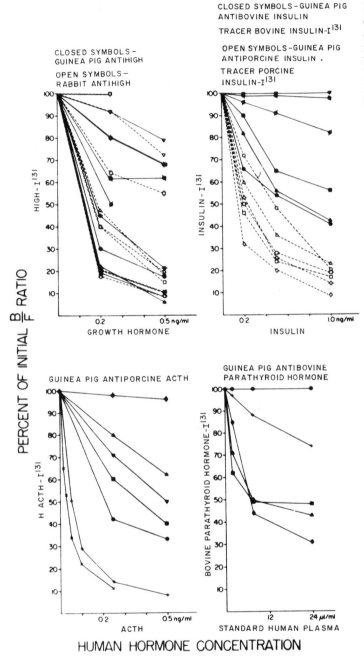

CLOSED SYMBOLS-GUINEA PIG
ANTIBOVINE INSULIN
TRACER BOVINE INSULIN-I^{131}

OPEN SYMBOLS-GUINEA PIG
ANTIPORCINE INSULIN .
TRACER PORCINE
INSULIN-I^{131}

CLOSED SYMBOLS-
GUINEA PIG ANTIHIGH
OPEN SYMBOLS-
RABBIT ANTIHIGH

GUINEA PIG ANTIPORCINE ACTH

GUINEA PIG ANTIBOVINE
PARATHYROID HORMONE

Fig. 8-7. Comparison of various antisera dose response curves to human growth hormone, insulin, ACTH and bovine parathyroid hormone. Each curve represents a different antiserum. (Yalow and Berson)[7,8]

The initial recognition of proinsulin was a consequence of its cross-reacting with insulin antisera[32] and the subsequent demonstration by Steiner that this cross-reacting substrate eluted from Sephadex columns in the 9,000 molecular weight region, in contrast to insulin which appeared in the 6,000 molecular weight region. The validity of the earlier observations on insulin secretory physiology was confirmed, however, following the demonstration that this "impurity" did not significantly alter determinations of plasma insulin concentration.[33,34] Some laboratories have developed antisera which are more specific for proinsulin than insulin,[35] and still other antisera for the connecting peptide fragment, permitting assay of these peptides in unextracted plasma without Sephadex fractionation, even in the presence of insulin antibodies.

The apparent observer difference in glucagon physiology based upon the early immunoassays for plasma glucagon can probably be explained in terms of varied antisera specificity and variable immunologic cross-reactivity of pancreatic and gut glucagon.[36-39] The identification of nonpancreatic glucagon was a consequence of the cross-reactivity of antisera to pancreatic glucagon, with a common amino acid sequence in the intestinal peptide.

As illustrated, each batch of antisera may have slightly different qualities, different structural recognition features (see Fig. 8-6), and different affinity constants (Fig. 8-7). Whereas different affinity constants and other minor assay-to-assay variants are accommodated by assaying known standards with each group of unknowns, this will not correct for antiserum variation if one antiserum reacts differently with the standard substrate (gland extract or synthetic source) and the unknown plasma substrate, as demonstrated for example by the variability of plasma disappearance rate of parathyroid hormone depending upon the antiserum used (see Fig. 8-6A).

These few illustrations demonstrate the virtually limitless selective recognition potential of antisera, and remind the reader of the need for confirmation of an antiserum's cognitive properties. In summary, whether antisera are purchased or prepared in the user's laboratory, data involving cross-reactivity (specificity) should be made available or determined by the user. Identical batches of antisera should be used from assay to assay of the same substrate.

Sensitivity. The sensitivity of the assay is determined both by the size of the tracer (i.e., chemical concentration of the labeled substrate; discussed earlier in the chapter)

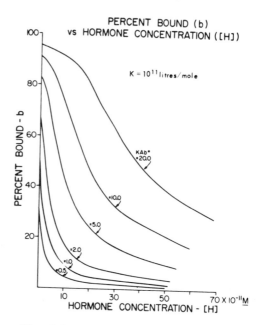

Fig. 8-8. Family of theoretical curves representing bound labeled hormone versus hormone concentration for different dilutions of an homogeneous antiserum with an equilibrium constant $K = 10^{11}$ L/mole. Note that KAb° → 1.0, the percent bound is 50 percent (i.e., B/F = 1) and the steepest slope is obtained for a given range of substrate concentrations. If the binding reagent is diluted further, the binding sites are too few for the assay range (limited by the concentration of the tracer). (Yalow and Berson)[12]

and the equilibrium constant of the highest affinity component of binding reagent.

To evaluate sensitivity, an appropriately dilute titer of the binding reagent must be used (see Fig. 8-3 and Fig. 8-8). This is determined by incubating serial dilutions of the binding reagent with the labeled substrate until a dilution is found which will bind approximately half of the labeled substrate (tracer). At this dilution, the capacity of the binding reagent is limited, and the more significant property of the binding reagent, the *sensitivity* (the ability to detect small changes in the substrate concentration) can be evaluated. To repeat, this *cannot* be done if the concentration of the tracer is too great (i.e., exceeds the binding reagent sensitivity) or if the binding reagent is not properly diluted (since less sensitive binding reagents with more capacity will bind the tracer. See Fig. 8-3, *A, B,* and *C*).

Following identification of a suitable dilution, binding reagents are incubated under assay conditions, with labeled substrate and different known concentrations of substrate. A standard curve is plotted, and the binding reagent yielding the greatest response (displacement of bound tracer) for the smallest increment in substrate concentration is identified as the most sensitive. This is conveniently done by inspection of the slope of the dose response (standard) curve; the steepest slope identifying the most sensitive binding reagent (see Fig. 8-7). Affinity may be expressed in terms of the equilibrium constant (K) derived from the multiple "k's" of the reaction

$$\text{Substrate} + \underset{\substack{\text{Binding}\\\text{Reagent}}}{} \overset{k1}{\underset{k2}{\rightleftharpoons}} \begin{array}{l}\text{Substrate-Reagent}\\\text{Complex}\end{array}$$

$$\begin{array}{l}\text{Labeled}\\\text{Substrate}\end{array} + \overset{k3}{\underset{k4}{\rightleftharpoons}} \begin{array}{l}\text{Labeled}\\\text{Substrate-Reagent}\\\text{Complex}\end{array}$$

It has been demonstrated that the minimal detectable substrate concentration approaches the reciprocal of the affinity constant, that is

$$[\text{Substrate}] \simeq \frac{1}{K},$$

if the dilution condition [Substrate] = [Binding Reagent°] is satisfied.*[5,12,40]

An extensive literature dealing with the mathematics of competitive binding radioassay has developed.[40,41,42,43] Of practical importance is the equation

$$B/F = K \, ([\text{B.R.}°] - B)$$

where [B.R.°] is the molar concentration of the binding reagent binding sites, B/F the ratio of bound-to-free labeled substrate, and K, the affinity constant. Since

$$B = b \, [S],$$

[S] being the total substrate concentration and b the fraction bound,

$$B/F = K([\text{B.R.}°] - b \, [S]).$$

This equation is recognizable as a specific form of the equation

$$y = mx + b$$

expressing a linear relationship between an independent and dependent variable. A plot of these linear theoretical relationships widely known as a Scatchard plot permits a determination of the affinity constant as the slope of the line, and the concentration of the binding sites as the X intercept. The steepest slope, determined by either the Scatchard plot or the usual B/F versus substrate concentration plot, identifies the binding reagent of highest affinity, and hence greatest sensitivity. Since immune binding reagents are actually heterogeneous mixtures of antibodies with different affinity constants, experimental data only approximates this linear relationship at appropriate dilutions of the binding reagent.

Naturally occurring circulating binding reagents have binding affinities in the physiologic range of the substances of interest, 1×10^9 l/mole,[19] but additional assay requirements for sample dilution may put the sensitivity of the assay beyond the range of the affinity constant. Recall that the limit of the detectable substrate concentration approaches the reciprocal of the affinity constant. In assays dependent upon circulating binding globulins, the extraction and drying of the sample which is a practical requirement for removing cross-reacting substrates and/or binding reagents (see p. 104, Availability and Production) also serves to maintain the sample concentration in the range of the sensitivity of the binding reagent. In radioimmunoassay of polypeptide hormones, the additional requirement for dilution of the plasma sample to reduce incu-

---

* This means that when the concentration of the binding reagent prior to reaction approaches the molar concentration of the substrate concentration to be measured, the limit of the measurable molar substrate concentration is the reciprocal of the affinity constant.

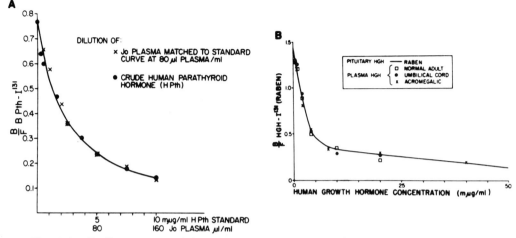

Fig. 8-9. Similar cross-reactivity (dose response) curves with antisera of gland-derived hormone and circulating hormone *A,* Parathyroid hormone (this finding was not observed with all antisera). *B,* Human growth hormone. (Berson and Yalow)[30]

bation damage is feasible only with the availability of antisera with affinity constants in the order of 1×10^{12} 1/mole,[40] which potentially can detect a substrate concentration as small as 1×10^{-12} moles/l. For the detection, therefore, of very small quantities of a substance, antisera offer the potential for greater sensitivity even for those compounds with naturally occurring binding reagents. In summary, therefore, in addition to potentially greater sensitivity, antisera, in contrast to naturally occurring binding reagents, are potentially more specific, usually do not require extraction and separation of the substrate, and have a more extensive potential applicability since they can be prepared to virtually any substrate.

Standard Substrate Preparations

The unknown substrate concentration is determined by comparing the *inhibition of binding* of the labeled substrate *by known quantities* of substrate, with the inhibition of binding *by unknown quantities* of the substrate in the sample to be assayed. Thus, it is *not* necessary that the *labeled substrate* and the *unlabeled substrate* be identical.[2,3,4] Arguments about the alteration of substrate identity by the introduction of a foreign atom (iodine) or side chain (iodotyrosyl moiety) are of little consequence, as long as the labeled derivative reacts with the binding reagent and is competitively inhibited by the substrate being assayed.[40,41,44]

Labeled peptide hormone from one species can frequently be used as the labeled substrate in assaying peptide hormones from another species, if appropriately reacting standards are used. Labeled substrates as structurally different as 3-0 succinyl-digoxin-tyrosine-^{125}I may be used as the tracer in the assay of plasma digoxin.[9]

In order to estimate correctly the concentration of the unknown, the unknown and standards must *react identically* with the binding reagent, even though they too may not be structurally identical. This is illustrated by the experience with human plasma insulin which may be assayed with either human or porcine insulin as standards since these 2 peptides *react* identically.[2,3,44] Human plasma, therefore, may be assayed even if human standards are unavailable, as long as reactivity of the known and unknown substrate are identical. The reactivity is demonstrable by preparing standard curves with different quantities of human plasma and comparing the curves obtained with the plasma "standards," with those from the available purified or relative standard. Indeed, this method is used to validate the assay of a plasma hormone by demonstrating that the circulating substrate reacts in a similar manner to tissue extracts (Fig. 8-9). Failure to confirm the expected cross-reactivity between tissue extracts has led to several new biologic observations. The immunochemical heterogeneity of parathyroid hormone[30] has already been mentioned. The demonstration that growth hormone activity in plasma from pregnant patients did not react over a range of dilutions in the same manner as nonpregnant patient's plasma or purified growth hormone, led to the observation of the structural relationship between human growth hormone and placental lactogen.[45]

Combination and Incubation of Assay Components

Duration of Incubation. In both immune and nonimmune systems, the rate of association (complex formation) is considerably greater than the dissociation rate. Since the incubation begins with dissociated components, equilibration is theoretically rapidly achieved even in dilute solutions. Since heat is generated during complex formation, cooling promotes equilibration. In experimental polypeptide-antibody interactions, however, equilibrium is frequently not achieved for several days, even under refrigerated incubation conditions. By contrast, nonpeptide substrate-binding reagent (immune and nonimmune) interactions have not empirically required prolonged incubation, frequently complexing sufficiently at dilutions of labeled substrate and binding reagent satisfactory for the required assay sensitivity within a few hours, even at room temperature.[28] Whereas shortened incubation times have the convenience of more rapid turnaround time, this technique should be applied cautiously since there is an increased potential for reduction of assay precision (reproducibility of result) due to experimental errors as a consequence of nonuniform sample incubation times, or dissociation of the complex during separation of bound and free labeled sub-

strate. The longer the incubation time, the less influence small inequalities in incubation time will have on the final bound fraction. Similarly, there is comparatively less opportunity for dissociation during separation (washing of complex or absorption of bound or free component on a solid phase absorbent), if the time for separation is short compared to the incubation period.

There is apparently little published experimental data, however, comparing the effect of longer incubation periods on the relative stability of the substrate-complexing reagent (antibody or nonimmune binding protein) complex. This problem lends itself to convenient evaluation in all laboratories equipped to do competitive binding radioassays. Optimal assay conditions can be determined and confirmed in clinical nuclear medicine laboratories regardless of whether these laboratories prepare their own reagents or purchase prepared kits.

Incubation Volume. Plasma with high concentrations of a substrate, outside the range of assay usefulness, must be assayed at greater dilution of plasma than samples which fall within the range. If the particular assay is sensitive to protein concentration at these dilutions, the total volume of plasma or serum is maintained by adding known substrate-free plasma. Occasionally, it is necessary to detect exceedingly small substrate concentrations, beyond the usual limit of assay sensitivity. This occurred, for example, when a plasma sample was fractionated into 20 or more samples by Sephadex column chromatography[33] followed by the determination of the substrate concentration in each fraction. This variation can be accommodated by incubating a larger than usual sample volume, and adjusting the volume of binding reagent and labeled substrate to maintain the same final concentration of these components regardless of the incubation volume. Alternately, extraction of a larger sample can be used to concentrate the substrate to be assayed.

In general, greater technical precision is afforded by working with larger incubation volumes. When assays relied on chromato-electrophoretic separation methods, sample size and counting statistics mandated small incubation volumes, generally up to 1.0 ml. With the availability of solid state and other test tube methods of separation (see below) larger incubation volumes (2.0-3.0 ml) are feasible. Consequently, the error due to pipette volume variability (i.e., $\pm$ 0.1 μL) is reduced proportionally. A 1.0 $\pm$ 0.1 μL volume of a standard (or other assay component) introduces a $\pm$ 10 percent volume variation, while greater assay volumes which permit the use of larger volume pipettes with the same order of accuracy, so that 10.0 $\pm$ 0.1 μL pipettes have an error of $\pm$ 1 percent of the total volume.

Other Factors. The rate of association of assay components (K value) is influenced by a variety of nonspecific factors (i.e., factors other than substrate and binding reagent structure). These factors include temperature, ionic environment, pH, and presence of various contaminants which interfere with the reactive portion of the molecule or degrade an assay component.

Given a plasma sample and a binding reagent with no other cross-reacting component, it is expected that the determination of concentration will be independent of the sample size (i.e., activity will be linear over a range of plasma dilutions). This is the case when the incubation mixture is sufficiently diluted so that the ionic strength of the incubation mixture is not significantly influenced by the plasma. If it is necessary to assay a more concentrated sample, the osmolality and even the protein concentration of the standard curve samples should be adjusted to approximate that of the unknowns. This is accomplished by adding reagent (hormone, drug, vitamin)-free plasma or albumin to these samples. When the sensitivity of an assay is adequate to determine the unknown concentration in 1:10 or greater dilution of plasma (100 μL plasma in a final incubation volume of 1.0 ml), these "nonspecific" protein and salt effects are usually of no consequence.

Incubations are usually performed in dilute buffer solution with a previously determined optimal pH in a range of 7.4 to 8.6.

The occasional interference by pharmaceuticals should be noted. Although there is some disagreement, heparin has no demonstrable effect during incubation in polypeptide hormone immunoassay systems. The polar character of this compound does, however, influence the adsorption of small acidic peptides by ion exchange resins used in the final separation of bound and free reagents.[14] The potential for interference with other small polar compounds should be kept in mind. Accordingly, it is best to evaluate the influence of other anticoagulants on each assay system, particularly if there is intra-assay variation, unless noninterference has been demonstrated previously. In vivo administration of pharmaceuticals to the patient usually does not affect the assay because of the dilution within the body. Endogenous antibodies following the therapeutic administration of polypeptide hormones will complex available substrate, yielding artifactually low or high results depending upon the method used for separation. The presence of such antibodies will be detected in the control.

The availability of semi-automatic pipetting equipment reduces experimental pipetting error when used properly. Since small air bubbles in the wrong place at the right time may significantly vary the amount of a sensitive assay component, great care should be used in setting up and monitoring time and laborsaving devices. The error introduced by small variations in the labeled substrate concentration can be accommodated over a range if both the free and bound fractions are counted. By counting a blank tube and comparing either the free or bound fraction to it (a convenient method which has grown in application with the use of automatic or semi-automatic calculating equipment), the laboratory loses a determinant of this type of error. Duplicate samples will detect a discrepancy between the 2 samples (if the error is random) and necessitate dis-

Table 8-4. Separation of Bound and Free Labeled-Substrate.

Partition of Free and Bound Labeled Substrate	Adsorption (Solid Phase) of Free Labeled-Substrate	Adsorption (Solid Phase) or Precipitation of Bound Labeled-Substrate
Chromatoelectrophoresis	Charcoal	Antibody precipitation, salts [$(NH_4)_2 SO_4$, Na_2SO_4]
Electrophoresis, paper	Talc	
Electrophoresis, starch gel	Silica (Quoso)	Antibody precipitation, second antibody
Gel filtration, Sephadex	Ion exchange resins (Amberlite, Biogel)	Millipore filters
		Sephadex bound binding reagent
Equilibrium dialysis	Diatomaceous earth	Antibody precipitation, organic solvent (polyethylene glycol)
	Cellulose	
	Sephadex	

carding both values and repeating the assay of that sample.

Since the assay is predicated upon the saturation of available binding sites, the greatest magnitude of error is produced with variation of the binding reagent concentration from one tube to another.

Separation of Assay Components

The final requirement for a successful competitive binding radioassay is a suitable technique for the separation of the bound (complexed) substrate and the free substrate (Table 8-4), followed by quantitation of the radioactivity in both fractions, or of either fraction and quantitation of tracer activity in control (total activity) tubes.[46] Most of the techniques are based upon differences in the molecular configuration of the bound substrate from the free substrate, as a consequence of the larger molecular weight protein coupled to it. In this regard it is important to confirm that adsorbent materials which recognize the free substrate do not *also* recognize the substrate component of the substrate-binding reagent complex.

Chromatoelectrophoretic separation of assay components was used in the early radioimmunoassays. The separation was based upon the affinity of the paper (usually cellulose, but ion exchange papers have also been used for other substrates) for the free antigen. The antigen-antibody complex migrates by hydrodynamic flow with the solvent front, as the solvent is evaporated from the center of the conducting bridge (buffer-soaked

paper). The advantage of this technique is that eluted iodide migrates ahead of the substrate-reagent complex, and is identified as a third peak or discarded, so that it does not contribute to an error in the estimation of either fraction. The technique is handicapped by both the limited volume of material that the paper strip can adsorb and hence, potentially poorer counting statistics, and the greater time and equipment required for separation. Although widely used during the early years of immunoassays, this technique has generally been replaced by test tube separation methods. Modest chromatographic, electrophoretic and chromatoelectrophoretic techniques should be available to "repair" an assay in difficulty, to confirm labeled substrate integrity, and to demonstrate incubation damage and free radioiodide eluted from the labeled tracer. Starch gel electrophoresis, Sephadex gel filtration and equilibrium dialysis have also been used as separation methods. These methods too are valuable approaches for unraveling assay riddles and providing the means of separation for assays without a convenient alternative, but because of the complexity and time involved do not lend themselves to efficient processing of large numbers of samples.

The test tube separation methods lend themselves to processing of large numbers of samples and to more convenient automated counting and calculating methods. Techniques based upon selective precipitation or adsorption of either the free or complexed substrate, however, will include in one or the other fraction, the eluted iodide which is

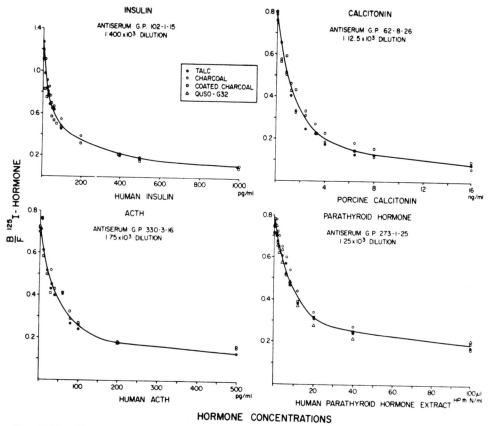

Fig. 8-10. Comparison of standard curves obtained in insulin, calcitonin, ACTH and parathyroid hormone assays using several different adsorbents for separation of bound and free labeled hormone. (Palmieri, G. M. A., Yalow, R. S., and Berson, S. A.: Horm. Metab. Res., *3*:301, 1971)[47]

separated as a third fraction in chromato-electrophoretic methods.

Substrate-binding reagent complexes may be precipitated by salts (ammonium sulfate, sodium sulfate), organic solvents (acetone, polyethylene glycol) or antibodies to the binding reagent. These techniques have been limited thus far to radioimmunoassays, although there is no theoretical reason for the failure to use them in nonimmune competitive binding radioassays.

Adsorption of the noncomplexed substrate is probably the most widely used separation method at this time. Powdered charcoal, talc, silica granules, diatomaceous earth, kaolin, magnesium silicate, and ion exchange resins are in use in a wide variety of radioassay systems. Ion exchange resins are

convenient for separation of more polar substrates.[23] In many assay systems (Fig. 8-10) the separation techniques are relatively interchangeable.[47,48] Charcoal probably has the widest use. Considerable discussion has developed concerning the necessity for coating the charcoal. In the presence of sera (nonextracted sample) there is no advantage to coating of the charcoal.[47]

Ion exchange resins also bind free iodine, resulting in erroneous estimation of the unbound fraction. Similarly, double antibody and protein precipitation leave the free iodide in the free fraction. Talc and silica do not bind the ionic iodide, and the radioactivity erroneously appears in the bound fraction. Despite this potential for artifact, the convenience, reproducibility and inexpensive cost of these agents make them more practical than chromatoelectrophoretic methods.

It is well to note that the protein concentration of the incubation mix affects the binding to charcoal and other solid phase adsorbents, such as talc and silica, and that equivalent volumes of sera or albumin should be present in all tubes, including controls and standards, even if it is necessary to add control sera prior to the separation step.[47] The adsorbents, and influence of protein, should be evaluated to ensure that the substrate end of the substrate-binding reagent complex does not also adsorb to the solid phase, resulting in false partition of the bound and free radioactivity.

In a variant of solid phase adsorption, the binding reagent or antibody is complexed to a solid phase (discs, particles or test tube walls) before incubation, resulting in the labeled tracer appearing in the solid phase as it is bound to the binding reagent. This method seems to offer advantages for the busy routine laboratory in which supervision may be limited. Although reported as an extremely simple procedure, Daughaday[46] has not found the coating of the tubes to be very convenient.

The double antibody technique of separation involves the addition to the incubation mixture, at the completion of the incubation period, of an antibody to the gamma globulin or serum of the animal species from which the assay binding reagent (usually an antibody) was prepared. This technique has been used widely and is a reliable test tube separation method. It is particularly useful in evaluating new assays before convenient, less expensive separation methods are identified. Disadvantages of the method are that it is expensive relative to other separation methods and an additional incubation period may be necessary to assure precipitation of the immune complex. Other methods that have been used include millipore filtering of the incubation mixture with filtration of complexed radioactivity, and Sephadex bound binding reagents permitting interaction of

components and separation in one step. This latter technique is commercially available in a competitive binding thyroxine assay. Polyethylene glycol precipitation of gamma globulin has proven useful in the immunoassay of several peptides. It is an inexpensive and technically simple method which can readily be used in· processing a large number of samples and readily adapted to automated techniques.

Standard Curves

Following separation and counting of the binding reagent-bound-labeled substrate and the free substrate, a standard curve is constructed and the values for the unknown samples are determined by comparison of the bound and free radioactivity to samples with known concentrations of the substrate (see Fig. 8-1). Correction for dilution of the plasma sample is made. As suggested earlier in the chapter, the data for the standard curve and unknowns lends itself to a variety of graph patterns, the choice of which usually depends upon the previous experience of the user. A considerable body of the immuno- and nonimmunoradioassay literature was developed using graph plots of bound/free, bound/total or percent bound versus substrate concentration. These 3 modes of expression (B/F, B/T and %B) are all quite identical except for the unit value of the ordinate. They are inversely proportional to the substrate concentration; the slope of the relationship expresses the affinity constant. A minority of the investigative literature, and most of the commercially developed kits, express the standard curve as the percent free, or total/bound versus substrate concentration, variables which are proportionally related, yielding a curve with a positive slope. These differences in plotting the standard curve are of no consequence except for the confusion that has been created among those who have not appreciated that the data can be handled in whichever way is most convenient for calculation and comparison with other laboratories and published observations.

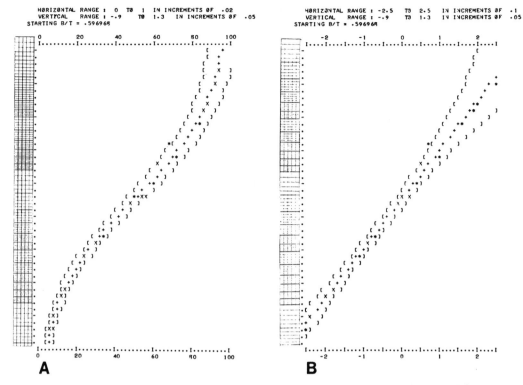

Fig. 8-11. Computer printout of dose response (standard) curves. *A*, Plot of B/B^0. versus $\log_{10}$ substrate concentration, *B*, plot of logit $(B/B^0.)$ versus $\log_{10}$ substrate concentration. (Rodbard, D. *In* Odell, W. D., and Daughaday, W. H.: J. B. Lippincott, 1971)[43]

With the growth of competitive radioassay applications and increasing number of samples, it has become desirable to seek a relationship between the substrate concentration and the dependent variable radioactivity partition data which lends itself to linear plots over a given range and makes automatic data processing, curve fitting, interpolation and extrapolation[42] more convenient. The so-called logit plot in which

$$\text{Logit } (B/B^\circ) = \log_e \frac{[B/B^\circ]}{[1 - B/B^\circ]}$$

is plotted as the dependent variable against the logarithm of the substrate concentration (Fig. 8-11) has been useful for this application. Obviously, although this may be convenient for automatic calculators and computers, it does not lend itself to convenient application in a small laboratory which depends upon manual calculation and determination of substrate concentration. In these locations, the traditional curvilinear plots of radioactivity versus the arithmetic plot of substrate concentration and visual interpolation of unknowns is more practical (Fig. 8-1).[48]

SUMMARY

This chapter has reviewed the "basic principles of competitive binding radioassay," and in so doing, has tried to find a line between the theoretical approach and the "cookbook" approach. Neither extreme seems necessary, since a considerable theoretical and practical bibliography already exists. Details of particular applications have been included to illustrate problems generic to this class of laboratory assay. Hopefully, in learning "how to set up" the assays included in this volume and which appear elsewhere in the medical literature, the reader is a little closer to understanding the "why".

References

1. Berson, S. A., Yalow, R. S., Bauman, A., Rothschild, M. A., and Newerly, K.: Insulin-^{131}I metabolism in human subjects: Demonstration of insulin binding globulin in the circulation of insulin-treated subjects. J. Clin. Invest., *35*:170, 1956.

2. Yalow, R. S., and Berson, S. A.: Assay of plasma insulin in human subjects by immunologic methods. Nature, *184*:1648, 1959.

3. Yalow, R. S., and Berson, S. A.: Immunoassay of endogenous plasma insulin in man. J. Clin. Invest., *39*:1157, 1960.

4. Berson, S. A., and Yalow, R. S.: Studies with insulin-binding antibody. Diabetes, *6*:402, 1957.

5. Berson, S. A., and Yalow, R. S.: Quantitative aspects of reaction between insulin and insulin-binding antibody. J. Clin. Invest., *38*:1996, 1959.

6. Hunter, W. M., and Greenwood, F. C.: Preparation of iodine-131 labelled human growth hormone of high specific activity. Nature, *194*:495, 1962.

7. Yalow, R. S., and Berson, S. A.: Topics on radioimmunoassay of peptide hormones. *In* Protein and Polypeptide Hormones: Proceedings of the International Symposium. Liege, Belgium, May 1968. Excerpta Medica, 1968.

8. Berson, S. A., and Yalow, R. S.: Principles of immunoassay of peptide hormone in plasma. *In* Astwood, E. B., and Cassidy, C. E.: Clinical Endocrinology. pp. 699-720. New York, Grune & Stratton, 1968.

9. Cerceo, E.: Advantages of gamma counting in radioimmunoassay of digoxin. Dialogos, *1*(No. 2):3, 1973.

10. Berson, S. A., and Yalow, R. S.: Iodoinsulin used to determine specific activity of iodine-131. Science, *154*:205, 1966.

11. Yalow, R. S., and Berson, S. A.: Labeling of proteins—problems and practice; Trans. Acad. Sci., *28*:1033, 1966.

12. Yalow, R. S., and Berson, S. A.: General aspects of radioimmunoassay procedures; *in* In Vitro Procedures with Radioisotopes in Medicine. IAEA, 1970.

13. Berson, S. A., and Yalow, R. S.: Species-specificity of human anti-beef, pork insulin serum. J. Clin. Invest., *38*:2017, 1959.

14. Yalow, R. S., and Berson, S. A.: Problems of validation of radioimmunoassays. *In* Odell, W. D., and Daughaday, W. H.: Principles of Competitive Protein-Binding Assays. Philadelphia, J. B. Lippincott, 1971.

15. Murphy, B. E. P.: Radioassays of non-antigenic hormones. Trans. Assoc. Amer. Physicians, *81*:92, 1968.

16. Roth, J.: Peptide Hormone Binding to Receptors: A Review of Direct Studies In Vitro. Metabolism, *22*:1059, 1973.

17. Korenman, S.: Measurement of Steroid Hormones Using Intracellular Receptors. Metabolism, *22*:1083, 1973.

18. Rothenberg, S. P.: A radioenzymatic assay for folic acid. Nature, *206*:1154, 1965.

19. Murphy, B. E. P.: Hormone assay using proteins in blood. *In* Odell, W. D., and Daughaday, W. H.: Principles of Competitive Protein-Binding Assays. Philadelphia, J. B. Lippincott, 1971.

20. Sterling, K., Bellabarba, D., Newman, E. S., and Brenner, M. A.: Determination of Triiodothyronine Concentration in Human Serum. J. Clin. Invest., *48*:1150, 1969.

21. Gharib, H., Ryan, R. J., Mayberry, W. E., and Hockert, T.: Radioimmunoassay for Triiodothyronine: Affinity and Specificity of Antibody. J. Clin. Endocrinol. Metab. *33*:509, 1971.

22. Lefkowitz, R. J., Roth, J., and Pastan, I.: Radioreceptor assay of ACTH: New approach to assays of polypeptide hormones in plasma. Science, *170*:633, 1970.

23. Yalow, R. S., and Berson, S. A.: Radioimmunoassay of Gastrin. Gastroenterology, *58*:1, 1970.

24. Berson, S. A., and Yalow, R. S.: Radioimmunoassay of ACTH. J. Clin. Invest., *47*:2725, 1968.

25. Glick, S. M., Kumarasen, P., Kagan, A., and Wheeler, M.: Radioimmunoassay of oxytocin. *In* Margoulis, M. (ed.): Protein and Polypeptide Hormones. Amsterdam, Excerpta Medica Foundation, 1968.

26. Abrahams, G. E., and Grover, P. K.: Covalent linkage of hormone haptens and steroid hormones to protein carriers for use in radioimmunoassay. *In* Odell, W. D., and Daughaday, W. H.: Principles of Competitive Protein-Binding Assays. Philadelphia, J. B. Lippincott, 1971.

27. Reiss, E., and Canterbury, J. B.: A radioimmunoassay for parathyroid hormone in man. Proc. Soc. Exp. Biol. Med., *128*:501, 1968.

28. Parkwer, C. W.: Nature of immunological responses and antigen-antibody interaction. *In* Odell, W. D., and Daughaday, W. H.: Principles of Competitive Protein-Binding Assays. Philadelphia, J. B. Lippincott, 1971.

29. Triiodothyronine Antibody Data Sheet, Wien Laboratories, Inc. Succasunna, N.J.

30. Berson, S. A., and Yalow, R. S.: Immuno-

chemical heterogeneity of parathyroid hormone. J. Clin. Endocrinol. Metab., *26*: 1037, 1968.

31. Arnaud, C. D.: Radioassay of the calciotropic hormones. Metabolism, *22*:1013, 1973.

32. Steiner, D. F., Cunningham, D., Spigelman, L., and Aten, B.: Insulin biosynthesis: Evidence for a precursor. Science, *157*: 697, 1967.

33. Goldsmith, S. J., Yalow, R. S., and Berson, S. A.: Significance of human plasma insulin Sephadex fractions. Diabetes, *18*:834, 1969.

34. Gorden, P., and Roth, J.: Plasma insulin: Fluctuations in the big insulin component in man after glucose and other stimuli. J. Clin. Invest., *48*:2225, 1969.

35. Melani, F., Ryan, W. G., Rubenstein, A. H., and Steiner, D. F.: Proinsulin secretion by a pancreatic beta cell adenoma: Proinsulin and C-peptide secretion. N. Eng. J. Med., *283*:713, 1970.

36. Unger, R. H., Eisentraut, A., McCall, M. S., *et al.*: Measurements of endogenous glucagon in plasma and the influence of blood glucose concentration upon its secretion. J. Clin. Invest., *41*:682, 1962.

37. Samols, E., Tyler, J., Marri, G., and Marks, V.: Stimulation of glucagon secretion oral glucose. Lancet, *2*:1257, 1965.

38. Lawrence, A. M.: Radioimmunoassayable glucagon levels in man: effects of starvation. Proc. Nat. Acad. Sci., *55*:316, 1966.

39. Heding, L. G.: Radioimmunological determination of pancreatic and gut glucagon in plasma. Diabetologica, *7*:10, 1971.

40. Yalow, R. S., and Berson, S. A.: Introduction and general considerations. *In* Odell, W. D., and Daughaday, W. H.: Principles

of Competitive Protein-Binding Assays. Philadelphia, J. B. Lippincott, 1971.

41. Eakins, R. P.: Radioimmunoassay, Protein binding and other saturation assay techniques. *In* The Yearbook of Nuclear Medicine. Chicago, Yearbook Medical Publication, 1973.

42. Feldman, H., and Rodbard, D.: Mathematical theory of radioimmunoassay. *In* Odell, W. D., and Daughaday, W. H.: Principles of Competitive Protein-Binding Assays. Philadelphia, J. B. Lippincott, 1971.

43. Rodbard, D.: Statistical aspects of radioimmunoassays. *In* Odell, W. D., and Daughaday, W. H.: Principles of Competitive Protein-Binding Assays. Philadelphia, J. B. Lippincott, 1971.

44. Yalow, R. S., and Berson, S. A.: Immunological specificity of human insulin: Application to immunoassay of insulin, J. Clin. Invest., *40*:2190, 1960.

45. Glick, S. M., Roth, J., Yalow, R. S., and Berson, S. A.: The regulation of growth hormone secretion. *In* Recent Progress in Hormone Research. vol. 21. New York, Academic Press, 1965.

46. Daughaday, W. H., and Jacobs, L. S.: Methods of separating antibody-bound from free antigen. *In* Odell, W. D., and Daughaday, W. H.: Principles of Competitive Protein-Binding Assays. Philadelphia, J. B. Lippincott, 1971.

47. Palmieri, G. M. A., Yalow, R. S., and Berson, S. A.: Adsorbent Techniques for the Separation of Antibody-bound from Free Peptide Hormones in Radioimmunoassay. Horm. Metab. Res., *3*:301, 1971.

48. Shelly, D. S., Brown, L. P., and Besch, P. K.: Radioimmunoassay. Clin. Chem., *19*: 146, 1973.

9 *Plasma Cortisol*

BENJAMIN ROTHFELD, M.D.

This chapter deals primarily with the determination of cortisol with the emphasis on plasma analysis.

Cortisol is produced by a specific area of the adrenal gland. This organ is divided into 2 portions—the medulla and the cortex. Because the medulla is intimately involved with the autonomic nervous system, it is not dealt with here. The cortex is divided into 3 portions—the zona glomerulosa, zona fasciculata, and zona reticularis. The zona glomerulosa, or outermost portion of the cortex, is involved in electrolyte balance through its production of aldosterone. The 2 inner portions, zona fasciculata and zona reticularis, are the areas in which cortisol is produced.[1]

NORMAL PHYSIOLOGY OF THE PITUITARY—ADRENAL AXIS

The portion of the adrenal as defined above is under the control of ACTH (adrenocorticotropic hormone) which is secreted by the anterior pituitary. Release of ACTH in turn is under the control of the corticotropin-releasing factor which is secreted by the hypothalamus. The plasma cortisol level affects release of ACTH in 2 ways: It has a direct effect on secretion of ACTH by the pituitary and an effect on release of the corticotropin-releasing factor by the hypothalamus. In both cases, high levels of plasma cortisol inhibit secretion of these substances and low levels facilitate their release. Normally there is a diurnal variation in the secretion of ACTH with a concomitant vari-

ation in the level of cortisol in the blood. In addition, under stress there is a rise in ACTH secretion and a concomitant rise in the plasma level of cortisol.

Chemistry of Compounds. The order of presentation of the various compounds (Fig. 9-1) is intended to make simpler the understanding of their chemistry. It has nothing to do with the way they are synthesized. At I the system for numbering steroids is shown as well as the lettering of the various rings. At II the compound corticosterone (compound B) is shown. From this compound, cortisol III may be derived by adding a hydroxyl group at the 17 position. Cortisone (compound E) shown at IV can be derived from cortisol by subtracting the hydrogen from the 11-position on the ring. 11-Deoxycortisol (compound S) can be derived from either cortisol or cortisone by subtracting the oxygen from the 11-carbon position.

The corticosteroids of interest here are characterized by a 2 carbon chain at the C-17 position. Additionally, they have a double bond between the C-4 and C-5, an oxygen at the 3-position and an hydroxyl group at the C-17 position. Also, there are methyl groups at the 18 and 19 positions. A hydroxyl group at the C-11 position confers the following biologic properties: inhibition of pituitary release of ACTH, regulation of gluconeogenesis, production of insulin resistance, lowering of peripheral blood eosinophils and lymphocytes, as well as negative nitrogen balance. Since compounds B and F have the necessary chemical properties they

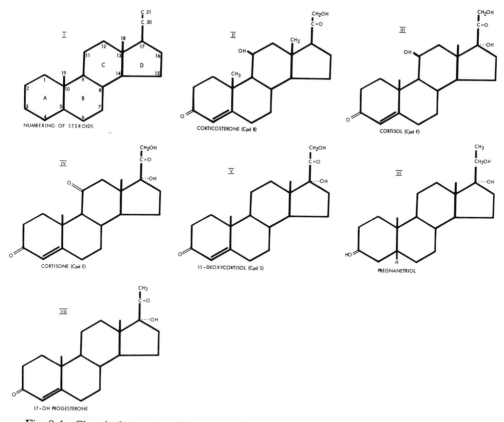

Fig. 9-1. Chemical structure of some steroids of importance in adrenal cortical physiology.

also have these biologic effects. Compound E does not have the biologic properties, but its ketone group at C-11 is readily reduced to a hydroxyl group, and so for practical purposes it has all the properties of compound F. Since compound S is lacking in oxygen in the C-11 position, it does not have these biologic properties.[2]

METHODS FOR DETERMINING CORTICOSTEROIDS

Practically all the methods for determination of corticosteroids are based on chemical rather than biologic techniques. For completeness the use of bioassay is mentioned, although it is rarely used for clinical purposes.

Bioassays use several methods: They may be based on the capacity of corticosteroids to induce glycogen deposition in the liver of adrenalectomized rats exposed to stress; or they may be based on their production of eosinopenia in the peripheral blood of experimental animals.[2]

Porter-Silber Technique. Of historical interest is the first chemical method which was introduced in 1948 by Corcoran and Page.[3] For the first time this allowed the chemical determination of corticosteroids in urine and plasma. The first really practical method for determination of corticosteroids was the Porter-Silber method.[4] This was based on the fact that certain corticosteroids reacted with phenylhydrazine and sulfuric acid to form a colored compound which could be measured spectrophotometrically. This reaction detects all corticoids having a dihydroxyacetone side chain at the [17]carbon atom. Since nonsteroids also react with this reagent, a preliminary purification of the material being tested is necessary. At first this required column chromatography; however, subsequently, the need for column chromatography has been replaced by the simpler technique of extraction into an organic solvent and is no longer part of many of the standard Porter-Silber techniques used.[5] Another modification of the Porter-Silber method is known as the Glenn-Nelson procedure,[6] which uses glucuronidase to split the conjugated steroids; thus avoiding the detrimental effects of strong acid hydrolysis. This method is more time-consuming than the standard method but is somewhat more specific.

The disadvantage of the Porter-Silber technique is that it requires relatively large amounts of plasma (5 cc), a minimum of 8 hours' incubation, and equipment microadapted for reading from a final volume of 0.2 cc. Additionally, it may be affected by nonsteroidal compounds or hemolysis.[7] These substances act by inhibiting or facilitating the development of the characteristic color reaction.

Fluorometric Technique. A technique which seems to be gaining in popularity is the fluorescent or fluorometric technique. It is based on the fact that certain steroids fluoresce when dissolved in ethanolic sulfuric acid and exposed to light of the appropriate wavelength.[8] At first, this method, like the Porter-Silber technique, required purification by column chromatography; however, it has subsequently been modified to eliminate this.[9] A further modification in this technique was made by Mattingly and is currently the most popular of the fluorescent techniques.[10]

The advantages of the fluorometric technique over the Porter-Silber technique are that it requires smaller quantities of plasma, it is easy to adapt to semiautomation, and it measures corticosterone (compound B). The disadvantages of the fluorometric technique are that very clean glassware is required; it may be upset by nonsteroid fluorescence usually found in plasma,[11] and it may be altered by the fluorescence of steroid drugs such as spironolactone.[5]

17-Ketogenic Steroid Technique. This method is an ingenious method for deter-

mining the 17-hydroxysteroids. In its original form it was based on estimating the 17-ketosteroids by the Zimmerman reaction involving color formation with metadinitrobenzene. The 17-hydroxycorticosteroids were then oxidized to 17-ketosteroids by using bismuthate. A second 17-ketosteroid determination was then done and the difference between the 2 determinations represented the 17-hydroxycorticosteroids.[12] A somewhat simpler technique involves exposing the urine to sodium borohydride to reduce the preformed 17-ketosteroids. The reaction with bismuthate is then carried out and only the newly formed 17-ketosteroids which were derived from the original 17-hydroxycorticosteroids are then measured.

The advantages of the 17-ketogenic steroid method over the Porter-Silber method are that the same color method may be used for both 17-ketosteroids and 17-ketogenic steroids, and this technique in addition to measuring 17-hydroxy, 20-ketosteroids, also measures 17-hydroxy, 20-hydroxysteroids such as cortol and cortolone. These latter are metabolites of cortisol which may be increased in hypothyroidism and liver disease. Since in these disorders the usual urinary metabolites of cortisol are reduced, the concomitant elevation of cortols and cortolones may help to avoid a faulty diagnosis based on estimation of 17-hydroxy, 20-ketosteroids alone. The disadvantages of the 17-ketogenic steroid method are that it is less specific than the Porter-Silber method and is only suitable on urinary samples.

RADIOASSAY OF CORTISOL

Radioassays are essentially the same as radioimmunoassays but employ specific binding proteins as receptors instead of antibodies. In both these situations the principle of competitive protein binding is used (Fig. 9-2). In this Figure it is assumed that there are a total of 10 receptors for the test substance. The normal state shown in the center has 5 units of test substance available to bind to the 10 receptors. In the hyper state, there are 9 such units and in the hypo state

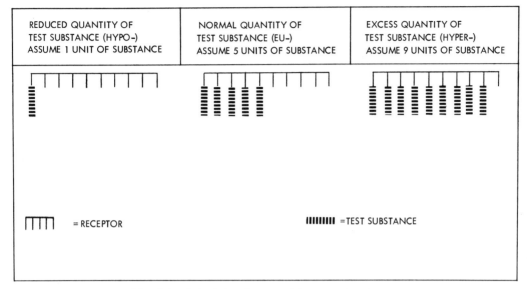

| REDUCED QUANTITY OF TEST SUBSTANCE (HYPO-) ASSUME 1 UNIT OF SUBSTANCE | NORMAL QUANTITY OF TEST SUBSTANCE (EU-) ASSUME 5 UNITS OF SUBSTANCE | EXCESS QUANTITY OF TEST SUBSTANCE (HYPER-) ASSUME 9 UNITS OF SUBSTANCE |

Fig. 9-2. Principle of competitive protein binding.

there is only 1 such unit available. It may thus be seen that if the test substance, which is nonradioactive, is mixed with the receptor substance and then the same test substance which has a radioactive tag is added, varying amounts of the radioactive labeled material will be bound. Since there is usually a dynamic equilibrium between the bound and unbound test material, ordinarily it doesn't matter whether the radioactive or nonradioactive material is added first to the receptor substance. In the hypo state, greater quantities and in the hyper state lesser quantities of tagged material will be bound.

In the analysis for cortisol the binding protein is cortisol binding globulin (CBG) which occurs normally in serum. The 3 basic steps in these assays are[13]: 1. Remove the binding proteins present in plasma; otherwise they may act in the same way as the assay protein which is subsequently added. 2. Mix the substance to be analyzed, with the solution containing the assay protein, in this case cortisol binding globulin, and a suitable tracer. The tracer most commonly used here is ^{3}H-cortisol. The conditions are so chosen that the cortisol binding globulin of the solution is just saturated with the tracer steroid. Since the steroid bound

to cortisol binding globulin (CBG) is in dynamic equilibrium with the unbound steroid, the steroid of the sample displaces a portion of the tracer and the remainder of the tracer, bound to CBG, falls. 3. Separate the protein bound and unbound fractions and determine the distribution of the tracer.

Both steps 1 and 3 can be done in various ways. Subsequently, the steroid of the sample is quantitated by comparing the displacement of the tracer with that caused by known amounts of steroids. A curve is drawn and the results read off.

Actually, over the years this method of radioassay has become simplified. The original method[14] involved ^{14}C-cortisol. Dialysis was the method used for separating the free from the bound cortisol. Although only 1 cc of plasma was required for this method, the time required for the test was 2 days.[14] This method was shortened to 2 hours when gel filtration using Sephadex was substituted for dialysis.[15] More recently a marked increase in sensitivity was obtained by using ^{3}H-steroids, and the technique has been further simplified by replacement of gel filtration with precipitation of the unbound fraction by adsorption to insoluble substances.[13] As mentioned above the first step (deproteiniza-

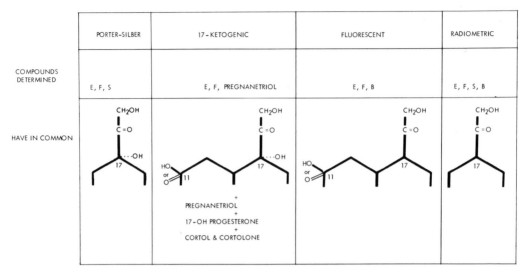

PORTER-SILBER	17-KETOGENIC	FLUORESCENT	RADIOMETRIC

COMPOUNDS DETERMINED

E, F, S	E, F, PREGNANETRIOL	E, F, B	E, F, S, B

HAVE IN COMMON

Fig. 9-3. Chemical determinants of the various assays.

tion) may be accomplished by various means, including heat, alcohol, or methylene chloride. Methylene chloride is a reliable means of separating corticosteroids from proteins but is technically more difficult than ethanol precipitation. For this reason ethanol precipitation has been a more popular technique. However, accuracy is probably improved by using methylene chloride. Additionally, methylene chloride has the advantage of being a good extracting agent for corticosteroids as well as precipitating protein.

In step 3 mentioned above, separation of the bound from the unbound cortisol, various techniques may be used, including dialysis, electrophoresis, gel filtration, ion exchange resins, protein precipitation, and the adsorption of the unbound fraction to insoluble particles. This latter method is currently the most popular. These particles may consist of Fuller's earth, Lloyds' reagent, florisil, or dextran-coated charcoal.

These adsorbents vary in their affinity for cortisol. Fuller's earth, Lloyd's reagent and dextran-coated charcoal have a relatively low affinity for cortisol. However, with florisil there is a problem, since its affinity for corticosterone (compound B) and also 11-deoxycortisol (compound S) is relatively weak

compared to its affinity for cortisol. Therefore, compounds B and S are measured using florisil to a greater extent than the other adsorbents.[13]

The adsorbents also may be affected by temperature. Dextran-coated charcoal is relatively little affected over a range of $10°$ to $45°C$. However, the other adsorbents which are all silicates seem to function best at $10°C$.[13]

Another variable in radioassays for cortisol is the fact that CBG from different species has different affinities for various steroids. Thus, CBG from the Rhesus monkey has a high affinity for compound B, dog CBG for compound F, and cat CBG for compounds E and S.[13]

The great advantage of radioassay for cortisol is that it is free from nonsteroidal interference. It is a very specific test for a very small group of biologically active steroids.[14,15] Another advantage is that it requires quite small amounts of plasma.

At the present time the disadvantage of this test is that it involves a tritium label and therefore requires liquid scintillation counting which is not available in all nuclear medicine laboratories.

With the evolution of techniques for determining 17-hydroxycorticosteroids there has been a concomitant reduction in the amount of plasma needed for the test.

SPECIFICITY OF THE VARIOUS TYPES OF ASSAY FOR CORTISOL

Porter-Silber Method. In addition to detecting compound F and its derivative, this method also measures compounds E and S and their tetrahydro derivatives.

17-Ketogenic Steroid Technique. In addition to the compounds measured by the Porter-Silber reaction, this reaction also measures pregnanetriol and 17-hydroxyprogesterone and also cortol and cortolone.

Fluorescent Techniques. These measure compounds E, F and their metabolites. Although it measures corticosterone (compound B), it does not measure compound S.[16]

Radioassay. In the absence of a preliminary chromatographic purification or carbon tetrachloride preextraction, these techniques in addition to picking up compound F also pick up compounds S and B. These preliminary steps, however, are not necessary in normal subjects, hypoadrenal patients, and in patients with Cushing's syndrome due to ACTH excess. They become necessary only in patients with adrenal tumors of certain types or specific enzyme defects.[17] (See Fig. 9-3.)[1]

COMPOUND F

Urinary Determination of Compound F. All the previously mentioned methods are, with some modifications in a few cases, applicable to urinary determination of compound F. In fact, the first of these methods was suitable only for urinary determinations until further study was made in their evolution. Normally in the urine, the predominant steroids derived from the adrenal cortex, aside from the 17-ketosteroids, are compounds E, F and their tetrahydro derivatives.

Although some of the metabolites of compound F have a slight effect on binding, they can be ignored in plasma, since they are present in concentrations only one to several times that of compound F. However in urine, metabolites and their tetrahydro de-

rivatives, are present in relatively large concentrations. Since the metabolites are water soluble but are not soluble in methylene chloride, they can be separated out by a preliminary extraction.[13]

A basic shortcoming of urinary determinations of urinary 17-hydroxycorticosteroids is that they do not reveal the level of 17-hydroxycorticosteroids in body fluids. Obesity increases urinary values but blood values are normal. In hyperthyroidism the urinary 17-hydroxycorticosteroid levels may be 2 times normal due to rapid turnover of these substances. In both these cases, however, the plasma levels are normal. Thus it is necessary to get either a plasma 17-hydroxycorticosteroid level or a urine free F level to decide whether the patient is being exposed to elevated plasma corticoid levels.[16] Another disadvantage of urinary 17-hydroxycorticosteroids, when compared with plasma cortisol levels, is that they cannot be used to follow closely rapid changes in the secretion and metabolism of cortisol.

Secretory Rate of Compound F. This may be determined isotopically. A known amount of labeled compound F is injected. Urine is then collected over a fixed period of time and is treated to liberate the conjugates. It is purified and its specific activity-radioactive content per microgram is determined. The amount of steroids secreted in the time covered by the urine collection is calculated by dividing the total dose administered by the specific activity of the isolated hormone. The value is increased in obesity and variably decreased in Addison's disease.[18] This technique is mainly of experimental interest and may be too involved for the average nuclear medicine laboratory to undertake.

Plasma F Levels in Studies of Normal Physiology. Although the presence of a diurnal variation in blood levels of plasma cortisol was known before radioassay developed, the greater sensitivity of radioassay and the smaller amounts of material required permitted a much more definitive exploration of the changes in plasma during the day. The earliest work in this area revealed that in normal persons the levels of 17-hydroxy-corticoids were at a maximum at about 8:00 A.M.; the lowest levels occurred in the evening about 11:00 P.M. and were approximately 50 percent of the maximal level.[19] This diurnal variation develops between 1 and 3 years of age and depends on parallel changes in ACTH secretion, which are probably related to changes in the hypothalamic corticotropin-releasing factor,[20,21,22,23] as well as on a normal sleep-activity cycle.[24] Additionally, it seems to be related to processes involved in dreaming and rapid eye movement during sleep.[25]

Actually, this normal diurnal variation seems ideally suited for human everyday needs. Thus, when a person arises to meet the stresses and strains of everyday life, his level of plasma cortisol is at a maximum and when he retires for sleep his plasma cortisol is at a minimum.

In elderly normal subjects the diurnal rhythm is maintained in a normal fashion. This is true even in individuals who sleep very poorly; although they remained in a darkened room during the night and stayed in bed, they carried out during the day the same activities as the other elderly subjects.[26]

Estrogens and Pregnancy: Effect on F Levels. Although a growing minority questions whether pregnancy should be listed under normal physiologic states, for the purposes of this chapter it is included. Since the effect of estrogens is quite similar to that of pregnancy this topic too is treated.

In a striking parallel with the changes in T-4 and thyroxine-binding globulin, the levels of transcortin as well as cortisol increase progressively during pregnancy.[27] While some authorities state that the free plasma F level increases in pregnancy,[28] others state that it shows no change.[29]

As might be expected, persons on estrogen therapy show elevation in plasma F levels. These elevations vary with the amount of estrogen the person is taking and in those on oral contraceptives containing only progesterone the F levels are normal. It has been found[29] that F levels may rise as early as

14 hours after the ingestion of the first estrogen tablet, and may go as high as 3 times normal. These levels usually return to normal within 2 weeks after the discontinuance of the estrogen-containing substances.

A study[27] comparing normal and pre-eclamptic pregnancies reveals that there was no difference in the plasma cortisol levels in the 2 groups. It was therefore felt unlikely that the fluid retention and hypertension of preeclampsia was related to abnormalities in plasma F levels.

It has been suggested that since in cases of fetal death and missed abortion the level of compound F drops considerably and rapidly, this might be used as an index of fetal viability.[29] Two precautions, however, must be observed[31]: (1) There is a brief small fall in the plasma F level about the fifth month of pregnancy; (2) Since there is a wide range of normal values in nonpregnant females, in any case of suspected missed abortion at least 2 determinations of plasma F should be done at weekly intervals. Of course, if the patient is being treated with estrogens during this period, this will affect the results. Actually, estimation of urinary estriol appears to be a more sensitive way of checking on fetal viability, since the changes in cortisol are most likely secondary to changes in levels of cortisol-binding globulin related to a fall in estrogen level.

Plasma F Levels in the Neonatal Period. At birth the F levels in cord blood are quite high.[31] This is probably related to the stress of birth and also high maternal levels of free plasma F, although the latter is controversial as mentioned above. Caesarian deliveries usually have lower F levels than vaginal deliveries. One researcher feels that the elevated F levels drop rapidly in the first 24 hours of life and remain at this new level for the first week.[32] Another feels that although the level is at a maximum on the first day of life, the drop is more gradual during the first week.[33] The difference between the two authorities may be based on the methods used, since the first used a competitive protein binding technique and the second used a Porter-Silber technique.

Comparing the competitive protein binding analysis with a double isotope derivative assay,[34] findings showed normal adults and children to have good correlation between the 2 tests. However, in neonates the Murphy technique gave definitely higher results. It was felt that among other things in the neonates, high levels of corticosterone could interfere with the test. Furthermore, although ordinarily progesterone does not interfere with the Murphy technique, when there are very high levels of this compound as in cord blood, there may be interference and this may account for very high free F levels in cord blood.[35]

Effects of Pharmacologic Agents. These effects are presented in order of increasing importance to the clinician.

1. *Topical steroids.* The effect of these on blood levels of compound F vary depending on whether they are measured by the method being used. Substances such as dexamethasone and its derivatives may result in diminution in blood F levels in competitive protein binding assay, since they are not measured. Thus, in a series of 19 cases who had been on such compounds for 3 to 14 weeks, 3 showed subnormal levels.[36] Patients on hydrocortisone ointment in some cases may show some elevation in blood levels. Thus, determination of plasma cortisol may be helpful in monitoring for absorption of topical steroids.

2. *Insulin.* In normal persons the standard *insulin tolerance test* produces a marked rise in plasma cortisol level. This depends on an intact hypothalamo-pituitary-adrenal axis. Needless to say, the validity of this test depends on the attainment of hypoglycemic levels during the study. It may be used as a test of the integrity of this axis.[37] The maximal compound F response occurred 60 to 90 minutes after the insulin injection.[38] In normals the plasma F level at least doubles at its peak. In patients with hypopituitarism the magnitude of the compound F response is greatly reduced.

3. *Response to ACTH.* This may be tested in 2 ways.[39]

(a) The 8-hour-ACTH test may be done in which 25 units of ACTH or 0.25 ml of synthetic cosyntropin in 1,000 cc of saline is given intravenously over an 8-hour period. Blood samples are taken at 1, 4 and 8 hours; and a 24-hour urine collection made. Both blood and urine samples should show at least a doubling over the basal value.

(b) A more rapid test is the plasma compound F response to ACTH in which an F level is drawn in the basal state. At 30 minutes and 60 minutes after an intramuscular injection of 25 units of ACTH or 0.25 ml of cosyntropin the F level should rise by at least 10 μg per 100 cc.[40]

4. *Dexamethasone.* The effect of this substance is to suppress normal production of compound F by the adrenal. The first suggested use of this was by administration of a dose of 0.5 mg every 6 hours for 8 doses —the low-dose dexamethasone suppression test. Another routine is to give 2 mg every 6 hours for 8 doses. Urine is collected before and after the administration of dexamethasone and checked for 17-hydroxycorticosteroid levels[40]—the high-dose dexamethasone suppression test. In normal persons the levels of steroid were dropped either to the lower end of normal or below normal. A newer version of this test involves determining compound F levels in the basal state. Then at 11:00 P.M. 1 mg of dexamethasone is given plus 1½ gr of Nembutal to assure a good night's rest. In normal persons the levels drop below 5 μg per 100 cc.

The overnight and low-dose dexamethasone suppression tests are designed to distinguish normal persons from those with Cushing's disease. The high-dose dexamethasone suppression test is done after the diagnosis of Cushing's disease is made to determine the etiology of the syndrome. Although there are exceptions, Cushing's due to adrenal hyperplasia suppresses, while that due to tumor does not.

Since there is some evidence that an appreciable number of normals may fail to suppress using the single dose of dexamethasone,[41] another variation has been suggested in which ½ mg dexamethasone is given every 6 hours for 2 days and then an 8:00 A.M. sample of blood is checked for compound F. This should be below 6 μg per 100 cc.[42] Failure of suppression in normals has been ascribed to the nonspecific stress of being in a hospital.

Dilantin may interfere with the dexamethasone suppression test because it interferes with dexamethasone absorption,[43] or because it enhances hepatic metabolism of dexamethasone by increasing its conjugation.[44]

USE OF PLASMA F DETERMINATIONS IN PATHOLOGIC STATES

Cushing's Disease

The typical case of Cushing's disease is easily recognized—buffalo hump type of obesity, plethora, hypertension, easy bruising, diabetes, hirsutism, purple abdominal striae, acne and behavioral abnormalities. Cushing's disease is much more often suspected than proven, however. Since many obese people are looking for a glandular cause for their overweight, this possibility is often raised.

The syndrome involved in Cushing's disease is produced by adrenal hyperplasia in 80 percent of the cases with occult, small pituitary adenomas present in a significant number of these. A single adrenal adenoma accounts for 15 percent of the cases and carcinoma of the adrenal cortex for the remaining 5 percent.[38]

Measurement of the plasma F level is helpful in the diagnosis of Cushing's disease but not as a single determination, because not all patients with Cushing's disease have abnormally high plasma F levels. Those in whom the disease has taken a mild form, or is cyclic or intermittent, or remits spontaneously even when it is due to an adrenal tumor, may have normal values. Furthermore, in normal persons the plasma F level may be temporarily raised by emotional and physical stress, or they may have question-

ably high values of plasma F because there is an overlap between the upper limit of normal plasma F and the lower range found in patients with Cushing's disease. Obese persons, too, may have high plasma F levels.

Three additional tests have been developed to determine the presence of Cushing's disease.

1. The *dexamethasone suppression test*. This, the oldest of these tests, involves giving the patient ½ mg of dexamethasone every 6 hours for a total of 8 doses. On this regimen—the low-dose dexamethasone suppression test—patients who are merely obese may be separated from those with Cushing's disease due to adrenal hyperplasia.[41] The former suppresses; the latter does not. By giving 2 mg every 6 hours for 8 doses—the high-dose dexamethasone suppression test—patients who have Cushing's disease secondary to adrenal hyperplasia show suppression of their urinary steroids; those with autonomous adrenal tumors do not.

Another way of doing this test involves drawing a basal plasma F level at 8:00 A.M., giving 1 mg of dexamethasone at 11:00 P.M., and then drawing another sample at 8:00 A.M. the next day.[47] On this regimen all normals suppressed below 5 μg per 100 cc. This was true of persons who were obese but who did not have Cushing's disease. In normals their plasma F levels fell to 50 percent of the control values, while in Cushing's disease none fell below 70 percent of the control value. Acutely ill patients and those on estrogens had higher plasma F levels after dexamethasone, and in some cases stayed above 20 μg per 100 cc. regardless of the underlying etiology. Other clinicians have found that in nervous, excitable patients there may not be suppression but that when these patients became calm there was definite suppression. Barbiturate sedation may be necessary in such patients.[45]

2. The *diurnal variation of plasma F test*. Normally there is a variation in plasma F level during the day—highest at 8:00 A.M. and lowest in the evening. The value at 11:00 P.M. is roughly half that at 8:00 A.M.

This normal variation is usually absent in Cushing's disease and may even be reversed, although an occasional patient with Cushing's disease may have normal diurnal variations. However, normal diurnal variation also may be lacking in patients with acute infections, severe pain, imminent death, various central nervous system lesions, diabetes mellitus with complications, and heart failure, so that abnormal diurnal variation alone is not enough to establish the diagnosis of Cushing's disease.[49-65]

3. *ACTH stimulation test.* This test is done as described earlier in this chapter. Responses may be classified as normal, supernormal, or subnormal. Usually when Cushing's disease is due to hyperplasia the response to ACTH is supernormal.[45,47] However, in some cases it may be normal,[47,67] as in Cushing's disease due to adrenal adenoma in which the response is more often than not normal, although not infrequently it may be less than normal.[45,47,61] In carcinoma of the adrenal it is subnormal.[69] Severely ill patients who do not have Cushing's disease may give a high response.[70]

Our technique for combining the various tests and studies for Cushing's disease is as follows: An 8:00 A.M. sample is drawn. This is followed by a 4:00 P.M. sample. At 11:00 P.M. 1 mg of dexamethasone is given and another basal sample drawn at 8:00 A.M. the next day. To avoid artifacts introduced by sleeplessness, Nembutal Gm. 0.1 may be given at 11:00 P.M. The 4:00 P.M. levels should be at least 35 percent less than the 8:00 A.M. level in the basal state. The 8:00 A.M. level the day after dexamethasone administration should be less than 5 μg per 100 cc. We feel that if both these levels and the original basal level are normal, the diagnosis of Cushing's disease may be safely excluded. An interesting technique for the diagnosis of Cushing's disease involves sampling the effluent of the adrenal veins for their content of compound F.

One set of investigators concluded that the most useful criteria for confirming Cushing's disease were a raised midnight plasma F level, raised basal urinary compound F level on at least 2 occasions, and failure of the morning plasma compound F level to suppress below 6 μg per 100 cc in response to 2 mg of dexamethasone per day for 48 hours.[42]

Addison's Disease and Addisonian Crisis

Addison's disease is no less striking in its clinical manifestations than is Cushing's disease. The typical manifestations are weakness, nausea, vomiting, diarrhea, increased skin pigmentation and nervousness. Adrenal crises are manifest by weakness, abdominal pain, high fever, confusion, nausea, vomiting and diarrhea.

Addison's disease most commonly is secondary to idiopathic adrenal atrophy or to tuberculous involvement of the adrenals. Adrenal crises may be secondary to acute adrenal destruction, cortisone withdrawal, or stress in the Addisonian patient.[16]

Like Cushing's disease, Addison's disease is uncommon. It is estimated that in the United States the death rate from Addison's disease is 4/100,000. The actual number of patients is probably higher than the recorded 5,000 cases in the United States, since many patients with unrecognized disease die in a crisis precipitated by some form of stress. The majority of cases occur between 20 and 50 years of age, the most productive time of life. This entity becomes of even more importance because of the not uncommon need to rule it out in persons who are underweight, anxious and weak and appear otherwise to be neurotic.

As in Cushing's disease, a single determination of plasma cortisol is not enough to separate all Addisonian cases from normals, since there is an overlap between the values in the 2 diseases.[72]

The plasma cortisol test may be ordered in various ways depending on the diagnostic possibilities being considered. Thus, in Addisonian crisis an immediate determination should suffice. A patient with hypotension, fever, nausea and vomiting due to causes other than an Addisonian crisis should have high values of plasma cortisol. He should be treated with dexamethasone as the major steroid and then ACTH stimulation tests may be done when his condition improves.

In Addison's disease an 8:00 A.M. plasma cortisol level may suffice. In both Addison's disease and crisis the level should be below normal. If any question of Addison's disease then persists, an ACTH stimulation test should be done. However, in Addison's disease ACTH may be hazardous since one may develop an anaphylactic reaction to it. Therefore, patients who are suspected of having Addison's disease should be treated with dexamethasone ½ mg bid on days when ACTH is being infused.[2] The dexamethasone does not alter the adrenal response to ACTH, and its metabolites do not contribute to the level of steroids. The ACTH may be administered as described above. Normal patients show a marked rise in their urinary compound F levels and also a definite rise in their plasma levels. After 60 minutes in normals the plasma F level should rise by at least 10 μg per 100 cc. In Addisonian cases there is little if any change in plasma or urinary levels.

Adrenogenital Syndromes

In these syndromes the plasma cortisol and urine-free cortisol levels may be low because of deficient production of compound F by the cortex. Sometimes in this situation the 17-ketogenic steroids are higher than the Porter-Silber values and higher than the radioassay, because pregnanetriol is measured in the 17-ketogenic steroids and not in the other tests.[2]

Renovascular Hypertension

In an interesting study, 12 of 16 patients with renovascular hypertension had abnormalities in their plasma cortisol levels.[69] In these cases the resting plasma F level was only 1.4 times greater than the evening level. In contrast, in this study, in normals the resting level was 3 times the evening level. These

abnormal results in the patients studied resulted from an abnormally high evening plasma cortisol and a somewhat depressed morning cortisol. In addition, on dexamethasone suppression only 5 of 12 patients had normal responses.

Three patients were studied, at least 6 months after surgery which resulted in normotension. All 3 at this time had normal diurnal variation and 2 of the 3 had normal dexamethasone suppression tests.

Before any surgery was done in 12 patients studied, 3 had elevated 17-hydroxycorticoids in the urine and in all patients studied the aldosterone level was normal. The renin levels were elevated in all patients.

The authors feel that the abnormal cortisol results are due to renin stimulating the adrenal cortex diffusely, rather than specifically affecting aldosterone.

Plasma Cortisol Levels and Nervous System Disease

Head injury. There is evidence that in conscious patients with lesions in the pretectal and hypothalamic regions there are abnormal circadian rhythms.[60] Certain authors feel that the loss of circadian rhythm may be the most sensitive index of hypothalamic damage, since this rhythm may be lost while adequate steroid response to artificially induced stress (pyrogens, insulin) or naturally induced stress (surgery) persists.[72] In view of the multitude of factors affecting circadian rhythm, it probably is wise not to place too much reliance on changes in it in such cases.

Chronic brain syndrome. If patients with this syndrome are free from congestive heart failure and diabetes there is no difference between their resting plasma cortisol levels and those of controls. However, the normal controls had a higher percentage of normal circadian rhythms than the patients with chronic brain syndrome. Possibly this is due to the abnormal sleep patterns that those with chronic brain syndrome have.[73]

The Effect of Change in the Sleep Cycle on Plasma F Levels

Both the sleep cycle and the pattern of light and dark may have marked effects on plasma F levels. It has been shown that an 8-hour shift in the timing of the sleep-wake cycle produces an 8-hour shift in the diurnal variation of plasma.[74]

Other workers have found that by changing the sleep cycle in normals to 12-, or 19- or 33-hour cycles a new rhythm synchronized with a new sleep-wake cycle developed with regard to the plasma F levels. No matter what the length of the cycle, the maximal concentration occurred at the time of awakening and the minimal in the early hours of sleep. Change for one day did not affect the diurnal variation. It usually took alteration at least one week before change occurred.[75] This study also showed that light is very important in diurnal variation. Blind patients may have diurnal cycles not normally synchronized with sleep.

As mentioned above, patients with chronic brain syndrome may maintain a normal diurnal pattern in spite of the fact that they did not sleep well at night (p. 126). It was felt in that study that the fact that the patients were kept in bed and in the dark during the normal sleep time enabled them to maintain their normal diurnal variation in plasma F levels.

PLASMA F LEVELS

Plasma F Levels in Mental Illness

Studies in chronic schizophrenics reveal that on the whole their resting F levels were within normal limits and there was a normal diurnal variation.[76] Patients who were more hyperactive and more acting-out tended to have higher resting levels than others, but they were still within the normal range.

In depressed patients the results by different authors have been quite variable, possibly due to methodologic differences. Thus some authors found that the resting plasma F levels tend to be at a higher range of normal.[77] Others[76] found no association between the plasma F levels, and the diagnosis and depth of depression. Normal diurnal variation has been found in depressives, although the authors found that dexamethasone suppression was not quite as marked as in normal individuals. That is, they found that in some of their patients the cortisol level did not go below 13. They made no mention, however, of how well their patients had rested the night before and perhaps this is the explanation of their anomalous results. Some found that the diurnal variation in depressives was greater than in normals due to their abnormally high resting plasma F levels.[78] When the patients improved, the diurnal variation became more normal.

In a study in manic patients it was found that 3 out of 7 had midnight levels higher than their 8:00 A.M. levels. At midnight these patients were awake and active.[79]

Plasma F Levels in Miscellaneous States

Terminal states. It has been found that in patients dying after a prolonged period of hypotension, their blood levels of cortisol were markedly elevated and were significantly higher than in patients after slowly progressive illnesses.[28] Therefore, irreversible shock is not associated with lack of biologically active corticosteroids in plasma. Also the terminal state does not seem to be associated ordinarily with adrenal exhaustion.

Abnormal levels of cortisol-binding globulin. Seal and his coworkers described cases with both high and low cortisol-binding globulin.[80,81] Their plasma 17-hydroxycorticoids levels were respectively above and below normal. However, their urinary 17-hydroxycorticoid excretion was normal and as in cases with abnormal levels of thyroxine-binding globulin, there was no evidence of endocrine abnormality. According to Seal,[82] families with either type of cortisol-binding globulin abnormality are very rare.[82]

Plasma F levels in alcoholics. For years it has been theorized that in acute and chronic alcoholic intoxication and also in the alcohol withdrawal state there might be adrenal insufficiency. Because of this, adrenal steroids have been advocated in these conditions. In a very thorough study this was investigated.[83] The authors studied alcoholics during a period of 11 to 29 consecutive days of experimentally induced ethanol intoxication. They found that with increase in the blood alcohol level there was progressive increase in the serum cortisol level, indicating a general dose-response relationship. Thus, alcohol intake seems to result in adrenal cortical activation. A radioassay was used in this study.

In this investigation a subject who showed withdrawal symptoms when his alcohol dosage was reduced developed peak cortisol levels. In subjects who stopped drinking without withdrawal symptoms, cortisol levels tended to return to baseline levels. Furthermore, with GI upsets and poor intake cortisol levels tended to rise. There was no evidence of adaptation or exhaustion of the cortisol response during drinking or after alcohol withdrawal.

A possibility for the high levels of cortisol in alcoholics is impairment of cortisol metabolism in the liver. However, hepatic function tests in these patients showed no evidence of progressive impairment. However, since these tests assessed only reserve and acute hepatic processes, it is possible that cortisol metabolism is still impaired here.

It seems that in this case as in so many others one good experiment is worth more than hours of armchair theorizing.

The development of the plasma cortisol assay like so many new techniques has opened new vistas. A number of old hypotheses have been destroyed. Hopefully new and fruitful hypotheses will soon be developed, based on this test.

References

1. Symington, T.: Functional Pathology of the Adrenal Gland. Williams & Wilkins, 1969.
2. Paschkis, C. E., Rakoff, A. and Cantarow, A.: Clin. Endocrinol., ed. 3, sect. 5. Hoeber Med. Div. of Harper and Rowe, 1967.
3. Corcoran, A. C., and Page, I. H.: Methods for the chemical determination of corticosteroids in urine and plasma. J. Lab. Clin. Med., 33:1326, 1948.
4. Porter, C. C., and Silber, R. H.: A quantitated color reaction for cortisol and related 17, 21 dihydroxy-20-ketosteroids. J. Biol. Chem., 185:201, 1950.
5. Silber, R. H., and Porter, C. C.: The determination of 17 - 21 dihydroxy-20-ketosteroids in urine and plasma. J. Biol. Chem., 210:923, 1954.
6. Glenn, E. M., and Nelson, D.: Method for fluorometric determination of hydroxysteroids. J. Clin. Endocrinol. Metab., 13:911, 1953.
7. Cryer, P., Sode, J., and Sabol, J.: The measurement of serum 11-hydroxycorticosteroids in the diagnosis of adrenal cortical disease. Med. Ann. D.C., 39:570, 1970.
8. Sweat, M. L.: Sulfuric acid induced fluorescence of corticosteroids. Anal. Chem., 26:773, 1954.
9. Silber, R. H., Busch, R. D., and Oslapas, R.: Practical procedures for estimation of corticosterone or cortisol. Clin. Chem., 4:278, 1958.
10. Mattingly, D.: Fluorometric technique for determination of 17 hydroxycorticoids. J. Clin. Pathol., 15:374, 1962.
11. James, B. H. T., Townsend, J., and Francis, R.: Comparison of fluorometric and isotopic procedures for determination of plasma cortisol. J. Clin. Endocrinol. Metab., 37:18, 1967.
12. Norymberski, J. K., Stubbs, R. D., and West, H. F.: Assessment of adrenal cortical activity by assay of 17 ketogenic steroids in urine. Lancet, 1:1276, 1953.
13. Murphy, B. E. P.: Some studies on the protein binding of steroids and their application to the routine micro and ultra micro measurement of various steroids in body fluids by competitive protein binding radioassay. J. Clin. Endocrinol., 27:973, 1967.
14. Murphy, B. E. P., Engelberg, W., and Pattee, C. J.: Method for determination of corticoids in plasma. J. Clin. Endocrinol., 23:293, 1963.
15. Murphy, B. E. P., and Pattee, C. J.: Modification of method for determining cortisol in plasma. J. Clin. Endocrinol., 24:919, 1964.
16. Forsham, P. H.: *In* Williams, R.: Textbook of Endocrinology, ed. 4, ch. 5. Philadelphia, W. B. Saunders, 1968.
17. Hsu, T. H., and Bledsoe, T.: Measurement of urinary free corticoids by competitive

protein binding radioassay in hypoadrenal states. J. Clin. Endocrinol. Metabol., *30*: 443, 1970.

18. Grollman, A.: Clinical Endocrinology and its Physiologic Basis. chap. 15 and 16. Philadelphia, J. B. Lippincott, 1964.

19. Bliss, E. L., Sanberg, A. A., and Nelson, D. H.: Normal levels of 17 hydroxycorticoids in the peripheral blood of man. J. Clin. Invest., *32*:818, 1953.

20. Franks, R. C.: Diurnal variation of plasma 17-hydroxycorticoids in children. J. Clin. Endocrinol. Metab., *27*:75, 1967.

21. Ney, R. L., Shimizu, N., and Nicholson, W.: Correlation of plasma ACTH Conc. with adrenal cortical response in normal human subjects, surgical patients, and patients with Cushing's disease. J. Clin. Invest., *42*:1669, 1963.

22. Graver, A. L., Ney, R. I., Nicholson, W. E., et al.: Natural history of pituitary adrenal recovery following long term suppression with corticosteroids. J. Clin. Endocrinol., *25*:11, 1965.

23. Nichols, C. P., and Tyler, F. H.: Diurnal variation in adrenal cortical function. Ann. Rev. Med., *18*:313, 1967.

24. Liddle, G. W.: An analysis of circadian rhythms in human adrenal cortical secretory activity. Trans. Amer. Clin. Climatol. Assoc., *77*:151, 1965.

25. Weitzman, E. D., Schaumburg, H., and Fishbein, W.: Plasma 17-hydroxycorticosteroid levels during sleep in man. J. Clin. Endocrinol., *26*:121, 1966.

26. Serio, M., Piolanti, P., Romano, S., et al.: The circadian rhythm of plasma cortisol in subjects over 70 years of age. J. Gerontol., *25*:95, 1970.

27. Copelman, J. J.: Plasma cortisol levels and cortisol binding in normal and preeclamptic pregnancies. Amer. J. Obstet. Gynecol., *108*:925, 1970.

28. Murray, D.: Cortisol binding to plasma proteins in man in health, stress and at death. J. Endocrinol., *39*:571, 1967.

29. Williamson, H., and Moody, L. O.: Plasma cortisol after one to 60 cycles of oral contraception. J. Reprod. Med., *5*:19, 1970.

30. Goldberg, S., Lewenthal, H., Gottfried, I., et al.: Free 11-hydroxycorticosteroids in plasma in normal pregnancy and in cases of fetal death and missed abortion. Amer. J. Obstet. Gynecol., *95*:892, 1966.

31. Migeon, C. J.: Cortisol production and metabolism in the neonate. J. Pediatr., *55*: 280, 1959.

32. Stevens, J. F.: Plasma cortisol levels in the neonate. Arch. Dis. Child., *45*:592, 1970.

33. Bayliss, R. I. S., Browne, J. C. M., Round, B. P., et al.: Plasma 17-hydroxycorticosteroids in pregnancy. Lancet, *1*:62, 1955.

34. Sturzaeta, N. F., Hillman, D., and Colle, E.: Measurement of plasma cortisol in children and adults: Comparison of double isotope derivative assay, competitive protein binding analysis and a modified competitive protein binding analysis. J. Clin. Endocrinol., *30*:185, 1970.

35. Rosenthal, H. E., Slaunwhite, W. R., Jr., et al.: Transcortin: A corticosteroid binding protein of plasma. X. Cortisol and progesterone interplay and unbound levels of these steroids in pregnancy. J. Clin. Endocrinol., *29*:352, 1969.

36. Feiwel, M., James, V. H. P., and Barnett, E. S.: Effect of potent topical steroids on plasma cortisol levels of infants and children with eczema. Lancet, *1*:485, 1969.

37. Serio, M., Tarquini, B., Contini, P., et al.: Plasma cortisol response to insulin and circadian rhythm in diabetic subjects. Diabetes, *17*:124, 1969.

38. Donald, R. A.: Plasma immuno reactive corticotropin and cortisol response to insulin hypoglycemia in normal subjects and patients with pituitary disease. J. Clin. Endocrinol., *32*:225, 1971.

39. Krupp, M., Chatton, H., and Margen, S.: Current diagnosis and therapy. pp. 614-625, Lange Medical Publications, 1971.

40. Liddle, G. W.: Test of pituitary-adrenal suppressibility in the diagnosis of Cushing's syndrome. J. Clin. Endocrinol., *20*:1539, 1960.

41. Connolly, C. K., Gore, M., Stanley, N., et al.: Dexamethasone suppression test. Br. Med. J., *2*:665, 1968.

42. Mattingly, D., and Tyler, C.: Plasma and urinary 11-hydroxycorticosteroids in the differential diagnosis of Cushing's syndrome. Br. Med. J., *3*:17, 1972.

43. Bledsoe, T.: Personal communication.

44. Jubiz, W. A., Meikoe, R. A., Levinson, S., et al.: Effect of chronic dilantin administration on metabolism of dexamethasone. N. Eng. J. Med., *283*:11, 1970.

45. Pavlatos, F. C., Smilo, R., and Forsham, P.: A rapid screening test for Cushing's disease. JAMA, *193*:720, 1965.

46. Sawin, C. T.: Measurement of plasma cortisol in the diagnosis of Cushing's Syndrome. Ann. Intern. Med., 68:624, 1968.

47. Nugent, C. A., Nichols, T., and Tyler, F.: Diagnosis of Cushing's syndrome. Arch. Intern. Med., *116*:172, 1965.
48. Lindsay, A. E., Nigeon, C. J., Nugent, C. A., *et al.*: The diagnostic value of plasma and urinary 17-hydroxycorticosteroid determinations in Cushing's syndrome. Amer. J. Med., *20*:15, 1956.
49. Ekman, H., Hakansson, B., McCarthy, J., *et al.*: Plasma 17-hydroxycorticosteroids in Cushing's syndrome. J. Clin. Endocrinol., *21*:684, 1961.
50. Brorson, I.: Concentration of corticosterone and hydrocortisone in the plasma of patients with Cushing's syndrome caused by hyperplasia or tumor of the adrenal cortex. Acta Chir. Scand., *127*:162, 1964.
51. Bliss, E. O., Sandberg, A. A., Nelson, B. H., *et al.*: The normal levels of 17-hydroxycorticosteroids in the peripheral blood of man. J. Clin. Invest., *32*:818, 1953.
52. McHardy, S., Harris, P. W., Lessof, M. H., *et al.*: Single dose dexamethasone suppression test for Cushing's syndrome. Br. Med. J., *2*:740, 1967.
53. Sholiton, L. J., Werk, E. E., and Marneli, R. T.: Diurnal variation of adrenal cortical function in nonendocrine disease states. Metabolism, *10*:632, 1961.
54. Espiner, E. A.: Urinary cortisol excretion in stress situations and in patients with Cushing's syndrome. J. Endocrinol., *35*:29, 1966.
55. Shenkin, H. A.: The effect of pain on the diurnal pattern of plasma corticoid level. Neurology, *14*:1112, 1964.
56. Sandberg, A. A., Eik-Nes, K., Migeon, C., *et al.*: Metabolism of adrenal steroids in dying patients. J. Clin. Endocrinol., *16*:1001, 1956.
57. Drewry, J., Unger, R., Caplan, N., *et al.*: The pituitary-adrenal axis in encephalitis. p. 91. Program 49th meeting of Endocrine Society (abstr.), Bal Harbor, Florida, 1967.
58. Kreiger, D. T.: Diurnal pattern of plasma 17 hydroxycorticosteroids in pretectal and temporal lobe disease. J. Clin. Endocrinol., *21*:695, 1961.
59. Kreiger, D. T., and Kreiger, H. P.: Circadian variation of the plasma 17 hydroxycorticosteroids in central nervous system disease. J. Clin. Endocrinol., *26*:929, 1966.
60. Oppenheimer, J. H., Fisher, L. V., and Jailer, J. W.: Disturbance of the pituitary-adrenal interrelationship in diseases of the central nervous system. J. Clin. Endocrinol., *21*:1023, 1961.
61. Hokfelt, D., and Luft, R.: The effect of suprasellar tumors on the regulation of adrenal cortical function. Acta Endocrinol., *32*:177, 1959.
62. Lentle, B. C., and Thomas, J. P.: Adrenal function and the complications of diabetes mellitus. Lancet, *2*:544, 1964.
63. Knapp, M. S., Keane, P. M., and Wright, J.: Circadian rhythm of plasma 11-hydroxycorticosteroids in depressive illness, congestive heart failure and Cushing's syndrome. Br. Med. J., *2*:27, 1967.
64. Connolly, C. K., and Wills, M. R.: Plasma cortisol levels in heart failure. Br. Med. J., *2*:25, 1967.
65. Ross, P. J., Marshall-Jones, P., and Friedman, M.: Cushing's syndrome: Diagnostic criterion. Quart. J. Med., *35*:149, 1966.
66. Hellman, L. F., Makada, F., Curti, J., *et al.*: Episodic nature of adrenal cortical secretion. J. Clin. Endocrinol. Metab., *30*:411, 1970.
67. Scott, H., Foster, J. H., Liddle, G., *et al.*: Cushing's syndrome due to adrenal cortical tumor: Eleven year review of 15 patients. Ann. Surg., *162*:505, 1965.
68. Weiss, E., Raybis, S., Nelson, D., *et al.*: Evaluation of stimulation and suppression tests in the etiologic diagnosis of Cushing's syndrome. Ann. Intern. Med., *71*:941, 1969.
69. Cave, R., Shires, L. D., Barrow, M. V., *et al.*: Abnormal diurnal variation of plasma cortisol in patients with renovascular hypertension. J. Clin. Endocrinol. Metabol., *27*:800, 1967.
70. Christy, N. P., Langson, D., and Jailer, J. W.: Studies in Cushing's syndrome. Amer. J. Med., *23*:910, 1967.
71. Cryer, P. E., Sode, J., Sabol, J., *et al.*: The measurement of serum 11-hydroxycorticosteroids in the diagnosis of adrenal cortical disease. Med. Ann. D.C., *39*:570, 1970.
72. Grad, B., Rosenberg, G., and Liberman, H.: Diurnal variation of the serum cortisol level of geriatric subjects. J. Gerontol., *26*:351, 1971.
73. Perkoff, G., Eik-nes, K., Nugent, C. A., *et al.*: Studies on the sleep-wake cycle. J. Endocrinol., *19*:432, 1959.
74. Orth, D. N., Island, D. P., and Liddle, G. W.: Experimental alteration of the circadian rhythm in plasma cortisol concentration in man. J. Clin. Endocrinol. Metabol., *27*:549, 1967.
75. Orth, D. N., and Island, D. P.: Light syn-

chronization of circadian rhythm in plasma cortisol concentration in man. J. Clin. Endocrinol., *29*:479, 1969.

76. Franzen, G.: Serum cortisol in chronic schizophrenia. A study of the diurnal rhythm in relation to psychiatric mental status. J. Psychosom. Res., *15*:367, 1971.

77. Bridges, P. K., and Jones, M. T.: The diurnal rhythm of plasma cortisol concentration in depression. Br. J. Psychiat., *112*: 1257, 1966.

78. Carrol, B. J., Martin, F. I. R., and Davis, B.: Resistance to suppression by dexamethasone of plasma 11-hydroxycorticosteroid levels in severe depressive illness. Br. Med. J., *3*:285, 1968.

79. Platman, S. R., and Sieve, R.: Lithium carbonate and plasma cortisol response in the affective disorders. Arch. Gen. Psychiat., *18*:591, 1968.

80. Lohrenz, F., Sloe, R. P., and Seal, U. S.: Idiopathic or genetic elevation of corticosteroid-binding globulin. J. Clin. Endocrinol. Metab., *28*:1073, 1968.

81. Lohrenz, F., Seal, U. S., and Sloe, R. P.: Adrenal function & serum protein concentrations in a kindred with decreased CBG concentration. J. Clin. Endocrinol. Metab., *27*:966, 1967.

82. Seal, U. S.: Personal communication.

83. Mendelson, J. H., Ogota, M., and Mello, N.: Adrenal function in Alcoholism: 1. Serum cortisol. Psychosom. Med., *33*:145, 1971.

10 Radioimmunoassays for Triiodothyronine and Thyroxine

CHARLES S. HOLLANDER, M.D. AND
LOUIS SHENKMAN, M.D.

INTRODUCTION

The past decade has seen major advances in the application of radioassays to the measurement of circulating thyroid hormones, significantly enhancing our understanding of thyroid pathophysiology. Utilizing these newer radioassay techniques, it is now possible to measure directly the concentrations of the circulating hormones themselves. Earlier methods (e.g., serum protein-bound iodine (PBI), thyroxine by column, and butanol extractable iodine) capitalized on the fact that the thyroid hormones were the principal iodine-containing organic compounds in blood.[1-5] The serum PBI was a major advance since it permitted for the first time a measurement, albeit indirect, of a thyroidal secretory product in blood.[6,7] Though technically demanding, for many years the serum PBI was the classic test for assessment of thyroidal activity. The major limitation of the assay, which has grown more important with the widespread use of iodine-containing compounds in clinical medicine, is that contamination by any form of iodine gives falsely elevated results.[8] The problem of inorganic iodine contamination was largely circumvented by the development of the butanol extractable iodine[3] and thyroxine by column techniques,[5] but organic iodine contamination remains a formidable technical problem.

In addition to these technical problems, it became apparent with the discovery of triiodothyronine (T3)[9] that measurements of organic iodine by whatever means do not accurately reflect thyroid function in all circumstances. The reason is that, although T3 is present in minute concentrations in the circulation, thereby making an insignificant contribution to the organic iodine-containing compounds in the blood, it is metabolically far more potent than is T4[10] because T3 has greater intrinsic metabolic activity, a faster turnover, and a larger volume of distribution.

It therefore became apparent that direct measurements of T3 and T4 were necessary for a proper understanding of the contribution of these compounds to thyroidal economy. It is of interest to note that the techniques of radioimmunoassay were not applied to the measurement of T3 and T4 until many years after they had been utilized for the assay of a variety of other hormones.

In 1965, Murphy successfully applied the competitive protein-binding technique to the measurement of thyroxine.[11] Variations of these techniques have become a standard method for the determination of serum thyroxine in man. Modifications of the competitive protein-binding analysis procedure have also been utilized to measure serum T3 levels, but this technique has now been largely supplanted by radioimmunoassay

Supported by U.S.P.H.S. grants ROI AM-14314 and FR96.

methods for T3.[12,13,14] Radioimmunoassays for T3 are now widely available and radioimmunoassays for T4 have also been developed.

In this chapter the applications of radioassay techniques are described, including competitive protein binding, and radioimmunoassay for measurement of T3 and T4, as well as the pathophysiological import of these observations.

COMPETITIVE PROTEIN-BINDING ANALYSIS (DISPLACEMENT ANALYSIS)

In the early 1960's, an ingenious new approach was introduced that circumvented the need for measuring iodine content and allowed for a direct estimation of the level of T4.[15] The test was based on the presence of a specific binding protein in serum for T4, thyroxine-binding globulin (TBG), which in this test system acts in a manner analogous to first antibody in a radioimmunoassay method. The basic features of the method as refined by Murphy and Pattee[11] are extraction of iodothyronine from serum and its binding proteins, and incubation of the extract with labeled T4 and a source of TBG in the presence of a nonspecific adsorbent. The extent of displacement from TBG onto the nonspecific adsorbent is then compared to a standard curve, permitting quantitation of the amount of T4 present.

A number of different nonspecific adsorbents have been utilized, including dextran and ion exchange resins. An additional modification that has been employed recently is the use of Sephadex G-25, which eliminates the need for chemical extraction.[16] This approach to the measurement of T4 has gained wide acceptance by virtue of its relative simplicity and the good correlation it affords with thyroid status.

Since T3 is present in much smaller amounts than T4 and since it has a far lower affinity for thyroxine-binding globulin, it does not interfere with the T4 assay. For these same reasons, the application of competitive protein-binding assay to the measurement of T3 has been less successful. The fact that T3 has a lesser affinity for TBG, and is present in much smaller amounts than T4, has entailed a careful and somewhat cumbersome separation of T3 from T4 in the process of which conversion of T4 to T3 has been shown to occur.[14] Because of these difficulties, the competitive protein-binding technique for measuring T3 has given way to radioimmunoassay.

RADIOIMMUNOASSAY FOR T3 AND T4

With the demonstration that antibodies can be raised to small molecules such as T3 and T4, radioimmunoassays for analysis of these hormones became feasible. As with other radioimmunoassays, the assays for T3 and T4 entail variations of 3 basic steps:

1. Preparation of specific anti-T3 or anti-T4 antibody.
2. Incubation of this antibody with isotopically labeled T3 or T4 and with standards or serum to be assayed.
3. Separation of antibody-bound T3 or T4 from free hormone.

In 1970, Brown, et al. reported the first successful production of anti-T3 antibody.[17] They employed the carbodiimide condensation product of T3 and succinylated poly-l-lysine as immunogen. Other workers subsequently produced suitable antigen by linking T3 to either bovine or human serum albumin by carbodiimide condensation.[18-21] A T3-fibrinogen complex has been utilized by Reichlin's group in raising anti-T3 antibody, and thyroglobulin has likewise been employed as immunogen by several groups.[22,23]

In general, the immunogen, emulsified in complete Freunds adjuvant, is injected both subcutaneously and into the foot pads of rabbits at monthly intervals. Most investigators have administered in the range of 0.4 to 1 mg of antigen at each injection time. Antibody can usually be detected in low titer after the first injection, although usable antibody in high titer is generally seen after 2 to 3 months.

Recently, some workers employed the

method of Vaitukaitis, et al.[24] for raising anti-T3 antibody whereby small amounts of antigen are injected into multiple sites. By this technique, usable antibody of high titer can be harvested after several weeks. Sera can either be lyophilized after harvesting or can be stored in the frozen state for future use.

To date, anti-T4 antibody has been raised by several groups utilizing techniques similar to those employed for anti-T3 antibody.[25,26,27] Both thyrogobulin and T4 bovine serum albumin conjugates have been successfully employed as immunogens. In general, the titers have been somewhat lower than for anti-T3 antibodies but are readily utilizable in a T4 radioimmunoassay.

A major methodologic hurdle in assaying either T3 or T4 is the presence in serum of proteins with high affinity for thyroid hormones (TBG, albumin and prealbumin). Since these proteins compete with anti-T3 or anti-T4 antibodies for T3 or T4, they either must be removed from the test serum or their capacity to bind thyroid hormones must be effectively blocked prior to incubation with antibody. This problem has been circumvented either by extracting the serum in order to remove the thyroid-binding proteins prior to assay, or by the addition of one of a variety of agents which have the capacity to block the interaction of thyroid hormones with serum proteins.

Several of the agents which have been found to displace T3 and T4 from binding proteins include salicylates, thimerosal, diphenylhydantoin, tetrachlorthyronine, the halogenated derivative of thyroxine, and the anion, 8-anilino, 1 naphthalene sulfonic acid (ANS).[18,20,21,23,25,28,29] Most current assays utilize one of the above agents, thereby permitting direct measurement in unextracted serum. With respect to the T3 assay, the blocking agents have the theoretical advantage of displacing more T3 from TBG than T4 and, therefore, tend to decrease the potential for cross-reactivity for T4 with T3 in the assay. Salicylates have been employed by Larsen for both T3 and T4 assays.[20,27]

Thimerosal has been utilized by Gharib, et al.[18] and by Huefner and Hesch in their T3 radioimmunoassays.[19] The latter group favors thimerosal because other agents decrease the specific binding of labeled hormone to the antibody. However, this effect is less pronounced in the presence of serum. We initially utilized tetrachlorthyronine for this purpose but, as we and others have found, unless purified, tetrachlorthyronine cross-reacts with anti-T3 antibody. Also, even highly purified tetrachlorthyronine cannot be used in the T4 assay. Therefore, we have since utilized ANS for both T3 and T4, as initially suggested by Chopra.[23,26] Beckers has also employed ANS for a T3 radioimmunoassay.[30] Huefner has shown that ANS is the most effective inhibitor of the binding of [125]I T3 to serum proteins but he prefers thimerosal, since he found that ANS also decreases the specific binding of the labeled hormone to the antibody.[31] However, we find, as has Huefner, that this inhibition of the antigen antibody reaction is less pronounced in the presence of serum and in our opinion does not constitute a major drawback. Lieblich and Utiger[21] have shown that dilantin can be employed for successfully blocking T3-TBG interaction and has the advantage of not inhibiting the antigen antibody reaction. Care must be taken with solubilization and an alkaline pH must be employed; its stability has also been questioned. However, despite these theoretical limitations, other groups have also utilized dilantin successfully as a blocker in their T3 assays.[22]

An alternative solution to the problem of TBG interference is to extract thyroid hormones from serum prior to radioimmunoassay. This has been done by Surks, et al. employing column chromatography with Sephadex G-25[32] and by Werner[33] and also Williams, et al.,[34] utilizing a prior ethanol extraction similar to that employed by Murphy in her competitive protein-binding assay.[11] Although this approach adds an additional step to the procedure, its proponents suggest that it does allow more accurate measurements, particularly in the hypo-thyroid range. Two methodologic problems in the extraction procedure are worthy of note. First, the extraction yield must be quantitated, and this can obviously be a source of error despite the fact that the yield with the Sephadex G-25 and ethanol extractions is reported to be of the order of 90 percent. Second, care must be taken to insure that no conversion of T4 to T3 occurs. Since T4 is present in far larger amounts than T3, even a minute percentage conversion can be a source of significant overestimation of T3. Such a problem was present in the early competitive protein-binding assays for T3.

Another methodologic variable of great import in the T3 and T4 radioimmunoassay is the vehicle in which the standards for the standard curve are diluted. If the standard curve is prepared in protein-free buffer, a higher bound-to-free ratio is observed than if the buffer contains protein. Carriers for such a standard curve have included hypothyroid sheep serum and 4 percent human serum albumin.[21,29] Theoretically, it is best to employ human serum and we, as well as Larsen,[20] and Beckers[30] have employed T3, T4-free serum prepared by a charcoal extraction procedure as a vehicle in which the standard curve is constructed. Since the standard curve obtained utilizing this approach has a lower bound-to-free ratio, the values obtained are lower than if the standard curve is prepared in protein-free buffer.

Cross-reaction. T3 and T4 molecules differ by only a single iodine atom. When these molecules are employed as immunogens, the potential for cross-reactivity against one or the other compound exists. In the case of the T4 assay, even if appreciable cross-reactivity existed between the anti-T4 antibody and T3, the effect on the observed T4 value is small, since the T3 concentration is very low relative to the T4 level in serum. In the case of the T3 radioimmunoassay, the differences in serum levels of T3 and T4 result in a significant overestimation of T3 unless the degree of cross-reactivity is ex-ceedingly small. Therefore, great care must be exercised in checking each T3 antiserum for its degree of cross-reactivity to purified T4. If cross-reactivity greater than 1 to 1,000 is found, the antibody probably should not be employed.

Combined T3 and T4 Radioimmunoassay

Utilizing the aforementioned principles, we have developed a rapid radioimmunoassay for measuring T3 and T4 in unextracted serum.[25] By combining the T3 and T4 antisera and by utilizing 2 isotopes, we have been able to measure both hormones simultaneously in the same test tube.

Materials. The materials required for this assay include antiserum to T3 and T4, T3-T4-free serum, nonradioactive standards for T3 and T4, $T3^{125}I$ and $T4^{131}I$ and ANS. Antiserum to T3 was produced in rabbits by injection of a T3-albumin conjugate prepared as described by Gharib, et al.[18] Antiserum to T4 was produced in analogous fashion. The presence and titer of antibody was determined as previously described.[25,28] The antiserum solution employed in this assay was prepared by mixing antiserum to T3 and antiserum to T4 in the same vessel with barbital diluent (0.08M sodium barbital, 0.1 Gm/100 ml bovine serum albumin, pH 8.4). The appropriate dilution must be individually determined for a given antibody.

Serum free of T3 and T4 (T3, T4-free serum) was prepared by incubating 100 ml of normal human serum with 20 Gm of Norit A charcoal* for 24 hours at 4°C. The resulting slurry was centrifuged 3 times at 20,000 rpm. This procedure removes over 99 percent of the T3 and T4 from serum, and does not affect total protein concentration, pH or T4-binding capacity. Nonradioactive standards of T3 and T4 were obtained from Sigma Chemical Corp. in the free acid form. T3 was dissolved in a mixture of ethanol and in HCl in a ratio of 2:1; T4 in 0.13M NaOH, 70 percent ethanol solution.

---

* Sigma Chemical Corp., St. Louis, Mo.

The standards were prepared in T3, T4-free serum.

T3 ^{125}I was obtained from the Abbott Laboratories* and T4 ^{131}I was initially obtained commercially from the same source, but now must be prepared utilizing chloramine-T in a standard iodinating procedure. The isotope mixture used in this assay was prepared by diluting both isotopes in barbital diluent in the same vessel at a concentration of 30 pg T3 ^{125}I and 50 pg of T4 ^{131}I per 100 λ of diluent; 8-anilino-l-naphthlenesulfonic acid (ANS)† was dissolved in barbital diluent. A concentration of 175 μg/0.2 ml was employed in assays in which serum or standards were diluted 1:4. In those cases involving serum samples or standards diluted 1:2, 350 μg/0.2 ml was used.

Assay Procedure

The assay procedure was performed in quadruplicate in 10 x 75 mm disposable glass tubes by the sequential addition of 0.1 ml of the unknown sample or standard (which had been diluted 1:2 or 1:4 in barbital diluent), 0.1 ml of the isotope solution, 0.2 ml of the ANS solution and 0.1 ml of the antibody solution. In those instances in which it was necessary to use a 1:2 dilution of hypothyroid serum to achieve maximal sensitivity, the ANS concentration was doubled to 350 μg/per tube, and the standard curve in T3, T4-free serum was run at a 1:2 dilution. For hyperthyroid sera suitable dilutions with T3, T4-free serum were employed. The assay mixture was agitated in a vortex mixer and incubated for 90 minutes at 37°C in a gently shaking water bath. After incubation, the samples were allowed to cool for 10 minutes in a 4°C cold room where the separation was carried out by the addition of 1 ml of a stock solution of dextran-charcoal.[35] The stock solution was prepared by mixing 5 Gm of Norit A charcoal and 0.5 Gm of dextran (MW 86,000)‡ in 600 ml of barbital diluent and constantly stirring with a magnetic stirrer to prevent settling during the addition procedure. The reaction mixture was agitated in a vortex mixer, incubated at 4° C for 20 minutes, and centrifuged at 1,000 × g for 15 minutes. The temperature at which the separation is performed is critical, since higher temperatures result in a time-dependent removal of antibody-bound T3 by the charcoal. At 4° C, the dextran-charcoal binding of hormone reached equilibrium within 15 minutes; 20 minutes was therefore selected for the second incubation. The supernatant containing the antibody-bound hormone was decanted off the hard charcoal pellet containing the free hormone. The two fractions were then counted in a 2-channel gamma counter* equipped with a 300-sample automatic changer.

Binding of serum proteins to T3 and T4 was accomplished by using barbital buffer to inhibit binding to thyroxine-binding prealbumin and ANS to inhibit binding to thyroxine-binding globulin (TBG). Figures 10-1 and 10-2 show typical standard curves for T3 and T4 prepared in buffer and also in T3, T4-free serum with and without ANS. The serum standard curves for both T3 and T4 obtained with ANS are almost identical to those obtained with buffer alone. Routinely a concentration of 175 μg per tube was selected because it was found that ANS at a concentration in excess of 150 μg per tube successfully inhibits TBG binding of T3 and T4 in hypothyroid, normal, pregnant and hyperthyroid subjects. The antigen-antibody reaction reaches equilibrium within 60 minutes at 37° C. We chose a 90-minute incubation time which was found to fall well within the plateau of the equilibrium curve.

Neither the anti-T3 nor the anti-T4 antisera used in this assay showed measurable cross-reaction with monoiodotyrosine, diiodotyrosine or ANS. The anti-T3 antiserum showed less than 1:5,000 cross-reaction with chromatographically-purified T4; the anti-T4 antiserum did not cross-react with T3. Re-

---

* North Chicago, Ill.
† Eastman Kodak Corp.
‡ K and K Labs, Hollywood, Calif.

---

* Nuclear Chicago

Fig. 10-1. The standard curve has been prepared by adding T3 to barbital diluent (●) and to T3, T4-free serum in the presence of ANS (○) and without ANS (□). Concentrations of 0, 12.5, 25, 50, 100, 200 and 400 pg of T3 per tube were prepared, representing T3 concentrations of 0, 50, 100, 200, 400, 800 and 1600 ng of T3/100 ml of serum. A parallel curve was obtained with dilutions of hyperthyroid serum (△). (Mitsuma, T., Colucci, J., Shenkman, L., and Hollander, C.: Rapid simultaneous radioimmunoassay for triiodothyronine and thyroxine in unextracted serum. Biochem. Biophys. Res. Commun., *46*:2107-2113, 1972)

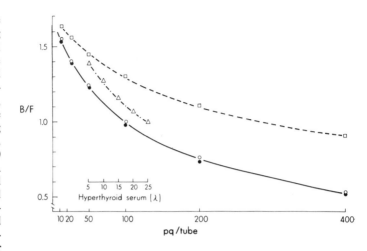

covery experiments performed by the addition of known amounts of T3 and T4 to T3, T4-free serum and normal serum demonstrated a recovery of 99.4 ± 2.9 percent for T3 and 100.8 ± 1.4 percent for T4. The T4 values obtained in this assay were compared with determinations on the identical specimens by competitive protein-binding analysis.* In 180 specimens, from 40 hypo-

* Boston Medical Laboratories

thyroid patients, 60 hyperthyroid subjects and 80 normal subjects, the agreement was excellent (coefficient of correlation: 0.99). Analysis of T3 and T4 in 5λ, 10λ, 20λ, and 25λ of hyperthyroid serum diluted to a 25λ volume in T3, T4-free serum yielded a curve superimposable upon standard curves obtained by the addition of T3 and T4 to T3, T4-free serum (see Figs. 10-1 and 10-2). Intra-assay reproducibility, assessed by measuring the identical sample 33 times was

Fig. 10-2. The standard curve has been prepared by adding T4 to barbital diluent (●) and to T3, T4-free serum in the presence of ANS (○) and without ANS (□). Concentrations of 0, 0.1, 0.5, 1, 2, 3, 4 and 5 ng of T4 per tube were prepared, representing concentrations of 0, 0.4, 2, 4, 8, 16 and 20 μg of T4/100 ml of serum. A parallel curve was obtained with dilutions of hyperthyroid serum (△). (Mitsuma, T., Colucci, J., Shenkman, L., and Hollander, C.: Rapid simultaneous radioimmunoassay for triiodothyronine and thyroxine in unextracted serum. Biochem. Biophys. Res. Commun., *46*: 2107-2113, 1972)

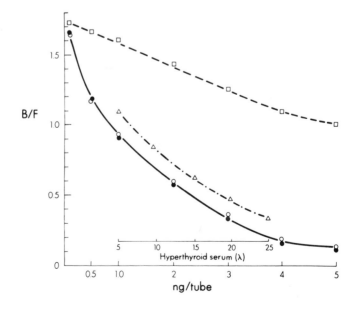

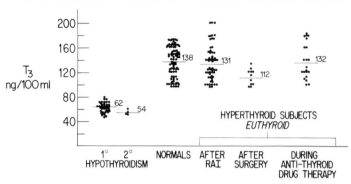

T3 LEVELS IN HYPOTHYROID AND NORMAL SUBJECTS
AND IN EUTHYROID PATIENTS WITH TREATED HYPERTHYROIDISM

Fig. 10-3. Patients with 1° and 2° hypothyroidism have T3 levels below normal. Hyperthyroid subjects who have been rendered euthyroid by either radioactive iodine (RAI), surgery or goitrogens have normal T3 levels.

4.4 percent for T3 and 4.1 percent for T4. Interassay variation, evaluated by determining 18 paired specimens in 2 successive assays was 6.8 percent for T3 and 7.4 percent for T4.

The results of our clinical observations are presented in Table 10-1. In 80 normal subjects, the mean T3 concentration was 138 ± 8.1 ng/100 ml (mean ± SEM) and mean T4 was 7.5 ± 0.5 μg/100 ml. In 60 patients with toxic diffuse goiter mean T3 was 494 ± 75 ng/100 ml and mean T4 was 16.0 ± 1.2 μg/100 ml. Forty hypothyroid subjects had a serum T3 which ranged from 48 ng/100 ml to 82 ng/100 ml and serum T4 varied from 0.2 μg/100 ml to 2.0 μg/ 100 ml.

The values for T3 found in normal, hypothyroid and hyperthyroid subjects are in good agreement with our own previously published results and with those of others. To further validate the T3 assay, we examined T3 levels in hyperthyroid patients who had been rendered euthyroid by surgery, antithyroid drugs and radioiodine and had normal T4 levels. As is seen in Figure 10-3, these patients had T3 levels within the normal range. The T4

determinations by this radioimmunoassay procedure agree well with those found by competitive protein-binding analysis. The combined T3, T4 method appears to be an accurate, sensitive and specific one, entails no serum extraction and permits the simultaneous measurements of T3 and T4 in 3 hours. These features render this assay highly desirable for both clinical and research applications.

Comparison of Various Radioimmunoassays for T3 and T4

As has already been pointed out, a number of different laboratories have developed radioimmunoassays for T3. A variety of approaches have been utilized for each of the steps involved and, despite rather considerable differences in methodology, the results of the various groups have been in general agreement. Our laboratory has obtained a normal range for T3 of 96 to 172 ng/100 ml. Larsen,[20] Chopra, et al.,[23] Huefner and Hesch,[19] Lieblich and Utiger,[21] Beckers,[30] Burger, et al.,[36] Docter, et al.,[37] and Reichlin's group have obtained similar results on unextracted serum. Others, in-

Table 10-1. T3 and T4 Levels in Normal, Hyperthyroid and Hypothyroid Subjects.

Subject	Number	T3 (ng/100 ml)	T4 (μg/100 ml)
Normal	80	138 ± 8.1 (mean ± 1 SEM)	7.5 ± 0.5 (mean ± 1 SEM)
Hyperthyroid	60	494 ± 75 (mean ± 1 SEM)	16.0 ± 1.2 (mean ± 1 SEM)
Hypothyroid	40	48-82 (range)	0.2-2.0 (range)

cluding Ekins' group,[34] Surks, et al.[32] and Werner's group[33] have obtained similar results utilizing a preliminary extraction with methanol or Sephadex G-25 chromatography. It is of interest that these results by radioimmunoassay agree closely with results obtained by gas liquid chromatography.[28,38] They also are in accord with the results of most competitive protein-binding assays in which either correction for conversion of T4 to T3 is made or in which care has been taken to minimize conversion.[14,39,40] Two groups have reported a somewhat higher normal range.[18,41] The differences noted between various laboratories may perhaps be related to methodologic differences or may reflect actual differences in thyroid hormone levels dependent on demographic characteristics of the populations studied. Differences in iodine intake, for example, can affect the relative rates of T3/T4 secretion, and thereby alter serum T3 concentrations. Recent studies by Rubenstein, et al.[33] have shown that T3 levels tend to fall with age. This variable may, perhaps, also contribute to some of the observed differences in the normal T3 range between various laboratories.

T3 concentrations found in hyperthyroid patients have been uniformly elevated and values ranging from 300 to 3,000 ng/100 ml have been reported. All reports to date indicate that T3 levels clearly distinguish the normal and hyperthyroid states and no overlap has been observed. Thus, a T3 determination by radioimmunoassay appears to be quite valuable in diagnosing hyperthyroidism. In hypothyroidism, however, the findings are less clear. Some groups found a clear-cut separation between hypothyroid and normal subjects[22,25,28,32] while others found a significant overlap.[21] Surks, et al.[32] obtained very low T3 values in hypothyroid subjects, and they suggest that a more accurate means of determining T3 levels in hypothyroidism is afforded by a preliminary extraction of serum prior to radioimmunoassay. These differences require resolution, since a normal T3 concentration in hypothyroidism is difficult to reconcile with the

concept of T3 as the active form of thyroid hormone unless alterations in free T3 levels or tissue concentrations of T3 are present.

Thus far, only a few radioimmunoassays for T4 have been reported. A radioimmunoassay for T4 in unextracted serum has been described by Chopra. He employed anti-T4 antibody produced by immunizing rabbits with human thyroglobulin, ANS as a blocker, and second antibody to separate bound from free T4.[26] The values obtained in this manner generally agreed with the results by competitive protein-binding analysis. However, serum T4 estimates by radioimmunoassay were higher than those by competitive protein-binding analysis in sera from several hyperthyroid patients and from a few euthyroid patients given TSH. The reasons for discrepancy are uncertain but could be related to the presence of T4 covalently linked to serum proteins. This discordance between competitive protein binding and radioimmunoassay has not been observed by us or by Larsen.[25,27]

Physiological Considerations

The development of methods for the measurement of circulating thyroxine whether indirectly by iodometry or, more specifically, by competitive protein-binding analysis has permitted a rather accurate analysis of thyroid status. Thus, thyroxine levels were found to be reliably elevated in the serum of patients with untreated hyperthyroidism and depressed in hypothyroidism prior to initiation of therapy. Moreover, T4 levels can be used to follow the results of therapy. Hyperthyroid patients rendered euthyroid by surgery, radioiodine or antithyroid drugs usually demonstrate a fall in T4 levels to normal as euthyroidism is achieved. Similarly, as hypothyroid patients are given replacement doses of T4, T4 levels rise to normal in parallel with attainment of euthyroidism.

It should be noted that T4 and T3 circulate largely bound to binding proteins in the serum.[42,43] Approximately 99.95 percent of T4 and 99.75 percent of T3 is bound for the most part to thyroxine-binding globulin or

TBG and, to a lesser extent, to thyroxine-binding prealbumin or TBPA and to albumin.[43] Although the free hormone levels are quite low, it seems likely that this overall fraction is the metabolically active form. One general exception to the parallelism of thyroid status and total T4 can be found in the patients with abnormalities in thyroid-binding proteins. It has been recognized that pregnancy and estrogen administration result in an elevation of TBG capacity and a concomitant rise in total T4. It is of some clinical import that ovulatory suppressants contain sufficient estrogen to produce these effects.[44] Similar changes in TBG have been noted in patients who have acute intermittent porphyria[45] and in the rare patient with congenitally elevated TBG levels. Although total serum T4 levels are elevated in patients with elevated TBG, they are nevertheless euthyroid since their free T4 levels are normal. Analogous changes in the opposite direction can be seen in subjects with decreased TBG capacity. Thus, subjects with congenital absence of TBG and patients receiving androgens or anabolic steroids can have low TBG capacity and low total T4 and yet be clinically euthyroid with normal free T4 levels.

Twelve years after T4 was initially demonstrated in plasma, Gross and Pitt-Rivers identified triiodothyronine (T3) as a second circulating iodoaminoacid.[46] It has been subsequently shown that T3, like T4, is a normal thyroidal secretory product.[47] Because of the ease with which T3 and T4 are labeled with radioiodine, many studies have been performed on the detailed kinetics and metabolism of these compounds, in man as well as in experimental animals.[48,49]

Approximately 80 μg of T4 are secreted daily in man and distributed in a volume of 10 L. The fact that only 10 percent of the extrathyroidal pool of the hormone is degraded per day is noteworthy and contrasts with the very rapid metabolism of the polypeptide and steroid hormones. This comparatively slow turnover of T4 is apparently related to the strong binding of T4 to serum proteins. Presumably because of its weaker association with serum proteins, T3 is more rapidly metabolized and has a larger volume of distribution than T4. T3 distributes in a volume of 50 L and about half of it is degraded daily. Thus, despite its low level in serum relative to T4, it has been estimated that T3 contributes a major portion of the calorigenic potency of the thyroid hormones.[49] Indeed, it has been suggested that T3 is the active thyroid hormone and that T4 serves merely as a precursor or prohormone.[50]

With the advent of the radioimmunoassay, it has become possible to examine more closely the physiologic and clinical significance of T3 in health and disease and to delineate those instances in which T3 appears to play a major role, including the following.

1. While iodide deprivation leads to a marked fall in serum T4, serum T3 levels in animals and in man remain comparatively normal.[51,52] This may be a reflection of high T3/T4 ratios in the thyroid gland as a result of iodine deficiency. It has been suggested that the relative hypersecretion of T3 may represent an important homeostatic mechanism in the face of inadequate iodine substrate.[53] Increased T3/T4 secretion ratios have also been noted in response to elevations of TSH[20,21] and since TSH levels probably rise in iodine deficiency this may be the explanation for the observed changes in T3 and T4.

2. In conventional hyperthyroidism, whether caused by toxic diffuse goiter (Graves' disease), toxic nodular goiter, or autonomously functioning adenoma, T3 concentrations are invariably elevated. In a series of 64 patients with the usual forms of thyrotoxicosis, we found that T3 concentration varied from 232 ng/100 ml to 1,700 ng/100 ml. This contrasts with the findings in normal and hypothyroid subjects, (see Fig. 10-3): 80 normal subjects had T3 concentrations ranging from 96 ng/100 ml to 172 ng/100 ml with a mean of 138 ng/

100 ml;[28] 45 patients with primary hypothyroidism had a mean serum T3 concentration of 62 ng/100 ml and 4 patients with hypothyroidism secondary to pituitary disease had a mean serum T3 concentration of 54 ng/100 ml. In general, patients with hypothyroidism had T3 levels which were approximately one-half those found in normals. Similar results have been noted by others.[20,29] However, as noted by others, some patients with hypothyroidism whom we have studied subsequently have had T3 levels which overlap the normal range. This point is of critical interest and is currently under intensive scrutiny. As is anticipated, the elevated T3 levels in hyperthyroid subjects fell to normal with the induction of the euthyroid state by surgery, radioiodine, or antithyroid drugs (see Fig. 10-3).[28]

3. Since first calling attention to the syndrome of T3 toxicosis (thyrotoxicosis caused by excessive secretion of T3 rather than T4), we have identified 40 additional patients in the course of 3 years.[54,55] Similar patients have been described by others.[14,56-59] Twenty-nine of our patients appeared to have Graves' disease; 8, autonomous adenoma; and 3, toxic multinodular goiter. These patients all had normal total and free T4 concentrations, normal thyroid-binding proteins, and a normal or elevated thyroidal uptake of radioiodine which could not be suppressed with exogenous thyroid hormone. All had elevated total T3 levels ranging from 228 to 2,000 ng/100 ml (Fig. 10-4) and high free T3 levels as well. The clinical picture and the response to therapy in patients with T3 toxicosis were indistinguishable from those with conventional thyrotoxicosis. More recently, we have seen this syndrome develop in children.[60] Moreover, we have noted several patients with a past history of conventional thyrotoxicosis who, after a euthyroid interval varying from several months to 30 years, developed a clinical recurrence of the thyrotoxic state with normal T4 but elevated T3 levels (Table 10-2).[61] It appears, therefore, that some patients with recurrent hyper-

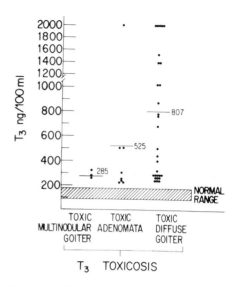

Fig. 10-4. The normal T3 range is depicted in the shaded area. All patients with T3 toxicosis, regardless of mode of presentation, had T3 levels above the normal range.

thyroidism may present as T3 toxicosis. This form of T3 toxicosis may be quite common, and, indeed, it may be the most frequently observed variant of isolated hypersecretion of T3. In addition, we have observed several patients with conventional hyperthyroidism who early in the course of antithyroid drug therapy remained clinically toxic despite a fall in their T4 levels to normal. It is interesting to note that in these patients, T3 levels had not yet fallen to normal, and probably accounted for the toxic state. There have also been reports of hyperthyroid patients who have been rendered euthyroid by either radioactive iodine or goitrogens and were then found to have low T4 but normal T3 levels.[62] In these patients, the euthyroid state was presumably being maintained by the normal levels of T3.

4. Perhaps of greatest potential clinical import is the observation that hyperthyroid patients may pass through a stage of T3 toxicosis before developing the usual form of thyrotoxicosis.[63] Over the past year we have had the opportunity to observe 10 hyperthyroid patients during the early phase of

Table 10-2. Recurrent Hyperthyroidism Presenting as Triiodothyronine (T3 Toxicosis).

Pa-tient	Sex	Age yr	Previous Therapy	Euthyroid Interval	Mode of Presentation*	Total T3 ng/100 ml	Free T3	Total T4 μg/100 ml	Free T4 ng/100 ml
1	F	58	Surgery	30 years	Autonomous adenoma	210	0.6	5.7	1.6
2	M	20	Surgery	5 years	Graves' disease	2,000	4.0	4.3	1.0
3	F	48	131I propyl-thiouracil	8 months	Graves' disease	272	0.5	7.5	1.4
4	F	83	131I	3 years	Autonomous adenoma	260	0.5	4.0	0.8
5	F	46	Methimazole	10 years	Graves' disease	280	0.9	5.6	1.2
6	F	19	Propyl-thiouracil	3 years	Graves' disease	1,120	2.3	6.2	1.2
7	F	74	Surgery	26 years	Graves' disease	640	1.3	7.2	2.0
8	M	74	131I	6 months	Graves' disease	240	1.2	6.2	1.5
9	F	75	131I	1 year	Graves' disease	320	0.9	6.0	1.6
10	M	55	Propyl-thiouracil	4 months	Graves' disease	210	1.6	5.0	1.1
Normal range						96-172	0.1-0.4	4-11	1.0-2.1

* In patients 2 through 10 initial and recurrent episodes of hyperthyroidism took the same form. Patient 1 had Graves' disease initially and presented with an autonomous adenoma 30 years later.

their disease. Although all had a clearly elevated serum T3 level, they were followed without therapy because their symptoms were relatively mild. After 1 to 10 months, 4 of these patients developed more overt thyrotoxicosis with classical physical and laboratory findings consistent with conventional toxic diffuse goiter, including a high serum T4 level. In these 4 instances, high circulating T3 levels were an early premonitory finding in toxic diffuse goiter. The other 6 patients remained symptomatic but failed to manifest an increased T4 over 12 to 18 months.

As further work is being done in this area, it is becoming apparent that T3 plays an important, if not the major role in determining thyroidal status. Indeed, the intriguing but speculative concept that T4 is a pro-hormone and acts by means of conversion to T3, initially raised by Gross and Pitt-Rivers in 1952,[50] is now receiving renewed attention.

References

1. Trevorrow, V.: Studies on the nature of the iodine in blood. J. Biol. Chem., *127*:737, 1939.
2. Riggs, D. S., Lavietes, P. H., and Man, E. B.: Investigations on the nature of blood iodine. J. Biol. Chem., *143*:363, 1942.
3. Man, E. B., Kydd, D. M., and Peters, J. P.: Butanol-extractable iodine of serum. J. Clin. Invest., *30*:531, 1951.
4. Wynn, J.: Organic iodine constituents in human serum. Arch. Biochem., *87*:120, 1960.
5. Pileggi, V. J., Lee, N. D., Golub, O. J., and Henry, R. J.: Determination of iodine compounds in serum. I. Serum thyroxine in the presence of some iodine contaminants. J. Clin. Endocrinol. Metab., *21*:1272, 1961.

6. Barker, S. B., Humphrey, M. J., and Soley, M. H.: Clinical determination of protein-bound iodine. J. Clin. Invest., *30*:55, 1951.

7. Sunderman, F. W., and Sunderman, F. W., Jr.: The clinical significance of measurements of protein-bound iodine. Amer. J. Clin. Pathol., *24*:885, 1954.

8. Davis, P. J.: Factors affecting the determination of serum protein-bound iodine. Amer. J. Med., *40*:918, 1966.

9. Gross, J., and Pitt-Rivers, R.: The identification of 3:5:3′-1-triiodothyronine in human plasma. Lancet, *1*:439, 1952.

10. Hollander, C. S., and Shenkman, L.: The physiologic significance of triiodothyronine. Amer. J. Med. Sci., *264*:5, 1973.

11. Murphy, B. E. P., and Pattee, C. J.: Determination of thyroxine utilizing the property of protein-binding. J. Clin. Endocrinol. Metab., *24*:187, 1964.

12. Nauman, J. A., Nauman, A., and Werner, S. C.: Total and free triiodothyronine in human serum. J. Clin. Invest., *46*:1346, 1967.

13. Sterling, K., Bellabarba, D., Newman, E. S., and Brenner, M. A.: Determination of triiodothyronine concentration in human serum. J. Clin. Invest., *48*:1150, 1969.

14. Larsen, P. R.: Technical aspects of the estimation of triiodothyronine in human serum: Evidence of conversion of thyroxine to triiodothyronine during assay. Metabolism, *20*:609, 1971.

15. Ekins, R. P.: The estimation of thyroxine in human plasma by an electrophoretic technique. Clin. Chim. Acta, *5*:453, 1960.

16. Green, W. L.: Separation of iodo compounds in serum by chromatography on Sephadex columns. J. Chromatogr., *72*:83, 1972.

17. Brown, B. L., Ekins, R. P., Ellis, S. M., and Reith, W. S.: Specific antibodies to triiodothyronine hormone. Nature, *226*:359, 1970.

18. Gharib, H., Ryan, R. J., Mayberry, W. E., and Hockert, T.: Radioimmunoassay for triiodothyronine (T3): I. Affinity and specificity of the antibody for T3. J. Clin. Endocrinol. Metab., *33*:509, 1971.

19. Huefner, M., and Hesch, R. D.: Results of a radioimmunoassay of triiodothyronine. Proceedings, European Thyroid Association, 1972.

20. Larsen, P. R.: Direct immunoassay of triiodothyronine in human serum. J. Clin. Invest., *51*:1939, 1972.

21. Lieblich, J., and Utiger, R. D.: Triiodothyronine radioimmunoassay. J. Clin. Invest., *51*:157, 1972.

22. Nejad, I. F., Bollinger, V. A., Mitnick, M. A., and Reichlin, S.: Importance of T3 (triiodothyronine) secretion in altered states of thyroid function in the rat: cold exposure, subtotal thyroidectomy, and hypophysectomy. Trans. Assoc. Amer. Phys., 1972 (in press).

23. Chopra, I. J., Ho, R. S., and Lam, R.: An improved radioimmunoassay of triiodothyronine in serum: Its application to clinical and physiological studies. J. Lab. Clin. Med., *80*:729, 1972.

24. Vaitukaitis, J., Robbins, J. B., Nieschlag, E., and Ross, G. T.: A method for producing specific antisera with small doses of immunogen. J. Clin. Endocrinol. Metab., *33*:988, 1971.

25. Mitsuma, T., Colucci, J., Shenkman, L., and Hollander, C. S.: Rapid simultaneous radioimmunoassay for triiodothyronine and thyroxine in unextracted serum. Biochem. Biophys. Res. Commun., *46*:2107, 1972.

26. Chopra, I.: A radioimmunoassay for measurement of thyroxine in unextracted serum. J. Clin. Endocrinol. Metab., *34*:938, 1972.

27. Larsen, P. R., Dockalova, J., Sipula, D., and Wu, F. M.: Immunoassay of thyroxine in unextracted human serum. J. Clin. Endocrinol. Metab., *37*:177, 1973.

28. Mitsuma, T., Nihei, N., Gershengorn, M. C., and Hollander, C. S.: Serum triiodothyronine: Measurements in human serum by radioimmunoassay with corroboration by gas liquid chromatography. J. Clin. Invest., *50*:2679, 1971.

29. Chopra, I. J., Solomon, D. H., and Beall, G. N.: Radioimmunoassay for measurements of triiodothyronine in human serum. J. Clin. Invest., 50:2033, 1971.

30. Beckers, C., Cornette, C., and Thalasso, M.: Serum triiodothyronine: importance of its determination in thyroid disorders and in the study of the hypothalamus-pituitary interplay. Proceedings, European Thyroid Association, 1972.

31. Huefner, M., and Hesch, R. D.: A comparison of different compounds for TBG-blocking used in radioimmunoassay for triiodothyronine. Clin. Chim. Acta, *44*:101, 1973.

32. Surks, M. I., Schadlow, A. R., and Oppenheimer, J. H.: A new radioimmunoassay for plasma 1-triiodothyronine: measurements in thyroid disease and in patients maintained on hormonal replacement. J. Clin. Invest., *51*:3104, 1972.

33. Rubenstein, H. A., Butler, Y. P., Jr., and Werner, S. C.: Progressive decrease in

serum triiodothyronine concentrations with human aging: Radioimmunoassay following extraction of serum. J. Clin. Endocrinol. Metab., *37*:247, 1973.

34. Williams, E. S., Pharoah, P., Lawton, N. F., Ekins, R., and Ellis, S. M.: Serum triiodothyronine concentration in subjects from an area of endemic goiter. Proceedings, European Thyroid Association, 1972. Published in Isr. J. Med. Sci., *8*:1871, 1973.

35. Mitsuma, T., Gershengorn, M. C., Colucci, J., and Hollander, C. S.: Radioimmunoassay of triiodothyronine in unextracted human serum. J. Clin. Endocrinol. Metab., 33:364, 1971.

36. Burger, A., Miller, B., Sakoloff, C., and Vallotton, M. B.: Thyroxine et triiodothyronine seriques. Schweiz. Med. Wochenschr, *102*:1280, 1972.

37. Docter, R., Hennemann, G., and Bernard, H.: A radioimmunoassay (RIA) for measurement of triiodothyronine (T3) in serum. Proceedings, European Thyroid Association, 1972.

38. Nihei, N., Gershengorn, H. C., Mitsuma, T., Stringham, L. R., *et al.*: Measurements of triiodothyronine and thyroxine in human serum by gas-liquid chromatography. Ann. Biochem., *43*:433, 1971.

39. Fisher, D. A., and Dussault, J. H.: Contribution of methodological artifacts to the measurement of T3 concentrations in serum. J. Clin. Endocrinol. Metab., *32*: 675, 1971.

40. Skovsted, L., and Christensen, L. K.: Determination of serum T3 by a non-radioimmunoassay procedure. Normal range and values in PTU-treated patients and other thyroid disorders. Abstr. No. 40. Proceedings, European Thyroid Assoc. Jerusalem, Israel, Sept. 17-21, 1973.

41. Sterling, K., and Milch, P. O.: Thermal inactivation of thyroxine-binding globulin for direct radioimmunoassay of triiodothyronine in serum. J. Clin. Invest., *52*(abstract): 82a, 1973.

42. Robbins, J., and Rall, J. E.: Patients associated with the thyroid hormones. Physiol. Rev., *40*:415, 1960.

43. Hollander, C. S., Odak, V. V., Prout, T. E., and Asper, S. P., Jr.: An evaluation of the role of prealbumin in the binding of thyroxine. J. Clin. Endocrinol. Metab., *22*: 617, 1962.

44. Hollander, C. S., Garcia, A. M., Sturgis, S. H., and Selenkow, H. A.: Effect of an ovulatory suppressant on the serum protein bound iodine and the red cell uptake of radioactive triiodothyronine. N. Eng. J. Med., *269*:501, 1963.

45. Hollander, C. S., Scott, R. L., Tschudy, D. P., Perloth, M., *et al.*: Increased protein-bound iodine and thyroxine binding globulin in acute intermittent porphyria. N. Eng. J. Med., *277*:995, 1967.

46. Gross, J., and Pitt-Rivers, R.: The identification of 3:5:3'-L-triiodothyronine in human plasma. Lancet, *1*:439, 1952.

47. Taurog, A., Wheat, J. D., and Chaikoff, I. L.: Nature of the ^{131}I compounds appearing in the thyroid vein after injection of iodine; [131]I. Endocrinology, *58*:121-131, 1956.

48. Rall, J. E., Robbins, J., and Lewallen, C. G.: The thyroid. *In* Pincus, G., Thimann, K. V., Astwood, E. B. (eds.): The Hormones. vol. V, p. 159. New York, Academic Press, 1964.

49. Robbins, J., and Rall, J. E.: The iodine-containing hormones. *In* Gray, C. H., Bacharach, A. C. (eds.): Hormones in Blood. ed. 2, p. 383. New York, Academic Press, 1967.

50. Gross, J., and Pitt-Rivers, R.: Physiologic activity of 3:5:3'-L-triiodothyronine. Lancet, *1*:593, 1952.

51. Greer, M. A., Grimm, Y., and Studer, H.: Qualitative changes in the secretion of thyroid hormones induced by iodine deficiency. Endocrinology, *83*:1193, 1968.

52. Hollander, C. S., Nihei, N., Mitsuma, T., *et al.*: Elevated serum triiodothyronine in association with altered available iodide in normal and hyperthyroid subjects. Clin. Res., *19*:560, 1971.

53. Hollander, C. S.: Discussion of Sterling, K.: Rec. Prog. Hor. Res., *26*:249, 1970.

54. Hollander, C. S.: On the nature of circulating thyroid hormone: clinical studies of triiodothyronine and thyroxine in serum using gas chromatographic methods. Trans. Assoc. Amer. Phys., *81*:76, 1968.

55. Hollander, C. S., Mitsuma, T., Nihei, N., *et al.*: Clinical and laboratory observations in cases of triiodothyronine toxicosis confirmed by radioimmunoassay. Lancet, *1*: 609, 1972.

56. Sterling, K., Refetoff, S., and Selenkow, H. A.: T3 thyrotoxicosis—thyrotoxicosis due to elevated serum triiodothyronine levels. JAMA, *213*:571, 1970.

57. Wahner, W. H., and Gorman, C. A.: Interpretation of serum triiodothyronine levels measured by Sterling technique. N. Eng. J. Med., *284*:225, 1971.

58. Sakurada, T., Saito, S., and Ingaki, K., *et al.*: Quantitative determination of total and

free triiodothyronine and thyroxine. Tohoku J. Exp. Med., *99*:179, 1969.

59. Ivy, H. K., Wahner, H. W., and Gorman, C. A.: Triiodothyronine (T3) toxicosis. Arch. Intern. Med., *128*:529, 1971.

60. Mitsuma, T., Owens, R., Shenkman, L., Reiter, E., and Hollander, C. S.: T3 toxicosis in childhood: Hyperthyroidism due to isolated hypersecretion of triiodothyronine. J. Pediatr., *81*:982, 1972.

61. Shenkman, L., Mitsuma, T., Blum, M., and Hollander, C. S.: Recurrent hyperthyroidism presenting as T3 toxicosis. Ann. Int. Med., *77*:410, 1972.

62. Sterling, K., Brenner, M. A., Newman, E. S., Odell, W. D., and Bellabarba, D.: The significance of triiodothyronine (T3) in maintenance of euthyrodism after treatment of hyperthyroidism. J. Clin. Endocrinol. Metab., *33*:729, 1971.

63. Hollander, C. S., Mitsuma, T., Shenkman, L., *et al.*: Hypertriiodothyroninaemia as a premonitory manifestation of thyrotoxicosis. Lancet, *2*:731, 1971.

11 Radioimmunoassay of Circulating Unconjugated Estrogens During Growth and Development in Normal and Abnormal Conditions

FREDERIC M. KENNY, M.D.
KITTI ANGSUSINGHA, M.D.
with the Technical Assistance of
CATHERINE RICHARDS, B.S. AND MILADA BRYCH, B.S.

INTRODUCTION

The recent availability of radioimmuno-assay (RIA) methods for determining peptide and steroid hormones permits physiologists, clinical investigators, and physicians to obtain answers to questions which until recently they were not able to ask because of the limitations of previous methodologies. Furthermore, the rapid transmission of a "research technique" to the clinical chemistry laboratory is illustrated by the increasing availability of estrogens by RIA to the practicing physician.

Prior to discussing the use of radioimmunoassay, a brief mention of other methods for determining estrogens is discussed. The majority of reports on urinary estrogens have utilized techniques involving hydrolysis of the specimen followed by extraction and separation of the phenolic fraction with quantitation by colorimetry (i.e., Kober color reaction).[1] More recently, gas-liquid chromatography (GLC) has been employed for quantitation. Kaplan and colleagues[2] employed thin layer (TLC) and anion exchange column chromatography of the phenolic extract, prior to quantitation by GLC, for low level urines. For specimens with high estrogen content (i.e., pregnancy) GLC was performed without prior conjugate extraction, TLC and column chromatography. A good correlation was found when the results were compared with those obtained by radioimmunoassay.[2] Increased sensitivity was obtained using electron-capture GLC.[3]

Previous methods for quantitation of circulating estrogens have required large serum

Supported in part by USPHS Grants FR-05507, RR-05416 and RR-84; Health Research and Services Foundation P-45; and the Renziehausen Fund.

Abbreviations

Estrone = E_1; 3-hydroxyestra-1, 3, 5 (10)-triene-17-one

Estradiol = E_2; estra-1, 3, 5 (10)-triene-3, 17β-diol

Estriol = estra-1, 3, 5 (10)-triene-3, 16α, 17β-triol

RIA = radioimmunoassay

GLC = gas-liquid chromatography

TLC = thin layer chromatography

FSH = follicle-stimulating hormone

LH = luteinizing hormone

or plasma samples, and were sufficiently laborious to preclude widespread application. Those methods included double isotope derivative,[4] fluorometric[5] and gas chromatographic[6] techniques.

In the past several years we have witnessed the development of a number of protein-binding and RIA systems for the determinations of steroid hormones.[7,8] In addition, uterine cytosol as a specific binder has been used to quantitate unconjugated estrogens by radioligand assay.[9]

The author has employed a method which was developed by Dr. J. Hotchkiss[10] and further modified by her. The antibody which we use (Ferin-Vande Wiele and Caldwell) cross-reacts with E_1, E_2, E_3, and other naturally occuring estrogens. This has the advantage of permitting quantitation of various estrogens which have been previously separated by Sephadex-LH 20 chromatography.

The specificity (or lack thereof) of a particular antiestrogen antibody is related to the nature of the steroid-protein conjugate used to immunize the animal (i.e., guinea pig, sheep, rabbit). The degree of specificity of the antibody appears to be increased by use of steroid-protein conjugate antigens, in which the steroid is attached to the protein (i.e., bovine-serum protein) at a position distal to the structurally unique region of the estrogen molecule. Thus, Exley and co-workers[11] report a 17β-estradiol-6-(0-carboxymethyl) oxime-bovine serum albumin antigen, used to raise antisera in rabbits. This antiserum enabled radioimmunoassay to be performed directly on extracted plasma samples without prior chromatographic separation.

Regarding the method of chromatographic separation, many workers have employed Sephadex-LH 20 for the separation of circulating estrogens. It was concluded that this is entirely suitable, since other naturally-occurring estrogens do not contribute significantly to the plasma estrone and estradiol levels when studying normal males and nonpregnant females.[12]

In this chapter, the authors report data obtained in normal boys and girls from infancy through adolescence, and contrast them with the results in various abnormal conditions encountered by physicians dealing with patients in this age group. In addition, our results in mothers at term and in the infant during the perinatal period are referenced.[13]

METHODS

Serum Estrogens. Serum estrogens were determined by radioimmunoassay.[13,14] Sephadex LH-20 chromatography was employed to isolate E_1 and E_2. The residue of diethyl ether extracts of 0.2 to 1.5 ml serum was applied to Sephadex LH-20 columns (0.5 x 6.5 cm) previously equilibrated with eluting solvent mixture (heptane:chloroform:methanol:water, 10:10:1.5:0.06). Chromatography of ^{14}C-labeled steroids showed that estrone emerged from the column in the 1.3 to 3.3 ml fraction, while estradiol emerged in the 4.3 to 8.3 ml fraction. These columns, used repeatedly for 6 months, were stored immersed in column solvent in a closed glass container when not in use, and were recalibrated monthly using ^{14}C-labeled estrogens.

This chromatographic step isolates and removes some of the compounds known to cross-react weakly with our antiserum to estradiol-17β-succinylbovine serum albumin raised in ewes, kindly supplied by Dr. Ferin and Dr. Vande Wiele.[15] Cholesterol emerges in the first milliliter of the eluate, and estriol emerges considerably later than estradiol.

Triplicate standard curves for estrone and estradiol (5-100 pg) were prepared in 12 x 75 mm disposable glass culture tubes in which 2 or 4 ml respectively of column solvent had previously been evaporated.

The radioimmunoassay was performed by sequential addition of 100 μl of estrogen antiserum (diluted 1:135,000 for the estrone assay and 1:180,000 for the estradiol assay) followed 30 minutes later by the addition of 100 μl of a tritiated estrone solution (estrone-2,4,6,7-^{3}H, SA = 95 c/mM,* approximately 10,000 cpm in 0.01M phosphate buffered saline containing 0.1% gela-

---

* New England Nuclear, Boston, Mass.

Table 11-1. Statistics Related to Levels of E_1 and E_2 in a Selected Group of Patients.

	Mean Levels of E_1*		Mean Levels of E_2			
	10-20	*<20*	*<5*	*5-10*	*10-20*	*>20*
Number of Patients	7	7	6	7	7	7
Average Number of Replicates/Patient	2.8	2.9	2.5	2.1	2.6	2.1
Mean	15.74	35.23	3.68	7.45	12.98	39.20
Range	10.1-21.6	18.7-62.3	.8-5.4	3.1-10.4	9.6-17.2	
Standard Deviation†	1.19	2.16	.66	1.55	1.30	1.77
Coefficient of Variation (%)	7.6	6.1	17.9	20.8	10.01	4.5

* Patients classified according to mean level.

† This value is the square root of the mean square of the pooled within patient variation (i.e., that variation among replications of measurements pooled over patients).

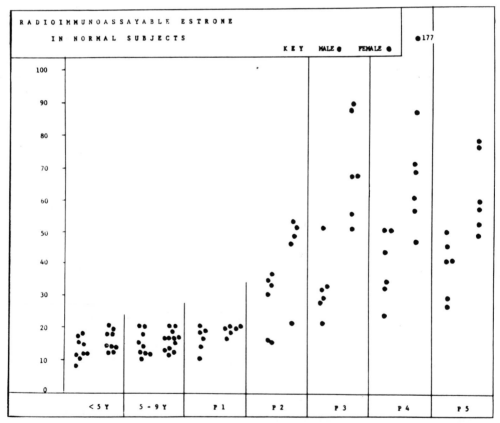

Fig. 11-1. Serum estrone in pg per ml of serum by age and secondary sexual development according to Tanner staging, where P1 indicates no sexual development; P5 is completed sexual development. Males are shown on the left, and females on the right for each age or Tanner stage.

There is no sex difference until Tanner Stage 2, when females begin to have higher values. Overlap between male and female values persists throughout adolescence for estrone.

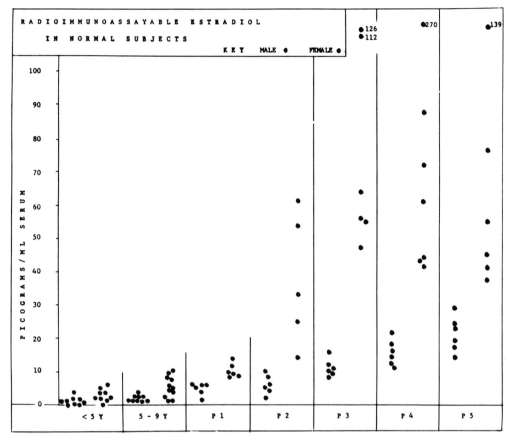

Fig. 11-2. Serum estradiol in pg per ml of serum. The format is identical to Fig. 11-1, with males on the left and females on the right for each age or Tanner stage grouping. It is evident that estradiol, the biologically most potent estrogen, rises gradually in males and females even prior to outward pubertal changes, and that the rise in females is greater. From the beginning to the completion of secondary sexual development, females had higher values with no overlap with those of the males.

tin). After overnight incubation of the samples at 4°C, separation of the antibody-bound and free steroid was performed.[10] The antibody-bound steroid was decanted into scintillation vials to which 10 ml of a toluene-based scintillation medium [7 Gm PPO* and 0.3 Gm bis-MSB† per 1 toluene] was added. The capped samples were shaken for 1 hour to ensure extraction of the radioactive steroid from the aqueous to the organic phase, and counted in a Packard model 3,320 liquid scintillation spectrometer with a tritium-counting efficiency of 50 to 55 percent.

Blanks. Blank values, determined by the extraction, chromatography and radioimmu-

noassay of appropriate aliquots of water, were equal to or slightly greater than 0 pg, but never equal to 5 pg of estrone and estradiol.

Sensitivity. Five pg of E_1 and E_2 were added in triplicate to water blank samples and processed using the described extraction and purification process. The results for E_1 were mean 5.1 with a range 4.8 to 5.3 pg; and for E_2 were 5.0 with a range 4.8 to 5.3 pg.

The reliability of the method as reflected by the standard deviation of the sampling error, decreases slightly with increasing amounts of E_1, and is essentially the same with increasing amounts of E_2 as shown in Table 11-1. The coefficient of variation

*Packard Instruments Co., Downers Grove, Ill.
†New England Nuclear, Boston, Mass.

ranged from 6.1 percent to 7.6 percent for E_1, and from 4.5 percent to 20.8 percent for E_2.

Recoveries. In each assay, duplicate 50 pg amounts of both estrone and estradiol were added to 200 to 1,000 μl aliquots of water and carried through the extraction, chromatography and radioimmunoassay steps to determine procedural losses. The average recovery of estrone was 80 percent, and of estradiol 83 percent. The mean difference in percent recovery between duplicates within a given assays was 6 percent for both estrogens with a range of 1 to 11 percent (N = 10).

Calculations. The standard curves for both estrone and estradiol were linearized using the logit transformation described by Rodbard.[16] The amount of material in the sample was read from the standard curve, the appropriate blank value subtracted, and the result corrected for procedural losses as determined in duplicate for each assay. The final data are expressed as picograms of steroid per milliliter serum.

Statistical Methods. Determination of the Spearman rank correlation was as described.[17]

RESULTS

Normal Prepubertal Subjects— Infancy to 10 Years

As shown in Figures 11-1 and 11-2 the values for E_2 overlap in both males and

Table 11-2. FSH, LH, Estrone and Estradiol in Prepubertal and Pubertal Males and Females.

	Males					Females			
					Tanner Stage I				
	FSH	*LH*	E_1	E_2			*FSH*	*LH*	E_1	E_2
Age 11-12; N = 6						Age 10-11; N = 6				
$\overline{X}$	120	20.8	15.8	4.8		$\overline{X}$	130	24.9	18.5	9.8
SEM	5	2.1	1.4	0.6		SEM	5	2.1	0.7	1.1
SD	15	4.2	3.2	1.5		SD	15	4.2	1.5	2.4
					Tanner Stage II					
Age 12-13; N = 6						Age 10-13; N = 5				
$\overline{X}$	165*	37.4*	27.4*	5.8		$\overline{X}$	230	33.3	44.6*	39.6*
SEM	15	4.2	3.9	1.1		SEM	70	4.2	5.5	7.8
SD	40	14.0	9.5	2.7		SD	140	8.3	12.3	17.4
					Tanner Stage III					
Age 12-13; N = 6						Age 12-13; N = 6				
$\overline{X}$	215	43.7	32.3	11 *		$\overline{X}$	260	85.3*	69.2*	76.7*
SEM	40	6.2	4.1	1.1		SEM	35	22.9	7.4	13.7
SD	105	14.6	10.1	2.8		SD	75	52.0	16.6	30.6
					Tanner Stage IV					
Age 13-14; N = 6						Age 12-13; N = 7				
$\overline{X}$	260	41.6	38.5	15.7*		$\overline{X}$	265	97.8	78.3	88.1
SEM	35	4.2	4.5	1.7		SEM	25	31.2	17.3	31.1
SD	80	8.3	10.0	3.8		SD	65	70.7	42.3	76.1
					Tanner Stage V					
Age 13; N = 6						Age 12-13; N = 6				
$\overline{X}$	210	52.0	38.2	21		$\overline{X}$	280	99.8	60.7	65.7
SEM	20	6.2	3.4	2.2		SEM	25	8.3	4.8	15.8
SD	40	12.5	7.7	4.9		SD	60	18.7	10.8	35.3

* A statistically significant ($P < 0.05$) increase over the corresponding mean value for the preceding Tanner stage.

females; however, some of the females have higher values than any of the males in each of the age groupings < 5, and 5 to 10 years. For E_1, there is no tendency for higher values in females in this age range.

Normal Prepubertal and Pubertal Subjects—10 Years to 13 Years (See Table 11-2)

Males. There was a 2.4-fold rise in E_1 and a 4.4-fold rise in E_2 from Stages I to V. The sharpest increase in E_1 was between Stages I and II; and for E_2 between Stages II and IV. The sharpest increases in FSH and LH were between Stages I and II. Spearman rank correlations were as follows: FSH, E_1 0.38; FSH, E_2 0.67; LH, E_1 0.37; LH, E_2 0.61, all significantly different from zero ($p < 0.05$).

As shown in Table 11-3, there were significant correlations between FSH, LH, E_1, and E_2 versus Tanner rating, chronologic age, and bone age ($p < 0.01$).

Females. There was a 3.3-fold increase in E_1 and a 6.8-fold rise in E_2 from Stages I to V. Estradiol was significantly ($p < 0.05$) greater in females at each stage. The difference in estrone between males and females was insignificant at Stage I, but was significantly higher in females in the remaining 4 stages ($p < 0.05$).

FSH and LH increased with each Tanner stage. The Spearman rank correlations were FSH, E_1, 0.43; FSH, E_2, 0.13; LH, E_1, 0.70; LH, E_2, 0.48; all except that for FSH and E_2 were significant ($p < 0.05$).

As shown in Table 11-3, there were significant correlations between LH, E_1, and E_2 versus Tanner rating, chronological age and bone age. FSH correlated significantly with Tanner rating. The data on normal subjects 10 to 13 years of age were reported.[14]

PHYSIOLOGIC INTERPRETATIONS OF CIRCULATING ESTRONE AND ESTRADIOL
Normal Prepubertal and Pubertal Subjects

The finding of an approximately twofold higher level of serum E_2 in the older prepubertal girls is consistent with our earlier report of an increased estrogen effect in pre-

Table 11-3. Spearman Rank Correlation Coefficients Between Specified Variables.

	FSH	LH	E_1	E_2
Males				
Tanner Rating	.6247*	.6587*	.6406*	.8978*
	30 †	29	30	30
Chronological Age	.4693*	.5024*	.6282*	.6448*
	30	29	30	30
Bone Age	.5968*	.6012*	.5705*	.7598*
	29	28	29	29
Females				
Tanner Rating	.3776‡	.7316*	.5394*	.4696*
	29	28	30	30
Chronological Age	.0631	.3257‡	.3160‡	.3557‡
	29	28	30	30
Bone Age	.2883	.6341*	.5797*	.5316*
	29	28	30	30
Both Sexes Combined				
Tanner Rating	.4905*	.7076*	.5588*	.5503*
	59	57	60	60
Chronological Age	.2425	.4065‡	.4012‡	.3774‡
	59	57	60	60
Bone Age	.4546*	.6425*	.5893*	.5662*
	58	56	59	59

* Statistically significantly different from zero at .01 level.
† Number of pairs of observations.
‡ Statistically significantly different from zero at the .05 but not .01 level.

pubertal girls than in boys in urethral cytology.[18] In that study the girls had more precornified and intermediate cells, and fewer non-nucleated cells than prepubertal males ($p \leq 10^{-4}$ in each instance). To our knowledge, that was the first report of a difference in sex hormone effect in prepubertal children. The urethral cytology could have reflected either increased estrogen in the females or androgen antagonism in the males, or both. Our new data are consistent with estrogen production by the prepubertal ovary.

Evidence for a rise in the levels of FSH and LH in male and female children prior to any evidence of secondary sexual development has been recently reviewed.[19] Our data are in accord with significant activity of the gonadotrophin-gonadal axis in prepubertal girls.

Estrone levels were not significantly different between prepubertal girls and boys. In adults, the adrenals contribute to the production of E_1 both by direct secretion,

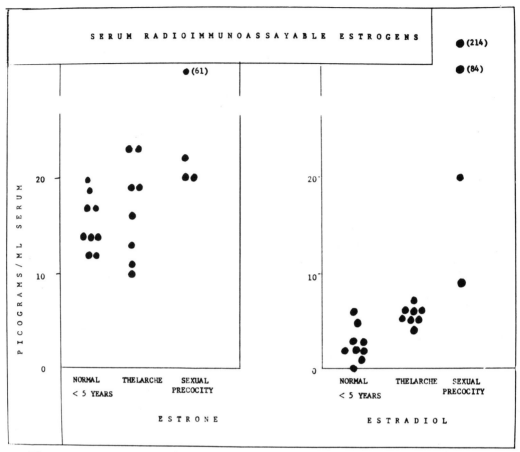

Fig. 11-3. Serum estrone (*left panel*) and estradiol (*right panel*) in from left to right: normal girls under 5 years; premature thelarche; sexual precocity. There was no difference in mean levels of estrone in premature thelarche versus normal. For estradiol, the values overlapped but the mean in premature thelarche was elevated (p <0.05).

Patients with sexual precocity had elevation of both estrogen values; the highest level of estradiol, 214 pg/ml, was in a girl with granulosa cell tumor.

and secretion of its immediate precursors androstenedione and dehydroandrosterone.[20] The adrenal contribution of prepubertal males can be expected to be similar to that of females, and can obscure any difference due to ovarian E_1 secretion.

The steady increase in estradiol during male adolescence can arise from several sources. Although studies in adolescent males have not yet been reported, in adult males E_2 is derived from at least 3 sources: (a) Longcope, et al.[21] estimate that approximately 50 percent of circulating E_2 arises from peripheral conversion of testosterone;

(b) testicular secretion can account for approximately 25 percent,[22] and (c) 5 percent can be attributed to peripheral conversion of estrone.[23]

Similarly, the rise in E_1 which we observed during adolescence can come from several sources. In adult males, the principal source of E_1 is the adrenal which contributes both by direct secretion of E_1 and by secretion of its precursors androstenedione and dehydroisoandrosterone.[22] Both of these steroids increase during adolescence. An additional small contribution from peripheral conversion of E_2 to E_1 can occur.[23]

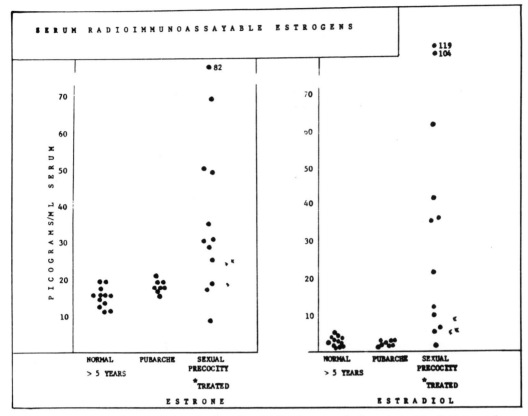

Fig. 11-4. The format is identical to Fig. 11-3. Age-matched control girls (*left*) in each panel are compared with girls aged 5 to 8 years with premature pubarche (*middle*) and sexual precocity (*right*). There is no alteration of estrone or estradiol in premature pubarche. Both E_1 and E_2 are elevated in sexually precocious girls, and both were decreased during therapy with depot-medroxyprogesterone acetate.

Our data on gonadotropins are in agreement with previous reports.[19] There was an increase in circulating FSH and LH in association with sexual maturation, the increase in LH was more marked than that for FSH. A more comprehensive report, based on a much larger group of youngsters, and comparing gonadotrophins and maturation, is in preparation.

Females. Circulating estradiol was higher than in males at each stage, and rose steadily to Tanner Stage IV, with an insignificant decrease at Stage V. A similar rise in E_2 during female puberty was reported by Jenner, et al.[24] In both their study and ours, pubertal stage and osseous maturation correlated better with E_2 than did chronologic age. In

adult women, it is likely that over 90 percent of circulating estradiol arises from ovarian secretion;[25] the increase during puberty is probably from that source. Therefore, the significant correlation between E_2 and LH and not with FSH is surprising.

Some explanations for this discrepancy can be considered. Postmenarchal girls in Groups III to V may have dissociation of FSH and E_2, since during the first half of the menstrual cycle FSH is relatively high, and E_2 low; the ratio is reversed in the second half. Furthermore, our sample size is relatively small.

The adrenal contributes to the plasma pool of estrone by direct secretion, and by providing precursors for peripheral conver-

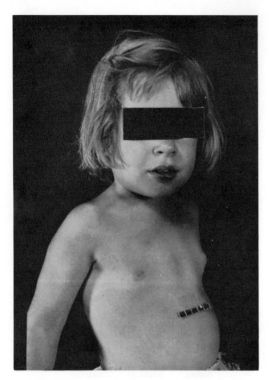

Fig. 11-5. Patient Nancy A seen at 19 months of age with premature thelarche. Breast measurements were 1.5 x 1.5 x 0.5 cms. The nipples were thinned and minimally pigmented. Breast enlargement persisted throughout childhood, but sexual precosity did not ensue.

sion, especially DHA and androstenedione.[20] Approximately 25 percent of circulating estrone was estimated to arise from peripheral conversion.[25] The higher values which we found in females Stage II to V than in males reflects ovarian contribution as well as peripheral conversion of E_2 to E_1.[23] This latter conversion results in a significant contribution to circulating E_2 in adult females, and a minor one in adult males.[23]

Abnormal Prepubertal and Pubertal Subjects

Premature Thelarche (Isolated Precocious Breast Development). This condition frequently encountered in the generalist's or pediatrician's office is described in the following case history.

Nancy A was seen at 19 months of age because of "breast development." There was

no pubic or axillary hair and no vaginal bleeding. There was no history of accidental estrogen ingestion, or of taking medications or vitamins which could have had estrogen contamination.

On physical exam the height was normal. The breasts measured 1.5 x 1.5 x .5 cms, and the nipples were thinned and minimally pigmented (Fig. 11-5). Rectal examination revealed that the uterus was not enlarged, there was no abnormal mass and the ovaries were not palpable. A urethral-cytology examination showed no increase in estrogen effect.[18] Follow-up to 9 years of age when she was discharged, revealed persistence of the breast enlargement but there was never early pubic hair or early menarche.

This patient is typical in that the precocious breast development was unaccompanied by any other evidence of premature secondary sexual development. In approximately two-thirds of the patients, the enlargement persists or increases; in the remainder, it disappears. Treatment consists of allaying the parents' anxiety. The child can wear "floppy" blouses so that the breast development is inapparent to classmates.

The evidence favors the concept that the condition is due to a slight activation of the normal CNS-gonadal axis which causes puberty. In support of this thesis, we have reported slight but statistically significant elevation of both FSH and LH,[26] and a similar mild but statistically significant increase in estrogen effect on urethral cytology in this condition.[18] The new data on elevation of circulating E_2 are consistent with these data. For clinical diagnosis, the urethral cytology is generally easier to perform but the serum estradiol level is more specific.

Sexual Precocity. In girls under 8 years of age, the appearance of isosexual secondary sexual development is abnormal. In reported series from endocrine clinic populations, the majority (75% or greater) of patients have a normal but early activation of the pubertal timing mechanism, which is sometimes a familial pattern.

In pathologic cases, ovarian tumors are

the most common lesion, and of these granulosa cell tumors[27] exceed theca cell tumors or choriocarcinomas. Feminizing adrenal tumors are infrequent. Intracranial lesions include pinealomas which presumably inactivate the inhibitory effect of pineal secretions on the gonadotropin-releasing mechanism. Among intracranial lesions, hamartoma of the tuber cinereum is seen. Craniopharyngiomas usually cause sexual infantilism. Albright's polyostotic fibrous dysplasia and Von Recklinghausen's neurofibromatosis are associated with sexual precocity.

Prior to a detailed work-up, a careful history of estrogen ingestion is sought. One mother who denied such a history initially, later volunteered the information that she had given her daughter the cellophane wrappers from oral contraceptives to play with. When the daughter stopped licking the wrappers, her "sexual precocity" regressed.

Clinically the girl has breast development, pubic and often axillary hair, with or without menses. The height and osseous maturation are advanced. Rectoabdominal examination (under sedation, if necessary), usually reveals an ovarian tumor if it is present. However, these are sometimes small and may be undetectable on initial examination.[27] In cases of pinealoma, paralysis of upward gaze may be present. Characteristic pigmented skin patches are concomitants of Albright's polyostotic fibrous dysplasia, and Von Recklinghausen's neurofibromatosis. In the latter condition, visual field cuts and pallor of the optic disc may be seen with lesions near the optic nerves.

Laboratory investigation includes determination of serum estrogens and gonadotropins, and estrogen effect on urethral cytology. All are increased in idiopathic cases and with the CNS lesions. Markedly elevated circulating estrogens, and low gonadotropins characterize functioning (i.e., granulosa cell tumors). With choriocarcinoma the pregnancy test is positive.

There is no consistently effective chemotherapy in terms of complete arrest of idio-

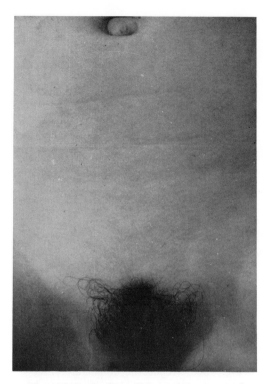

Fig. 11-6. Patient SN at 4½ years of age with premature pubarche. Abundant pubic hair was the only evidence of secondary sexual development. Other than an increase in pubic hair, no other secondary sexual development was observed by the time she was discharged from follow-up at 8 years of age.

pathic sexual precocity. Medroxyprogesterone acetate fails to consistently arrest osseous maturation, although it usually curtails menses. As shown in Figure 11-4, the circulating levels of estrone and estradiol were lower in patients so treated.

Premature Pubarche (Adrenarche). This condition consists of the precocious appearance of sexual hair, without breast development or other evidence of estrogen effect. A typical history is that of SN a female who was seen at 4½ years of age because of the appearance of moderate pubic hair growth. There was no other evidence of secondary sexual development.

On physical examination there was no abnormality other than the moderate pubic hair (Fig. 11-6). There were moderate pre-

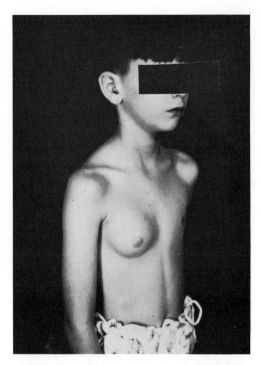

Fig. 11-7. Prepubertal unilateral gynecomastia in an 8-year-old boy. The condition was idiopathic in this case, and in 6 other prepubertal males in our clinic during a period of 10 years. No instances of feminizing adrenal or testicular tumors were encountered during that time.

putial folds, although the corpus of the clitoris was not large.

The urinary excretion of 17-ketosteroids, dehydroisoandrosterone and pregnanetriol were normal (ruling out congenital adrenal hyperplasia or virilizing tumor). The bone age was not advanced.

When discharged from follow-up at 8 years of age, the pubic hair had increased, but there was no other evidence of virilization or feminization.

The cause of the adrenal component of puberty is obscure, but it usually coincides with the CNS-gonadal activation of male and female adolescence. Premature pubarche results when the adrenal and CNS mechanisms are dissociated. Rosenfield[28] described elevation of dehydroandrosterone sulfate, accompanied by parallel but slight increases in unbound testosterone into the

low adult female range in 6 of 7 girls with this condition. In those girls, the production of pubertal adrenal 17-ketosteroids was ACTH dependent.

Our finding of normal circulating estrone and estradiol (see Fig. 11-4) indicates that the ovary is uninvolved; our report of normal prepubertal levels of FSH and LH in premature adrenarche[26] shows that they play no role.

It is important to differentiate the condition from virilization due to adrenal or other androgen-secreting tumors or androgen ingestion. In those conditions, more marked virilizing signs (i.e., clitoral hypertrophy, muscularity, facial hair and deepened voice) are seen.

Gynecomastia in Prepubertal and Pubertal Males. In prepubertal males, the appearance of gynecomastia is uncommon and can be due to feminizing adrenal or testicular tumors, as well as to accidental ingestion of estrogen. However, during a period of 10 years, the author has encountered 7 instances of idiopathic gynecomastia in boys 2 to 7 years of age[29] (see Fig. 11-7). Four boys, 5 to 10 years of age, with no male secondary sexual development, had isolated unilateral or bilateral gynecomastia. Their mean values for both E_1 and E_2 (18 $\pm$ 8 SD and 4 $\pm$ 3 SD pg/ml respectively) were normal.

The etiology of the condition in males is obscure; however, in two instances urinary estrogen excretion was increased. In the 4 boys who presented after our serum estrogen assay was operative, normal values for E_1 and E_2 were obtained. It is possible that at the time the samples were taken we had missed the event which led to elevation of circulating estrogen. As mentioned under the section on premature thelarche, once breast enlargement occurs, it tends to persist.

Adolescent male gynecomastia is common, and palpable breast tissue which does not usually extend beyond the areola is present in about one-third of normal pubertal males. Three adolescent males, 4 to 17 years of age (Tanner Stages 4 and 5) had mean estrone 32 $\pm$ 3 SD pg/ml and estradiol

17 $\pm$ 4 SD pg/ml, not significantly different from those of normal males at comparable Tanner stages. Others have failed to detect an increase in urinary estrogen excretion in this condition.[29] Our finding of normal circulating E_1 and E_2 in the few patients studied is confirmatory. Serum prolactin is not increased.[30] The etiology remains elusive, although an increased estrogen/androgen ratio, or elevation of nonsex steroid-binding globulin-bound estradiol have not yet been excluded.

Pathological causes for adolescent gynecomastia include testicular and adrenal feminizing tumors. The former are nearly always palpable. High levels of urinary and serum estrogens are anticipated in either case, although we have not had the opportunity to study such patients. It should be recalled also that Klinefelter's syndrome is relatively common (approximately 1 to 500 phenotypic males). Therefore, the association of adolescent male gynecomastia with relatively small testes warrants obtaining a buccal smear for sex chromatin.

In adult males, gynecomastia may be associated with recovery from malnutrition, and hepatic cirrhosis and digitalis-treated congestive cardiac failure. It is seen in hyperthyroidism when it is associated with an increase in the absolute concentration of estradiol unbound to sex hormone-binding globulin.[31] Drugs which affect central nervous system function (phenothiazines, meprobamate, reserpine) as well as spironolactone may result in gynecomastia. Hodgkin's disease and bronchogenic carcinoma are sometimes accompanied by gynecomastia.

Tumors situated in the mammary area (neurofibromata, lipomata, carcinoma) may simulate gynecomastia. In obesity, it may be difficult to differentiate the normal "wormy" feel of breast tissue, from the lumpy consistency of adiposity in that area.

Failure of Secondary Sex Development in Females. At the time of this writing, the average age of menarche is between 12 and 13 years. Breast development and pubic hair antedate that event by several years. A delay in appearance of secondary sexual characteristics may occur in normal females until the late teens and there may be a family history of similar delay.

The most common cause of failure of secondary sexual development is Turner's syndrome (gonadal dysgenesis). The XO variety occurs in 1/2,000 phenotypic females. However, in our clinic, approximately half of the patients have less readily detectable mosaic forms, and the classical stigmata are less frequently present. In these patients, the finding of low circulating estradiol in conjunction with elevated circulating gonadotropins is confirmatory of ovarian absence or inadequacy. Six patients with Turner's syndrome, ranging in age from 11 to 15 years had lower levels of E_1 (mean 15 $\pm$ 5 SD, range 9-24 pg/ml) and very low levels of E_2 (mean 1.7 $\pm$ 1 SD, range < 1-4 pg/ml) in comparison to controls matched for age.

In hypopituitary hypogonadism, both estradiol and gonadotropins are low. The association of anosmia (or hyposmia) and hypogonadotrophic hypogonadism (Kallman's syndrome) occurs in both males and females.[32.]

URINARY ESTROGEN DETERMINATIONS DURING PREGNANCY

It has been recognized for over a decade that measurement of urinary estrogen levels assists in the evaluation of high-risk pregnancies. This topic has recently been reviewed.[33,34] Early in gestation, low urinary estriol (below 100 μg/24 hr) was useful in predicting abortion which occurred one or more weeks after the test.[34] In late pregnancy, the definition of the lower limit of normal for estriol is a line connecting 2 mg per 24 hours at 20 weeks, 8 mg at 30 weeks, and 12 mg at 40 weeks and later. Low levels were encountered in anemic (hemoglobin less than 10 Gm/100 ml) mothers, as well as in those with hypertension and multiple prenatal complications. Fetal mortality and low-birth-weight-for-gestation age were also seen.

Since estriol excretion may be low for several weeks without abnormal clinical findings, serial measurements should be made for completeness of evaluation. Therefore, those authors suggest routine urinary estriol screening at 30 and 36 weeks' gestation, with follow-up of low values.[34]

Summary

RIA of estrogens provides the investigator and the clinician with a sensitive, precise method for elucidation of normal and abnormal physiological mechanisms during growth and development. It is applicable to the study of both serum and urine specimens. Urinary estrogens during growth and development will be the topic of a subsequent more detailed report; our data have already appeared in abstract form.[35,36]

The authors are grateful to R. Julane Hotchkiss for advice in the RIA of estrogens; and to Lois Pischke and Donna Borchert for valuable secretarial assistance.

References

1. Brown, J. B., MacLeod, S. C., Macnaughtan, C., Smith, M. A., and Smyth, B.: A rapid method for estimating oestrogens in urine using a semi-automatic extractor. J. Endocrinol., *42*:5, 1968.

2. Kaplan, H. G., Aoki, T., Sansone, A., *et al.*: Comparison of urinary estrogen values determined by radioimmunoassay and gas liquid chromatography. Amer. J. Obstet. and Gynecol., *113*:956, 1972.

3. Knorr, D. W. R., Kirschner, M. A., and Taylor, J. P.: Estimation of estrone and estradiol in low level urines using electron-capture gas liquid chromatography. J. Clin. Endocrinol., *31*:409, 1970.

4. Baird, D. T.: A method for the measurement of estrone and estradiol-17β in peripheral human blood and other biological fluids using ^{35}S pipsyl chloride. J. Clin. Endocrinol., *28*:244, 1965.

5. Ichii, S., Forchielli, E., Perloff, W. H., and Dorfman, R. I.: Determination of plasma estrone and estradiol-17β. Anal. Biochem., *5*:422, 1963.

6. Wotiz, H. H., Charransol, G., and Smith, I. N.: Gas chromatographic measurement of plasma estrogens using an electron capture detector. Steroids, *10*:127, 1967.

7. Midgley, A. R., and Niswander, G. D.: In Diczfalusy, E. (ed.): Karolinska Symposia on Research Methods in Reproductive Endocrinology. p. 320. Steroid Assay by Protein Binding, Bogtrykksriet Forum, Copenhagen, 1970.

8. Peron, F. G., and Caldwell, B. G. (eds.): Immunologic Methods in Steroid Determination. New York, Appleton-Century-Crofts, 1970.

9. Tulchinsky, D., and Korenman, S. G.: A radio-ligand assay for plasma estrone; normal values and variations during the menstrual cycle. J. Clin. Endocrinol. Metab., *31*:76, 1970.

10. Hotchkiss, J., Atkinson, L. E., and Knobil, E.: Time course of serum estrogen and luteinizing hormone (LH) concentration during the menstrual cycle of the rhesus monkey. Endocrinology, *89*:177, 1971.

11. Exley, D., Johnson, M. W., and Dean, P. D. G.: Antisera highly specific for 17β-oestradiol. Steroids, *18*:605, 1971.

12. Wright, K., Robinson, H., Collins, D. C., and Preedy, J. R. K.: Investigation of a radioimmunoassay for plasma estrone and estradiol 17-β in males and nonpregnant females. Comparison with an independent method using fluorimetry. J. Clin. Endocrinol. Metab., *36*:165, 1973.

13. Kenny, F. M., Angsusingha, K., Stinson, D., and Hotchkiss, J.: Unconjugated estrogens in the perinatal period. Pediatr. Res., *7*:826, 1973.

14. Angsusingha, K., Kenny, F. M., Nankin, H., and Taylor, F. H.: Unconjugated estrone, estradiol, and FSH and LH in prepubertal and pubertal males and females. J. Clin. Endocrinol., *39*:63, 1974.

15. Ferin, M., Zimmering, P. E., Lieberman, S., and Vande Wiele, R. L.: Inactivation of the biological effects of exogenous and endogenous estrogens by antibodies to 17β-estradiol. Endocrinology, *83*:565, 1968.

16. Rodbard, D., Bridson, W., and Rayford, P. L.: Rapid calculation of radioimmunoassay results. J. Lab. Clin. Med., *74*:770, 1969.

17. Siegel, S. (ed.): Non Parametric Statistics for Behavioral Services. p. 202. New York, McGraw-Hill, 1956.

18. Preeyasombat, C., and Kenny, F. M.: Urethral cytology in normal children and in various abnormal conditions. Pediatrics, *38*:436, 1966.

19. Root, A. W.: Endocrinology of puberty I: Normal sexual maturation. J. Pediatr., *83*:1, 1973.

20. Saez, J. M., Morera, A. M., Dazord, A., and Bertrand, J.: Adrenal and testicular contribution to plasma estrogens. J. Endocrinol., *55*:41, 1972.

21. Longcope, C., Kato, T., and Horton, R.: Conversion of blood androgens to estrogens in normal adult men and women. J. Clin. Invest., *48*:2191, 1969.

22. Kelch, R. P., Jenner, M. R., Weinstein, R., Kaplan, S. L., and Grumbach, M. M.: Estradiol and testosterone secretion by human, simian, and canine testes in males with hypogonadism and in male pseudohermaphrodites with the feminizing testes syndrome. J. Clin. Invest., *51*:824, 1972.

23. Longcope, C., Layne, D. S., and Tait, J. F.: Metabolic clearance rates and interconversions of estrone and 17β-estradiol in normal males and females. J. Clin. Invest., *47*:93, 1968.

24. Jenner, M. R., Kelch, R. P., Kaplan, S. L., and Grumbach, M. D.: Estradiol and testosterone secretion by human, simian and canine testes, in male pseudohermaphrodites with hypogonadism and feminizing testes syndrome. J. Clin. Endocrinol., *34*: 521, 1972.

25. Baird, D. T., Horton, R., Longcope, C., and Tait, J. F.: Steroid pre-hormones. Perspect. Biol. Med., *11*:384, 1968.

26. Kenny, F. M., Midgley, A. R., Jaffe, R. B., Garces, L. Y., Vazquez, A., and Taylor, F. T.: Radioimmunoassayable Serum LH and FSH in girls with sexual precocity, premature thelarche and adrenarche. J. Clin. Endocrinol., *29*:1272, 1969.

27. Iturzaeta, N., Kenny, F. M., and Sieber, W.: Precocious pseudopuberty due to granulosa cell tumor in three girls. Amer. J. Dis. Child., *114*:29, 1967.

28. Rosenfield, R. L.: Plasma 17-ketosteroids and 17-beta hydroxysteroids in girls with premature development of sexual hair. J. Pediatr., *79*:768, 1971.

29. Latorre, H., and Kenny, F. M.: Idiopathic gynecomastia in seven preadolescent males: elevation of urinary estrogen excretion in two cases. Amer. J. Dis. Child., *126*:771, 1974.

30. Turkington, R. W.: Serum prolactin levels in patients with gynecomastia. J. Clin. Endocrinol. Metab., *34*:62, 1972.

31. Chopra, I. J., Abraham, G. E., Chopra, U., et al.: Alterations in circulating estradiol-17β in male patients with Grave's disease. N. Eng. J. Med., *286*:124, 1972.

32. Tagatz, G., Fialkow, P. J., Smith, E., and Spadoni, L.: Hypogonadism associated with anosmia in the female. N. Eng. J. Med., *283*:1326, 1970.

33. Brown, J. B., and Beischer, N. A.: Current status of estrogen assay in gynecology and obstetrics. Part I. Estrogen assays in gynecology and early pregnancy. Obstet. Gynecol. Survey, *27*:205, 1972.

34. Beischer, N. A., and Brown, J. B.: Part II. Estrogen assays in late pregnancy. Obstet. Gynecol. Survey, *27*:303, 1972.

35. deLevie, M., Richards, C., Brych, M., and Kenny, F. M.: Radioimmunoassay of urinary estrone and estradiol in normal and abnormal conditions from infancy through adolescence. Pediatr. Res. (abstr.), *7*:328, 1973.

36. Kenny, F. M., Radfar, N., Angsusingha, K., and deLevie, M.: Radioimmunoassayable serum and urinary estrone and estradiol and percent of dialyzable estradiol from infancy through adolescence: evidence for activity of the human prepubertal ovary. The Endocrine Society, Program and Abstracts, p. A-57, 1974.

12 Determination of Androgens in Biological Fluids

MARVIN A. KIRSCHNER, M.D.

INTRODUCTION

It has been approximately 10 years since the first sensitive assay system to measure testosterone in biological fluids was reported.[1,2] During this decade, many types of assays have been reported, reflecting advances in instrumentation and refinements in the in vitro nuclear techniques. Table 12-1 shows these evolutionary changes in testosterone methodology, noting the vast improvements in assay sensitivity and working time that have taken place.[1-8] Virtually all methods to measure androgens in biological fluids involve the use of radionuclides to monitor losses during the sample purification. Many of the methods, particularly the newer ones, employ radiotracer-protein interactions (radioligand analyses).

The following discussion reviews the varying methods that have been used to measure testosterone and other C_{19} steroids in biological fluids, and considers the more common procedures in use today. The clinical application of these measurements in assessing gonadal function in men, and virilized states in women, are then considered.

GENERAL CONSIDERATIONS

Although testosterone is probably the most important secreted androgen, it is but one of a series of closely related C_{19} steroids known to be present in human and other biological fluids. The structural configuration of testosterone and its closely related "androgens" are indicated in Figure 12-1. It is apparent from the structural similarities of these compounds that successful measurement of testosterone or any of these substances must carefully exclude the others. This may be accomplished by (a) an absolutely specific detection system, which identifies and measures the steroid of interest in the presence of these potential and/or real contaminants, or (b) preliminary purification of the biologic sample prior to assay in sensitive but "nonspecific" detection systems. In the methods devised to date, there have been no detection systems which are absolutely specific for testosterone; thus, the various procedures require preliminary purification of the sample prior to assay. Specificity of these methods depends on the combination of chromatographic purification followed by a "relatively specific" detection system.

Measurement of Testosterone by Enzymatic Conversion to Estrogen

This approach represented the first "modern-day" attempt to quantify testosterone in biological fluids.[1,2] This method involved extraction of plasma, chromatographic isolation of testosterone and then conversion of testosterone to estradiol by incubation with a placental microsomal enzyme preparation. The estradiol thus formed was quantified by fluorometry.

This method was indeed cumbersome, time-consuming and never achieved widespread use. The values obtained by this approach did, however, establish that testosterone was present in human plasma in submicrogram quantities and correlated reason-

Table 12-1. Evolution of Methods to Measure Testosterone in Biological Fluids.

Year	Author	Principle	Use of Radionuclides	Time required	Quantity of plasma required
1961	Finkelstein	Enzyme conversion to estrogens Measure estrogens by fluorimetry	To monitor purification losses		20 ml
1963	Riondel	Double isotope derivative method	To monitor purification losses Second tracer is derivatizing reagent	2-3 weeks	10 ml
1965	Kirschner	Double isotope derivative method GLC for purification	Same as above	7-10 days	20 ml
1964	Brownie	Electron-capture GLC	To monitor procedural losses	4-5 days	10 ml
1968	Kirschner	Electron-capture GLC high-affinity derivatives	To monitor procedural losses	2-3 days	4-10 ml
1967	Murphy	Competitive protein binding, using testosterone-binding globulin	To monitor procedural losses For competitive displacement curves	1-2 days	5 ml
1970	Furuyama	Radioimmunoassay, using antibody versus testosterone	To monitor procedural losses For competitive displacement curves	1-2 days	1-2 ml

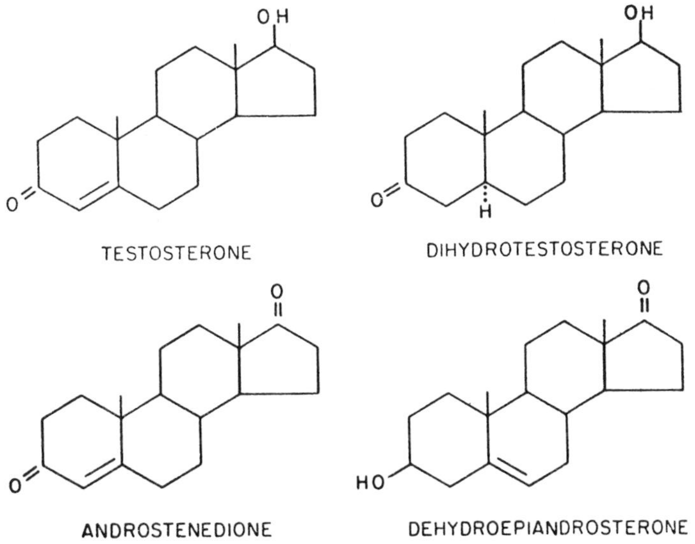

Fig. 12-1. Structural formulae of testosterone and closely related $C_{19}O_2$ steroids.

TESTOSTERONE

DIHYDROTESTOSTERONE

ANDROSTENEDIONE

DEHYDROEPIANDROSTERONE

ably well with the clinical state of virilism. This approach was superseded shortly thereafter by double-isotope derivative methods.

Double-Istotope Derivative Methods

This analytic approach was the first widely used method to measure testosterone and other $C_{19}O_2$ compounds in biological fluids.[3,4,9-15] The principles of this approach as outlined by Kliman and Peterson[16] are demonstrated in Figure 12-2. At the outset, ^{3}H-testosterone is added to the sample to monitor purification losses. The plasma sample is extracted with ether and testosterone is purified from contaminants by multiple chromatographic steps. A derivative of testosterone is then prepared using a second, tracer-labeling reagent of known specific activity. The most commonly used reagent for derivatization is ^{14}C-acetic anhydride, which reacts with hydroxyl groups on the steroid molecule to form a ^{14}C-acetate.

Following the acetylation, several additional chromatographic "clean-up steps" are required to remove other hydroxyl-containing substances that may have reacted to form ^{14}C-acetates. Radiochemical purity is achieved when ^{3}H/^{14}C in the testosterone sample remains constant through at least the final 2 purification steps. Since the ^{14}C-acetic anhydride reacts with testosterone on an equimolar basis (see Fig. 12-2), the ^{14}C counts contained in the final purified sample indicate the moles of testosterone in this sample. This is corrected for procedural losses, as monitored by the ^{3}H-counts in the sample, yielding the amount of testosterone contained in the original plasma sample.

In several laboratories, ^{35}S-thiosemicarbazide has been used as the derivatizing agent.[3,12] ^{35}S-thiosemicarbazones are formed at sites of ketonic functional groups (3-keto). The product is purified to a constant ^{3}H/^{35}S ratio, and the subsequent calculations are similar to the above.

Limitations. There are several limitations to the use of this method:

1. It is cumbersome and requires multiple chromatographic steps both before and after the derivative is prepared. Working time is generally several weeks. In later procedures, some of the purification steps have been reduced by using gas-liquid chromatography with fraction collection.[4]

2. It is costly. ^{14}C-labeled acetic anhydride or ^{35}S-thiosemicarbazide of high-specific activity are prohibitively expensive, making this method unacceptable for routine assays.

3. It is less sensitive than more recent approaches. Because of the relatively low-specific activity of the ^{14}C-acetic anhydride, these methods cannot measure beyond nanogram levels. Thus, to measure testosterone in low-level samples, as much as 10 to 20 ml of plasma may be required. Switching the labels (^{3}H-acetic anhydride and ^{14}C-testosterone) provides higher specific activities of the derivatizing reagent, but use of ^{14}C-labeled testosterone results in significant amounts of testosterone being added to the sample. ^{35}S-thiosemicarbazide has not been widely used because of the apparent instability of this reagent.

Gas Liquid Chromatography

Much interest was generated during the mid-1960's in the potential use of gas-liquid chromatography (GLC) for measuring androgens in biological fluids. Since GLC sys-

MEASUREMENT OF TESTOSTERONE

DOUBLE ISOTOPE DERIVATIVE METHOD

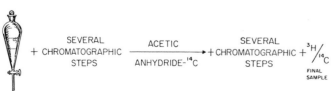

Fig. 12-2. Determination of testosterone using double isotope derivative method. ^{3}H-testosterone is added at the onset to monitor procedural losses. ^{14}C-acetic anhydride is used as derivatizing agent. (See text for details.)

Fig. 12-3. Determination of testosterone in biological fluids, using electron-capture GLC. Testosterone hepta-fluorobutyrate (HFB) is prepared, purified and quantified by GLC. (See text for details.)

MEASUREMENT OF TESTOSTERONE

ELECTRON−CAPTURE GLC

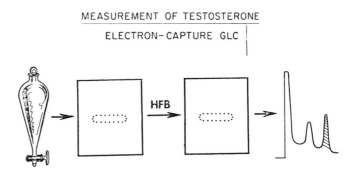

tems generally have greater resolving power than traditional paper or thin-layer chromatography, it was hoped that multiple chromatographic steps required for sample purification would be reduced. Further, the sensitivity of GLC detection systems, particularly the electron-capture detectors seemed adequate for the measurements required.[5,6,17,18]

The procedure for determining testosterone in biological fluids, using electron-capture GLC is shown in Figure 12-3. ^{3}H-tracer is added to the sample at the outset to monitor methodologic losses, and the sample is extracted with ether. Preliminary purification of the sample is achieved by thin-layer chromatography. The eluate is then dried and a suitable derivative is prepared to enhance the electron-capturing properties of testosterone. The most commonly used derivative for this purpose is the hepta-fluorobutyrate (HFB), which is easily prepared by adding heptafluorobutyric anhydride to the benzene-dissolved testosterone sample, and incubating in a sand bath at 60°C for 30 minutes. Following this reaction, excess reagents are blown off with nitrogen, and a second TLC step is usually necessary to remove other hydroxyl-containing impurities which may also have reacted with the reagent. The second TLC also serves to remove any 3-enol heptafluoro-butyrate of testosterone which may have formed during the chemical reaction. Following the second TLC step, the dried sample is taken up with benzene. An aliquot is removed for counting to monitor recovery. A duplicate aliquot is injected into the GLC

system containing a polar silicone polymer stationary phase such as 3% QF-1, XE-60, or OV-225. A representative GLC tracing is presented in Figure 12-4. To insure proper aliquoting at the final stages, an internal standard may be used.

To determine the amount of testosterone in the sample from the GLC tracing, the area responses under the respective testosterone-HFB and internal standard samples are determined. A standard curve relating the ratio of testo-HFB/internal standard versus nanogram of testosterone is con-

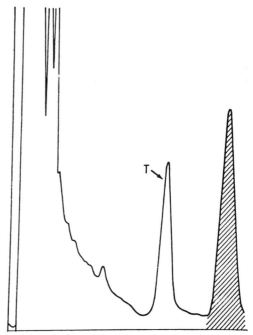

Fig. 12-4. GLC tracing showing testosterone (T) in a 4ml extract of male plasma. Shaded area represents internal standard testosterone-HFN.

Table 12-2. Reactivity of Various Natural Steroids in Competitive Protein-Binding Assays Using TEBG, and Radioimmunoassays Using Antibody to Testosterone-3-oxo-Conjugates.

	Competitive Protein-Binding (TEBG-rich Serum)	Radioimmunoassay (3-oxo-conjugates of Testosterone)
Testosterone	100%	100%
Dihydrotestosterone	260-340	5-100
Epitestosterone	<0	0.1
5α Androstane-3α, 17β-diol	160	<0.5
5α Androstane-3α, 17β-diol	160	<0.5-3.0
Androstenedione	<1	0.3-5.0
Dehydroepiandrosterone	<5	<0.1
Δ⁵-Androstenediol	50	0.1-1.5
Estrone	<1-20	<0.1
Estradiol	20-60	<0.1
Estriol	5	<0.1
Progesterone	<5	<0.1
17-Hydroxyprogesterone	<5	<0.1
Cortisol	<3	<0.1

structed. The amount of testosterone in a given unknown sample is determined by obtaining the ratio of area responses of testosterone-HFB/internal standard and interpolating the quantity of testosterone from this standard curve. The value obtained is corrected for procedural losses to yield the amount of testosterone contained in the original sample.

Recently, other more potent electron-capture derivatives of testosterone have been explored in an attempt to increase the sensitivity of the method. The hexadecafluoronanoate (HFN) derivative is a polyfluoride derivative which can be made from the acyl chloride.[18] Use of this derivative has resulted in some simplification of the GLC-electron capture method to measure testosterone.[18]

Limitations. Although this method represents a considerable advance over double-isotope derivative methods, GLC with electron-capture detection requires sophisticated electronic hardware operating at maximal sensitivity. Such systems are susceptible to easy breakdown, and require diligent dedication and frequent trouble-shooting. This method is not readily suitable for a routine chemistry laboratory. For low-level determinations, 10 to 20 ml of plasma are required, along with several days of work. The most recent modification using HFN derivatives improves the sensitivity so that 5 ml of plasma can be used and working time is somewhat decreased.

Competitive Protein Binding

With the observation that sex hormones, testosterone and estradiol are transported in the blood of most animal species by a carrier protein, testosterone estradiol binding globulin (TEBG), there was much interest in utilizing this "specific protein" in a radioligand-type of assay.[7,19-24] A competition reaction between ³H-testosterone and increasing quantities of unlabeled testosterone for this binding protein was easily demonstrated in in vitro incubations and provided the basic reaction for a competitive protein-binding type of assay (CPB).

In developing a CPB assay, large quantities of TEBG or plasma rich in TEBG are desired. High titers of TEBG can be obtained by using plasma from estrogen-treated patients or pregnant women. Since a variety of C_{18} and C_{19}-steroids bind to TEBG (Table 12-2), it became apparent that preliminary purification of the sample was necessary to obtain a true value for testosterone.

The determination of testosterone by CPB assay is outlined in Figure 12-5. The sample is extracted with ether after addition of tracer-labeled testosterone to monitor procedural losses. Following extraction, the sample is purified by TLC prior to incubation with TEBG. In performing the assay, preincubation of the unknown sample with ³H-testosterone and TEBG-rich plasma is carried out at 37°C for 30 minutes followed by overnight incubation at 4°C. After completion of the equilibrium reaction, separation of the protein-bound versus unbound testosterone is accomplished by adding saturated ammonium sulfate, which precipitates protein-bound testosterone, or by adding 0.5 percent dextran-coated charcoal, florisil or other adsorbing agents which remove the unbound (free) testosterone. The remaining sample, representing free or bound testosterone respectively is added to a counting vial along with phosphor solution, and counted in order to determine the percent ^{3}H-bound testosterone. At this point it is necessary to consider the ^{3}H-testosterone tracer added to the plasma sample at the outset of the procedure for the purpose of monitoring procedural losses. This is done as follows: The total counts in the assay tube equals the counts of ^{3}H-testosterone added to establish the equilibrium reaction with TEBG + the counts of ^{3}H-testosterone contained in the aliquot of plasma extract. This latter value is obtained by taking a duplicate aliquot of the purified plasma sample for counting. Since these 2 sources of ^{3}H-testosterone distribute themselves between bound and free in the same manner as the unlabeled sample being determined, the percent ^{3}H-bound to protein = cpm precipitated by $(NH_4)_2SO_4$/ cpm of ^{3}H-testosterone added to assay tube + cpm ^{3}H-testosterone in plasma sample (determined from the duplicate aliquot of purified plasma sample). By relating the protein-bound testosterone in the unknown sample to the standard displacement curve, the nan-

ograms of testosterone contained in the unknown sample are then determined. This standard curve is constructed with each assay. The value for testosterone obtained from this CPB assay is then corrected for recovery, yielding the quantity of testosterone contained in the original plasma sample.

Limitations. Although CPB assay is considerably easier to perform and more readily adapted to routine laboratory use than the preceding methods, this approach has largely been preempted by even simpler, more predictable radioimmunoassays. Since relatively large amounts of TEBG-bearing serum are generally required for this assay, it is necessary to replenish the supply of protein every few weeks, with its associated restandardizations, etc. Further, the protein seems more labile in prolonged storage compared to the excellent stability of antibodies. Sensitivity and specificity of this method, although acceptable, are not as good as that provided by radioimmunoassay. As noted in Table 12-1, assay of testosterone in female plasma or other biological samples using this method requires the same working time as radioimmunoassay. In general, 2 to 5 ml of plasma are required for this assay.

Radioimmunoassay

Although testosterone and other steroids are not antigenic, when chemically complexed with a large molecule (e.g., albumin, hemocyanin or thyroglobulin), it serves as an excellent hapten for the generation of antibodies which can then be used as a "specific protein" for a radioligand assay (radioim-

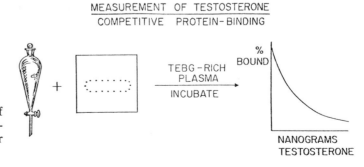

MEASUREMENT OF TESTOSTERONE
COMPETITIVE PROTEIN-BINDING

Fig. 12-5. Determination of testosterone using competitive-protein binding. (See text for details.)

munoassay).[8,25-30] The antibodies to testosterone thus produced have very high affinity constants, are stable for long periods of storage in the deep-freeze, and can be used in extremely high dilutions so that a single yield of rabbit antiserum is usually capable of supplying antibody for the projected lifetime of the laboratory.

The specificity of antibodies raised against testosterone by different methods of conjugation varies somewhat, but in general, the antibodies raised against 3-oxo-conjugates are more specific than those raised against 17-conjugates of testosterone.[25] As noted in Table 12-2, most antibodies to the 3-oxo-conjugate of testosterone cross-react with dihydrotestosterone, but do not cross-react with Δ^5-3βol compounds, estrogens, progestins or corticoids.

Although specificity of testosterone antibodies is quite high, most radioimmunoassay methods to date still employ solvent extraction and some preliminary purification prior to the assay. Sephadex LH-20 or celite partition chromatography provide simple, rapid clean-up, rendering the testosterone-containing fraction free of known cross-reacting substances. An outline of the testosterone assay system used in our laboratory is shown in Figure 12-6. The plasma sample is extracted with ether, after addition of ³H-testosterone to monitor procedural losses. The extract is put through a small 5 ml Sephadex LH-20 column, using isooctane:benzene:methanol, 85:10:5. In this system, the testosterone fraction elutes at 45 to 60 ml, dihydrotestosterone elutes at 30 to 40 ml and androstenedione elutes at 15 to 28 ml. The dried eluate is reacted with antibody over-night at 4°C, or 1 hour at room tempraeture followed by 1 hour at 4°C. Separation of bound versus free testosterone is accomplished with 0.5 percent dextran-coated charcoal. Following centrifugation of the charcoal, the supernate containing the protein-bound testosterone is poured into counting vials and counted in a solution of 3 ml dioxane and 10 ml of PPO-POPOP solution. The dioxane is used to facilitate solution of the protein-bound testosterone.

The sensitivity of the standard curve using testosterone antibody is approximately 10 times that achieved by use of TEBG in a competitive protein-binding assay.

Limitations. Although this method is the simplest and most sensitive approach devised to date, plasma extraction and preliminary purification are still required. The development of antibodies entirely specific for testosterone might enable the assay to be performed on unextracted plasma, and thus approach the ease and rapidity of radioimmunoassays currently in use for protein hormones.

Other Androgens

Although double-isotope derivative methods, electron-capture GLC and competitive protein-binding assays have been reported for the measurement of other C_{19} compounds, these more complex and time-consuming methods are rapidly being replaced by specific radioimmunoassay methods. As described in the previous section, none of the antibodies generated to date seems to be entirely specific for the compound to be measured, thus requiring preliminary extraction of the sample and chromatography prior

MEASUREMENT OF TESTOSTERONE
RADIOIMMUNOASSAY

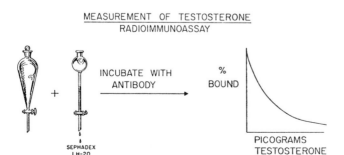

Fig. 12-6. Determination of testosterone using radioimmunoassay. Preliminary purification is achieved, using a Sephadex LH-20 column. (See text for details.)

Table 12-3. Radioimmunoassay Methods for Measurement of Lesser $C_{19}O_2$ Steroidal Compounds.

Steroid	Author	Antibody	Procedure	Normal Values (ng/100 ml)
Dehydroepi-androsterone (DHEA)	Nieschlag[31]	Versus DHEA-17-albumin	Extraction + TLC + assay	M = 532 ± 134 F = 403 ± 216
Dehydroepi-androsterone-sulfate (DHEA-SO₄)	Nieschlag[31]	Versus DHEA-17-albumin	Solvolysis + extraction + TLC + assay	M = 195 ± 47 μg% F = 196 ± 72 μg%
Androstenediol (Δ⁵-diol)	Loriaux[32]	Versus DHEA-17-albumin (cross-reaction)	Extraction + TLC + assay	M = 161 ± 52 F = 100 ± 84
Androstenedione	Thorney-craft[33]	Versus Testosterone-17-albumin (cross-reaction)	Extraction + celite column + assay	M = 115 ± 35 F = 141 ± 30
	Kirschner[34]	Versus Testosterone-3-oxo-conjugate	Extraction + Sephadex LH-20 + borohydride + testosterone assay	M = 60-200 F = 100-250
Androsterone	Youssefne-jadian[35]	Versus Androsterone-17-oxo-conjugate	Extraction + assay	M = 46 ± 28 F = 54 ± 32
Dihydro-testosterone	Ito[36]	Competitive protein-binding, using TEBG	Extraction + chromatography + CPB + assay	M = 54 ± 19 F = 14.8 ± 5.4

to the assay procedure. A rapidly growing list of radioligand methods for the lesser C_{19} androgenic compounds is presented in Table 12-3.[31-36] Note that a given antibody may be useful for measuring more than one substance, providing the sample has been adequately purified from contaminants, prior to the assay (i.e., antibody to measure plasma DHEA may be used to measure other Δ⁵ compounds after they have been adequately purified). Similarly, it should be possible to quantify dihydrotestosterone in plasma, using cross-reacting antibodies to testosterone.

Determination of androstenedione (androst-4-ene-3, 17-dione) in biological fluids merits special attention, since it is the major prehormone of testosterone in women, and thus its determination is often desired in assessing clinical states of virilism. Androstenedione is readily converted to testoster-

one by enzymatic reduction, or even simpler, by borohydride reduction at the 17 position. Thus, many methods reported for measuring androstenedione in biological fluids involve extraction, chromatographic isolation of the androstenedione-containing fraction and then reduction to testosterone with borohydride. Testosterone is then quantified by the detection system used in the respective laboratory. In our present radioimmunoassay system, androstenedione, dihydrotestosterone and testosterone may be determined from a single plasma sample by collecting the appropriate fractions from a Sephadex LH-20 column (see previous section). The androstenedione fraction is reduced with borohydride and treated thereafter as testosterone.[34] In the method of Thorneycraft,[33] androstenedione is isolated and measured directly, utilizing a cross-reacting antibody to testosterone-17-

albumin. More recently, an antibody raised against androstenedione-6-oxo-albumin has been reported to be entirely specific for androstenedione, enabling this steroid to be assayed without chromatography and without chemical transformation to testosterone.

As of this time, there is no published method for radioimmunoassay of dihydrotestosterone.

CLINICAL USES OF ANDROGEN DETERMINATIONS

In Men

Testosterone production rates in normal men average 7 mg per day, of which 90 to 95 percent is secreted directly by the testes. Approximately 50 percent of this is metabolized to the 17-ketosteroids, androsterone and etiocholanolone, which are then excreted in the urine. As noted in Table 12-4, total 17-ketosteroid excretion in normal men ranges from 10 to 15 mg per day, and thus it is apparent that testosterone accounts for only 25 percent of the total 17-ketosteroid metabolites excreted in the urine of normal men. Previous studies by Camacho and Migeon[37,38] have shown that approximately 1 percent of testosterone is excreted in the urine as testosterone glucuronide; thus normal men excrete approximately 70 μg per day of this metabolite. Plasma testosterone concentrations in normal men range from 400 to 1,000 ng/100 ml, with highest values noted in younger men, 20 to 40 years of age, and a gradual decline in these levels through the subsequent decades of life.[39] Most laboratories agree that there is diurnal variation in plasma testosterone levels in men similar to that of cortisol, although of smaller magnitude.

Testosterone secretion by the testes appears to be governed by luteinizing hormone (LH) in a negative feedback-inhibition system. Testosterone secretion is stimulated by LH (and HCG) and is inhibited by exogenous androgens such as fluoxymesterone or 2α methyl dihydrotestosterone.[40,41] Recent studies by Boyar[42] indicate that early adolescence is characterized by major discharges in

Table 12-4. Parameters of Androgen Production in Normal Men and Women.

	Men	*Women*
Testosterone production rate	7 mg/day	0.23 mg/day
Urinary 17-ketosteroid excretion	10-15 mg/day	5-10 mg/day
Urinary testosterone excretion	70 μg/day	5 μg/day
Plasma testosterone concentration	700 ng/100 ml	35 ng/100 ml

LH and concomitant increments in plasma testosterone levels during periods of deep sleep. In later stages of puberty and in adult men, early deep sleep is not associated with surges of testosterone secretion. Although testosterone secretion responds within minutes to LH, and LH responds within minutes to the polypeptide releasing hormone, LH-RH,[43-45] there are no known physiologic situations where plasma testosterone rises acutely, except during sleep in adolescence. Male arousal and coitus is not associated with changes in plasma levels of testosterone or the pituitary-trophic hormones.[46]

Testosterone measurements have been most useful in evaluating hypogonadal states, particularly when combined with estimation of gonadotrophin excretion or plasma LH levels. In primary gonadal failure, such as Klinefelter's syndrome, low plasma testosterone levels are combined with elevated gonadotrophin excretion.[40,47] In men with pituitary disorders, such as acromegaly, hypogonadism is associated with low gonadotrophins and low testosterone levels which can be stimulated by exogenous gonadotropin.[48] Gonadal deficiency states such as Kallman's syndrome, testicular feminization, myotonic dystrophy, hepatic cirrhosis, and various pseudohermaphrodite syndromes have been greatly clarified by testosterone measurements.[40,48-53] Of more limited value, however, has been the assessment of testosterone blood levels in male impotence and in men with aberrant sexual behavior. In most cases testosterone parameters are normal, unless underlying gonadal disease is co-existent.[54-58]

Of great interest has been the observation that men with gonadotrophin-producing neoplasms (choriocarcinoma, teratocarcinoma, etc.) whose testes are under continuous intensive, gonadotrophic stimulation, do not demonstrate elevated testosterone blood levels or production rates. Plasma testosterone levels in these men are normal, or low, and it appears that the Leydig cells of these patients have a peculiar refractoriness to the excessive production of trophic hormone.[59]

In Women

The normal testosterone production rate in women is 230 ± 73 μg per day (Table 12-4). Approximately half of this small amount is excreted as 17-ketosteroids, thus making it apparent that testosterone production contributes insignificantly to the total 17-KS excretion. It follows that 17-ketosteroid determinations are a very poor index of androgen production in women. Further, as noted in Table 12-4, urinary testosterone glucuronide excretion in normal women is approximately twice that expected. This apparent discrepancy was explained by Korenman[60] who showed that prehormones could be metabolized directly to testosterone glucuronide, without entering the plasma testosterone pool. Thus, in women, urinary testosterone does not accurately reflect the plasma testosterone production rate.

Plasma testosterone concentrations in normal women average 35 ng/100 ml, with the range of normal extending from 20 to 70 ng%.[61,62] As illustrated in Figure 12-7, testosterone in women comes from 3 distinct sources. Testosterone is secreted in small quantities by both adrenals and ovaries,[63] and in normal women 50 to 60 percent of daily testosterone production arises from peripheral metabolism of prehormones, chiefly androstenedione.[61,62] This latter steroid, is normally produced at the rate of 2 to 4 mg per day and androstenedione plasma concen-

trations vary from 100 to 250 ng/100 ml. Although androstenedione has minimal inherent androgenic activity, it is readily transformed to testosterone (4-5%) by various nonendocrine tissues, accounting for a major portion of the daily testosterone production rate in women. It thus becomes important to determine androstenedione concentrations in blood of women with abnormal androgen production. Other $C_{19}O_2$ steroids such as dehydroepiandrosterone and Δ^5-androstenediol are only minimally converted to testosterone in the peripheral circulation and account for only 6 percent of

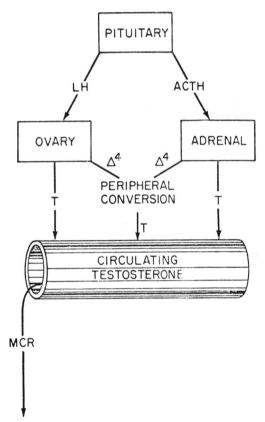

Fig. 12-7. Representation of the origin and disposition of testosterone in women. Testosterone is secreted by the ovaries and adrenals. Approximately 50 percent of testosterone arises by peripheral metabolism of androstenedione (Δ^4). The plasma level of testosterone is determined by rate of entry from the above 3 sources, and rate of exit (metabolic clearance rate).

Table 12-5. Factors Effecting Metabolic Clearance Rates of Testosterone.

Increased Metabolic Clearance Rates	Decreased Metabolic Clearance Rates
Hypothyroidism	Hyperthyroidism
Virilization	Aging
Androgen treatment	Pregnancy
Dexamethasone treatment	Estrogen treatment
Large adrenal, ovarian	Barbiturate treatment
and testicular tumors	Erect posture
Progestins	Hypogonadism

the total testosterone produced in women.[34]

As noted in Figure 12-7, the plasma testosterone concentration depends on production rates of testosterone from 3 sources, as well as the rate of clearance of testosterone from the blood (metabolic clearance rate). Clearance of testosterone in normal women appears to take place entirely in the liver; however, in various states of virilism, extrahepatic tissues participate in testosterone clearance.[64] The metabolic clearance rate of testosterone may be altered by 50 to 100 percent in a variety of clinical conditions; primarily those which alter the binding protein, TEBG, or conditions associated with androgen overproduction (Table 12-5).[63] It is thus necessary to consider these factors which influence testosterone clearance when evaluating the significance of a plasma testosterone determination. Since most clinical facilities currently do not have the capability of measuring the metabolic clearance rates of testosterone, alternate attempts to assess functional androgen levels have been made. Several laboratories have determined the proportion of circulating testosterone which is bound to carrier protein, TEBG versus the free or unbound testosterone. These determinations of testosterone-binding index, or binding capacity have an excellent negative correlation with the metabolic clearance rate, as shown by Vermeulen.[65] When binding capacity is elevated (as after estrogen therapy), clearance is decreased; when the binding index is decreased, MCR_T is increased. Thus, determination of binding index or binding capacity may be a useful indicator of clearance.

Virilizing States. Virilization in women is associated with exogenous administration of androgens and with endogenous overproduction of testosterone. Testosterone production rates in 62 women with varying degrees of virilism are shown in Figure 12-8. Increased body hair and hirsutism represent mild (early) features of increased testosterone production. As the virilizing process becomes more severe, other features such as menstrual abnormalities, clitorimegaly, temporal balding and deepening of the voice may occur.

As noted in the previous section, the testosterone production rate is the product of the plasma testosterone concentration and metabolic clearance rate (P_B^T = plasma T × MCR_T). Studies from a variety of laboratories indicate that approximately 25 percent of women with varying degrees of virilism have plasma testosterone concentrations that fall within the normal female range (false-negatives).[61,63,64,66] In these cases, increased testosterone production rate is associated with normal plasma testosterone levels and increased metabolic clearance rate. Measurement of testosterone and its major prohormone, androstenedione in peripheral blood have been useful in determining the degree of androgen abnormality in most virilized women. Measurement of these compounds in ovarian and adrenal venous effluents by means of percutaneous catheterization or by direct venous sampling at the time of surgical exploration have been most useful in localizing the sites of androgen excess.[66] In patients with adrenal tumors or hyperplasia associated with virilism, localization of androgen production to the diseased adrenal

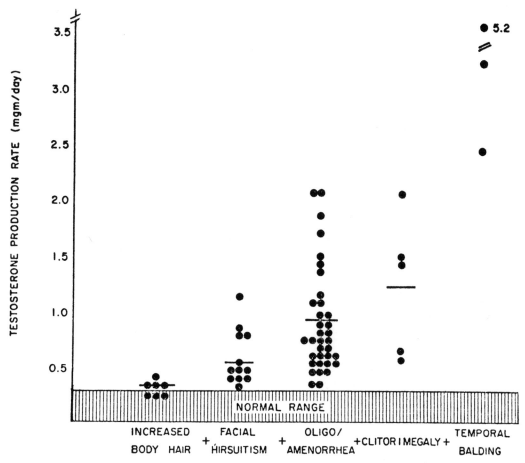

Fig. 12-8. Testosterone production rates in 62 consecutive women with varying degrees of virilism. With increasing signs of virilism, testosterone production rate increases.

is readily demonstrated.[63] Similarly, when virilism is associated with ovarian tumors, hilar cell hyperplasia, or stromal hyperthecosis, localization of androgen production to the ovary has been demonstrated.[63]

In women with idiopathic hirsutism, percutaneous catheterization of ovarian and adrenal veins has permitted us to localize the site of excessive androgen production to the ovaries in 20 of 28 patients. In 7 patients both ovaries and adrenals participated in the androgen overproduction; and in only 1 case was the excessive androgen production localized to the adrenal, as noted in Table 12-6. Of great interest was the obser-

Table 12-6. Origin of Excess Androgens in 28 Women with Idiopathic Hirsutism. (Deterimned by adrenal and ovarian vein catheterizations)

	No. of Patients	No. of Patients Showing Suppression of Androgens after Dexamethasone*
Ovarian	20	6
Ovarian and adrenal	7	7
Adrenal	1	1

* At least a 50 percent decrease in both plasma testosterone and androstenedione after 4 days of dexamethasone, 1 mg q.i.d.

vation that approximately one-third of the patients with ovarian over-production of androgens exhibited a 50 percent decrease in plasma testosterone and androstenedione concentrations when placed on exogenous glucocorticoids. In all patients where the adrenal gland was involved in androgen overproduction, glucocorticoids suppressed these androgens, as expected. The above data cast doubt on the validity of "corticoid suppression tests" to localize the site(s) of androgen overproduction in women with hirsutism. This does not, however, diminish the usefulness of these suppression tests in determining whether use of exogenous glucocorticoids are worthwhile in the long-term management of the virilized woman.

References

1. Finkelstein, M., Forchielli, E., and Dorfman, R. I.: Estimation of testosterone in human plasma. J. Clin. Endocrol. Metab., *21*:98, 1961.
2. Forchielli, E., Sorcini, G., Nightingale, M. S., Brust, N., *et al.*: Testosterone in human plasma. Ann. Biochem., *5*:416, 1963.
3. Riondel, A., Tait, J. F., Gut, M., Tait, S. A. S., *et al.*: Estimation of testosterone in human peripheral blood using ^{35}S-thiosemicarbazide. J. Clin. Endocrol. Metab., *23*:620, 1963.
4. Kirschner, M. A., Lipsett, M. B., and Collins, D. R.: Plasma ketosteroids and testosterone in man: A study of the pituitary-testicular axis. J. Clin. Invest., *44*:657, 1965.
5. Brownie, A. C., Van der Molen, H. J., Nishizawa, E. E., and Eik-Nes, K. B.: Determination of testosterone in human peripheral blood using gas-liquid chromatography with electron-capture detection. J. Clin. Endocrinol. Metab., *24*:1091, 1964.
6. Kirschner, M. A., and Coffman, G. D.: Measurement of plasma testosterone and Δ^4-androstenedione using electron-capture gas-liquid chromatography. J. Clin. Endocrinol. Metab., *28*:1347, 1968.
7. Murphy, B. E. P.: Protein binding and the assay of nonantigenic hormones. Recent Progr. Horm. Res., *25*:563, 1969.
8. Furuyama, S., Mayes, D. M., and Nugent, C. A.: A radioimmunoassay for plasma testosterone. Steroids, *16*:415, 1970.
9. Hudson, B., Coghlan, J., Dulmanis, A., Wintour, M., and Ekkel, I.: Estimation of testosterone in biological fluids. 1. Testosterone in plasma. Aust. J. Exp. Biol. Med. Sci., *41*:235, 1963.
10. Burger, H. G., Kent, J. R., and Kellie, A. E.: Determination of testosterone in human peripheral and adrenal venous plasma. J. Clin. Endocrol. Metab., *24*:432, 1964.
11. Coppage, W. S., and Cooner, A. E.: Testosterone in human plasma. N. Eng. J. Med., *273*:902, 1965.
12. Lim, N. Y., and Brooks, R. V.: A modification of the ^{35}S-thiosemicarbazide method for the estimation of plasma testosterone. Steroids, *6*:561, 1965.
13. Rivarola, M. A., and Migeon, C. J.: Determination of testosterone and androst-4-ene-3, 17-dione concentration in human plasma. Steroids, *7*:103, 1966.
14. Bardin, C. W., and Lipsett, M. B:. Estimation of testosterone and androstenedione in human peripheral plasma. Steroids, *9*:71, 1967.
15. Gandy, H. M., and Peterson, R. E.: Measurement of testosterone and 17-ketosteroids in plasma by the double isotope dilution derivative technique. J. Clin. Endocrinol. Metab., *28*:949, 1968.
16. Kliman, B., and Peterson, R.: Double isotope derivative assay of aldosterone in biological extracts. J. Biol. Chem., *235*:1639, 1960.
17. Sarda, I. R., Pochi, P., Strauss, J. S., and Wotiz, H. H.: Determination of plasma testosterone as the heptafluorobutyrate using gas liquid chromatography with electron-capture detection. Steroids, *12*:607, 1968.
18. Kirschner, M. A., and Taylor, J. P.: New derivatives for electron-capture gas chromatography of steroids: A simplified procedure for measuring plasma testosterone. Ann. Biochem., *30*:346, 1969.
19. Horton, R., Kato, T., and Sherins, R.: A rapid method for the estimation of testosterone in male plasma. Steroids, *10*:245, 1967.
20. Hullberg, M. C., Zorn, E. M., and Wieland, R. G.: A sensitive testosterone assay by protein-binding. Steroids, *12*:241, 1968.
21. Kato, T., and Horton, R.: A rapid method for the estimation of testosterone in female plasma. Steroids, *12*:631, 1968.
22. Mayes, D. M., and Nugent, C. A.: Determination of plasma testosterone by the use of competitive protein binding. J. Clin. Endocrinol. Metab., *28*:1169, 1968.
23. Rosenfield, R. L., Eberlein, W. R., and Bongiovanni, A. M.: Measurement of

plasma testosterone by means of competitive protein binding analysis. J. Clin. Endocrinol. Metab., *29*:854, 1969.

24. Vermeulen, A., and Verdonck, L.: Testosterone assays by competitive protein binding. Karolinska Symposium on Research Methods in Reproductive Endocrinology, *2*:239, 1970.

25. Niswender, G. D., and Midgley, A. R.: Hapten-radioimmunoassay for steroid hormones. *In* Poron, F. G., and Caldwell, B. V.: Immunologic Methods in Steroid Determination. ch. 8. New York, Appleton-Century-Crofts, 1960.

26. Chen, J. C., Zorn, E. M., Hellberg, M. C., and Wieland, R. C.: Antibodies to testosterone-3-bovine serum albumin, applied to assay of serum 17β-ol androgens. Clin. Chem., *17*:585, 1971.

27. Nieschlag, E., and Loriaux, D. L.: Radioimmunoassay for plasma testosterone. Z. Klin. Chem. Klin. Biochem., *10*:164, 1972.

28. Dufau, M. L., Catt, K. J., Tsurnhara, T., and Ryan, D.: Radioimmunoassay of plasma testosterone. Clin. Chim. Acta, *37*:109, 1972.

29. Forest, M. G., Cathiard, A. M., and Bertrand, J. A.: Total and unbound testosterone levels in the newborn and in normal and hypogonadal children: Use of a sensitive radioimmunoassay for testosterone. J. Clin. Endocrinol. Metab., *36*:1132, 1973.

30. Hillier, S. G., Brownsey, B. G., and Cameron, E. H. D.: Some observations on the determination of testosterone in human plasma by radioimmunoassay using antisera raised against testosterone-3-BSA and testosterone 11-α-BSA. Steroids, *21*:735, 1973.

31. Nieschlag, E., Loriaux, D. L., and Lipsett, M. B.: Radioligand assay for Δ^5-3β-hydroxysteroids. 1) 3β-hydroxy-5-androstene-17-one and its 3-sulfate. Steroids, *19*:669, 1972.

32. Loriaux, D. L., and Lipsett, M. B.: Radioligand assay for Δ^5-3β hydroxysteroids and 5-androstene-3β, 17β-diol and 3β, 17α-dihydroxy-5-pregnene-20-one. Steroids, *19*:681, 1972.

33. Thorneycraft, I. H., Ribeiro, W. O., and Stone, S. C.: A radioimmunoassay of androstenedione. Steroids, *21*:111, 1973.

34. Kirschner, M. A., Sinhamahapatra, S., Zucker, I. R., Loriaux, D. L., and Nieschlag, E.: The production, origin and role of dehydroepiandrosterone and Δ^5-androstenediol as androgen prehormones in hirsute women. J. Clin. Endocrinol. Metab., *37*:83, 1973.

35. Youssefnejadian, E., Collins, W. P., and Sommerville, I. F.: Radioimmunoassay of plasma androsterone. Steroids, *27*:63, 1973.

36. Ito, T., and Horton, R.: Dihydrotestosterone in human peripheral plasma. J. Clin. Endocrinol. Metab., *31*:362, 1970.

37. Camacho, A., and Migeon, C. J.: Isolation, Identification and quantitation of testosterone in the urines of normal adults and in patients with endocrine disorders. J. Clin. Endocrinol. Metab., *23*:301, 1963.

38. Camacho, A., and Migeon, C. J.: Studies on the origin of testosterone in urine of normal adult subjects and patients with ovarian endocrine disorders. J. Clin. Invest., *43*:1083, 1964.

39. Kent, J. R., and Acone, A. B.: *In* Vermeulen, A., and Exley, D. (eds.): Androgen in Normal and Pathological Condition. Excerpta Medica Foundation International Congress Series, Amsterdam, *101*:31, 1966.

40. Lipsett, M. B., Wilson, H., Kirschner, M. A., Korenman, S. G., et al.: Studies on leydig cell physiology and pathology: Secretion and metabolism of testosterone. Recent Progr. Horm. Res., *22*:245, 1966.

41. Lipsett, M. B., Migeon, C. J., Kirschner, M. A., and Bradin, C. W.: Physiologic basis of disorders of androgen metabolism. Ann. Intern. Med., *68*:1327, 1968.

42. Boyar, R.: Personal communication.

43. Kastin, A. J., Schally, A. V., Gual, C., and Arimura, A.: Release of LH and FSH after administration of synthetic LH-releasing hormone. J. Clin. Endocrinol. Metab., *34*:753, 1972.

44. Isurugi, K., Wakabayashi, K., Fukutani, K., Takayasu, H., et al.: Responses of serum luteinizing hormone and follicle-stimulating hormone levels to synthetic luteinizing hormone-releasing hormone (LH-RH) in various forms of testicular disorders. J. Clin. Endocrinol. Metab., *37*:533, 1973.

45. Roth, J. C., Grumbach, M. M., and Kaplan, S. L.: Effect of synthetic luteinizing hormone-releasing factor in serum testosterone and Gonadotropins in prepubertal, pubertal and adult males. J. Clin. Endocrinol. Metab., *37*:680, 1973.

46. Stearns, E. L., Winter, J. S. D., and Faiman, C.: Effect of coitus on gonadotropin, prolactin and sex steroid levels in man. J. Clin. Endocrinol. Metab., *37*:687, 1973.

47. Paulsen, C. A., Gordon, D. L., Carpenter, R. W., Gandy, H. M., and Drucker, W. D.: Klinefelter's syndrome and its variants: A hormonal and chromosomal study. Recent Progr. Horm. Res., *24*:321, 1968.

growing body of evidence implicating Na[+], K[+]-activated "transport" ATPase in the mechanism of cardiac glycoside action.[31-35] Direct evidence has been obtained in studies of the squid giant axon and red blood cells that this enzyme system, presumed to be located within the plasma membrane, is inhibited by cardioactive steroids only when the latter are present at the external cell surface.[36,37] Thus, if an important mediator of digitalis effect lies in close proximity to the external cell surface, this site should be maximally responsive to serum digitalis concentrations.

Recent experiments in animals have borne out the expectations of a close relationship between plasma digoxin concentrations and electrophysiologic effects on the heart. Changes in automaticity reflected by provocation of repetitive ventricular responses by low-energy endocardial stimuli were significantly related to plasma digoxin concentration.[38] Serum digoxin concentration was also significantly related over a wide range to acetyl strophanthidin tolerance in a canine experimental model.[38] As shown in Figure 13-1 over a range from 0 to 14 ng/ml, serum digoxin concentration was inversely correlated with acetyl strophanthidin tolerance; for each 1.0 ng/ml increase in digoxin level, a mean value of 5.2 μg/kg

less acetyl strophanthidin was needed to evoke ventricular tachycardia.

DIGITALIS ASSAY TECHNIQUES

The literature related to quantitation of serum or plasma digitalis glycoside concentrations has expanded rapidly in recent years. Table 13-1 lists the various approaches which have been employed, followed by the drug(s) to which each method has been applied and relevant references.

Prior to the development of radioisotope technology and improved immunochemical methodology, chemical methods were employed to measure relatively large quantities of cardiac glycosides (μg to mg range). The standard U.S.P. assay system for digitoxin involves measurement of the optical density at 495 mμ after reaction of digitoxin with alkaline picrate.[39] Sample preparation is time consuming, and the sensitivity is such that the method is suitable only for samples in the milligram range. The U.S.P. assay for digoxin is also a colorimetric procedure in which digoxin is reacted with alkaline dinitrobenzene.[39] The activated methylene group in the lactone ring results in a colored product which is read at 620 mμ. Again, the method is exacting and relatively insensitive.

Jelliffe developed improved methods for the chemical determination of microgram

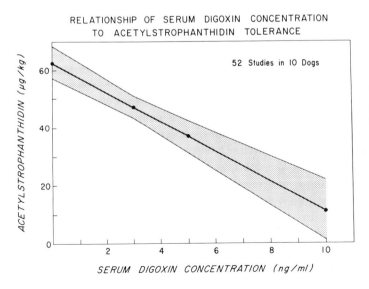

RELATIONSHIP OF SERUM DIGOXIN CONCENTRATION
TO ACETYLSTROPHANTHIDIN TOLERANCE

52 Studies in 10 Dogs

Fig. 13-1. Relation between serum digoxin concentration and acetylstrophanthidin tolerance in a canine experimental model. Serum digoxin concentration is inversely correlated with the amount of acetylstrophanthidin required to evoke ventricular tachycardia. The shaded area defines 95 percent confidence limits. (Data plotted from Barr, et al. Pharmacol. Exp. Ther., *180*:710, 1972)[38]

quantities of digitoxin and digoxin which could be used for studies of urinary excretion of these drugs.[40] This procedure employs chloroform extraction, successive alkali and water washes, thin-layer chromatographic isolation, elution, and xanthydrol quantification. This method has not been used for serum determinations.

The remainder of this section is concerned with methods of high sensitivity which are capable of quantitating the minute concentrations of digitalis compounds present in the serum of patients receiving usual therapeutic doses.

Much of the development of earlier techniques such as the various bioassay methods, including the duck embryo bioassay, has been reviewed by Friedman, St. George, and Bine.[42] The refinements introduced by these authors allowed the detection of digitoxin and lanatoside C concentrations as low as 5 ng/ml.[42,68]

During the 1950's, it became possible to label cardiac glycosides with ^{14}C and tritium (^{3}H). Administration of these labeled cardiac glycosides to experimental animals and human volunteers yielded useful information on the pharmacokinetics of these drugs.[43] In addition, development of radioisotope technology laid the groundwork for almost all of the assay techniques to be discussed subsequently.

Double-Isotope Derivative Assay. This assay for digitoxin developed by Lukas and Peterson[12] has been applied to measurements of digitoxin in plasma, whole blood, urine, and stool. ^{3}H-digitoxin is used to monitor procedural losses of digitoxin, while acetyl anhydride − 1 − ^{14}C is used to convert digitoxin to the triacetate. The method is capable of detecting 10 ng of digitoxin, and has been employed in studies of various aspects of digitoxin pharmacokinetics.[12,13]

A major asset of this method is its high specificity. Glycoside levels less than 1 ng/ml cannot be detected, and relatively large volumes of plasma are required for assay.

Gas-Liquid Chromatography. Watson and Kalman[46] developed a gas-liquid chromato-

Table 13-1. Approaches to Digitalis Concentration Determination.

I. **CHEMICAL METHODS OF LIMITED SENSITIVITY (MICROGRAM TO MILLIGRAM RANGE)***

  A. Alkaline Picrate: digitoxin[39]

  B. Alkaline Dinitrobenzene: digoxin[39]

  C. Xanthydrol: digitoxin and digoxin[40]

II. **MICROMETHODS SUITABLE FOR MEASUREMENT OF NANOGRAM QUANTITIES**

  A. Duck Embryo Bioassay: lanatoside C[41]; digitoxin[42]

  B. Radioisotope Labeling: digitoxin[43]; digoxin[43]; ouabain[43,44,45]

  C. Physicochemical Methods

    1. Double isotope dilution derivative: digitoxin[12,13]

    2. Gas-liquid chromatography: digoxin[46]

  D. Na$^+$, K$^+$ − Activated ATPase Inhibition

    1. Red cell rubidium uptake inhibition

      a. ^{86}Rb radioactivity measurement: digitoxin[25,47,48,49,50] digoxin[15,47,48,50-52]

      b. Atomic absorption spectrophotometry of nonradioactive rubidium: digitoxin[53,54]; lanatoside C[53,54]

    2. Microsomal Na$^+$, K$^+$ − activated ATPase inhibition: digitoxin[14,55]; digoxin[56]

  E. Competitive Protein Binding

    1. Radioimmunoassay: digoxin[19,20,22,24,57-60]; digitoxin[61,62]; deslanoside[63]; ouabain[64,65]; acetyl strophanthidin[66]

    2. ATPase enzymatic isotopic displacement: digoxin and digitoxin[67]

* An exhaustive review of these methods is beyond the scope of this discussion.

graphic method for assay of digoxin. Like the double-isotope derivative digitoxin assay discussed above, an initial extraction step is necessary. An internal ^{3}H-digoxin standard is added to the plasma sample to quantitate losses and methylene chloride extraction carried out, followed by preliminary purification on a florisil column and thin-layer chromatography on silica gel G. The hepafluorobutyrate derivative is then formed and the extract chromatographed again on silica gel. Gas-liquid chromatography is then carried out with electron-capture detection to enhance sensitivity. As in the case of the double derivative isotope method for digitoxin, this method has a high degree of specificity which has proved useful in the study of metabolic patterns.[69] As little as 0.2 ng/ml of digoxin can be detected.

[86]Rb Uptake Inhibition Assay. The discovery of Schatzmann[70] that cardiac glycosides are potent inhibitors of cellular monovalent cation transport laid the groundwork for the red blood cell ^{86}Rb uptake inhibition assay introduced by Lowenstein.[47] Initially modified by Lowenstein and Corrill[48] the method has been further developed by other workers for both digoxin[15,51,52] and digitoxin[25,49,71] assay. Serum or plasma samples are extracted with water-immiscible organic solvents, and the extract is assayed for ability to inhibit red blood cell ^{86}Rb uptake. [86]Rubidium, a potassium analog, is actively pumped into red cells and is used because of its relatively convenient radioactive half-life. Unknown samples are estimated by comparison with a standard curve defined with known amounts of the glycoside to be measured. Several important variables in this type of assay system have been defined by Bertler and Redfors[15] and by Gjerdrum.[49] Although some investigators have reported values for plasma digoxin concentrations with this technique which tend to be somewhat higher than those obtained by other methods,[51] more recent reports[16,72] reflect good agreement with the methods to be discussed subsequently. Since an extraction step is required, care must be given to the details of the extraction procedure to insure uniform recovery of standards and unknown samples. Metabolites of digoxin and digitoxin also cause inhibition of ^{86}Rb by red blood cells.[73]

An interesting variant of the red cell ^{86}Rb uptake inhibition assay is the method described by Bourdon and Mercier.[53] Inhibition of red cell Rb+-uptake by extracted cardiac glycosides forms the basis of this procedure, but quantitation of Rb+ concentrations is accomplished by atomic absorption spectrophotometry rather than counting of gamma radiation from [86]Rb.

Inhibition of Na+, K+-activated ATPase. This technique, originally described for digitoxin,[55] again employs the inhibitory properties of cardiac glycosides toward Na+, K+-activated ATPase. Plasma samples are first extracted with methylene dichloride and the extracts are included in a buffer system containing ATP and partially purified microsomal Na+, K+-activated ATPase prepared from pork brain. Increasing amounts of digitoxin result in increasing inhibition of the cleavage of ATP; enzymatic activity is quantitated by a colorimetric assay of inorganic phosphate liberated. The sensitivity of the method is adequate over the range of plasma digitoxin concentrations of clinical interest.

This method has been extended to the measurement of plasma digoxin concentrations.[56] The enhanced sensitivity necessary to measure clinically relevant plasma digoxin levels was obtained by incubating the plasma extract to be assayed with pork brain Na+, K+-ATPase in the absence of K+. Binding of cardiac glycosides to the enzyme with consequent inhibition of ATPase activity is maximal when K+ is absent during the incubation step, and this modification allowed a sensitivity of 0.3 ng/ml to be achieved. As the authors point out, although the procedure is less precise than radioimmunoassay and more time consuming, it has the advantage of applicability in the clinical laboratory which lacks radioisotope counting equipment.

Competitive Binding to Na+, K+-ATPase. Competitive binding of cardiac glycosides to Na+, K+-ATPase has been used by Brooker and Jelliffe[67] to measure digoxin and digitoxin concentrations. Reported results agree well with those obtained by radioimmunoassay. Five milliliters of serum is extracted with chloroform and the extract allowed to compete with ^{3}H-ouabain for specific binding sites on guinea pig brain Na+, K+ATPase. ^{3}H-ouabain bound to the enzyme is separated by centrifugation, and the amount of unbound ³H-ouabain displaced from the binding site by cardiac glycosides in the sample is measured by liquid scintillation counting. Correction for extraction efficiency of various cardiac glycosides must be made, but was found to be relatively constant at 89.2 ± 4.9% (1 S.D.) for digoxin and 46.9 ± 4.4% for digitoxin. This method is potentially applicable to any cardiac glycoside which can be reproducibly extracted from serum. The sensitivity of this method allows detection of 0.2 ng/ml.

RADIOIMMUNOASSAY

Our own experience is based on a radioimmunoassay approach.[57] In contrast to some of the previously described methods for measuring serum digitalis levels, the radioimmunoassay technique is quite applicable for practical, routine clinical use. Radioimmunoassay methods are capable of high sensitivity, accuracy, and rapidity. They can be carried out on 0.1 ml or less of serum, and require no extraction step. Large numbers of specimens can be processed within several hours.

The cardiac glycosides are not immunogenic by themselves, and to obtain antibodies it is necessary to couple these drugs as haptens to protein carriers. Butler and Chen[74] immunized rabbits with conjugates of digoxin and serum albumin, and antibodies were obtained which were shown to bind digoxin.

Antiserums obtained in this way have been characterized in detail.[63]

Radioimmunoassays employing antibodies that bind digoxin,[63] digitoxin,[61] ouabain,[64,65] and acetyl strophanthidin[66] have been useful in our own studies. Appropriately selected antisera have, exceptionally high affinity and specificity for the cardiac glycoside of interest, allowing the measurement of subnanogram amounts. The specificity of antibodies studied to date has been directed largely at determinants on the C-D ring end of the steroid portion of the molecule, and to a much lesser extent at the glycoside moiety. An antiserum selected for use in the digoxin-assay[57] bound digoxin with an affinity about fiftyfold greater than digitoxin, although the latter differs only in the absence of a single hydroxyl group at position 12 in the C ring of the steroid moiety.[63] Deslanoside, which has an identical steroid-lactone structure to digoxin but differs in the presence of a fourth sugar, glucose, on the oligosaccharide portion of the molecule, has nearly identical affinity.[63] There is no significant interference by either endogenous steroids from mammalian species or other drugs when properly selected antisera are employed.

The radioimmunoassay technique which has evolved in our laboratory[22,57,58,61,65,75,76] is briefly summarized in Figure 13-2. In this case an aliquot of serum containing un-

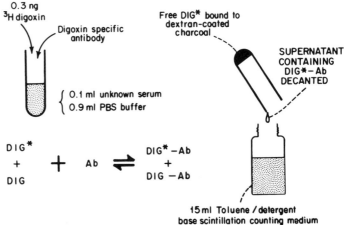

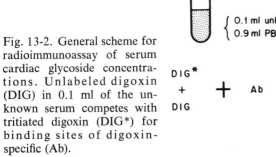

Fig. 13-2. General scheme for radioimmunoassay of serum cardiac glycoside concentrations. Unlabeled digoxin (DIG) in 0.1 ml of the unknown serum competes with tritiated digoxin (DIG*) for binding sites of digoxin-specific (Ab).

labeled digoxin (without prior extraction) is adjusted to a convenient volume with phosphate buffered saline (PBS) and an appropriate tracer quantity of ³H-digoxin is added. The amount of tracer used is determined by the range of digoxin concentrations which one wishes to measure, and this in turn depends upon the size of the serum aliquot used. For resolution of digoxin concentrations over the clinically relevant range from 0.2 to 20 ng/ml, a tracer quantity of about 2 to 3 ng is suitable. Thus, for 0.1 ml aliquots of serum 0.3 ng of tracer is used. The high specific activity of commercially available ³H-digoxin provides adequate counting rates for these small amounts of tracer. After thorough mixing, an amount of digoxin-specific antiserum is added which will bind about 40 to 50 percent of tracer counts in the absence of an unlabeled drug. This amount of antibody is selected to strike an optimal balance between sensitivity and precision. During incubation, an equilibrium is established (see Fig. 13-2) in which the amount of ³H-digoxin bound to antibody combining sites depends upon the amount of unlabeled digoxin in the sample.

Dextran-coated charcoal is then added to separate antibody-bound from free ³H-digoxin. Care should be taken to expose both known samples used to construct the standard curve and unknown samples to charcoal for similar lengths of time, since the equilibrium shown in Figure 13-2 may be pulled toward the left as free digoxin is bound to the charcoal. This tendency proves to be of little consequence when very high-affinity antibodies are used, but becomes an increasing problem with lower affinity antisera. After centrifugation to remove the charcoal, antibody-bound ³H-digoxin remaining in the supernatant phase is transferred to scintillation counting vials containing a toluene-detergent base-counting fluid. Samples are then counted (usually for 2 minutes) in a liquid scintillation spectrometer equipped with a ²²⁶Radium external standard for quenching correction. When results are urgently needed, a sample can be run in 1 hour without serious compromise of accuracy.

Figure 13-3 shows a typical standard curve obtained with known, gravimetrically determined amounts of crystalline digoxin. Because of the relatively large number of samples assayed daily in our laboratory, we have developed a simple computer program which corrects raw counts per minute for background and quenching, and plots the reciprocal count rate against a linear scale of digoxin concentration. The limited heterogeneity of antibody-binding site affinities in

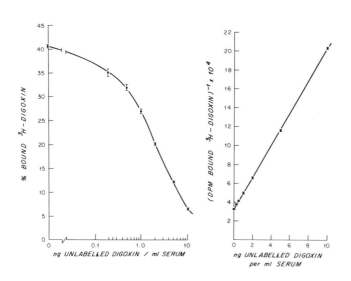

Fig. 13-3. Standard curves obtained by the procedure outlined in Fig. 13-2. *Left panel:* Percent of ³H-digoxin tracer bound by the antibody is plotted against a logarithmic scale of unlabeled digoxin concentration in the sample. Horizontal lines indicate ranges of duplicate determinations. It is apparent that a 0.2 ng/ml concentration is readily measurable in the 0.1 ml sample. *Right panel:* The same data are plotted as reciprocal antibody-bound counts (corrected for background and quenching) against a linear scale of unlabeled digoxin concentration. The rectilinear plot obtained is well suited to computer usage.

the antisera used results in a rectilinear plot (Fig. 13-3). The computer plots this line by least squares linear regression analysis, compares count rates for unknown samples, and prints out the concentration value. This computer program has been published elsewhere.[77] A single technician is able to assay up to 50 samples in duplicate in a normal working day.

The specificity of this assay system has been assessed by hapten inhibition experiments (Fig. 13-4). None of the endogenous steroid compounds tested produced measurable displacement of ³H-digoxin from antibody-binding sites of this antiserum unless present in greater than one-thousandfold molar excess.

This assay system can also be used for the determination of serum deslanoside concentrations. Known amounts of deslanoside are used to construct the standard curve, and tritiated digoxin is used as a tracer. Analogous methods are used for digitoxin,[61] ouabain,[64] and acetylstrophanthidin[66] measurement.

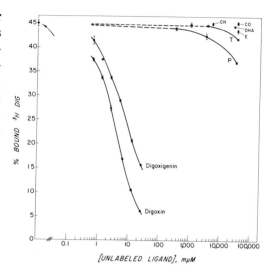

Fig. 13-4. Specificity of a selected rabbit digoxin-specific antiserum. ³H-digoxin is displaced from antibody binding sites to the extent shown by unlabeled digoxin, digoxigenin, cholesterol (CH), cortisol (CO), dehydroepiandrosterone (DHA), 17β-estradiol (E), progesterone (P), and testosterone (T). The endogenous steroid compounds cause significant displacement only when present in concentrations greater than 1,000-fold above those of digoxin.

Technical Pitfalls of Radioimmunoassay

There are a number of potential pitfalls which appear to have befallen some investigators who have employed radioimmunoassay techniques for the measurement of cardiac glycosides.[76,78] Erroneous results may occur if careful attention is not given to selection of antisera, assurance of purity of standards and tracers, and counting techniques.[76,77,79] Since assay results are no more accurate than the preparation of standards for the plotting of the standard curve, it is important to test crystalline digoxin for purity by thin-layer chromatography or some other sensitive analytical technique. The standard is then dried to constant weight before careful gravimetric preparation of standards. Fresh standards should be made up every few weeks. Purity of tracer tritiated digoxin is monitored as well, since there is significant variation from lot to lot from commercial suppliers. Loss of sensitivity at digoxin levels below 1 ng/ml due to deteri-

oration of the labeled antigen has been reported.[80] The presence of preexisting radioactivity in a serum sample is a relatively frequent cause of confusion. This is usually the result of a scanning procedure utilizing a gamma-emitting isotope and may be recognized by setting one channel of the liquid scintillation spectrometer to detect selectively these higher energy photons. When identified, the problem may be dealt with by prior extraction of the cardiac glycoside or by the method outlined by Butler.[81] Errors in counting also occur when correction for quenching by bile pigments or hemoglobin is neglected.

The most important and probably the most common source of error in cardiac glycoside radioimmunoassay procedures is the use of inadequate antibody preparations. Some investigators have failed to appreciate the importance of thorough characterization of antibodies prior to use in radioimmuno-assay procedures. Failure to select antisera of sufficient specificity may result in significant interference by endogeneous or exogeneously administered steroids or steroid antagonists such as spironolactone. An antibody with relatively rapid dissociation kinetics of the antibody-cardiac glycoside complex may also yield spurious results, particularly if charcoal contact times are not held constant for known and unknown samples.[76] Due to disturbance of antibody-hapten equilibrium, the antibody-bound fraction progressively decreases with increasing duration of exposure to charcoal in the assay, yielding inaccurate results.[77]

The specificity of an antibody may be defined in terms of the relative affinities for the homologous hapten and a potentially cross-reacting hapten at equilibrium. Antisera which have adequate specificity at equilibrium for use in radioimmunoassay systems may afford problems in cross-reactivity when the incubation is stopped short of equilibrium. At such times apparent specificity is influenced by the ratio of the association rate constants of haptens competing for antibody-binding sites, and this ratio may be substantially different from the ratio of their equilibrium constants. This phenomenon was graphically demonstrated with a ouabain-specific antibody that showed considerably greater apparent cross-reactivity with digoxin and digitoxin at 5 minutes' incubation than it did after 18 hours.[77] Some of these problems have been identified in certain commercial antisera that are made available without adequate characterization.

Another not uncommon source of error in clinical situations is the use of test systems designed for digoxin in evaluating patients on digitoxin or digitalis leaf.

It should also be pointed out that serum cardiac glycoside concentrations are only clinically meaningful if sufficient time has elapsed since the last dose to allow equilibration between plasma and tissue compartments. In practical terms, blood samples for cardiac glycoside assay should generally not be drawn until at least 5 to 6 hours after the last dose.

For hospital laboratories which do not wish to prepare their own antisera, availability of components in commercial kit form now exists. This allows for more widespread use of this method in clinical practice. Recognition of the technical pitfalls cited above is, of course, of great importance. The commercial availability of a digoxin analog with a radioactive-iodine label suitable for use as a tracer in the system has further extended the availability of the digoxin radioimmunoassay method to the laboratory with gamma-counting equipment but lacking a liquid scintillation counter. Park, et al.,[26] utilizing one of these latter kits, found the minimal detectable amount of digoxin in a 0.05 ml serum sample to be 0.4 ng/ml. Ten replicate analyses gave a 2-standard deviation of $\pm 7.1\%$ (within day reproducibility) whereas the 2-standard deviation for 14 assays performed over a month's period was $\pm 30\%$ (day-to-day reproducibility).

RELATIONSHIP BETWEEN SERUM CARDIAC GLYCOSIDE CONCENTRATION AND DIGITALIS INTOXICATION

During the past several years, a number of studies utilizing different assay methods have been carried out. These reflect substantial agreement concerning serum or plasma digoxin and digitoxin levels in patients receiving usual doses of these drugs. Tables 13-2 and 13-3 show mean serum digoxin and digitoxin concentrations in a number of groups of patients independently studied. Although not shown in these tables, the administered dose is generally well correlated with plasma concentration when appropriate factors, such as body size and renal function, are taken into account.[12,14,15,18,19,21,22,24,58] As expected, larger doses of digoxin were associated with higher serum concentrations of the drug. In the case of digoxin, impairment of renal function is associated with higher serum concentrations at any given dose level.[5,21,24,82] Plasma digi-

Table 13-2. Serum or Plasma Digoxin Concentrations: Nontoxic and Toxic Patients.

Authors (Ref.)	Method	Mean Conc. Nontoxic	Mean Conc. Toxic	Statistical Significance
Beller, et al.[5]	Radioimmunoassay	1.0	2.3	Yes
Bertler and Redfors[16]	[86]Rb uptake	0.9	2.4	Yes
Brooker and Jelliffe[67]	Enzymatic displacement	1.4	3.1	Yes
Burnett and Conklin[56]	ATPase inhibition	1.2	5.7	Yes
Chamberlain, et al.[19]	Radioimmunoassay	1.4	3.1	Yes
Evered and Chapman[21]	Radioimmunoassay	1.38	3.36	Yes
Fogelman, et al.[83A]	Radioimmunoassay	1.4	1.7	No
Grahame-Smith and Everest[51]	[86]Rb uptake	2.4	5.7	Yes
Hoeschen and Proveda[24]	Radioimmunoassay	0.8-1.3	2.8	Yes
Iisalo, Dahl, and Sundquist[84]	Radioimmunoassay	1.2	3.1	Yes
Johnston, Pinkus, and Down[85]	Radioimmunoassay	1.0	3.15	Yes
Lader, Bye, and Marsden[72]	Radioimmunoassay	1.1	2.2	Yes
Morrison, Killip, and Stason[18]	Radioimmunoassay	0.76	3.35	Not stated
Oliver, Parker, and Parker[60]	Radioimmunoassay	1.6	3.0	Yes
Park, et al.[26]	Radioimmunoassay	1.1	3.8	Yes
Smith, Butler, and Haber[63]	Radioimmunoassay	1.3	3.3	Yes
Smith and Haber[22]	Radioimmunoassay	1.4	3.7	Yes
Whiting, et al.[82]	Radioimmunoassay	1.4	3.5	Yes
Zeegers, et al.[86]	Radioimmunoassay	1.6	4.4	Yes

Table 13-3. Serum or Plasma Digitoxin Concentrations: Nontoxic and Toxic Patients.

Authors (Ref.)	Method	Mean Conc. Nontoxic	Mean Conc. Toxic	Statistical Significance
Beller, et al.[5]	Radioimmunoassay	20	34	Yes
Bentley, et al.[14]	ATPase inhibition	23	39	Yes
Brooker and Jelliffe[67]	Enzymatic displacement	31.8	48.8	Not stated
Lukas and Peterson[12]	Double isotope dilution derivative	20	43-67 (range)	Not stated
Morrison and Killip[17]	Radioimmunoassay	25 (0.1 mg/day) 44 (0.2 mg/day)	53	Yes
Rasmussen, et al.[25]	[86]Rb uptake	16.6	48.7	Not stated
Ritzmann, et al.[50]	[86]Rb uptake	19	39-51 (range)	Not stated
Smith[61]	Radioimmunoassay	17	34	Yes

toxin concentrations are, however, poorly correlated with renal function.[5,25,61] Patients taking digitalis leaf have apparent serum digitoxin concentrations similar to those taking crystalline digitoxin,[5,14,61] which is not surprising since digitoxin is the major active constituent of digitalis leaf.[11]

Some of the variation in mean serum digitalis levels in nontoxic patients is attributable to differing times at which serum was obtained for determination. For example, the relatively low mean serum digoxin concentration of 1.0 ng/ml in nontoxic patients observed by Beller, et al.,[5] is probably due in large part to the fact that some patients had received no digoxin for up to 48 hours prior to the time of serum sampling. It is reassuring to note that mean values for non-toxic patients tend to cluster closely around the mean steady state blood level of 1.4 ± 0.3 (SD) ng/ml found by Marcus, et al.[83] in a study of normal volunteers receiving 0.5 mg of tritiated digoxin per day.

Studies in Clinically Digitalis-toxic Patients

The relationship between serum digitalis concentrations and digitalis effects in toxic and nontoxic patients has attracted the interest of a number of investigators recently. This is a particularly complex subject because of a multiplicity of variables which influence cardiac responses to digitalis glycosides.[87] Factors of known importance include serum potassium, sodium, calcium, and magnesium levels, acid-base balance, hypoxemia, thyroid functional status, and autonomic nervous system influences. Additional drugs, particularly those with anti-arrhythmic properties, may exert modifying effects. The nature and severity of underlying heart disease is also of great importance in determining response to digitalis.[88] Studies of the relationship between serum digoxin concentration and occurrence of digitalis intoxication are also summarized in Table 13-2. Despite the multiple variable known to influence cardiac response to digitalis glycosides, it can be seen that significantly higher mean serum digoxin concentrations were observed in toxic patients compared with nontoxic patients in nearly all studies published to date. Mean serum digoxin levels of toxic patients tend to be about two- to threefold higher than those of patients without toxicity. It must be pointed out, however, that overlap clearly occurs between serum levels of toxic and nontoxic patients. It is apparent that no arbitrary level can be chosen which clearly differentiates toxic from nontoxic serum digoxin concentrations. This is not surprising when one considers that there is no specific "digitalis toxic" rhythm disturbance which does not occur as a result of

heart disease alone in patients who have never received digitalis.

In our own experience, one of the most important single factors predisposing to digoxin toxicity has been impaired renal function. Mean blood urea nitrogen concentration and incidence of uremia were both significantly higher in toxic hospitalized patients than in nontoxic.[22] Toxic patients in this series also tended to be older, a finding which may well have exerted its influence, at least in part, through diminished glomerular filtration rate and hence decreased digoxin excretion.[89] A high incidence of renal functional impairment was also evident in digoxin-toxic patients studied prospectively.[5]

Similar consideration applies to the evaluation of serum digitoxin concentrations. The results of a number of studies of serum or plasma digitoxin concentrations are summarized in Table 13-3. As in the case of digoxin, significant differences in mean concentrations have been observed between groups of patients with and without cardiac toxicity. Mean serum digitoxin levels in nontoxic patients are approximately tenfold higher than those of digoxin, presumably due to the substantially greater serum protein-binding of digitoxin.[90] Overlapping of serum digitoxin values among toxic and nontoxic patients has been noted[5,14,61] and, if anything, tends to be greater than in the case of digoxin. Patients on usual maintenance doses of digitalis leaf usually have serum digitoxin concentrations comparable to those of patients on usual maintenance digitoxin doses.[5,61,80] In contrast to digoxin toxic patients, no significant difference in serum creatinine or BUN was found between toxic patients receiving digitoxin or digitalis leaf and nontoxic patients on these drugs. This difference is illustrated in Figure 13-5 from the prospective study by Beller, et al.[5] in which mean serum creatinine concentration was significantly higher only in digoxin toxic patients when compared to a nontoxic digitalized group.

Although cardiac digitalis toxicity lends itself to certain relatively precise definitions of endpoint, it is more difficult to correlate therapeutic effects with serum levels in man. Chamberlain, et al.[19] showed that there was a correlation between slowing of ventricular rate in patients with atrial fibrillation and plasma digoxin levels when patients were studied who had rapid rates prior to treatment. As previously mentioned, another measure of the degree of digitalization is the cumulative dose of acetyl strophanthidin required to reach a toxic endpoint.[87,90] Barr, et al.[92] found a significant inverse correlation in a series of hospitalized patients between the dose of acetyl strophanthidin tolerated and the preexisting serum digoxin concentration, but pointed out that substantial variation in acetyl strophanthidin sensitivity was demonstrated by certain patients with similar serum digoxin levels, indicating a continuing need to correlate serum digoxin concentration with independent means of assessing myocardial sensitivity to cardiac glycosides.

DIGITALIS RADIOIMMUNOASSAY IN STUDIES OF THE CLINICAL PHARMACOLOGY OF CARDIAC GLYCOSIDES

Serum digitalis measurements have been useful in the investigation of various special problems in the clinical pharmacology and toxicology of cardiac glycosides including digoxin bioavailability studies.[88,93-106]

Cardiopulmonary Bypass. It has been suggested that certain patients exhibit increased sensitivity to digitalis in the immediate period following cardiopulmonary bypass. Digoxin handling by patients undergoing cardiopulmonary bypass has been investigated by the use of radioimmunoassay methods. Coltart, et al.[93] demonstrated negligible losses of digoxin from the body during bypass. Hemodilution resulted in an initial fall in mean serum digoxin concentration from 1.5 ng/ml to 1.1 ng/ml after 2 hours of bypass, but this returned to an average of 1.7 ng/ml on the first postoperative day. The amount of digoxin left in the discard reservoir bottle at the end of bypass amounted to no more than 3 μg. Morrison and Kilip[18]

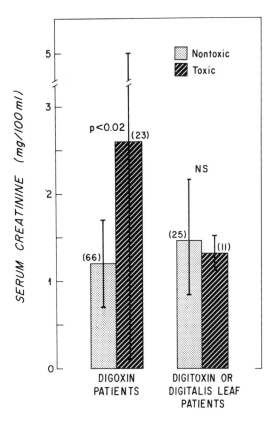

Fig. 13-5. Mean serum creatinine concentrations in nontoxic and toxic patients receiving digoxin (*left*) or digitoxin or digitalis leaf (*right*). A significant difference (P<0.02) in mean serum creatinine concentration was observed only in patients on digoxin. (Beller, G., et al.: N. Eng. J. Med., *284*:989, 1971)[5]

reported a similar experience in a group of chronically digitalized patients undergoing open-heart surgery. They found that after the initial fall during bypass, serum digitalis rebounded, rising to or surpassing the preoperative value in 21 of the 24 patients studied. Eight patients receiving maintenance digoxin developed arrhythmias postbypass at or near the peak of the rebound. Mean serum digoxin at the time of the rhythm disturbance was 1.3 ± 0.2 (SD) ng/ml which was significantly higher than the value of 0.7 ± 0.3 ng/ml found in patients without arrhythmia. These authors suggested that since the arrhythmias occurred at serum levels lower than those observed in digoxin-toxic patients not undergoing by-pass, and since the arrhythmias disappeared as serum levels declined, increased myocardial sensitivity to the arrhythmogenic effects of the glycoside occurs in the first 24 hours following cardiopulmonary bypass. The metabolic consequences of bypass might contribute to this observed increased sensitivity.

Studies in Pediatric Patients. Digoxin dosages commonly used in neonates, infants, and children are substantially larger than those in adults on a basis of milligrams per kilogram of body weight or milligrams per square meter of body surface area. Rogers, et al.[98] found that on this higher dosage schedule mean serum digoxin concentration 5 to 8 hours after the last maintenance dose was 2.0 ± 0.9 (SD) ng/ml in children, a value significantly higher than that of adults (1.3 ± 0.4). Despite the higher concentration, which ranged up to 4.3 ng/ml, no case of cardiac rhythm disturbance suggesting digoxin toxicity was documented.

Serum Digoxin Levels and Intestinal Malabsorption. The availability of radioimmunoassay methods for measuring serum digoxin concentration has provided an opportunity to investigate digoxin absorption in patients with malabsorption syndromes. These patients have been shown to have poor and erratic gastrointestinal absorption of digoxin. Heizer, et al.[96] found that 9 patients with sprue, short bowel syndrome, radiation enteritis, or hypermotility syndrome had a mean serum digoxin level of only 0.4 ng/ml while receiving a 0.25 mg daily maintenance dose. Two patients with steatorrhea secondary to pancreatic insufficiency maintained serum digoxin levels comparable to those of normal control subjects, suggesting that abnormal mucosa rather than steatorrhea per se caused the abnormality in absorption.

Digoxin Bioavailability Studies. With the availability of methods for measuring clinically relevant serum digoxin concentrations, large variations in gastrointestinal absorption of digoxin from tablets of identical nominal digoxin content have been reported.[100-104]

Lindenbaum, et al.[100] documented pronounced differences in serum digoxin levels over a 5-hour period after ingestion of digoxin tablets from different manufacturers. One product gave peak serum concentrations that were 7 times higher than those obtained with another, and substantial variation between different lots of the same brand was documented. These findings have been confirmed by the subsequent studies cited previously. More recently it has been suggested that human bioavailability studies be incorporated into the requirements of drug-regulating agencies.[101] Greenblatt, et al.[106] provided evidence that urinary excretion after intravenous infusion of digoxin is a suitable standard for bioavailability. In addition, recent experience with a technique for determining the rate of dissolution of digoxin from tablets suggests a useful in vitro method of predicting human bioavailability.[105]

CONCLUSIONS

Recent technical advances and availability of commercial radioimmunoassay kits have placed measurement of clinically relevant serum or plasma cardiac glycoside concentrations within reach of the well-equipped clinical laboratory. The rapidly expanding literature on serum digitalis levels provides a basis for ongoing examination of the role of these measurements in clinical practice. To date, results of these studies indicate that mean digoxin and digitoxin levels are significantly higher in patients with electrocardiographic evidence of toxicity compared with nontoxic patients. It must be emphasized, however, that because of the overlap in serum digitalis concentrations and the multifactorial nature of digitalis intoxication, sole dependence on these levels for establishing the diagnosis of digitalis toxicity is not warranted. Serum level data should be interpreted in the overall clinical context. Type and extent of underlying cardiac disease appear to be particularly important determinants of the effect of any given serum or myocardial digitalis concentration. Suspected manifestations of digitalis intoxication in the absence of an adequate history, fluctuating renal function, the presence of overt or suspected malabsorption, and use of preparations of uncertain bioavailability are among those circumstances in which knowledge of the serum level is most helpful. More broadly, it is our feeling that the measurement of serum cardiac glycoside concentrations is indicated whenever an unanticipated response to these drugs (either suspected toxicity or absence of an expected therapeutic effect) is encountered. In addition, serum digitalis measurements have been highly useful in the investigation of various special problems in the clinical pharmacology and toxicology of cardiac glycosides,[18,88,93-98] including digoxin bioavailability studies.[99-106]

References

1. Giuffra, I. J., and Tseng, H. L.: Some clinical aspects of digitalis intoxication. N.Y. State J. Med., *52*:581, 1952.
2. Rodensky, P. L., and Wasserman, F.: Observations on digitalis intoxication. Arch. Intern. Med., *108*:171, 1961.
3. Schott, A.: Observations on digitalis intoxication—a plea. Postgrad. Med. J. *40*: 628, 1964.
4. Gotsman, M. S., and Schrire, V.: Toxicity —a frequent complication of digitalis therapy. S. Afr. Med. J., *40*:590, 1966.
5. Beller, G. A., Smith, T. W., Abelmann, W. H., et al.: Digitalis intoxication: A prospective clinical study with serum level correlations. N. Eng. J. Med., *284*:989, 1971.
6. Shapiro, S., Stone, D., Lewis, G. P., and Jick, H.: The epidemiology of digoxin: A study in three Boston hospitals. J. Chronic Dis., *22*:361, 1969.
7. Boston Collaborative Drug Surveillance Program: Relation between digoxin arrhythmias and ABO blood groups. Circulation, *45*:352, 1972.
8. Howard, D., Smith, C. I., Stewart, G., et al.: A prospective survey of the incidence of cardiac intoxication with digitalis in patients being admitted to hospital and correlation with serum digoxin levels. Aust. N.Z. J. Med., *3*:279, 1973.
9. Henderson, R. R., Bessey, P. O., Jr., Abelmann, W., and Stason, W. B.: Serum digoxin levels in a cardiac out-patient population. A prospective clinical study. Circulation, *44*:177, 1971.
10. Moe, G. K., and Farah, A. E.: Digitalis and allied cardiac glycosides. *In* Goodman, L. S., and Gilman, A.: The Pharmacologic Basic of Therapeutics. p. 677. New York, MacMillan, 1970.
11. Lely, A. H., and Enter, C. van: Noncardiac symptoms of digitalis intoxication. Amer. Heart J., *83*:149, 1972.
12. Lukas, D. S., and Peterson, R. E.: Double isotope dilution derivative assay of digitoxin in plasma, urine and stool of patients maintained on the drug. J. Clin. Invest., *45*:782, 1966.
13. Lukas, D. S.: Some aspects of the distribution and disposition of digitoxin in man. Ann. N.Y. Acad. Sci., *179*:338, 1971.
14. Bentley, J. D., Burnett, G. H., Conklin, R. L., and Wasserburger, R. H.: Clinical application of serum digitoxin levels—a simplified plasma determination. Circulation, *41*:67, 1970.
15. Bertler, A., and Redfors, A.: An improved method of estimating digoxin in human plasma. Clin. Pharmacol. Ther., *11*:665, 1970.
16. Bertler, A., and Redfors, A.: Plasma levels of digoxin in relation to toxicity. Acta. Pharmacol. Toxicol., *29*:III:281, 1971.
17. Morrison, J., and Killip, T.: Radioimmunoassay of digitoxin. Clin. Res., *18*: 668, 1970.
18. Morrison, J., Killip, T., and Stason, W. B.: Serum digoxin levels in patients undergoing cardiopulmonary bypass. Circulation, *42*:III:110, 1970.
19. Chamberlain, D. A., White, R. J., Howard, M. R., and Smith, T. W.: Plasma digoxin concentrations in patients with atrial fibrillation. Br. Med. J. *3*:429, 1970.
20. Evered, D. C., Chapman, C., and Hayter, C. J.: Measurement of plasma digoxin concentration by radioimmunoassay. Br. Med. J., *3*:427, 1970.
21. Evered, D. C., and Chapman, C.: Plasma digoxin concentrations and digoxin toxicity in hospital patients. Br. Heart J., *33*: 540, 1971.
22. Smith, T. W., and Haber, E.: Digoxin intoxication: The relationship of clinical presentation to serum digoxin concentration. J. Clin. Invest., *49*:2377, 1970.
23. Brown, D. D., and Abraham, G. N.: Plasma digoxin levels in normal human volunteers. Circulation, *44*:II:146, 1971.

24. Hoeschen, R. J., and Proveda, V.: Serum digoxin by radioimmunoassay. Can. Med. Assoc. J., *105*:170, 1971.

25. Rasmussen, K., Jervell, J., and Storstein, O.: Clinical use of a bio-assay of serum digitoxin activity. Eur. J. Clin. Pharmacol. *3*:236, 1971.

26. Park, H. M., Chen, I. W., Manitasas, G. T., Lowey, A., and Saenger, E. L.: Clinical elevation of radioimmunoassay of digoxin. J. Nucl. Med., *14*:531, 1973.

27. Doherty, J. E., and Perkins, W. H.: Tissue concentration and turnover of tritiated digoxin in dogs. Amer. J. Cardiol., *17*:47, 1966.

28. Doherty, J. E., Perkins, W. H., and Flanigan, W. J.: The distribution and concentration of tritiated digoxin in human tissues. Ann. Intern. Med. *66*:116, 1967.

29. Marks, B. H.: Factors that affect the accumulation of digitalis glycosides by the heart. *In* Marks, B. H., and Weissler, A. M. (eds.): Basic and Clinical Pharmacology of Digitalis. p. 69. Springfield, (Ill.), Charles C Thomas, 1972.

30. Kuschinsky, K., Lahrtz, H., Lüllman, H., and van Zwieter, P. A.: Accumulation and release of ^{3}H-digoxin by guinea-pig heart muscle. Br. J. Pharmacol., *30*:317, 1967.

31. Repke, K.: Metabolism of cardiac glycosides. *In* Wilbrandt, W. (ed.): Proc. 1st Int. Pharm. Meeting. p. 47, vol. 3. Oxford, Pergamon Press, 1963.

32. Akera, T., Larsen, F. S., and Brody, T. M.: Correlation of cardiac sodium—and potassium—activated ATPase activity with ouabain—induced inotropic stimulation. J. Pharmacol. Exp. Ther., *173*:145, 1970.

33. Besch, H. R., Jr., Allen, J. C., Glick, G., and Schwartz, A.: Correlation between the inotropic action of ouabain and its effects on subcellular enzyme systems from canine myocardium. J. Pharmacol. Exp. Ther., *171*:1, 1970.

34. Langer, G. A.: The intrinsic control of myocardial contraction—ionic factors. N. Eng. J. Med., *285*:1065, 1971.

35. Smith, T. W., Wagner, H., Jr., Markis, J. E., and Young, M.: Studies on the localization of the cardiac glycoside receptor. J. Clin. Invest., *51*:1777, 1972.

36. Caldwell, P. C., and Keynes, R. D.: The effect of ouabain on the efflux of sodium from a squid giant axon. J. Physiol., *148*: 8P, 1959.

37. Hoffman, J. F.: The red cell membrane and the transport of sodium and potassium. Amer. J. Med., *41*:666, 1966.

38. Barr, I., Smith, T. W., Klein, M. D., *et al.*: Correlation of the electrophysiologic action of digoxin with serum digoxin concentration. J. Parmacol. Exp. Ther., *180*: 710, 1972.

39. The United States Pharmacopeia. p. 191. rev. 17, 1965.

40. Jelliffe, R. W.: A chemical determination of urinary digitoxin and digoxin in man. J. Lab. Clin. Med., *67*:694, 1966.

41. Friedman, M., and Bine, R., Jr.: A study of the rate of disappearance of a digitalis glycoside (lanotoside C) from the blood of man. J. Clin. Invest., *28*:32, 1949.

42. Friedman, M., St. George, S., and Bine, R., Jr.: The behavior and fate of digitoxin in the experimental animal and man. Medicine (Baltimore), *33*:15, 1954.

43. Doherty, J. E.: The clinical pharmacology of digitalis glycosides: a review. Amer. J. Med. Sci., *255*:382, 1968.

44. Marks, B. H., Dutta, S., Gauthier, J., and Elliot, D.: Distribution in plasma, uptake by the heart, and excretion of ^{3}H-ouabain in human subjects. J. Pharmacol. Exp. Ther., *145*:351, 1964.

45. Lullmann, H., and Zwieten, P. A., van: The kinetic behavior of cardiac glycosides in vivo, measured by isotope techniques. J. Pharmacol., *21*:1, 1969.

46. Watson, E., and Kalman, S. M.: Assay of digoxin in plasma by gas chromatography. J. Chromatogr., *56*:209, 1971.

47. Lowenstein, J. M.: A method for measuring plasma levels of digitalis glycosides. Circulation, *31*:228, 1965.

48. Lowenstein, J. M., and Corrill, E. M.: An improved method for measuring plasma and tissue concentrations of digitalis glycosides. J. Lab. Clin. Med., *67*:1048, 1966.

49. Gjerdrum, K.: Determination of digitalis in blood. Acta Med. Scand., *187*:371, 1970.

50. Ritzmann, L. W., Bangs, C. C., Coiner, D., *et al.*: Serum glycoside levels in digitalis toxicity. Circulation, *40*:III:170, 1969.

51. Grahame-Smith, D. G., and Everest, M. S.: Measurement of digoxin in plasma and its use in diagnosis of digoxin intoxication. Br. Med. J., *1*:826, 1969.

52. Binnion, P. F., Morgan, L. M., Stevenson, H. M., and Fletcher, E.: Plasma and myocardial digoxin concentrations in patients on oral therapy. Br. Heart J., *31*:636, 1969.

53. Bourdon, R., and Mercier, M.: Dosage des heterosides cardiotoniques dans les liquides biologiques par spectrophoto-

metric d'absorption atomique. Ann. Biol. Clin., *27*:651, 1969.

54. Pebay-Peyroula, F., Gaultier, M., and Nicaise, A. M.: Assay of digitalis glycosides: Its application in clinical toxicology. Clin. Tox., *4*:419, 1971.

55. Burnett, G. H., and Conklin, R. L.: The enzymatic assay of plasma digitoxin levels. J. Lab. Clin. Med., *71*:1040, 1968.

56. Burnett, G. H., and Conklin, R. L.: The enzymatic assay of plasma digoxin. J. Lab. Clin. Med., *78*:779, 1971.

57. Smith, T. W., Butler, V. P., Jr., and Haber, E.: Determination of therapeutic and toxic serum digoxin concentrations by radioimmunoassay. N. Eng. J. Med., *281*:1212, 1969.

58. Smith, T. W.: The clinical use of serum cardiac glycoside concentration measurements. Amer. Heart J., 82:833, 1971.

59. Larbig, D., and Kochsick, K.: Radioimmunochemische Bestimmung von digoxin in menschlichen serum. Klin Wochenschr., *49*:1031, 1971.

60. Oliver, G. C., Parker, B. M., and Parker, C. W.: Radioimmunoassay for digoxin. Technic and clinical application. Amer. J. Med., *51*:186, 1971.

61. Smith, T. W.: Radioimmunoassay for serum digitoxin concentration: Methodology and clinical experience. J. Pharmacol. Exp. Ther., *175*:352, 1970.

62. Oliver, G. C., Jr., Parker, B. M., Brasfield, D. L., and Parker, C. W.: The measurement of digitoxin in human serum by radioimmunoassay. J. Clin. Invest., *47*:1035, 1968.

63. Smith, T. W., Butler, V. P., Jr., and Haber, E.: Characterization of antibodies of high affinity and specificity for the digitalis glycoside digoxin. Biochemistry, *9*:331, 1970.

64. Selden, R., and Smith, T. W.: Ouabain pharmacokinetics in dog and man: Determination by radioimmunoassay. Circulation, *45*:1176, 1972.

65. Smith, T. W.: Ouabain specific antibodies: Immunochemical properties and reversal of Na$^+$, K$^+$ — activated adenosine triphosphatase inhibition. J. Clin. Invest., *51*:1583, 1972.

66. Selden, R., Klein, M. D., and Smith, T. W.: Plasma concentration and urinary excretion kinetics of acetyl strophanthidin. Circulation, *47*:744, 1973.

67. Brooker, G., and Jelliffe, R. W.: Serum cardiac glycoside assay based upon displacement of ^{3}H-ouabain from Na-K-ATPase. Circulation, *45*:20, 1972.

68. Friedman, M., and Bine, R., Jr.: Employment of the embryonic duck heart for the detection of minute amounts of a digitalis glycoside (Lanatoside C). Proc. Soc. Exp. Biol. Med., *64*:162, 1947.

69. Watson, E., Clark, D. R., and Kalman, S. M.: Identification by gas chromatography —Mass spectroscopy of dihydrodigoxin— a metabolite of digoxin in man. J. Pharmacol. Exp. Ther., *184*:424, 1973.

70. Schatzmann, H. J.: Hertzglykoside als Hemmstoffe fur den aktiven kallumund Narruim—transport durch die Erythrocytenmembran. Helv. Physiol. Pharmacol. Acta, *11*:346, 1953.

71. Coiner, D., Bangs, C. C., Walsh, J. R., and Ritzmann, L. W.: Serum cardiac glycoside assay method and possible clinical use. J. Nucl. Med., *9*:377, 1968.

72. Lader, S., Bye, A., and Marsden, P.: The measurement of plasma digoxin concentration: A comparison of two methods. Eur. J. Clin. Pharmacol., *5*:22, 1972.

73. Kaufman, J. M., and Belpire, F. M.: The influence of metabolites of digoxin and digitoxin on the ^{86}Rb uptake assay. Eur. J. Clin. Pharmacol., *6*:54, 1973.

74. Butler, V. P., Jr., and Chen, J. P.: Digoxin-specific antibodies. Proc. Natl. Acad. Sci. (USA), *57*:71, 1967.

75. Smith, T. W., and Haber, E.: The current status of cardiac glycoside assay techniques. *In* Yu, P. N., and Goodwin, J. F. (eds.): Progress in Cardiology. p. 49. Philadelphia, Lea & Febiger, 1973.

76. Smith, T. W., and Haber, E.: Clinical value of the radioimmunoassay of the digitalis glycosides. Pharmacol. Rev., *25*:219, 1973.

77. Smith, T. W., Kaplan, E.: Radioimmunoassay of cardiac glycosides: Progress and pitfalls. *In* Diagnostic Nuclear Cardiology, (Johns Hopkins Symposium on Nuclear Cardiology), St. Louis, C. V. Mosby, (In press).

78. Butler, V. P., Jr.: Assays of digitalis in the blood. Progr. Cardiovasc. Dis., *14*:571, 1972.

79. Smith, T. W.: Measurement of cardiac glycoside concentrations in serum or plasma: Technical problems and clinical implications. Techniques in Radioimmunoassay (Hahnemann Symposium on Nuclear Medicine) (In press).

80. Schall, R. F.: Digoxin radioimmunoassay: dealing with a loss of sensitivity. Clin. Chem., *19*:688, 1973.

81. Butler, V. P., Jr.: Digoxin radioimmunoassay. Lancet, *1*:186, 1971.

82. Whiting, B., Sumner, D. J., and Goldberg, A.: An assessment of digoxin radioimmunoassay. Scot. Med. J., *18*:69, 1973.

83. Marcus, F. I., Burkhalter, L., Cuccia, C., et al.: Administration of tritiated digoxin with and without a loading dose: a metabolic study. Circulation, *34*:865, 1966.

83A. Fogelman, A. M., LaMont, J. T., Finkelstein, S., et al.: Fallibility of plasmadigoxin in differentiating toxic from nontoxic patients. Lancet, *2*:727, 1971.

84. Iisalo, E., Dahl, M., and Sunquist, H.: Serum digoxin in adults and children. Int. J. Clin. Pharmacol., *7*:219, 1973.

85. Johnston, C. I., Pinkus, N. B., and Down, M.: Plasma digoxin levels in digitalized and toxic patients. Med. J. Aust., *1*:863, 1972.

86. Zeegers, J. J. W., Maas, J. H. J., and Willebrands, A. F.: The radioimmunoassay of digoxin. Clin. Chim. Acta, *44*: 109, 1973.

87. Surawicz, B., and Mortelmans, S.: Factors affecting individual tolerance to digitalis. *In* Fisch, C., and Surawicz, B. (eds.): Digitalis. p. 127. New York, Grune & Stratton, 1969.

88. Smith, T. W., and Willerson, J. T.: Suicidal and accidental digoxin ingestion: Report of five cases with serum digoxin level correlations. Circulation, *44*:29, 1971.

89. Ewy, G. A., Kapadia, G. G., Yao, L., Lullin, M., and Marcus, F. I.: Digoxin metabolism in the elderly. Circulation, *39*:449, 1969.

90. Lukas, D. S., and DeMartino, A. G.: Binding of digitoxin and some related cardenolides to human plasma proteins. J. Clin. Invest., *48*:1041, 1969.

91. Lown, B., and Levine, S. A.: Current Concepts in Digitalis Therapy. p. 164. Boston, Little, Brown & Co., 1954.

92. Barr, I., Klein, M. D., Lown, B., et al.: Correlation of serum digoxin level with acetyl strophanthidin tolerance. Ann. Intern. Med., *74*:817, 1971.

93. Coltart, D. J., Chamberlain, D. A., Howard, M. R., et al.: The effect of cardiopulmonary bypass on plasma digoxin concentrations. Br. Heart J., *33*:334, 1971.

94. Coltart, D. J., Watson, D., and Howard, M. R.: Effect of exchange transfusions on plasma digoxin levels. Arch. Dis. Child., *47*:814, 1972.

95. Goldfinger, S. E., Heizer, W. D., and Smith, T. W.: Malabsorption of digoxin in malabsorption syndromes. Gastroenterology, *58*:952, 1970.

96. Heizer, W. D., Smith, T. W., and Goldfinger, S. E.: Absorption of digoxin patients with malabsorption syndrome. N. Eng. J. Med., *285*:257, 1971.

97. White, R. J., Chamberlain, D. A., Howard, M., and Smith, T. W.: Plasma concentrations of digoxin after oral administration in the fasting and postprandial state. Br. Med. J., *1*:380, 1971.

98. Rogers, M. C., Willerson, J. T., Goldblatt, A., Smith, T. W.: Serum digoxin concentrations in the human fetus, neonate, and infant. N. Eng. J. Med., *287*:1010, 1972.

99. Lindenbaum, J., Maulitz, R. M., Saha, J. R., et al.: Impairment of digoxin absorption by neomycin. Clin. Res., *20*:410, 1970.

100. Lindenbaum, J., Mellow, M. H., Blackstone, M. D., and Butler, V. P., Jr.: Variation in biological availability of digoxin from four preparations. N. Eng. J. Med., *285*:1344, 1971.

101. Shaw, T. R. D., Howard, M. R., and Hamer, J.: Variation in the biological availability of digoxin. Lancet, *2*:303, 1972.

102. Huffman, D. H., and Azarnoff, D. L.: Absorption of orally given digoxin preparations. JAMA, *222*:957, 1972.

103. Falch, D., Teinen, A., and Bjerkelund, C. J.: Comparative study of the absorption, plasma levels, and urinary excretion of the "new" and the "old" Lanoxin. Br. Med. J., *209*:695, 1973.

104. Wagner, J. G., Christensen, M., Sakmar, E., and Young, M.: Equivalence lack in digoxin plasma levels. JAMA, *224*:199, 1973.

105. Lindenbaum, J., Butler, V. P., Murphy, J. E., and Cresswell, R. M.: Correlation of digoxin tablet dissolution rate with biological availability. Lancet, *1*:1215, 1973.

106. Greenblatt, D. J., Duhme, D. W., Koch-Weser, J., and Smith, T. W.: Evaluation of digoxin bioavailability in single dose studies. N. Eng. J. Med., *289*:651, 1973.

14 *Growth Hormone*

DAVID RABINOWITZ, M.D. AND
THOMAS J. MERIMEE, M.D.

Knowledge of the physiology of human growth hormone (hGH) has accumulated at a notable rate over the past 10 years. Knobil and his coworkers showed that only human and simian growth hormone (GH) were active in the monkey, and this was subsequently also shown in intact man.[1] In 1963, Roth, Glick, Yalow and Berson published a note in "Science" demonstrating the use of a new radioimmunoassay for hGH. They also made the first meaningful observations on stimulation of hGH release in normal man (a) by insulin-induced hypoglycemia and (b) by prolonged starvation.[2,3] These 2 classical observations were the forerunners of scores of articles on hGH release. There has now emerged the unexpected picture of hGH levels in serum exhibiting wide fluctuations. An impressively large and varied list of stimuli other than hypoglycemia trigger release of hGH, and, to bedevil further the investigator, it became clear that the circulating concentration of hGH was at times high even in the absence of a known stimulus (so-called spontaneous or agnogenic tides of hGH release).[4,5]

In this review, we shall consider control of hGH release; peripheral physiologic actions of hGH; appropriate clinical tests of the integrity of hGH release and their applications and useful practical aspects of the hGH radioimmunoassay.

Physiology of hGH Release

It is difficult to reconcile all the data presently in the literature concerning release of hGH in man. Our attempts to synthesize available information have been greatly aided by the thoughtful review of J. B. Martin, to whom we are indebted for further helpful discussions.[6]

The α-cell of the adenohypophysis synthesizes hGH, stores the hormone, and releases it into the peripheral circulation under appropriate conditions. The α-cell appears to be under the control of at least 2 opposing groups of stimuli: inhibitory and excitatory. The former may be mediated by growth hormone release inhibitory factor, GHRIF or somatostatin, the later by growth hormone releasing factor, GHRF.[7-10] While progress has been made in isolating a GHRF active in a number of animal systems, this material has proven to be essentially inactive in man. On the other hand a GHRIF, or somatostatin has been isolated from the hypothalamus, the polypeptide has been synthesized and this has been shown to be effective in inhibiting hGH release in man.

Let us now examine more closely the nature of excitatory stimuli for hGH release. GHRF is probably synthesized by peptidergic neurones in the arcuate nucleus (AN) and then secreted along axons which terminate near the median eminence (ME). There appear to be 3 classes of stimuli acting on GHRF: dopaminergic, norepinephrinergic and serotoninergic.

1. Dopamine may be the neurotransmitter for excitatory stimuli reaching the arcuate nucleus. Indeed, administration of L-dopa leads to a rise in serum hGH in man. It is

thought that L-dopa is taken up by terminals in the region of the AN where it is converted to dopamine by the enzyme L-dopa-decarboxylase. Increased storage of transmitter is followed by release of transmitter, and activation of release of GHRF into the portal system. Chlorpromazine may inhibit hGH release by acting as a postsynaptic inhibitor at the site of the dopamine receptor.

2. Norepinephrine may be the neurotransmitter for excitatory stimuli of hGH release which reach the ventro-medial nucleus (VMN) of the hypothalamus. Thus when lesions are placed in the VMN of the rat, there is clear suppression of GH release.[11] The VMN may possess a "glucoreceptor," and its stimulation is achieved by hypoglycemia, by a falling blood glucose concentration, or by intracellular deprivation of glucose. These positive stimuli to the glucoreceptor appear to be mediated by an α-adrenergic receptor.[12] Thus, blunting of excitatory stimuli can be achieved by the administration of phentolamine, an inhibitor of α-adrenergic transmission. Inhibition of firing of VMN may also be achieved by inducing hyperglycemia, and by β-adrenergic stimulation. There is inferential evidence that stimuli other than glucopenia may also act at the ventro-medial nucleus (e.g., glucagon, vasopressin and l-arginine-HCl).

3. A third system involved in the control of hGH release is the limbic system. Sleep is a potent stimulus for hGH release. Slow-wave sleep appears to require the generation of serotonin, and the limbic system plays an important part in slow-wave sleep. It has been suggested that the limbic system may also be involved in sleep-initiated hGH release.

The locus of action of many stimuli remains unclear (e.g., stress, exercise, protein depletion). The mode whereby glucocorticoids, high-circulating FFA levels, or states of obesity induce inhibition of hGH release is similarly unclear. It is theoretically possible that these effects could be produced by modulation of GHRIF (Somatostatin), which

is discussed below. It is useful to mention 2 hormones which have a strong modifying influence on hGH release: estrogen and progesterone.[13,16] Estrogens appear to "sensitize" the pituitary to a number of provocative agents. For example, mild ambulation is associated with a higher level of hGH in females than in males. Similarly, males who are "nonresponders" to l-arginine-HCl show a brisk response to the amino acid after pretreatment with estrogen. Furthermore, among young females, the amino acid is a more powerful secretogogue in the preovulatory period when estradiol levels are high compared to the time of menstrual flow when circulating estradiol levels are at their nadir.

Progesterone by contrast has an inhibitory influence on hGH release. Simon, et al., showed that medroxyprogesterone acetate (MPA) suppressed the hGH rise produced by insulin, and possibly also by l-arginine-HCl. Finkelstein, *et al.*[17] compared growth hormone secretory patterns at different ages, by measuring samples every 20 minutes for a 24-hour period. Results were: prepubertal children, 91 μg per 24 hours; adolescents 690 μg; young adults 385 μg; in older adults (47-62 years) secretion decreased, often approaching zero. Thus, there appears to be an age-related change in spontaneous hGH secretion.

Somatostatin

This polypeptide is highly effective in inhibiting GH release from in vitro pituitary systems. Yen, *et al.*, have established its effectiveness in man: infusion of Somatostatin blunts hGH release to the stimuli of insulin-hypoglycemia and of arginine. Somatostatin appears to have other wide-ranging and complex effects. It induces a fall in blood-glucose levels and in serum-insulin levels; it blunts TSH rise after TRH. This area is expanding rapidly. At present it is not possible to assess the relative importance of GHRF and of Somatostatin on the overall economy of hGH release in man.

Peripheral Actions of hGH

Human growth hormone appears to have 2 apparently paradoxical kinds of actions: diabetogenic (or anti-insulin) and anabolic (or insulin-like).[18,19,20]

1. The diabetogenic effects of hGH include (a) inhibition of glucose translocation into skeletal muscle and adipose tissue, (b) enhancement of FFA release from adipose tissue, and (c) antagonism of insulin's action on glucose movement into peripheral tissues, chiefly muscle and adipose tissue. These effects can be observed in part acutely in the human forearm during the intra-arterial injection of hGH. However, their full expression generally requires a period of hours after hGH administration and may reflect the prerequisite that hGH be modified in vivo.

In the pancreatectomized, or otherwise insulin-compromised animal, the diabetogenic effects of growth hormone may lead to severe hyperglycemia, hyperlipacidemia (elevation of serum-FFA levels) and ketosis. These effects are considerably less dramatic in the intact animal, which is probably a consequence of an important action of growth hormone on the pancreatic islet: growth hormone not only induces insulin resistance by virtue of its "diabetogenic" effect, but also has an insulinotropic effect. That is, with hGH pretreatment, insulin secretogogues effect a much greater rise in serum insulin compared to the control non-hGH treated state. This effect on insulin secretion is substantially reduced in states of compromised pancreatic β-cell function. We can summarize these effects by the statement that hGH therapy induces insulin resistance and hyperinsulinism. The latter partially or completely compensates for the former, unless the pancreatic islet cannot respond optimally, in which case a frank diabetic picture can ensue.

The usefulness to body economy of an anti-insulin effect of hGH would be to spare glucose, and to encourage the burning of fat as FFA as fuel for peripheral tissues, chiefly skeletal muscle. Such an action would be appropriate under conditions of glucopenia, for example starvation. Indeed, hGH levels do rise during periods of starvation, but this does not necessarily imply a role for hGH in the physiology of starvation.

2. The second effect of hGH is its anabolic or insulin-like action. We can define an anabolic effect as an action which leads to nitrogen retention in the intact animals. This has clearly been shown for growth hormone in many animal species. Furthermore, clear effects of growth hormone have also been demonstrated on protein metabolism in in vitro systems. Knobil and his colleagues showed that growth hormone enhanced uptake of α-amino isobutyric acid (AIB) into excised hemidiaphragm. Subsequently, the same group demonstrated the same phenomenon with respect to ^{14}C-leucine and to other natural amino acids. Not only did growth hormone enhance amino-acid transport into muscle but also incorporation of label into protein was accelerated.[1]

We shall presently attempt to reconcile these apparently disparate actions in one hormone. We must emphasize that, in general, the anti-insulin effects of growth hormone are delayed. Second, although anabolic effects of growth hormone can be shown in in vitro systems in the absence of

Table 14-1. A Useful Mnemonic for Rationally Categorizing Actions of hGH.

hGH

ANABOLIC	DIABETOGENIC
(or insulin-like)	(or contra-insulin)

INSULIN

* hGH has both "anabolic" and "diabetogenic" properties. It is proposed that the former are dominant in the presence of insulin; the diabetogenic actions obtain when insulin levels are insignificant.

insulin, growth hormone fails to induce nitrogen retention in vivo in the insulin-compromised animals. We suggested some years ago that the conflicting actions of the hormone may be reconciled by the model shown in Table 14-1. The hypothesis suggests that in circumstances of insulin lack, hGH will act chiefly as a diabetogenic factor; that is, blunting of glucose uptake, and stimulation of lipolysis. Conversely, in the presence of appropriate levels of insulin, hGH will act in concert with insulin as an anabolic hormone; insulin does indeed obliterate the lipolytic action of hGH. This formula certainly cannot reconcile all that we know about hGH; it still, nevertheless, retains usefulness, despite the following perplexing aspects of the hormone's actions: the so-called early insulin-like action,[21] the insulinotropic effects of growth hormone and the actions of growth hormone in mediating the generation of somatomedin.

Early Insulin-like Actions

When hGH is given intravenously to man in concentrations of 4 mg or greater, blood glucose and serum FFA levels fall acutely.[21] This effect is not consequent upon any measurable rise in serum-insulin levels; it appears to be mediated by a change in cell permeability, chiefly of muscle and adipose tissue, to glucose. We suspect that this may be a pharmacologic effect of hGH, for which there may be no physiologic counterpart.

Insulinotropic Effect. There is compelling evidence for an insulinotropic effect of growth hormone in many species. This generally requires pretreatment, so to speak, of the pancreatic islet with growth hormone for a period of hours. The "primed" islet will then respond to stimulation by some secretogogues with exaggerated insulin release. Thus hyperinsulinism, which follows glucose and arginine but not tolbutamide or glucagon, is potentiated.

Somatomedin. Many effects of growth hormone cannot be demonstrated in vitro, or require very large local concentrations to elicit the effect. For example, since growth hormone is necessary for longitudinal growth, in vitro effects of the hormone were sought on cartilage metabolism; such experiments yielded negative results. Ellis[22] then made the observation that growth hormone pretreatment of the animal resulted in the appearance in serum of a factor (sulfation factor, SF) which enhanced sulfate incorporation into cartilage. Daughaday, Salmon[23] and their colleagues greatly advanced knowledge in this area. This SF also enhanced leucine incorporation into protein, collagen synthesis, uridine incorporation into RNA, and thymidine incorporation into DNA. The SF activity first rises in serum 3 hours after hGH injection and remains elevated for 9 to 24 hours, at which time serum-hGH levels have already returned to basal levels. Van Wyk[24] has made progress in establishing the structure of SF or Somatomedin as it is now called; he has also shown that Somatomedin competes with insulin for binding to an insulin receptor. Somatomedin shares in fact many of the properties of nonsuppressible insulin-like activity (NSILA).

It is useful to view the physiology of hGH from the following angle: hGH has both diabetogenic and anabolic effects. The former results in glucose sparing and lipid combustion. Indeed, states of hypoglycemia, glucopenia and starvation result in a rise in serum hGH levels, and the diabetogenic actions of hGH are important to body economy under these circumstances. The anabolic effects of hGH lead to enhanced amino acid incorporation into protein and the "presence" of insulin appears to be important for this action at least in vivo. In fact, many amino acids, including l-arginine-HCl do trigger release of both hGH and insulin whose synergistic effect on protein synthesis is appropriate under these conditions. This relatively simple scheme is unfortunately a vast oversimplification, and should be viewed as no more than a mnemonic with the many caveats and exceptions that we have mentioned.

Practical Applications

In the light of the physiology we have just discussed, the physician faces a large number of choices in seeking an adequate test for the integrity of hGH release. Today we assess the latter, almost exclusively by measuring concentration of hGH in plasma, either in "random samples" or after suitable provocation. The former method is suitable only in children. Thompson, *et al.*,[25] employ a constant withdrawal pump to obtain an integrated cencentration of hGH, and in conjunction with evaluation of the plasma disappearance rate of hGH, they are able to calculate hGH production rates. This approach is not readily applicable on a routine basis although these data are the most useful. Since we thus generally rely on plasma levels, we have somewhat arbitrarily—in fact, based on cumulative experience—reached a consensus as to what constitutes "low" levels: values which rise above 5 ng/ml serum. It is more difficult to define "normal" or "high" values since hGH levels fluctuate so widely. It is perhaps best to define "high" values as levels which remain elevated constantly above 5 ng/ml even under conditions which should suppress hGH levels, for example hyperglycemia.

At the practical level, we have used the following approach: we take 3 blood samples respectively drawn randomly, at sleep and after 5 minutes of brisk exercise. If these samples fail to show adequate hGH levels we perform the following 2 tests: (a) The insulin tolerance test: With the subject in the fasting state, a control blood sample is drawn, and then insulin (0.10 u/kg) is injected intravenously, with further bloods being drawn at 15, 30, 45, 60 and 90 minutes. (b) The arginine infusion test: L-arginine-HCl (0.5 Gm per kg) is infused as a 5 percent or 10 percent solution over 30 minutes. Blood samples are drawn with the time schedule indicated for insulin. All males are pretreated with stilbesterol for 3 days (2.5 mg, b.i.d.) prior to the arginine

test, which ensures maximal "responsiveness" to arginine. It is possible to combine the 2 tests on one morning, first infusing arginine and giving the insulin 1 hour or so later.

These tests will in most cases answer the question: Is hGH release adequate? A number of other tests are also satisfactory: oral administration of L-dopa (0.5-1 Gm);[26] or intramuscular injection of glucagon (1 mg) are reliable.[27] A recent report however showed that, whereas all but 7 percent of young persons given 0.5 Gm L-dopa showed a satisfactory hGH response, 36 percent of older persons and 77 percent of depressed persons had inadequate hGH responses.[28]

When the integrity of hGH release is not in question, but rather the problem of whether this release is autonomous or not, we attempt to attenuate hGH release physiologically. An oral glucose load generally suppresses hGH levels except under unusual circumstances (chronic renal disease, chronic liver disease, some patients with cancer) and most classically in acromegaly.

Technical Aspects of the hGH RIA

The principles of the radioimmunoassay were set forth by Berson and Yalow and are embodied in the following equation.[29]

$$[H]^* + [Ab] \rightleftharpoons [H^*Ab] ----- (1)$$
$$+$$
$$\text{cold}$$
$$\text{hormone}$$

For our purposes, we require pure unlabeled hGH which can be "labeled" with [125]Iodine or [131]Iodine. We require also suitable anti-hGH antiserum. Appropriate concentrations of labeled hormone ([H]*) and of antiserum ([Ab]) are incubated and allowed to reach equilibrium. As indicated, at equilibrium the labeled hormone is in part "free" and in part is "bound" to antibody. The bound hormone is still in solution but relatively simple means are available for distinguishing "free" and "bound" hormone.

When the same amounts of labeled hormone and of antibody are reacted, in the presence of unlabeled hormone, the latter competes with the tracer for binding sites on the antibody. The net result is that, at equilibrium, less labeled hormone are bound to antibody, relatively more remain "free." Indeed, the fraction of labeled hormone bound to antibody is inversely related to the mass of unlabeled hormone added to the particular tube. This enables us to construct a dose-response curve which plots fraction of labeled hGH bound to antibody versus concentration of unlabeled hGH present. An unknown (e.g., serum sample) added to the constant amounts of tracer and antibody can be determined by referring the observed fractional binding of tracer to the standard dose-response curve.

At the practical level, the assay requires:

1. A purified source of hGH, suitable for labeling.

2. Antiserum to hGH with sufficient affinity for hGH such that competition (displacement) with tracer will be found at physiologic levels of unlabeled hGH.

3. An adequate means of separating "free hormone" and hormone bound to antiserum.

Human growth hormone is provided by the National Pituitary Agency. Iodination is readily achieved by the method of Greenwood, *et al.,*[30] as modified by Roth.[31] For this method to be effective, the volume of the reaction mixture should be small, and the oxidizing agent, chloramine T, should be added in appropriate stoichiometric quantities. A typical reaction mixture would be:

hGH, 5 μg in 5 μl
0.3 M PO$_4$ buffer, 10 μl
0.2 M NaH$_2$PO$_4$, 5 μl
Na-^{125}Iodide, 5 μl (100 μC/μl)

Chloramine T (5 μl of a 30 μg/ml solution) is added and the mixture is agitated vigorously. An aliquot is taken, and the fraction of labeled iodine which is precipitated by 10 percent trichloracetic acid can be employed as a useful index of the efficiency of iodination. If one wishes to reach a specific activity of 50 μC/μg in the examples given, one needs 50 percent precipitation of radioiodine. If the fraction is lower, a further aliquot or aliquots of chloramine T (5 μl) can be added, and the TCA step repeated. The labeled hormone can be fractionated on Sephadex G-75 which readily separates protein from free iodine. Thereafter, an appropriate tracer quantity can be selected for the assay (for example 0.1 ng of hGH which will contain sufficient counts when the hormone has been labeled to a specific activity of 50 μC/μg).

Incubations of tracer, antibody with or without unlabeled hormone, can be made for 5 days at 4°C. Methods for separating "bound" from "free" hormone[31-36] fall into 2 large classes: (1) Methods based on adsorption of the free hormone and (2) Methods based on precipitating the antibody-bound hormone. In the former, charcoal or talc is added to the tube and to this free hormone adheres. The charcoal or talc can be precipitated and thus the "free" hormone can be separated and counted. These systems are rather simple, but require rigorous attention to detail—concentrations of talc and/or charcoal, attention to constancy of protein concentration in all tubes. Different batches of these reagents may behave quite disparately, and should be individually evaluated. The single antibody system can also be employed in a so-called solid-phase assay. This approach was introduced by Catt, and utilizes adsorption of antibody to a solid surface (e.g., the walls of a plastic test tube). Labeled hormone binds to the latter, which binding is inhibited by the presence of unlabeled hormone in the tube. Separation of "bound" tracer from "free" is achieved by decanting the solution from the tube, and counting the remaining radioactivity.

The alternative approach relies on the addition of a second antibody directed against the hGH antiserum (e.g., goat anti-rabbit antiserum) and added in sufficient concentration to produce precipitation. Thus "bound" hormone can by centrifugation be separated and counted.

Clinical Syndromes in Which hGH Measurements are Useful

Human growth hormone levels have been measured in many different syndromes. While eventually such levels may prove useful in a variety of clinical situations, practical applications of the hGH RIA are limited largely to evaluation of states of dwarfism,[37-41] and of suspected excessive hGH production.

Confronted with the clinical problem of short stature, the differential diagnosis is determined by the clinical appraisal. If short stature is severe ($< $ 3rd percentile) and if body proportions are normal, the question of hGH deficiency arises. Deficiency of hGH may occur as part of the spectrum of hypopituitarism or as an isolated defect. Hypopituitarism can be secondary to known pituitary disease (e.g., chromophobe tumors, craniopharyngioma or more rarely granulomatous or vascular disease) or can be "idiopathic." Clinical clues may derive from symptoms suggesting a space-occupying mass in the pituitary (headache, visual disturbances, optic atrophy, x-ray evidence of a large sella), or from failure of other pituitary hormones (TSH, ACTH, gonadotropins). In isolated hGH deficiency, there are no ancillary features, and patients present with shortness of stature. In our own series, the syndrome was heritable, mostly as an autosomal recessive syndrome, occasionally as an autosomal dominant. Sporadic examples of the syndrome are also observed. Birth weight is generally normal, and even length is usually only modestly decreased. However, growth retardation is often noticed early. In some patients there may be episodes of hypoglycemia. The patient has normal or near-normal body proportions. The skin is soft and wrinkled, the voice is often high-pitched, even squeaky. Sexual development is normal, although it may be delayed.

The laboratory features reflect absence of circulating hGH. Subjects are sensitive to exogenous insulin, and show "hypoglycemic unresponsiveness"; that is, blood glucose falls after insulin and does not recover over a period of 90 minutes. Despite severe hypoglycemia, hGH levels are 0 or less than 5 ng/ml. Subjects placed on total starvation for 3 days develop hypoglycemia, but postabsorptive glucose levels are not usually subnormal.

Of considerable interest are the results of glucose tolerance tests (GTT) in this syndrome. As a group, there is glucose intolerance. A glucose load elicits a poor insulin response. Indeed, insulinopenia is characteristic of these patients, reflecting the absence of the physiologic insulinotropic role of hGH. Insulinopenia can be construed as a regulatory device which reduces the hazard of hypoglycemia in the absence of hGH. Administration of hGH profoundly changes insulin secretion: normal or exaggerated insulin responses to glucose and to arginine occur within 3 to 4 days of hGH therapy. Also, subjects respond to exogenous hGH with predictable metabolic changes: positive nitrogen balance, hypercalciuria and a fall in serum urea nitrogen.

Diagnosis can be confirmed by showing failure of hGH levels to rise after insulin and after arginine. Several caveats are in order. First, the obese state is associated with poor hGH responsiveness to provocative stimuli; usually, however, on multiple sampling 1 or 2 values in the normal range are found. Second, there remains controversy whether partial hGH deficiency exists. Our present view is that appropriate methods for conclusively showing the existence of such a syndrome are not yet at hand. Third, there is a syndrome of dwarfism in which hGH levels are normal or high, and in which the subjects do not respond to exogenous hGH (the Laron dwarf).[40] The hGH in these subjects is not distinguishable immunologically from that of control subjects. Since Somatomedin levels do not rise after hGH administration in these subjects, the defect may be in the pathway whereby hGH leads to Somatomedin generation. Fourth, there are probably several syndromes in which hGH release and Somatomedin generation are intact but in which the end organ response may be impaired. One such syndrome has been reasonably defined, namely, the short stature characteristic of the Babinga pygmies.[41]

Human growth hormone measurements are also useful in states of hGH excess. Thus acromegaly may be defined as a clinical syndrome characterized by excessive and inappropriate secretion of hGH. In order to demonstrate this, it is necessary to show continued secretion of hGH in the face of a stimulus which normally inhibits hGH release. The simplest way of performing this is by giving an oral glucose load. We reemphasize that syndromes other than acromegaly may show a similar failure of inhibition. Furthermore, there is not always a good correlation between hGH levels and the clinical status of the acromegalic.

Other Approaches to hGH Measurements

Roth and his colleagues showed conclusively that polypeptide hormones react with receptors on the surface of cells, and that this reaction can be quantified.[31] Receptors show great specificity: uptake of hormone can be inhibited by unlabeled hormone in a manner similar to that discussed above for RIA. This approach should prove useful in probing phenomena which may be closer to the bioactivity of the hormone than is the RIA.

Thus Lesniak, Roth, *et al.,* have shown the presence of hGH receptors in cultured lymphocytes.[42,43] They have shown large differences in "radioreceptors" compared to "radioimmunoassayable" activity in different batches of hGH. Since plasma hGH is heterogeneous (both a "big" and a "little" hGH are present) Gorden, *et al.,* evaluated the activities of these moieties.[44] They report equal RIA activity in the 2 fractions but reduced radioreceptor activity of "big" hGH. These interesting observations suggest new approaches to examination of hGH activity in serum.

Summary

In this review we have summarized aspects of physiologic effects of hGH, and control of hGH release in man, and have proposed a model relating these 2 areas. The hGH radioimmunoassay technique has been discussed from both a theoretical and practical perspective, and we have briefly reviewed those clinical syndromes in which it may be useful.

References

1. Knobil, E.: The pituitary growth hormone: an adventure in physiology. Physiologist, *9*:25, 1966.
2. Roth, J., Glick, S. M., Yalow, R. S., and Berson, S. A.: Hypoglycemia: a potent stimulus to secretion of growth hormone. Science, *140*:987, 1963.
3. Glick, S. M., Roth, J., Yalow, R. S., *et al.*: The regulation of growth hormone secretion. Recent Prog. Hor. Res., *21*:241, 1965.
4. Glick, S. M., and Goldsmith, S.: Proc. Int. Symp. Growth Hormone. Milan, Amsterdam, Excerpta Medica, p. 84. 1967.
5. Spitz, I., Gonen, B., and Rabinowitz, D.: Growth and growth hormone. Amsterdam, Excerpta Medica, p. 379. 1972.
6. Martin, J. B.: Neural regulation of growth hormone secretion. N. Eng. J. Med., *288*: 1384, 1973.
7. Schally, A. V., Arimura, A., Bowers, C. Y., *et al.*: Hypothalamic neural hormones regulated anterior pituitary function. Recent Progr. Hormone Res., *24*:497, 1968.
8. Abrams, R. L., Parker, M. L., Blanco, S., *et al.*: Hypothalamic regulation of growth hormone secretion. Endocrinology, *78*: 605, 1966.
9. Brazeau, P., Vale, W., Burgus, R., *et al.*: Hypothalamic polypeptide that inhibits the secretion of immunoreactive pituitary growth hormone. Science, *179*:77, 1973.
10. Siler, T. M., Vandenberg, G., and Yen, S. S. C.: Inhibition of growth hormone release in humans by somatostatin. J. Clin. Endocrinol. Metab., *37*:632, 1973.
11. Frohman, L. A., and Bernardis, L. L.: Growth hormone and insulin levels in weanling rats with ventromedial hypothalamic lesions. Endocrinology, *82*:1125, 1968.
12. Blackard, W. G., and Heidingsfelder, S. A.: Adrenergic receptor control mechanism for growth hormone secretion. J. Clin. Invest., *47*:1407, 1968.

13. Frantz, A. G., and Rabkin, M. T.: Human growth hormone: clinical measurement, response to hypoglycemia and suppression by cortical steroids. N. Eng. J. Med., *271*: 1375, 1964.

14. Rabinowitz, D., Merimee, T. J., Nelson, J. K., Schultz, R. B., and Burgess, J. A.: Proc. Int. Symp. Growth Hormone, Milan, Amsterdam, Excerpta Medica, p. 105. 1967.

15. Frantz, A. G., and Rabkin, M. T.: Effects of estrogen and sex difference on secretion of human growth hormone. J. Clin. Endocrinol. Metab., *25*:1470, 1965.

16. Simon, S., Schiffer, M., Glick, S. M., *et al.*: Effect of medroxyprogesterone acetate upon stimulated release of growth hormone in man. J. Clin. Endocrinol. Metab., *27*:1633, 1967.

17. Finkelstein, J. W., Roffwarg, H. P., Boyar, R. M., *et al.*: Age-related change in a 24-hour spontaneous secretion of growth hormone. J. Clin. Endocrinol. Metab., *35*:665, 1972.

18. Pearson, O. H., Dominguez, J. M., Greenberg, E., *et al.*: Diabetogenic and hypoglycemic effects of human growth hormone. Trans. Assoc. Amer. Physicians, *73*:217, 1960.

19. Young, F. G.: Growth and the diabetogenic action of anterior pituitary preparations. Br. Med. J., *2*:897, 1941.

20. Daughaday, W. H., and Kipnis, D. M.: The growth promoting and anti-insulin action of somatotropin. Recent Prog. Hor. Res., *22*:49, 1966.

21. Zahnd, G. R., Steinke, J., and Renold, A. E.: Early metabolic effects of human growth hormone. Proc. Soc. Exp. Biol. Med., *105*:455, 1960.

22. Ellis, S., Huble, J., and Simpson, M. E.: Influence of hypophysectomy and growth hormone on cartilage sulfate metabolism. Proc. Soc. Exp. Biol. Med., *84*:603, 1953.

23. Salmon, W. D., and Daughaday, W. M.: A hormonally controlled serum factor which stimulates sulfate incorporation by cartilage in vitro. J. Lab. Clin. Med., *49*:825, 1957.

24. Van den Brande, J. L., Van Wyk, J. J., Hall, J., and Weaver, R. P.: Further purification and characterization of sulfation factor and thymidine factor from acromegalic factor. J. Clin. Endocrinol. Metab., *32*:389, 1971.

25. Thompson, R. G., Rodriguez, A., Kowarski, A., and Blizzard, R. M.: Growth hormone: metabolic clearance rates, integrated concentrations and production rates of normal adults and the effect of prednisone. J. Clin. Invest., *51*:3193, 1972.

26. Boyd, A. E., Lebowitz, H. E., and Pfeiffer, J. G.: Stimulation of human growth hormone secretion by l-DOPA. N. Eng. J. Med., *283*:1425, 1970.

27. Mitchell, M. L., Byrne, M. J., Sanchez, Y., and Sawin, C. T.: Detection of growth hormone deficiency: the glucagon stimulation test. N. Eng. J. Med., *282*:539, 1972.

28. Sachar, E. J., Mushrush, G., Perlow, M., *et al.*: Growth hormone responses to l-DOPA in depressed patients. Science, *178*:1304, 1972.

29. Berson, S. A., and Yalow, R. S.: The hormones. vol. 4, p. 557. New York, Academic Press, 1964.

30. Greenwood, F. C., Hunter, W. M., and Glover, J. S.: The preparation of ^{131}I labeled human growth hormone of high specific radioactivity. Biochem. J., *89*:114, 1963.

31. Roth, J.: Peptide hormone binding to receptors: a review of direct studies in vitro. Metabolism, *22*:1059, 1973.

32. Moloney, M., and Devlin, J. G.: Comparison of three methods for human growth hormone immunoassay. Ir. J. Med. Sci., *8*:469, 1969.

33. Meek, J. C., Stoskopf, M. M., and Bolinger, R. E.: Optimization of radioimmunoassay for human growth hormone by the charcoal-dextran technique. Clin. Chem., *16*: 845, 1970.

34. Hales, C. N., and Randle, P. J.: Immunoassay of insulin with insulin-antibody precipitate. Biochem. J., *88*:137, 1963.

35. Ewer, R. W., and Deiss, W. P.: Clinical experience with human growth hormone immunoassay via two antibody method. Arch. Intern. Med., *124*:461, 1969.

36. Catt, K. J., Tregear, G. W., Burger, H. G., *et al.*: Antibody-coated tube method for radioimmunoassay for human growth hormone. Clin. Chim. Acta, *27*:267, 1970.

37. Rimoin, D. L., Merimee, T. J., Rabinowitz, D., *et al.*: Genetic aspects of clinical endocrinology. Recent Progr. Hormone Res., *24*:365, 1968.

38. Kaplan, S. L., Abrams, C. A. L., Bell, J. J., *et al.*: Growth and growth hormone. I. Changes in serum level of growth hormone following hypoglycemia in 134 children with growth retardation. Pediatr. Res., *2*: 43, 1968.

39. Rabinowitz, D., and Merimee, T. J.: Isolated human growth hormone deficiency and related disorders. Isr. J. Med. Sci., 9:1601, 1973.

40. Laron, Z., Pertzelan, A., and Karp, M.: Pituitary dwarfism with high serum levels of growth hormone. Isr. J. Med. Sci., 4: 883, 1968.

41. Rimoin, D. L., Merimee, T. J., Rabinowitz, D., *et al.*: Peripheral subresponsiveness to human growth hormone in the African pygmies. N. Eng. J. Med., 281:1383, 1969.

42. Lesniak, M. A., Roth, J., Gorden, P., *et al.*: Human growth hormone radioreceptor assay using cultured human lymphocytes. Nature (New Biol.), 241:20, 1973.

43. Gorden, P., Gavin, J. R., Kahn, C. R., *et al.*: Application of radioreceptor assay to circulating insulin, growth hormone and to the tissue receptors in animals and man. Pharmacol. Rev., 25:179, 1973.

44. Gorden, P., Lesniak, M. A., Hendricks, C. M., *et al.*: "Big" growth hormone components from human plasma: decreased reactivity demonstrated by radioreceptor assay. Science, 182:829, 1973.

15 *Thyrotropin*

E. Chester Ridgway, M.D., Ione A. Kourides, M.D.
and Farahe Maloof, M.D.

The high prevalence of thyroid disease and the sensitive and subtle negative feedback relationship between the thyroid and pituitary gland make an accurate measurement of human thyrotropin (hTSH) in biological fluids an important clinical tool. Early urinary bioassay attempts to measure hTSH suffered from insensitivity and non-specificity. With the purification of hTSH by Condliffe[1] and the development of antibodies to hTSH in laboratory animals,[2] a specific radioimmunoassay for hTSH based on the immunoassay principles of Berson and Yalow[3] was possible. The first hTSH radioimmunoassay of Utiger[4] and Odell, Wilber, and Paul[5] provided sufficient sensitivity to be clinically useful in detecting abnormal elevations of hTSH. Utilization of these assay techniques by many investigators[6-10] has been enormously useful in defining abnormal thyroid function. Although elevated hTSH concentrations were clearly

distinguished from normal concentrations of hTSH, distinction between normal and low concentrations of hTSH was not possible until several modifications were made in the immunoassay.[11,12] The following discussion will describe how sensitive radioimmunoassay techniques have been used to determine the serum concentrations, metabolic clearance rates, production rates, and pituitary reserve of hTSH in various states of thyroid pathology. In addition, the development of a radioimmunoassay to measure the free beta subunit of hTSH will be discussed.

Radioimmunoassay of hTSH. Purified hTSH for iodination and rabbit anti-hTSH have been obtained from the National Institute of Arthritis, Metabolism, and Digestive Diseases. The rabbit anti-hTSH was used at a dilution of 1:200,000, at which 50 percent of labeled hTSH was bound. The standard for the assay was obtained from the Medical Research Council, Mill Hill, England; each μU of MRC Standard B contained 0.5 ng of hTSH. Purified hTSH was labeled with ^{125}I to a specific activity of 50 to 100 μCi per μg by the chloramine-T method of Hunter and Greenwood.[13] Labeled hTSH was separated from inorganic ^{125}I and non-immunoreactive hormone by gel chromatography on a 90 $\times$ 1.5 cm column of Sephadex G-100. The radioimmunoassay standard curve was derived by preincubating duplicate hTSH standards, containing 200 μl of hTSH-suppressed serum (obtained from individuals whose serum hTSH was

Supported by grants from the USPHS AM 16791 and CA 12749 and the Am. Phil. Soc. 1-9 C.S. 36.

The authors acknowledge Dr. B. D. Weintraub and Dr. R. N. Re for their invaluable contributions to this work; the National Institute of Arthritis, Metabolism, and Digestive Diseases for hTSH, anti-hTSH, and hLH and to the Medical Research Council, Mill Hill, England for hTSH Standard B and hLH-β; Dr. J. Hickman for hCG; Dr. O. Bahl for hCG-α and hCG-β; Dr. G. Hennen for hLH-α; a number of our associates for expert technical and secretarial assistance: R. K. DiBlasi, C. T. Graeber, N. Kessner, L. Lorenz, M. L. Martorana, H. Mover, M. C. Rack, and R. Rich; to Dr. Michael Anderson and Janice Dorn of Abbott Laboratories for the TRH.

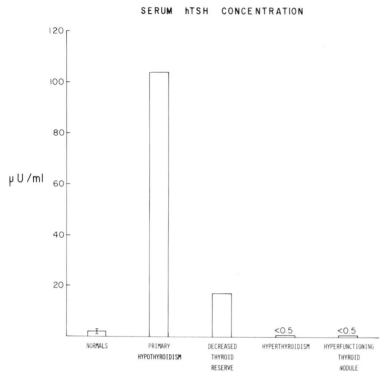

SERUM hTSH CONCENTRATION

Fig. 15-1. Serum thyro-
tropin concentration in
various thyroid dis-
orders.

suppressed by exogenous thyroid hormone), with anti-hTSH and buffer* for 48 to 72 hours at 4°C prior to the addition of approximately 0.05 ng hTSH-^{125}I. After a further 72-hour incubation at 4°C, antibody-bound labeled and unlabeled hTSH were precipitated 20 to 24 hours after the addition of an appropriate amount of goat anti-rabbit gamma globulin. The tubes were then centrifuged, the supernatants decanted, and the precipitates counted in a standard auto-gamma spectrometer. Less than 2 percent of the radioactivity was nonspecifically precipitated in tubes without anti-hTSH, and 80 to 90 percent was precipitated with excess anti-hTSH. These assay techniques differ from previous assays by utilization of highly purified labeled hTSH with a low specific activity, incubation of standards in hTSH-suppressed serum, and nonequilibrium incubation in order to improve sensitivity. The

sensitivity of the assay was from 0.25 to 1.0 µU/ml of serum with normal subjects having a mean serum hTSH concentration of 1.67 ± 0.68 µU/ml (SD). Less than 10 percent of normal subjects had levels which were not detectable, whereas greater than 90 percent of hyperthyroid patients had hTSH concentrations which were not detectable.

Clinical Studies. Previous investigators reported the normal range for serum hTSH to be from 0 to 10 µU/ml, and thus distinction between low and normal serum concentrations of hTSH was not possible.[4-10] Utilizing the modifications just described, normal serum concentrations of hTSH can now be differentiated from low serum concentrations.[11,12] Pathology of the hypothalamus or pituitary resulting in hypothyroidism usually is associated with low serum concentrations of hTSH.[6-8,14-18] Alternatively, when failure of the thyroid produces hypothyroidism, the serum hTSH concentrations is nearly always markedly elevated (Fig. 15-1).[4-10]

As the assay sensitivity for hTSH has

---

* The buffer contained 0.05 M sodium phosphate at pH 7.4 with 0.1 percent human albumin, 8 µl normal rabbit serum, and 5 I.U. of human chorionic gonadotropin per assay tube.

improved, more subtle forms of primary thyroid failure have been observed. Patients with Hashimoto's thyroiditis or treated Graves' disease may have "decreased thyroid reserve" before any of the signs or symptoms of hypothyroidism develop and before the radioactive iodine uptake or serum concen- trations of thyroxine and triiodothyronine decrease to below the normal range. These patients have "decreased thyroid reserve" because they fail to respond to bovine TSH injections with an increase in the radioactive iodine uptake, serum thyroxine, or serum triiodothyronine. They usually have serum

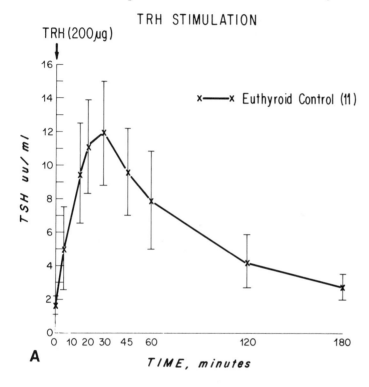

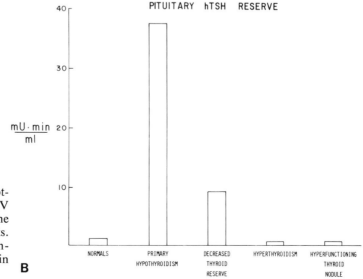

Fig. 15-2. Pituitary thyrotropin reserve. *A*, After IV thyrotropin-releasing hormone (200 *μ*g) in normal subjects. *B*, After IV thyrotropin-releasing hormone (200 *μ*g) in various thyroid disorders.

hTSH concentrations which are midway between normal patients and patients with primary hypothyroidism (see Fig. 15-1).[19-22] Thus, in the evaluation and care of such patients a slightly elevated serum hTSH concentration is the first indication of "decreased thyroid reserve." Furthermore, it has been shown that some of these patients progress to overt primary hypothyroidism suggesting that the elevated serum hTSH concentration may be predictive of impending primary thyroidal failure.[20,21]

Patients with hyperthyroidism and high serum concentrations of thyroid hormones usually have undetectable serum hTSH concentrations (see Fig. 15-1). This combination suggests that the high serum thyroid hormones suppress pituitary secretion of hTSH.[6,8,11,12] The pituitary hTSH suppression exists regardless of whether the high levels of thyroid hormone are due to Graves' disease, a toxic hyperfunctioning nodule, or exogenous administration of thyroid hormones.[12] Recently it has been shown that undetectable serum hTSH concentrations exist in certain conditions with serum concentrations of thyroid hormone that are well within an acceptable but wide "normal range." Patients with a hyperfunctioning thyroid nodule[12] or Graves' disease[23-25] who are apparently "euthyroid" with normal serum concentrations of thyroid hormone may have undetectable serum hTSH concentrations. This suggests that the pituitary is exquisitely sensitive to small increments in the circulating concentrations of thyroid hormone,[12,26] which are not sufficient to produce the usual signs and symptoms of hyperthyroidism.

An elevated serum hTSH concentration has rarely been associated with clinical hyperthyroidism and elevated levels of thyroid hormone.[27-32] Hamilton, Adams, and Maloof[28] recently described a patient with a pituitary adenoma and clinical hyperthyroidism with an elevated serum hTSH concentration, who had a remission of hyperthyroidism following partial hypophysectomy and pituitary irradiation.

Pituitary Thyrotropin Reserve. Evaluation of pituitary thyrotropin reserve has recently been made possible by the isolation, purification, and synthesis of the hypothalamic thyrotropin-releasing hormone (TRH), 1-pyroglutamyl-1-histidyl-l-proline amide.[33-35] TRH stimulation in humans[14-17,36-39] has added considerable information about the physiological regulation of the thyroid gland in health and disease. In normal subjects intravenous (Fig. 15-2*A*) or oral administration of TRH causes release of hTSH into the serum. This response is dose related, tends to be greater in females than males, and is inversely related to age in men.[38] The intravenous dose of TRH required to produce a maximal hTSH response has not been definitely established and is apparently between 100 and 500 μg of TRH depending on the investigator.[14,37-40] Exact quantitation of the hTSH response can be accomplished by measuring the total area under the hTSH curve after administration of intravenous TRH and expressing this pituitary thyrotropin reserve (PTSHR) as

$$\frac{mU \cdot min}{ml}.$$

In normal subjects after 200 ug of IV TRH, the PTSHR has been determined to be

$$1.1 \pm 0.3 \frac{mU \cdot min}{ml}$$

(Fig. 15-2*B*). In patients with primary hypothyroidism there is a further increment in hTSH above the elevated basal hTSH concentration such that the total mean PTSHR was

$$37.7 \pm 25.4 \frac{mU \cdot min}{ml}$$

(Fig. 15-2*B*). Although these patients have clinical hypothyroidism with low concentrations of circulating thyroid hormones and high basal concentrations of hTSH, the pituitary can still be stimulated to release even more hTSH. Measuring PTSHR in patients with primary hypothyroidism has also been useful in determining the appropriate replacement or suppressive dose of thyroid hormone. Adequate replacement doses of thyroid hormone were thought to

Fig. 15-3. *A*, Sequential studies with IV thyrotropin-releasing hormone (200 μg) in a hypothyroid patient given increasing doses of l-thyroxine. *B*, Pituitary thyrotropin reserve after IV thyrotropin-releasing hormone (200 μg) in a patient with decreased thyroid reserve.

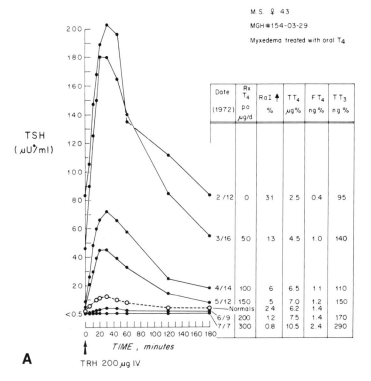

M.S. ♀ 43

MGH #154-03-29

Myxedema treated with oral T4

Date (1972)	Rx T$_4$ po μg/d	RaI ↑ %	TT$_4$ μg%	FT$_4$ ng%	TT$_3$ ng%
2/12	0	31	2.5	0.4	95
3/16	50	13	4.5	1.0	140
4/14	100	6	6.5	1.1	110
5/12	150	5	7.0	1.2	150
Normals		2.4	6.2	1.4	
6/9	200	1.2	7.5	1.4	170
7/7	300	0.8	10.5	2.4	290

TSH (μU/ml)

TIME, minutes

TRH 200 μg IV

A

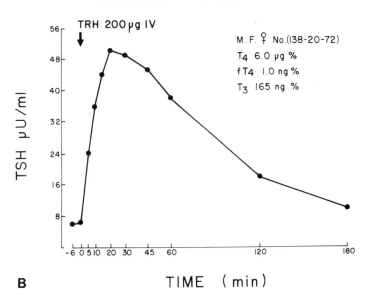

DECREASED THYROID RESERVE

TRH 200 μg IV

M.F. ♀ No.(138-20-72)

T$_4$ 6.0 μg %

fT$_4$ 1.0 ng %

T$_3$ 165 ng %

TSH μU/ml

TIME (min)

B

be equivalent to 1 to 3 gr of desiccated thyroid or 100 to 300 μg of l-thyroxine and suppressive doses to be 300 μg of l-thyroxine. Utilization of sequential TRH studies[12,26] during increasing thyroid hormone replacement determines more precisely the correct replacement dose for a given patient. These studies have shown that pituitary hTSH reserve may become normalized at doses of 150 to 200 μg of l-thyroxine per day. Furthermore, sequential TRH studies in hypothyroid patients have shown that both the serum hTSH concentration and the PTSHR may become unmeasurable at doses of l-thyroxine below the maximum of 300 μg per day and at serum thyroxine and triiodothyronine concentrations which are well within the normal range (Fig. 15-3*A*). Precise documentation of appropriate replacement dosage has obvious clinical utility in the hypothyroid patient in whom excessive thyroid hormone replacement should be avoided. Such studies also document the physiological fact that circulating thyroid hormones exert their negative feedback at the level of the pituitary and not the hypothalamus. In patients with "decreased thyroid reserve" the elevated basal serum hTSH concentrations imply an augmentation of pituitary hTSH reserve. When TRH stimulation is performed in such patients, PTSHR is elevated at

$$9.4 \pm 5.8 \, \frac{mU \cdot min}{ml},$$

approximately 10 times normal (Figs. 15-2*B*, and 15-3*B*).[22]

The TRH-stimulation test is perhaps most useful in evaluating the undetectable basal concentrations of hTSH usually seen in hyperthyroidism, in hypothalamic and pituitary hypothyroidism, and in 10 percent of normal controls. In patients with elevated serum thyroid hormone concentrations and clinical *hyperthyroidism,* the PTSHR is undetectable (Fig. 15-4*A*), confirming that the undetectable basal hTSH concentration indicates pituitary hTSH suppression.[12,36-39,41,42] Furthermore, in patients with concentrations of thyroid hormone in the normal range who have a hyperfunctioning thyroid nodule (Fig. 15-2*B*)[12,43] or euthyroid Graves' disease,[23,24,25] the PTSHR may also be undetectable or low, again confirming pituitary hTSH suppression. Alternatively, when the patient has clinical *hypothyroidism* and low concentrations of serum hTSH, the TRH-stimulation test can be used to localize the site of the pathology. In patients with pituitary disease (secondary hypothyroidism), the PTSHR is usually undetectable,[14-18] whereas in patients with hypothalamic disease (tertiary hypothy-

roidism), the PTSHR is easily detectable (Fig. 15-4*B*). The reported hTSH response to TRH in patients with supposed hypothalamic hypothyroidism shows either a normal response or an enhanced, prolonged response.[16,17,18,44,45,46] These varied responses, which warrant clarification, are probably related to the inability to define specifically defects in the hypothalamus on a clinical or laboratory basis. The anencephalic fetus, that has the only anatomical documentation of hypothalamic deficiency, has an enhanced, prolonged hTSH response to TRH.[47,48] In an adult female who had a pituitary tumor and anatomical demonstration of hypothalamic compression, the hTSH response to TRH was likewise enhanced and prolonged.[49]

In summary, TRH stimulation as a test of PTSHR has been very useful in

1. Determining normal pituitary hTSH reserve.

2. Establishing correct replacement and suppressive doses of exogenous thyroid hormone.

3. Confirming that elevated serum hTSH concentrations in patients with "decreased thyroid reserve" are associated with an augmentation of PTSHR.

4. Confirming a low basal hTSH concentration in a variety of thyroid disorders and to define the reason for it.

5. Localizing the defect in hypothyroidism due to central nervous system disease to either the pituitary or hypothalamus.

Metabolic Clearance Rates of hTSH. Iodination of hTSH with ^{131}I in tracer quantities has allowed investigators to study the metabolism of the labeled hormone in humans without using the large quantities of unlabeled hormone which cause biologic perturbations. Metabolism of hTSH was first studied by following the disappearance of a single intravenous bolus of labeled hTSH.[50,51] HTSH was found to be distributed in multiple compartments and had an initial half-life of 54 minutes. Because of the problems inherent in studying multiple exponential functions by this single injection technique, more recent data have been generated utilizing the constant infusion to equi-

Fig. 15-4. Pituitary thyrotropin reserve. *A*, After IV
thyrotropin-releasing hormone
(200 μg) in hyperthyroid patients as compared to normal
subjects. Shaded area indicates
values below limit of detectability in radioimmunoassay.
B, After IV thyrotropin-
releasing hormone (500 μg) in
a patient with hypothalamic
hypothyroidism.

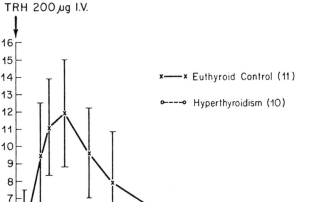

TRH STIMULATION

TRH 200 μg I.V.

x——x Euthyroid Control (11)

o----o Hyperthyroidism (10)

A

TIME, minutes

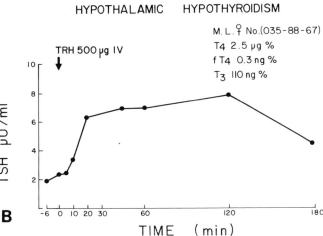

HYPOTHALAMIC HYPOTHYROIDISM

M.L.♀ No.(035-88-67)
T4 2.5 μg %
f T4 0.3 ng %
T3 110 ng %

TRH 500 μg IV

B

TIME (min)

librium method of Tait.[52] In this method[22]
hTSH-^{131}I was purified utilizing a 90 × 1.5
cm column of Sephadex G-100 and sterilized by millipore filtration. The labeled
hormone was then infused into patients at a
constant rate until equilibrium had been
achieved and constant serum concentrations
of hTSH-^{131}I were found. Since the infusion
rate and serum concentration were constant
and measurable at equilibrium, the metabolic
clearance rate of hTSH-^{131}I could be calculated by the formula:

$$\text{hTSH-}^{131}\text{I MCR} = \frac{\text{hTSH-}^{131}\text{I infusion rate}}{\text{hTSH-}^{131}\text{I serum concentration}}$$

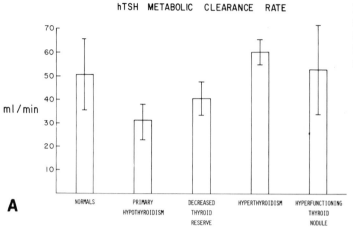

hTSH METABOLIC CLEARANCE RATE

ml / min

A

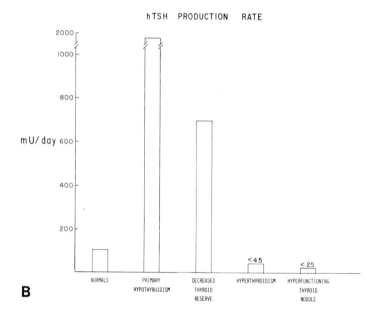

hTSH PRODUCTION RATE

mU/ day

B

Fig. 15-5. *A*, Metabolic clearance rate of hTSH in various thyroid disorders. *B*, Production rates of hTSH in various thyroid disorders.

The important assumptions of this method are the achievement of equilibrium during the time of infusion and the similarity of the metabolic clearances of labeled and unlabeled hormone. Both these assumptions have been shown to be valid for labeled hTSH.[22,53] Utilizing this technique in humans,[22] normal subjects have been shown to have metabolic clearance rates (MCR) of 50.1 ± 15.6 ml per minute (Fig. 15-5*A*). Males had significantly higher MCR (51.6 ml/min) than females (43.0 ml/min), although this apparent sex difference disappeared when the MCR were corrected for surface area. Males (25.8 ml/min/m^2) and females (25.2 ml/min/m^2) then had similar MCR per m^2. The MCR varied directly with the serum concentration of thyroid hormones so that hypothyroid patients had MCR of 30.9 ml per minute, patients with "decreased thyroid reserve" had MCR of 40.1 ml per minute, and hyperthyroid patients had MCR of 60.1 ml per minute. The correlation coefficient between the hTSH MCR and serum thyroxine and serum triiodothyronine has been shown to be highly significant (p<0.001).

Production Rates of hTSH. Since the production rate (PR) of any hormone is the product of its total metabolic clearance and serum concentration, the hTSH PR can be calculated from the observed MCR and serum concentration of hTSH.[22] In expressing the PR as amount per unit of time, one assumes that both the MCR and serum concentration remain constant during the unit of time. During a 24-hour period the serum concentration of hTSH remains relatively constant without any diurnal variation except for one very small and brief increase during the early morning hours, recently shown by sensitive radioimmunoassay techniques.[42,54] If this small early morning rise in serum hTSH concentration is not considered, normal subjects have hTSH PR of 104.3 ± 41.4 mU/d (Fig. 15-5B), somewhat lower than previous estimates.[50,51] Patients with primary hypothyroidism have elevated hTSH PR of 4440 mU/d. Furthermore, patients with "decreased thyroid reserve" have hTSH PR nearly 10 times higher than normals (956 mU/d), but lower than patients with primary hypothyroidism. Patients with hyperthyroidism usually have undetectable hTSH PR. In addition, patients with a hyperfunctioning thyroid nodule, but concentrations of thyroid hormone in the normal range, also have undetectable hTSH PR. Thus, hTSH serum concentrations and PR vary inversely with the circulating level of thyroid hormones, and both increase with primary thyroid failure. Furthermore, there is a highly significant correlation ($p < 0.001$) between the serum concentration and PR of hTSH in primary thyroid failure confirming the adequacy of hTSH serum concentration as an indicator of increased pituitary hTSH secretion throughout the spectrum of primary thyroid failure.

Control of Serum hTSH Concentration. In this text attention has been drawn to the stimulatory effect of TRH on both pituitary hTSH secretion and the serum concentration of hTSH. Conversely, circulating thyroxine and triiodothyronine exert an inhibitory effect on pituitary hTSH secretion and ultimately the serum concentration of hTSH.

Furthermore, increasing thyroid hormone concentration primarily inhibits hTSH production, as well as accelerating the metabolic clearance of hTSH. These effects are additive in lowering the serum concentration of hTSH. Recently it has been shown that corticosteroids in high doses also reduce both the serum concentration and the pituitary reserve of hTSH.[14,55,56,57] Preliminary studies have extended these findings by showing decrease in the production rate of hTSH and acceleration of the metabolic clearance rate with large doses of dexamethasone.[58] Thus, high doses of corticosteroids and thyroid hormone have similar effects on pituitary hTSH secretion.

Additionally, hTSH is elevated on exposure to cold. This is probably mediated through thyrotropin-releasing hormone. This response is more marked in human neonates than in human adults. In human adults the response is relatively blunted and probably not clinically important.[59] The elevated levels of hTSH found in chronic hypothyroidism may be suppressed by l-DOPA.[60] Conversely hTSH was elevated in a substantial number of patients on lithium carbonate, possibly related to small depressions in the serum thyroxine concentrations.[61]

Site of hTSH Metabolic Clearance. The exact site of hTSH clearance in humans is not known. Most pituitary and placental glycoproteins are cleared at least partially by the kidney and excreted in a biologically active form.[62] Early bioassay data on urinary hTSH measurements did suggest that this glycoprotein was also excreted in a biologically active form.[63,64] Unfortunately, radioimmunoassay confirmation of these data is still lacking. In humans there is a reduced MCR hTSH in chronic renal insufficiency,[51] and a significant correlation ($p < 0.001$) does exist between the endogenous creatinine clearance and the metabolic clearance rate of hTSH in patients with normal renal function.[22]

In the dog, recent experiments utilizing labeled hTSH have shown that there is a statistically significant arteriovenous difference of labeled hTSH across the kidney, but not across the liver, thyroid, or skeletal muscle.[53] Using the observed arteriovenous difference across the kidney, one can show that the calculated renal clearance of labeled hTSH is sufficient to completely account for the observed metabolic clearance of labeled hTSH. Whether this renal clearance of

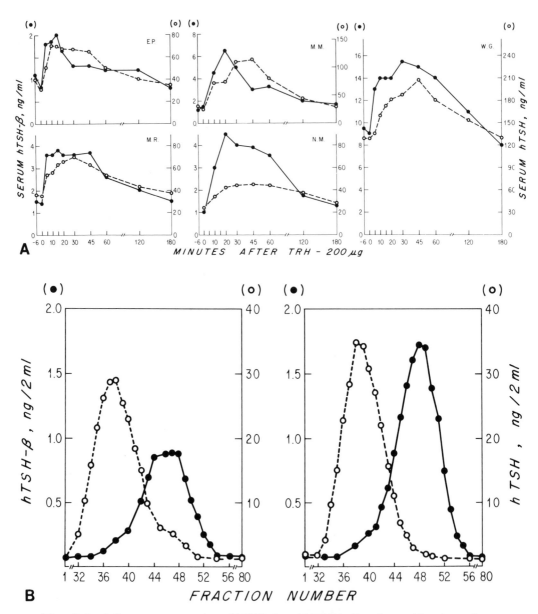

Fig. 15-6. *A,* Serum concentration of hTSH-β and hTSH in 5 patients with primary hypothyroidism following administration of IV thyrotropin-releasing hormone (200 μg). (From JCEM, *37*:836, 1973) *B,* Fractionation of serum of a hypothyroid patient. The left panel shows the separation of 2 ml of serum before TRH on a column of Sephadex G-100. The right panel shows the separation of 1.5 ml of serum pooled from samples 10 to 45 minutes after TRH. There are 2 separate peaks of hTSH-β and hTSH as measured in their respective radioimmunoassays. After TRH the increment in hTSH-β is proportionally greater than that of hTSH. (From J. Clin. Endocrinol. Metab., *37*:836, 1973)

labeled hTSH involves degradation to subunits or merely excretion of intact hTSH is still unsettled.

Subunits of hTSH. HTSH, like the other human glycoprotein hormones, luteinizing hormone (hLH), follicle-stimulating hormone (hFSH), and chorionic gonadotropin (hCG), has recently been found to contain 2 dissimilar, noncovalently bound subunits. The subunit structure of these hormones was discovered after techniques had been developed to dissociate the subunits using such agents as propionic acid or urea.[65-73] The alpha subunits of these 4 hormones are very similar, whereas the beta subunits are distinct and confer biologic and immunologic specificity to each hormone.[65,68,74,75,76]

The alpha and beta subunits of hTSH (hTSH-α and hTSH-β) are of approximately equal molecular weight. If hTSH-α differs from the alpha subunits of the other glycoprotein hormones, the differences probably occur in the carbohydrate portion of the molecule or in a few amino acids.[77,78,79] However, hTSH-β has major differences in amino acid composition from the other beta subunits.[65,80,81,82] Both subunits of hTSH appear essential for biologic activity. However, the alpha subunit of any of the glycoprotein hormones, even from a different species, will combine with the beta subunit of TSH to yield TSH biologic activity.[83]

In order to understand more fully the synthesis, secretion, and metabolism of intact hTSH, radioimmunoassays for the individual subunits have been developed after dissociation of hTSH with propionic acid and purification of the subunits by gel and ion exchange chromatography.[75] The hTSH-β radioimmunoassay could detect 0.25 to 0.5 ng/ml hTSH-β in serum. HTSH and hTSH-α each displayed only a 1 percent cross-reactivity in this beta assay, and hLH and hCG and their beta subunits demonstrated virtually no cross-reactivity.[75] Although it has been shown that the beta subunit determines the immunologic specificity of the intact hormone,[74,84] it appears from the insignificant cross-reaction of hTSH in this hTSH-β immunoassay that there must

be determinants on the beta subunit that are not exposed because of the conformation of intact hTSH. Thus an immunoassay specific for the beta subunit of hTSH can be developed even though intact hTSH contains the same beta subunit.

Once the subunits of hTSH were purified, the cross-reactivity of hTSH-α and hTSH-β and the subunits of hLH and hCG in the hTSH radioimmunoassay was investigated. Although the very similar alpha subunits of hTSH, hLH, and hCG were immunologically identical in their insignificant cross-reactivity in the hTSH assay, it was the cross-reactivity of the less similar beta subunits of hLH and hCG that appeared to determine the cross-reactivity of intact hLH and hCG in the hTSH assay. In addition, hTSH-β demonstrated a 15 percent cross-reactivity in the hTSH assay. In spite of this significant cross-reactivity, no sera examined have been found to contain hTSH-β in sufficient quantity to invalidate the hTSH level measured by radioimmunoassay.

Because the beta subunit is the immunologically specific subunit, work to date has centered on the measurement of hTSH-β in serum. Normal subjects have been found to have undetectable hTSH-β (<0.5 ng/ml). Patients with primary hypothyroidism have significant concentrations of hTSH-β in serum with a range from < 0.5 to 9.5 ng/ml, representing from < 3 to 7 percent of the hTSH by mass. Hypothyroid patients studied at multiple time intervals after the administration of IV TRH (200 μg) showed increases in hTSH-β at the earliest time point studied (5 or 10 min). All patients demonstrated greater percent increases in hTSH-β than in hTSH at the earliest time points (Fig. 15-6A); they also had earlier peak responses of hTSH-β compared to those of hTSH.[85] Although the hTSH levels in primary hypothyroidism may be very elevated, the hTSH-β measured was not caused by the small cross-reactivity of hTSH in the beta assay. After determining the hTSH level, each serum was diluted so that there was insufficient hTSH remaining to cause significant cross-reaction in the beta assay.

In order to validate the measurement of hTSH-β in unfractionated serum, the serum of 1 hypothyroid patient both before and after TRH was fractionated by gel chromatography on Sephadex G-100 (Fig. 15-6*B*). In both cases there were 2 separate peaks of hTSH-β and hTSH; there was also good agreement between unfractionated and fractionated serum in determination of hTSH-β and hTSH concentrations.[85]

Dr. John Pierce in 1971 in his Eli Lilly lecture[65] asked the following provocative and intriguing questions: (1) What are the mechanisms controlling the biosynthesis, storage and release of TSH? (2) Is only the intact hormone released by the thyroid releasing hormone or are the individual subunits under some sort of control? (3) Will the similarity of immunological response of each intact hormone and its β chain hinder efforts to determine if an excess of hormone-specific chain is present in any pathological condition? Radioimmunoassays for hTSH-β have now been developed with sufficient specificity to measure hTSH-β accurately in the presence of elevated serum concentrations of hTSH. Free circulating hTSH-β has been detected in primary hypothyroidism. The more rapid rise and earlier peak of hTSH-β relative to hTSH in serum of such patients after TRH suggests that hTSH-β is secreted from the pituitary rather than derived from peripheral dissociation of hTSH. Further studies are currently in progress to determine definitively whether subunits of hTSH are secreted from the pituitary. The role of subunits in the biosynthesis of intact hTSH and the possibility of degradation of hTSH to subunits at the time of clearance from the circulation remain important areas of investigation.

References

1. Condliffe, P. G.: Purification of human thyrotropin. Endocrinology, *72*:893, 1963.
2. Utiger, R. D., Odell, W. D., and Condliffe, P. G.: Immunologic studies of purified human and bovine thyrotropin. Endocrinology, *73*:359, 1963.
3. Berson, S. A., and Yalow, R. S.: Immunoassay of protein hormones. *In* Pincus, G., Thumarin, K. V., and Astwood, E. B. (eds.): The Hormones: Physiology, Chemistry and Applications. vol. 4, p. 557. New York, Academic Press, 1964.
4. Utiger, R. D.: Radioimmunoassay of human plasma thyrotropin. J. Clin. Invest., *44*: 1277, 1965.
5. Odell, W. D., Wilber, J. F., and Paul, W. E.: Radioimmunoassay of thyrotropin in human serum. J. Clin. Endocrinol. Metab., *25*:1179, 1965.
6. Odell, W. D., Wilber, J. F., and Utiger, R. D.: Studies of thyrotropin physiology by means of radioimmunoassay. Recent Progr. Horm. Res., *23*:47, 1967.
7. Mayberry, W. E., Gharib, H., Bilstad, J. M., *et al.*: Radioimmunoassay for human thyrotropin. Ann. Intern. Med., *74*:471, 1971.
8. Hershman, J. M., and Pittman, J. A.: Utility of the radioimmunoassay of serum thyrotropin in man. Ann. Intern. Med., *74*:481, 1971.
9. Hershman, J. M., and Pittman, J. A.: Control of thyrotropin secretion in man. N. Eng. J. Med., *285*:997, 1971.
10. Nelson, J. C., Johnson, D. E., and Odell, W. D.: Serum TSH levels and the thyroidal response to TSH stimulation in patients with thyroid disease. Ann. Intern. Med., *76*:47, 1972.
11. Patel, Y. C., Burger, H. G., and Hudson, B.: Radioimmunoassay of serum thyrotropin: sensitivity and specificity. J. Clin. Endocrinol. Metab., *33*:768, 1971.
12. Ridgway, E. C., Weintraub, B. D., Cevallos, J. L., *et al.*: Suppression of pituitary TSH secretion in the patient with a hyperfunctioning thyroid nodule. J. Clin. Invest., *52*:2783, 1973.
13. Hunter, W. M., and Greenwood, F. C.: Preparation of iodine-[131] labelled human growth hormone of high specific activity. Nature (London), *194*:495, 1962.
14. Haigler, E. D., Pittman, J. A., Hershman, J. M., *et al.*: Direct evaluation of pituitary thyrotropin reserve utilizing synthetic thyrotropin releasing hormone. J. Clin. Endocrinol. Metab., *33*:573, 1971.
15. Fleischer, N., Lorente, M., Kirkland, J., *et al.*: Synthetic thyrotropin releasing factor as a test of pituitary thyrotropin reserve. J. Clin. Endocrinol. Metab., *34*:617, 1972.
16. Schalch, D. S., Gonzalez-Barcena, D., Kastin, A. J., *et al.*: Abnormalities in the release of TSH in response to thyrotropin releasing hormone (TRH) in patients with disorders of the pituitary, hypothalamus

and basal ganglia. J. Clin. Endocrinol. Metab., *35*:609, 1972.

17. Faglia, G., Beck-Peccoz, P., Ferrari, C., *et al.*: Plasma thyrotropin response to thyrotropin releasing hormone in patients with pituitary and hypothalamic disorders. J. Clin. Endocrinol. Metab., *37*:595, 1973.

18. Patel, Y. C., and Burger, H. G.: Serum thyrotropin (TSH) in pituitary and/or hypothalamic hypothyroidism: normal or elevated basal levels and paradoxical responses to thyrotropin-releasing hormone. J. Clin. Endocrinol. Metab., *37*:190, 1973.

19. Utiger, R. D.: Plasma TSH in health and disease: immunoassay studies. *In* Gual, C., and Ebling, F. J. G. (eds.): Progress in Endocrinology. p. 1186. Excerpta Medica Foundation, Amsterdam, 1968.

20. Maloof, F., Cevallos, J. L., Adams, L., *et al.*: The use of the radioimmunoassay of TSH in the early detection of hypothyroidism. Forty-seventh Meeting Amer. Thyroid Assoc., (abstr.) p. 39, 1971.

21. Shenkman, L., Mitsuma, T., and Hollander, C. S.: Methods for detecting incipient primary hypothyroidism, a comparative study. J. Clin. Endocrinol. Metab., *36*:1074, 1973.

22. Ridgway, E. C., Weintraub, B. D., and Maloof, F.: Metabolic clearance and production rates of human thyrotropin. J. Clin. Invest., *53*:895, 1974.

23. Lawton, N. F., Ekins, R. P., and Nabarro, J. D. N.: Failure of pituitary response to thyrotropin-releasing hormone in euthyroid Graves' disease. Lancet, *2*:14, 1971.

24. Cooper, D., Ridgway, E. C., Lorenz, L., *et al.*: The thyroid-pituitary-hypothalamic axis in euthyroid patients with Graves' ophthalmopathy. Clin. Res. (abstr.), *20*:864, 1972.

25. Chopra, I. J., Chopra, U., and Orgiazzi, J.: Abnormalities of the hypothalamo-hypophyseal-thyroid axis in patients with Graves' ophthalmopathy. J. Clin. Endocrinol. Metab., *37*:955, 1973.

26. Snyder, P. J., and Utiger, R. D.: Inhibition of thyrotropin to thyrotropin-releasing hormone by small quantities of thyroid hormones. J. Clin. Invest., *51*:2077, 1972.

27. Lamberg, B. A., Pipatti, J., Gordin, A., *et al.*: Chromophobe pituitary adenoma with acromegaly and TSH-induced hyperthyroidism associated with parathyroid adenoma. Acta Endocrinol., *60*:157, 1969.

28. Hamilton, C. R., Adams, L. C., and Maloof, F.: Hyperthyroidism due to thyrotropin producing, pituitary chromophobe adenoma. N. Eng. J. Med., *283*:1077, 1970.

29. Utiger, R. D.: (Editorial) Thyrotropin RIA: another test of thyroid function. Ann. Intern. Med., *74*:627, 1971.

30. Hamilton, C. R., and Maloof, F.: Acromegaly and toxic goiter. J. Clin. Endocrinol. Metab., *35*:659, 1972.

31. Faglia, G., Ferrari, C., Neri, U., *et al.*: High plasma thyrotropin levels in two patients with pituitary tumours. Acta Endocrinol., *69*:649, 1972.

32. Emerson, C. H., and Utiger, R. D.: Hyperthyroidism and excessive thyrotropin secretion. N. Eng. J. Med., *287*:328, 1972.

33. Bøler, J., Enzmann, F., Folkers, K., *et al.*: The identity of chemical and hormonal properties of the thyrotropin releasing hormone and pyroglutamyl-histidyl-proline amide. Biochem. Biophys. Res. Commun., *37*:705, 1969.

34. Burgus, R., Dunn, R. F., Desiderio, D., *et al.*: Structure moleculaire du facteur hypothalamique hypophysiotrope TRF d'origine ovine: mise en evidence par spectrometrie de masse de la sequence PGA-His-Pro-Nitz., Cr. Acad. Sci. [D] (Paris), *259*:1970, 1969.

35. Schally, A. V., Arimura, A., Bowers, C. Y., *et al.*: Purification of hypothalamic releasing hormones of human origin. J. Clin. Endocrinol. Metab., *31*:291, 1970.

36. Ormston, B. J., Kilborn, J. R., Garry, R., *et al.*: Further observations on the effect of synthetic thyrotropin releasing hormone in man. Br. Med. J., *2*:199, 1971.

37. Anderson, M. S., Bowers, C. Y., Kastin, A. J., *et al.*: Synthetic thyrotropin releasing hormone: a potent stimulator of thyrotropin secretion in man. N. Eng. J. Med., *285*:1279, 1971.

38. Snyder, P. J., and Utiger, R. D.: Response to thyrotropin releasing hormone in normal man. J. Clin. Endocrinol. Metab., *34*:380, 1972.

39. Gual, C., Kastin, A. J., and Schally, A. V.: Clinical experience with hypothalamic releasing hormones. Part I. Thyrotropin-releasing hormone. Recent Progr. Horm. Res., *28*:173, 1972.

40. Karlberg, B., and Almquist, S.: Effects of increasing doses of pyroglutamyl-histidyl-proline amide on serum thyrotropin in normal subjects. Acta Endocrinol., *70*:196, 1972.

41. Shenkman, L., Mitsuma, T., and Hollander, C. S.: Modulation of pituitary responsiveness to thyrotropin releasing hormone by triiodothyronine. J. Clin. Invest., *52*:205, 1973.

42. Vanhaelst, L., Van Canter, E., Degaute, J. P., *et al.*: Circadian variations of serum thyrotropin levels in man. J. Clin. Endocrinol. Metab., *35*:479, 1972.

43. Karlberg, B. E.: Thyroid nodule autonomy; its demonstration by the thyrotropin releasing hormone (TRH) stimulation test. Acta Endocrinol., *73*:689, 1973.

44. Pittman, J. A., Haigler, E. D., Hershman, J. H., *et al.*: Hypothalamic hypothyroidism. N. Eng. J. Med., *285*:844, 1971.

45. Costom, B. H., Grumbach, M. M., and Kaplan, S. L.: Effect of thyrotropin releasing factor on serum thyroid-stimulating hormone. An approach to distinguishing hypothalamic and pituitary forms of idiopathic hypopituitary dwarfism. J. Clin. Invest., *50*:2219, 1971.

46. Hall, R., Ormston, B. J., Besser, G. M., *et al.*: The thyrotropin-releasing hormone test in diseases of the pituitary and hypothalamus. Lancet, *1*:759, 1972.

47. Hayek, A., Driscoll, S. C., and Warshaw, J. B.: Endocrine studies in anencephaly. J. Clin. Invest., *52*:1636, 1973.

48. Allen, J. P., Greer, M. A., McGilvra, R., *et al.*: Endocrine function in an anencephalic infant. J. Clin. Endocrinol. Metab., *38*:94, 1974.

49. Case Records of the Massachusetts General Hospital. Case 14-1972. N. Eng. J. Med., *286*:767, 1972.

50. Odell, W. D., Utiger, R. D., Wilber, J. F., *et al.*: Estimation of the secretion rate of thyrotropin in man. J. Clin. Invest., *46*:953, 1967.

51. Beckers, C., Machiels, J., Soyez, C., *et al.*: Metabolic clearance rate of thyroid-stimulating hormone in man. Horm. Metab. Res., *3*:34, 1971.

52. Tait, J. F.: Review: the use of isotopic steroids for the measurement of production rates *in vivo*. J. Clin. Endocrinol. Metab., *23*:1285, 1963.

53. Ridgway, E. C., Singer, F. R., Weintraub, B. D., *et al.*: Metabolic clearance of human thyrotropin in the dog. Endocrinology, (In press, 1974).

54. Patel, Y. C., Alford, F. P., and Burger, H. G.: The 24-hour plasma thyrotropin profile. Clin. Sci., *43*:71, 1972.

55. Otsuki, M., Dakoda, M., and Baba, S.: Influence of glucocorticoids on TRH induced TSH response in man. J. Clin. Endocrinol. Metab., *36*:95, 1973.

56. Faglia, G., Ferrari, C., Beck-Peccoz, P., *et al.*: Reduced plasma thyrotropin response to thyrotropin releasing hormone after dexa-

methasone administration in normal subjects. Horm. Metab. Res., *5*:289, 1973.

57. Dussault, J. H.: The effect of dexamethasone on TSH and h-Pr secretion after TRH stimulation. Clin. Res. (abstr.), *21*:1025, 1973.

58. Re, R. N., Kourides, I. A., Ridgway, E. C., *et al.*: Glucocorticoid effect on TSH and prolactin secretion. Clin. Res. (abstr.), *22*: 347a, 1974.

59. Hershman, J. H., and Pittman, J. A.: Control of thyrotropin secretion of man. New Eng. J. Med., *285*:997, 1971.

60. Rapoport, B., Refetoff, S., Fang, V. S., *et al.*: Suppression of serum thyrotropin (TSH) by L-Dopa in chronic hypothyroidism: interrelationships in the regulation of TSH and prolactin secretion. J. Clin. Endocrinol. Metab., *36*:256, 1973.

61. Emerson, C., Dyson, W. L., and Utiger, R. D.: Serum thyrotropin and thyroxine concentrations in patients receiving lithium carbonate. J. Clin. Endocrinol. Metab., *36*: 338, 1973.

62. Van Hell, H., Schuurs, A. H. W. M., and den-Hollander, F. C.: Purification and some properties of human urinary FSH and LH. *In* Saxena, B. B., Beling, C. G., and Gandy, H. M. (eds.): Gonadotropins. p. 185. New York, John Wiley & Sons, 1972.

63. Hertz, S., and Oastler, E. G.: Assay of blood and urine for thyrotropic hormone in thyrotoxicosis and myxedema. Endocrinology, *20*:520, 1963.

64. Rawson, R. W., and Starr, P.: Direct measurement of height of thyroid epithelium: a method of assay of thyrotropic substance; clinical application. Arch. Intern. Med., *61*:726, 1938.

65. Pierce, J. G.: Eli Lilly Lecture: The subunits of pituitary thyrotropin—their relationship to other glycoprotein hormones. Endocrinology, *89*:1331, 1971.

66. Pierce, J. G., Liao, T., Howard, S. M., *et al.*: Studies on the structure of thyrotropin: its relationship to luteinizing hormone. Recent Progr. Horm. Res., *27*:165, 1971.

67. Liao, T., and Pierce, J. G.: The presence of a common type of subunit in bovine thyroid-stimulating and luteinizing hormones. J. Biol. Chem., *245*:3275, 1970.

68. Cornell, J. S., and Pierce, J. G.: The subunits of human pituitary thyroid-stimulating hormone. J. Biol. Chem., *248*:4327, 1973.

69. Sairam, M. R., and Li, C. H.: Human pituitary thyrotropin: Isolation and chemical characterization of its subunits. Bio-

chem. Biophys. Res. Commun., *51*:336, 1973.

70. Swaminathan, N., and Bahl, O. P.: Dissociation and recombination of the subunits of human chorionic gonadotropin. Biochem. Biophys. Res. Commun., *40*:422, 1970.

71. Morgan, F. J., and Canfield, R. E.: Nature of the subunits of human chorionic gonadotropin. Endocrinology, *88*:1045, 1971.

72. Closset, J., Hennen, G., and Lequin, R. M.: Isolation and properties of human luteinizing hormone subunits. FEBS Letters, *21*: 325, 1972.

73. Saxena, B. B., and Ratham, P.: Dissociation phenomenon and subunit nature of follicle-stimulating hormone from human pituitary glands. J. Biol. Chem., *246*:3549, 1971.

74. Vaitukaitis, J. L., Ross, G. T., Reichert, L. E., Jr., *et al.*: Immunologic basis for within and between species cross-reactivity of luteinizing hormone. Endocrinology, *91*: 1337, 1972.

75. Kourides, I. A., Weintraub, B. D., Levko, M. A., *et al.*: Alpha and beta subunits of human thyrotropin: purification and development of specific radioimmunoassays. Endocrinology, *94*:1411, 1974.

76. Vaitukaitis, J. L., Ross, G. T., Pierce, J. G., *et al.*: Generation of specific antisera with the hormone-specific β-subunit of hTSH or hFSH. J. Clin. Endocrinol. Metab., *37*: 653, 1973.

77. Sairam, M. R., Papkoff, H., and Li, C. H.: Human pituitary interstitial cell stimulating hormone: primary structure of the α subunit. Biochem. Biophys. Res. Commun., *48*:530, 1972.

78. Bellisario, R., Carlsen, R. B., and Bahl, O. P.: Human chorionic gonadotropin. J. Biol. Chem., *248*:6796, 1973.

79. Bahl, O. P., Carlsen, R. B., Bellisario, R., *et al.*: Human chorionic gonadotropin: amino acid sequence of the α and β subunits. Biochem. Biophys. Res. Commun., *48*:416, 1972.

80. Morgan, F. J., Birken, S., and Canfield, R. E.: Comparison of chorionic gonadotropin and luteinizing hormone: a note on a proposed significant structural difference in the beta subunit. FEBS Letters, *31*:101, 1973.

81. Carlsen, R. B., Bahl, O. P., and Swaminathan, N.: Human chorionic gonadotropin. J. Biol. Chem., *248*:6810, 1973.

82. Shome, B., and Parlow, A. F.: Human TSH subunits: radioimmunoassay and primary structure of the beta subunit. Endocrinology, *23*:A-60 (abstr.), 1973.

83. Pierce, J. G., Bahl, O. P., Cornell, J. S., *et al.*: Biologically active hormones prepared by recombination of the α chain of human chorionic gonadotropin and the hormone-specific chain of bovine thyrotropin or of bovine luteinizing hormone. J. Biol. Chem., *246*:2321, 1971.

84. Vaitukaitis, J. L., Braunstein, G. D., and Ross, G. T.: A radioimmunoassay which specifically measures human chorionic gonadotropin in the presence of human luteinizing hormone. Amer. J. Obstet. Gynecol., *113*:751, 1972.

85. Kourides, I. A., Weintraub, B. D., Ridgway, E. C., *et al.*: Increase in the beta subunit of human TSH in hypothyroid serum after thyrotropin releasing hormone. J. Clin. Endocrinol. Metab., *37*:836, 1973.

16 *Gonadotropins*

BENJAMIN ROTHFELD, M.D., T. H. HSU, M.D.,
AND RONALD STEELE, PH.D.

This chapter is devoted primarily to a discussion of follicle-stimulating hormone (FSH), luteinizing hormone (LH), which is also known as interstitial cell stimulating hormone (ICSH), and human chorionic gonadotropin (hCG). Additionally, there is some discussion on human placental lactogen (HPL) and gonadotropin-releasing hormone (Gn-RH).

FSH, LH, AND hCG

Bioassay. The early work and much of the information with regard to the above hormones was based on bioassay.

The usual method for bioassay of FSH is to inject the material to be tested into immature female rats or mice and then subsequently to weigh the ovaries or uterus. Actually LH also plays a role in this test. The most widely used bio-assay for LH involves measurement of ovarian ascorbic acid depletion in the rat after injection of the unknown material. Here immature intact pseudo-pregnant rats are used and given the test material intravenously. Another method involves the injection of the material to be assayed into hypophysectomized male rats. The increase in the weight of the ventral prostate is then measured.[1] Another bioassay for LH involves the rat ovarian hyperemia method. However, like the other bioassays it does not distinguish LH from hCG.

In most bioassays the disadvantages are that the precision of the method is usually not as great as desired, and also there is a fair amount of overlap between normal and abnormal clinical states.

Chemistry. Like thyrotropin (TSH), FSH, LH and hCG are all glycoproteins consisting of a protein core with carbohydrate side chains. They are similar in their physicochemical properties as shown below.[2-6]

All 4 glycoprotein hormones consist of 2 nonidentical subunits, by convention designated as alpha and beta. The alpha subunits show strong homology for different hormones and among animal species. The beta subunit is hormone specific, and responsible for target organ specificity and the immunological properties of the glycoprotein hormones. For example, ovine LH alpha subunit and bovine LH alpha subunit amino acid sequence are identical to that of bovine TSH alpha subunit. The presence of a common alpha subunit provides an explanation for the major problem of cross-reactivity encountered in glycoprotein hormone radioimmunoassay. Antisera to the beta subunits may therefore provide the most specific agents for radioimmunoassay of the intact hormone.[7,8] Sialic acid apparently protects gonadotropins from metabolic degradation but is not essential for target organ recognition.[9] The significance of the difference in sialic acid content in gonadotropins is discussed below.

RADIOIMMUNOASSAY

Roughly 5 years after the initial report[9] concerning application of radioimmunoassay

Table 16-1. Biochemical Characteristics of Human Glycoprotein Hormones

Hormones	Mol Wt	Sub Unit	Carbohydrate Content	Sialic Acid Content	Amino Acid Sequence
FSH	36,000	α & β	25%	5%	Not known
LH	30,000	α & β	25%	1%	Established for ovine, human not known
TSH	26,000	α & β	10%	2%	Established
hCG	56,000	α & β	40%	9%	Established

to hormone studies in man, the first reports regarding use of RIA for gonadotropins in man appeared.[11,12,13]

A disadvantage of radioimmunoassay noted quite early was the fact that there was cross-reactivity between hCG, FSH, LH and thyroid-stimulating hormone (TSH). From a practical point of view, however, the cross-reactivity of TSH did not present a major problem in studies of gonadotropin. Cross-reactivity between FSH, LH and hCG has presented a greater problem. By chance, antisera with relatively high activities against FSH or LH can be obtained by immunizing either rabbits or guinea pigs. The fact that LH and hCG are so similar is taken advantage of in preparing FSH antisera. That is, the antisera may be preabsorbed with hCG removing the LH antibodies and hopefully leaving an antiserum specific for FSH. The great majority of FSH radioimmunoassays have utilized hCG preabsorption.[14] The close similarity between LH and hCG however makes the development of separate antisera for them much more difficult. This is discussed below.

The usual principles of radioimmunoassay are carried out in studies of FSH, LH, and hCG. A major problem, which is particularly prevalent in gonadotropin assays, is the production of a high specific activity radioiodinated gonadotropin with little or no loss of immunoreactivity. There is a tendency during iodination for the gonadotropins to dissociate into subunits which are not totally separable from the intact hormone by chromatographic systems commonly used.[15] The net result is a loss of immunoreactivity which does not invalidate the assay but may lessen its sensitivity and precision.[16] To date radioiodination has been performed almost exclusively by the chloramine-T method of iodide oxidation.[17] Most recently an enzymatic iodination procedure which produces material suitable for radioimmunoassays has been described for FSH, LH, and hCG; however, its particular merits remain to be evaluated.[18]

A variety of procedures have been utilized to separate bound from free hormones in gonadotropin assays. Chromatoelectrophoresis, double antibody, solid phase, organic solvents, ion exchange, and adsorption chromatography have all been used.[19] A method of separation advocated as somewhat simpler has been the use of dioxane.[20] However, this method is only effective in the presence of low protein concentrations and therefore requires the use of a highly sensitive gonadotropin antiserum capable of detecting normal gonadotropin values in small volumes of plasma. Many gonadotropin antiserums do not provide this sensitivity. Because it can be used with any available antiserum and labeled antigen, the double antibody method of separation is most widely used.

An advantage of the radioimmunoassay for gonadotropins, which it shares with other radioimmunoassays, is that it is a practical test, has good precision and considerable sensitivity. Additionally, it makes possible the development of hormone specific, species-nonspecific assays. Thus, there is an RIA with which it is possible to assay LH in the sera of sheep, rats, pigs, cattle, monkeys, horses, etc.[22] Moreover, it is possible to develop heterologous assays where the label tracer is from a species different from that used to develop the antisera.[23] Needless to say, this possibility makes RIA's for gonadotropins potentially much more flexible.

An application of the basic knowledge about the subunits of the various gonadotropins was the use of the β-subunit to develop antisera. By this means it was possible to develop antisera quite specfic for hCG, making it possible to distinguish this from LH in sera. This method used a rabbit antisera developed against the β-subunit of hCG and then a sheep antirabbit serum to separate bound from free.[24] This antisera in addition to not cross-reacting with LH, did not cross-react with FSH and TSH in their physiologic concentrations. By this means it is also possible to develop specific antisera for LH, FSH and TSH.[25]

Furthermore, there has been some work in this area involving radioreceptor assays. For example, the interstitial cell fraction from rat testes has been used to study the binding of hCG and LH.[26]

RIA VERSUS BIOASSAY

When RIA was first introduced into the study of gonadotropins there was some question about its validity as compared to bioassay. A recent study compared the results of application of an RIA for FSH with the ovarian augmentation method and also with the uterine weight method.[27] They found a good correlation between RIA and ovarian augmentation. Both these tests are designed to measure FSH. The correlation with the uterine weight method was almost as good in spite of the fact that this method is not specific for FSH but measures the total effect of FSH and LH.

However, in much of the work in this area there is not a good correlation between the two approaches. This discrepancy may result from the endogenous hormone existing in various forms which differ in chemical and physical nature, alterations of the hormone resulting from extraction and/or storage, and nonhormonal factors or other hormones effecting the assay system. It is possible that the presence of subunits in the body fluids could account for some of the discrepancy, since the isolated LH and hCG subunits have little or no biological activity, while the isolated beta subunits of LH and hCG demonstrate considerable immunologic activity.[28,29] Detection of the isolated beta subunit of hCG in human plasma has been reported.[28]

There is some provocative work, which has not yet been confirmed, indicating that under some conditions there might be a qualitative change in the FSH and perhaps other gonadotropins stimulated under certain conditions. It has been suggested that this might lead to a change in these hormones as tested by bioassay but not as measured by RIA.[30] Furthermore, immunologically active urinary hCG has been extracted as 3 species of differing molecular size.[31]

Extraction of gonadotropins can alter their biological and immunological activities.[32,33] The sialic acid portion of the glycoproteins is necessary for the biological activity of FSH and hCG, but not LH, which contains little sialic acid. Thus, the biologically active sites for hCG and LH are different but their biological activity can be measured by the same bioassays.[34] The immunological activity of the gonadotropins is not altered by removal of sialic acid. Since sialic acid is easily removed, it is not difficult to understand why with certain procedures the biological activity might be destroyed without affecting the immunological activity. If the purification procedure prior to bioassay does not remove the sialic acid from intact molecules, but instead removes partially desialytated but less active molecules of FSH or of hCG, the biological activity of material to be analyzed will increase steadily.[25] Since the immunologic activity does not increase concomitantly this too will lead to a discrepancy between the two tests.

Another reason for differences might be related to gonadotropin inhibitors in urine. This is a very confusing area. It seems to have its greatest importance in bioassays. Here may be involved general toxicity to the experimental animal. Factors which may affect RIA as well as bioassay are enzymes in urine which destroy FSH and LH before the analysis and result in formation of inactive products of the glycoproteins which may compete for binding sites. It is possible to get different results between the bioassay and the RIA depending on which inhibitors are involved.[1]

Bioassays are time-consuming and the number of samples which can be assayed is limited by the number of animals available. Not infrequently, repeated estimations have to be done in a given subject. All in all, since radioimmunoassay does not have the limitations that bioassay has it is a preferable means of investigation in most situations.

Bioassay therefore has less and less of a role to play in work involving gonadotropins. The one place where it still seems to have a role appears to be in cases where biological activity is of importance and there is some question how well RIA is measuring this activity. Good agreement between biological and immunological activity is important in plasma determinations in which the results are to be utilized to assess the extent to which the target organs are being stimulated. This appears to be especially true in study preparations for medical and veterinary use.[35] Primarily, 24-hour urinary gonadotropin determinations are conducted to estimate production rates. For such studies maintenance of biological activity in urinary extracts is not essential, however it is essential that immunological activity be maintained in order to assure that the immunological activity quantitatively varies with hormone production. On the whole the tedious and nonspecific bioassay work has virtually been

replaced by RIA. This is also true for the difficult double-isotope dilution assay procedures.

PHYSIOLOGY

It is impossible in a chapter like this to give a detailed account of the knowledge about gonadotropins. Basically, the function of FSH is related to maturation of spermatozoa or ova. The function of LH is related to production of the sex hormones by the testes or the ovary. A brief summary of the findings in the 4 physiologic states of maturation, menstruation, pregnancy, menopause and the pathologic state of castration will give a general idea of the findings to be expected in these conditions.

Maturation. In prepubertal boys and girls the mean FSH and LH levels are approximately half that of the adult value.[2] With the approach of puberty the level of both of these hormones rises. In girls, values of FSH rises more rapidly than in boys. Conversely in boys LH rises more rapidly.[36] The values of FSH and LH rise with advancing puberty and gradually stabilize within the ranges characteristic of adult reproductive life. Recent work has shown that secretion of LH in any case is episodic in man.[37] Apparently this is not true in children but develops with maturity and probably represents a maturation of the hypothalamus.[38] This episodic secretion is at first sleep related but later occurs throughout the entire 24-hour cycle.

Menstruation. During the cycle, FSH levels are elevated at the onset of the follicular phase. They subsequently fall and then begin to rise again reaching a peak near the midcycle. Levels of LH rise slowly during the late follicular phase but there is a preovulatory LH and FSH surge on about the fourteenth day of the menstrual cycle in most cases. This may be related to the peak of estradiol, progesterone and 17-hydroxyprogesterone which occurs just before this peak.[39]

If pregnancy occurs, FSH and LH rise above basal levels. The FSH stabilizes during the rest of pregnancy and returns to basal levels within a few days of delivery. LH appears high but conceivably this may be due to a cross-reaction with hCG. Early in pregnancy hCG becomes elevated and remains so throughout pregnancy.[2]

With the onset of the menopause FSH increases greatly but there is little or no increase in LH.[40]

Castration. As might be expected in castration also, FSH increases greatly but LH less so.[40]

Normal FSH and LH Levels.

The mean levels of FSH and LH in prepubertal boys and girls range from 3 to 10 mouse international units per cc (mIu/cc) or 1 to 3 mug/cc.

With maturity these values rise to 6 to 25 mIu per cc or 2 to 8 ng/cc. As discussed above with menstruation FSH and LH rise to a peak at midcycle.

A crucial function is played by hCG in the maintenance of normal pregnancy. It is secreted by the trophoblastic epithelium of the placental villus. It is normally present in the serum of the mother and fetus during pregnancy and immediately postpartum. Also, hCG has a role in maintenance of normal corpus luteum function during pregnancy.

STORAGE

Like most proteins FSH, LH and hCG are not stable when freeze-dried or frozen and thawed. In addition if urine is dealt with there is no completely satisfactory way of storing it. At 4° C bacterial growth is slowed but not stopped, and so there may be enzymatic destruction of the glycoproteins. Glacial acetic acid if used as a preservative may remove sialic acid or carbohydrate from the glycoprotein and thereby cause denaturation of the gonadotropins. The best answer with either serum or urine is to run the test as soon as possible after collection. Where urine is involved extraction should be done as soon as possible by one of the following methods: acetone; tannic acid; zinc precipita-

tion; acetone precipitation. Plasma may be extracted by means of ethanol precipitation; acetone precipitation or zinc precipitation.[1] However, radioimmunoassays for plasma gonadotropins invariably utilize unextracted plasma which has been stored at minus 10 to 20° C. If several hormone determinations are to be made, it is preferable that the plasma be stored in aliquots to prevent added freezing and thawing.

CLINICAL APPLICATIONS

Because of the rapid fluctuation in plasma gonadotropin levels, a single such level is not necessarily diagnostic. Either multiple samples must be taken or 24-hour urinary collections made. If studies are done on urine the precautions mentioned above should be observed. On the whole there is good correlation between urinary gonadotropins and plasma gonadotropin measurements. It is possible (though not yet established firmly) that a 24-hour urine sample will be more reliable than single plasma estimates.[41]

Measurement of gonadotropins has its main applications in the differential diagnosis of hypogonadism, the diagnosis and follow-up of treated choriocarcinoma, in hydatidiform mole, the monitoring of ovulation induction and the diagnosis of pregnancy.

Physiological facts lay the ground work for the clinical evaluation of hypogonadism by determining blood or urine concentrations of gonadotropins. Hypogonadotropic hypogonadism roughly corresponds to a hypothalamic-pituitary disorder. A low gonadotropin is diagnostic of hypopituitarism only when there is concomitant evidence of deficiency of the gonadal steroid or other gonadal secretory products. When the measurements of FSH and LH on a single specimen of blood is at the lower part of normal range, studies using clomiphene citrate and/or Gn-RH stimulation may be required. Clomiphene causes release of gonadotropin probably by competing with gonadal steroids at the receptor site in the hypothalamus. In response to a dosage of 50 mg twice a day for

5 days, the average adult male or female increases serum gonadotropin concentration on day five to 30 percent above baseline value. Rarely a false-negative response in patients subsequently proven to be normal has been obtained. Purified Gn-RH of porcine origin as well as synthetic Gn-RH have been shown to stimulate release of both LH and FSH in human beings.[42] Theoretically, the exogenous administration of Gn-RH is an ideal way to evaluate pituitary gonadotropin reserve. However, since there is still uncertainty whether Gn-RH is the sole gonadotropin-releasing factor and the chronically unstimulated pituitary gonadotrope may require repeated Gn-RH stimulation before it regains its responsiveness to one pulse of Gn-RH, results are not always clear cut. The use of Gn-RH in the evaluation of pituitary gonadotropin function is now still under active investigation.

Hypergonadotropic hypogonadism is associated with testicular or ovarian failure. Recent studies seem to indicate an inverse correlation between sperm count and serum FSH concentration. In males with Sertoli-cell failure (testicular germinal aplasia), an elevation of serum FSH is a common finding. The Leydig cells are intact and testosterone and LH levels are normal. In Klinefelter's syndrome (seminiferous tubule dysgenesis), testicular agenesis or severe testicular failure, serum levels of LH and FSH are elevated to values typical for castrates.

In the same way it is not possible to rely completely on gonadotropin levels whether determined by bioassay or radioimmunoassay in deciding on replacement therapy. Thus in a study there were a number of persons with high or normal levels of gonadotropins who, nevertheless, were treated with gonadotropins and who responded as measured by steroid production or subsequent pregnancy. In some of these persons both the bioassay and the RIA were in agreement and in some they were not. Nevertheless, there were some responses in all groups.[27] The authors, in agreement with others, feel that gonadotropin determinations are useful in screening patients before treatment with gonadotropins but that isolated high or normal values by either method may not indicate permanent ovarian failure.[43] They recommended that on the basis of their study of 71 patients at least 3 bioassays be done on urine collected at weekly intervals before reaching a definite diagnosis. They believe that an occasional high level of gonadotropin is not a contraindication to treatment with these substances.

Amenorrhea and anovulatory menstrual cycles are most commonly due to hypothalamic dysfunction. The hypogonadotropic amenorrhea and anovulatory cycles due to the absence of the LH ovulatory surge may be detected by serial gonadotropin assay. The polycystic ovary syndrome is also considered as a hypothalamic disorder. LH is elevated in at least 50 percent of the cases, but FSH typically remains at the levels of the normal follicular phase. Primary ovarian failure causes elevation of gonadotropin. In Turner's syndrome, the ovaries typically are unable to produce adequate sex steroids and do not have germinative activity. LH and FSH rise to postmenopausal levels at the time of expected puberty. LH is abnormally high even before the age of puberty.[44] Menopause is due to age-dependent cessation of ovarian function. By virtue of a feedback mechanism, the intact hypothalamic-pituitary axis will compensate by increasing the release of FSH and LH as in the case of castrates.

As to hCG, the primary use for this assay is in diagnosing pregnancy. Additionally, following the level of hCG is of help in the diagnosis and follow-up therapy of hydatidiform mole or chorionic carcinoma.

As mentioned above, recently a highly sensitive RIA for hCG has been developed. By means of this it is possible to determine hCG in the presence of LH. Before the development of this test, it was difficult to diagnose pregnancy by hormonal studies before the eleventh day following ovulation, because the levels of hCG did not rise to above the mean LH level until that time.[45]

With the development of this new test it is now possible to diagnose pregnancy by means of an hCG assay much earlier.[46]

Using this more sensitive assay it has been found that 60 of 828 patients seen with nontrophoblastic neoplasm had detectable hCG.[47] The authors found a high frequency of positive responses in those patients with carcinoma of the stomach, liver, pancreas, breast and with multiple myeloma and melanoma. In one article the author suggests that the specificity and ease of performance using this test seem to make it of value for screening high-risk populations for early detection of hCG-producing tumors.[25]

RELEASING HORMONES

Although these hormones are currently confined to the research area some mention will be made of them. In the past few years evidence has accumulated that the hypothalamus is involved in the elaboration of hormones having to do with the release of FSH and LH. At first there seemed to be evidence that two separate hormones were involved. However, more recently the evidence seems to point to the fact that one hormone originally known as luteinizing hormone-releasing hormone (LH-RH) is responsible for the release of both these substances.[48] More recently this has been called gonadotropin-releasing hormone (Gn-RH).

The bioassay for Gn-RH consists of injecting ovariectomized-progesterone-estrogen-thyroxine-treated rats with serum extracts of Gn-RH and utilizing radioimmunoassay for detection of LH in the rat plasma. This method has detected measurable Gn-RH in a methanol extract of 40 ml of human serum taken during the pre- or postovulatory phase of the menstrual cycle.[49] In addition to requiring large volumes of plasma, the bioassay lacks precision. The preinjection levels of LH and FSH vary considerably from one test animal to another and such variation markedly affects the sensitivity of the bioassay.[50] A radioimmunoassay has been described which can detect Gn-RH in serum of normal sheep.[51] The antiserum

used in this assay has not been utilized in human studies. The only reported radioimmunoassay utilized for detection of Gn-RH in human plasma failed to detect serum Gn-RH even during the midcycle.[52] In addition to the presumably low levels of Gn-RH in peripheral plasma, the major problem in detecting Gn-RH in the plasma is its possible inactivation by the plasma itself. Rapid inactivation of bioassayable synthetic Gn-RH by rat, dog, guinea pig, sheep, and human plasma has been reported.[53]

HUMAN PLACENTAL LACTOGEN (HPL)

History

In the late 1950's and early 1960's a number of investigators isolated a prolactin-like substance from placentas.[54,55,56] In 1962 a polypeptide which had both lactogenic actions and seemed to cross-react with human growth hormone was isolated.[57] This is what is now known as HPL. Because of its actions it has also been called human chorionic somatomammatropin.

Chemistry and Physiology

HPL is a polypeptide hormone which is secreted by the placenta and has immunochemical similarities to human growth hormone.

Physiologic Properties. HPL seems to have somatotropic, prolactin-like and luteotropic properties. Thus with food deprivation, HPL concentration increases.[58] Since the postulated role of HPL in pregnancy is to spare maternal utilization of glucose by stimulating fat mobilization, one would expect HPL to increase with fasting. In rabbits and mice HPL produces breast development and lactational changes, similar to the effect of prolactin. This effect has also been noted in rhesus monkeys. However, there is no effect in hypopituitary dwarfs, and therefore one cannot be very definite as to the role of HPL in breast development in pregnant humans.[59] HPL also increases aldosterone excretion and erythropoiesis. For many of the above reasons HPL has been called "the metabolic hormone of pregnancy."[60] However, since infusion of HPL into nonpregnant females does not produce many of the changes observed during pregnancy, it is well not to make too many definite assumptions about the effect of HPL. Probably HPL plays a definite role in pregnancy only in interaction with estrogen, progesterone, and cortisone.[61]

HPL is secreted almost entirely into the maternal circulation. The plasma level in the fetus is only 1 percent of that in the mother at term. There is no circadian rhythm. Its half-life in the plasma of pregnant females is less than 30 minutes.[62]

Since the half-life of HPL in plasma is less than 30 minutes in contrast to that of hCG (24 to 48 hours), HPL falls more rapidly with placental damage than hCG.

HPL is not uncommonly confused with prolactin.[63] They are similar in that they both rise early in pregnancy. However HPL is not found in nonpregnant women and prolactin is and varies during the menstrual cycle. HPL rises to a peak about the time of delivery and then rapidly disappears. Prolactin rises early in the puerperium. With nursing it continues to increase and reaches a maximum between the sixth and sixtieth days after delivery. HPL rises steadily in maternal serum and reaches its peak just before delivery. It reaches levels higher than that of any other known protein hormone at any time and may be as much as 1,000 times the level of human growth hormone. Because of its very high level, the problem of false reaction with human growth hormone is not a serious one. By diluting serum, the interference from growth hormone can be eliminated. On the whole the level of HPL correlates with the weight of the placenta. This explains its steadily increasing levels through pregnancy. Additionally, it seems to explain the high levels found in twin pregnancies and also in diabetic pregnancies.[64] As mentioned above, the level of HPL drops rapidly after delivery of the placenta.

Actually detection of HPL and its distinction from HGH and prolactin is most widely done by means of radioimmunoassay. Bioassays do not distinguish these various hormones. Presence of high levels of HPL late in pregnancy permit the use of very dilute specimens in RIA, and as a result endogenous human growth hormone has little effect on the results obtained.[65]

Practical Value of HPL

A number of workers using independent RIA methods have delineated identical normal ranges in pregnancy. They are all in agreement that in the fourth quartile of pregnancy the value of HPL should be 4 μg/cc or greater. This general agreement on normal values seems to enhance the utility of the test.[67] It is also of interest to note that some workers in titling HPL the "watchdog of fetal distress" advocate its use as a screening test to give forewarning of fetal distress or neonatal asphyxia after an apparently normal pregnancy.[68] They felt that there is a 56 percent chance of perinatal complications if the hormone concentration is in the fetal danger zone (more than 2 S.D. below normal on at least one occasion). Other workers have also pointed out that HPL may be of value since there may be no clinical signs of fetal distress although the fetus is doing poorly. These workers in a prospective study checked the level of HPL between the thirty-fifth and fortieth weeks of pregnancy. They found that if there were 3 or more levels below 4 μg/cc, there was a 71 percent risk of fetal distress or neonatal asphyxia. Levels above 5 μg/cc were associated with a very low level of these complications. These authors suggested that since the assay is simple and a large number of samples can be processed, HPL should be a routine screening test in pregnancy.[69]

There is some conflict as to the prognostic value of HPL alone in pregnancy. Some workers feel that it is impossible to predict the outcome of the pregnancy from measurements of HPL alone.[61] Others place much greater faith in HPL determination. Thus one set of workers[70] suggests that abnormally low levels of HPL may be an indication for evacuating the uterus in the presence of vaginal bleeding. This seems to the current authors to put a somewhat excessive amount of faith in this test.

Comparison with Urinary Estriol

It was felt by some that HPL cannot replace urinary estriol since HPL measures only placental function while estriol measures both fetal and placental function.[64] That is, estriol measures both the ability of the fetal adrenals to produce 16-alphadehydroepian-drosterone and the ability of the placenta to convert this to estriol. Nevertheless, in the author's opinion the simplicity of the determination of HPL gives it a definite advantage as a screening test. There is no question that estriol gives more definitive information.

Use in Tumors

HPL in the serum of patients suffering from benign or malignant trophoblastic disease varies depending on the stage of the disease. With increasing malignancy its level diminishes. The finding of low HPL and high hCG in trophoblastic disease may help in differentiating neoplasia from normal or term gestation.[61] Another use of HPL is in following the course of trophoblastic tumors. Its much shorter half-life, compared to that of hCG, appears to give it somewhat of an advantage in following the effect of various therapeutic agents in these disorders.

References

1. Stevenson, P. M., and Loraine, J. A.: Pituitary gonadotrophins—chemistry, extraction and immunoassay. Adv. Clin. Chem., *14*:1, 1971.
2. Saxena, B. B., Rathnam, P., and Romnler, A.: Human FSH and LH: current status. Endocrinol. Exp., *7*:19, 1973.
3. Saxena, B. B., and Rathnam, P.: Purification of follicle-stimulating hormone from human pituitary glands. J. Biol. Chem., *242*:3769, 1967.
4. Rathnam, P., and Saxena, B. B.: Isolation character of LH. J. Biol. Chem., *245*:3725, 1970.
5. Reichert, L. E., and Lawson, G. M.: Molecular weight relationships among the subunits of human glycoprotein hormones. Endocrinology, *92*:1034, 1973.
6. Catt, K. J.: Dufau, M. L., and Tsuruhara, T.: Absence of intrinsic biological activity in LH and hCG subunits. J. Clin. Endocrinol. Metab., *36*:73, 1973.
7. Kettelsleggers, J. M., Franchimont, P., and Hennen, G.: *In* Margoulies, M., and Grenwood, F. C. (eds.): Structure-activity Relationships of Protein and Polypeptide Hormones. Excerpta Medica ICS, *241*:148, 1971.
8. Ross, G. T., Vaitukaitis, J. L., and Robbins, J. B.: *In* Margoulies, M., and Grenwood, F. C. (eds.): Structure-activity Relationships of Protein and Polypeptide Hormones. Excerpta Medica ICS, *241*:153, 1971.
9. Tsuruhara, T., Van Hall, E. V., Dufau, M. L., and Catt, K. J.: Ovarian binding of intact and disialytated hCG in vivo and in vitro. J. Clin. Endocrinol. Metab., *91*:463, 1972.
10. Yalow, R. S., and Berson, S. A.: Immunoassay of endogenous plasma insulin in man. J. Clin. Invest., *39*:1157, 1960.
11. Midgley, A. R.: RIA for human chorionic gonadotrophins and luteining hormones. Fed. Proc., *24*:162, 1965.
12. Odell, W., Ross, G., and Rayford, P.: RIA for LH. Metabolism, *15*:287, 1966.
13. Faiman, C., and Ryan, R.: RIA for human FSH. J. Clin. Endocrinol. Metab., *27*:444, 1967.
14. Midgley, A. R., Niswender, G. B., Gay, V. L., *et al.*: Use of antibodies for characterization of gonadotrophins and steroids. Recent Progr. Horm. Res., *27*:235, 1971.
15. Van Orden, D. E.: The analysis and fractionation of LH[125]I by gel filtration. Proc. Soc. Exp. Biol. Med., *139*:267, 1972.
16. Hunter, W. M.: Assessment of radioodinated Hormone Preparations. Acta Endocr. (suppl.) (Kbh), *142*:134, 1969.
17. Greenwood, F. C., Hunter, W. M., and Glover, J. S.: The preparation of ^{131}I-labelled human growth hormone of high specific radioactivity. Biochem. J., *89*:114, 1963.
18. Miyachi, Y., Vaitukaitis, J. L., Nieschlag, E., and Lipsett, M. B.: Enzymatic radioiodination of gonadotropins. J. Clin. Endocrinol. Metab., *34*:22, 1972.
19. Saxena, B. B., *et al.*: RIA, FSH, & LH. Acta Endocrinol. S, *142*:185, 1969.
20. Thomas, K., and Ferin, J.: *In* Saxena, B. B., *et al.* (eds.): Gonadotrophins. New York, John Wiley & Sons, 1972.
21. Sand, T., and Torjesen, P. A.: Dextran-coated charcoal used in the RIA of LH. Acta Endocrinol., *73*:444, 1973.

22. Niswender, G. V., Midgley, A. R., and Reichert, L. E.: Radioimmunologic studies with various luteinizing hormones. *In* Rosenberg, E. (ed.): Gonadotrophins. p. 299. 1968.

23. L'Hermite, M., and Midgley, A. R.: RIA of human FSH with antisera to the ovine hormone. J. Clin. Endocrinol. Metab., *33*:68, 1971.

24. Vaitukaitis, J. L., Braunstein, G. D., and Ross, G. T.: A RIA which specifically measures hCG in the presence of human LH. Amer. J. Obstet. Gynecol., *113*:751, 1972.

25. Vaitukaitis, J. L., and Ross, G. T. Recent advances and evaluation of gonadotrophic hormones. Ann. Rev. Med., *24*:295, 1973.

26. Catt, K. J., Dufau, M. L., and Tsuruhara, T.: Radioligand receptor assay of LH and hCG. J. Clin. Endocrinol. Metab., *34*:123, 1972.

27. Butt, W. R., and Lynch, S. S.: Estimation of urinary gonadotrophins by bioassay and by RIA. J. Endocrinol., *51*:993, 1971.

28. Weintraub, B. D., and Rosen, S. W.: Ectopic production of the isolated beta subunit of human chorionic gonadotrophin. J. Clin. Invest., *52*:3135, 1973.

29. Reichert, L. E., Ward, D. N., Niswender, G. D., and Midgley, A. R.: On the isolation and characterization of subunits of human pituitary luteinizing hormone. *In* Butt, W. R., Crooke, A. C., and Ryle, M. (eds.): Gonadotropins and Ovarian Development. p. 149. Chigago, Williams & Wilkins, 1970.

30. Diebel, N. D., Yamamoto, M., and Bogdanove, E. M.: Discrepancy between RIA and bioassay for rat FSH: Evidence that androgen treatment and withdrawal can alter bioassay-immunoassay ratios. Endocrinology, *92*:1065, 1973.

31. Kaplan, G. N., Maffezoli, R. D., and Chrambach, A.: Characterization of human chorionic gonadotropin and luteinizing hormone contained in urinary extracts by polyacrylamide gel electrophoresis. J. Clin. Endocrinol. Metab., *34*:370, 1972.

32. Butt, W. R., Lynch, S. S., Chaplin, M. F., Gray, C. J., and Kennedy, J. F.: The effects of chemical modifications on the biological and radioimmunological activity of pituitary follicle stimulating hormone. *In* Butt, W. R., Crooke, A. C., and Ryle, M. (eds.): Gonadotropins and Ovarian Development. p. 171. Chicago, Williams & Wilkins, 1970.

33. Stevens, V. C., Anderson, D. G., and Powell, J. E.: Comparison of the characteristics of human pituitary and urinary FSH and LH during purification. *In* Butt, W. R., Crooke, A. C., and Ryle, M. (eds.): Gona- dotropins and Ovarian Development. p. 22. Chicago, Williams & Wilkins, 1970.

34. Wilde, C. E.: The Correlation Between Immunological and Biological Estimation of hCG in Body Fluids. Acta Endocrinol. (suppl.) (Kbh), *142*:360, 1969.

35. Barth, R., and Kim, N. H.: Human gonadotrophins—A review of recent developments. Can. Med. Assoc. J., *102*:1173.

36. Job, J. C., Garnier, P. E., Chaussain, J. L., *et al.*, quoted by Franchimont, P., Burger, H., and Legros, J. J.: Impact of radioassay techniques on the field of sex hormones. Metabolism, *22*:1007, 1973.

37. Naftolin, F., Yen, S. S. C., and Tsai, C. C.: Rapid cycling of plasma gonadotrophins in normal man as demonstrated by frequent sampling. Nature (New Biology), *236*:92, 1972.

38. Boyar, R. M., Finkelstein, J., Roffwarg, H., *et al.*; Identification of puberty by synchro- nization of LH release with sleep. J. Clin. Invest., *51*:(abstr.)1308, 41, 1972.

39. Burger, H., Catt, J., and Brown, J.: Rela- tionship between plasma LH and urinary estrogen excretion during the menstrual cycle. J. Clin. Endocrinol. Metab., *28*:1508, 1968.

40. Daughaday, W. H.: Williams Textbook of Endocrinology. ed. 4, chap. 2. Philadel- phia, W. B. Saunders, 1968.

41. Franchimont, P., Burger, H., and Legros, J. J.: Impact of radioassay techniques on the field of sex hormones. Metabolism, *22*: 1003, 1973.

42. Kastin, A. J., Schally, A. V., Gaul, C., Midgley, A. R., Jr., *et al.*: Stimulation of LH release in men and women by LH- releasing hormone purified from porcine hypothalamic. J. Clin. Endocrinol. Metab., *29*:1046, 1969.

43. Sutaria, B., and Crooke, A. C.: Selection of patients for treatment with human gonado- trophin. Int. J. Fertil., *16*:42, 1971.

44. Migeon, C.: Personal communication, 1972.

45. Marshall, J. R., Hammond, C. B., Ross, G. T., *et al.*: Obst. Gynecol., *32*:760, 1968.

46. Kosasa, T., Levesque, L., Goldstein, D. B. T., *et al.*: Early detection of implantation using a RIA specific for hCG. J. Clin. Endocrinol. Metab., *36*:622, 1973.

47. Braunstein, G. D., Vaitukaitis, J. L., Car- bone, P. P., *et al.*: Ectopic production of hCG by neoplasma. Ann. Intern. Med., *78*: 39, 1973.

48. Arimura, A., Kastin, A. J., Schally, A. V.: In Saxena, B. B., *et al.*: (eds.): Gonado- trophins. New York, John Wiley & Sons, 1972.

49. Malacara, J. M., Seyler, L. E., and Reichlin, S.: Luteinizing hormone releasing factor activity in peripheral blood from women during the midcycle luteinizing hormone ovulatory surge. J. Clin. Endocrinol. Metab., *34*:271, 1972.

50. Blackwell, R., Amoss, M., Vale, W., Burgus, R., Rivier, J., *et al.*: Concomitant release of FSH and LH induced by native and synthetic LRF. Amer. J. Physiol., *224*:170, 1973.

51. Nett, T. M., Akbar, A. M., Niswender, G. D., *et al.*: A RIA for gonadotrophin-releasing hormone in serum. J. Clin. Endocrinol. Metab., *36*:880, 1973.

52. Barker, H. M., Isles, T. E., Fraser, H. M., and Gunn, A.: Radioimmunoassay of luteinizing hormone releasing hormone. Nature, *242*:527, 1973.

53. Sandow, J., Enzmann, F., Schroeder, H. G., and Vogel, H. G.: Inactivation of LR-RH by the plasma of various species. Naunyn Schmiedebergs Arch. Pharmakol. (suppl.), *274*:95, 1972.

54. Contopoulos, A. N., and Simpson, M. E.: Growth promoting activity of pregnant rat plasma after hypophysectomy and after thyroidectomy. Endocrinology, *64*:1023, 1959.

55. Higashi, K.: Studies on the prolactin-like substance in human placenta. Endocrinol. Japan, *8*:288, 1961.

56. Ito, Y., and Higashi, K.: Studies on the prolactin-like substance in human placenta. Endocrinol. Japan, *8*:279, 1961.

57. Josimovich, J. B., MacLaren, J. A.: Presence in human placenta and term serum of highly lactogenic substance immunologically related to pituitary growth hormone. Endocrinology, *71*:209, 1962.

58. Tyson, J. E., Austin, K. L., Farinholt, J. W.: Prolonged food deprivation in pregnancy. Amer. J. Obstet. Gynecol., *109*:1080, 1971.

59. Friesen, H. G.: Human placental lactogen in human pituitary prolactin. Clin. Obstet. Gynecol., *14*:669, 1971.

60. Grumbach, M., and Caplan, S. L.: Ann. N.Y. Acad. Sci., *148*:501, 1968.

61. A First Conference and Workshop in HPL. Obstet. Gynecol. Survey, *25*:207, 1970.

62. Genazzani, A. R., Aubert, M. L., Casoli, M., *et al.*: Use of HPL RIA to predict outcoming cases of threatened abortion. Lancet, *2*:1385, 1969.

63. Friesen, H. G.: HPL and human pituitary prolactin. Clin. Obstet. Gynecol., *14*:669, 1971.

64. Saxena, B. N., Emerson, K., and Selenkow, H.: Serum HPL levels as an index of placental function. N. Eng. J. Med., *281*:225, 1969.

65. Grant, D. V., Caplan, S. L., and Grumbach, N. N.: Studies on the cross-reaction between human growth hormone and human chorionic somato-mammatrophin in RIA assay systems. J. Clin. Endocrinol. Metab., *32*: 88, 1971.

66. Theptisal, H., Mishell, V., and Nakmura, R.: Comparison of a rapid new method of hemagglutination inhibition assay of HPL with micro-complement fixation and RIA. J. Clin. Endocrinol. Metab., *32*:382, 1971.

67. Zuckerman, J. E.: HPL in the management of high risk pregnancy. Lancet, *1*:200, 1973.

68. England, P., Fergusson, J. C., Lorrimer, V., *et al.*: HPL: The watchdog of fetal distress. Lancet, *1*:5, 1974.

69. Letchworth, A. T., and Chard, T.: HPL levels as a screening test for fetal distress and neonatal asphyxia. Lancet, *1*:704, 1972.

70. Niven, P., Landon, J., and Chard, T.: HPL levels as a guide to the outcome of threatened abortion. Br. Med. J., *3*:799, 1972.

17 Radioimmunoassay of Gastrin

JOHN H. WALSH, M.D.

INTRODUCTION

It was known for many years that extracts of gastric mucosa were capable of stimulating gastric acid secretion, but for some time this activity was felt to be due to the presence of histamine in the extracts. In 1938 Komarov showed that the stimulant was distinct from histamine.[1] The presence of a circulating stimulant of acid secretion was demonstrated by Grossman in dogs with totally denervated gastric pouches.[2] Then Gregory and Tracy isolated, characterized and synthesized gastrin.[3] Subsequently, many experiments have been performed in dogs having various types of gastric pouches and many of the factors responsible for the control of gastrin release have been defined. However, gastric secretion is controlled by complex interactions between nervous reflexes and circulating stimulants and inhibitors,[4] so that many conclusions about the release of gastrin which were based on measurement of acid secretion can only be inferential.

In 1955 Zollinger and Ellison described the syndrome (which now bears their name, Z-E syndrome, ZES), as consisting of fulminant peptic ulcer disease, and massive gastric acid hypersecretion associated with nonbeta cell tumors of the pancreatic islets.[5] A few years later gastrin was extracted from several ZE tumors.[6] It also was shown that the serum of patients with ZES contained a substance with gastrin-like properties (i.e., it stimulated acid secretion in the rat).[7] More recently hypergastrinemia has been demonstrated by RIA in these patients.[8]

Chemical analysis of the gastrin purified by Gregory and Tracy revealed that it was a linear peptide consisting of 17 amino acids.[9] Two forms were identified which differed only in the presence (gastrin-II) or absence (gastrin-I) of a sulfate substitution in the tyrosine residue. Subsequently, gastrins from several other species were defined chemically and were found to have no more than 2 residues different from hog gastrin (Table 17-1).[10] The human gastrin was synthesized and was made available for biological studies and also was used for immunization of animals to raise antibodies.

The availability of pure gastrin for labeling and of reasonable quantities for immunization inevitably led to development of radioimmunoassay methods for measurement of gastrin. The first assay suitable for measurement of gastrin in normal serum was described by McGuigan.[11] In rapid succession several other laboratories including that of Yalow and Berson[12] also reported successful gastrin RIA methods.[13,14,15,16] In all these assays pure heptadecapeptide gastrin was employed for labeling and as standard, although some of the antibodies were raised against crude gastrin preparations and some against conjugated gastrin molecules. Recently it has become apparent that circulating gastrin is more heterogeneous than originally was realized and that gastrin molecules may differ in the size of the peptide chain as well as in the presence or absence of a sul-

231

Table 17-1. Structures of Gastrins and Related Peptides.

	1	2	3	4	5	6	7	8	9	10	11	12	13	14	15	16	17
Human G-17-I	*Pyr-Gly-Pro-Trp-Leu-Glu-Glu-Glu-Glu-Glu-Ala-Tyr-Gly-Trp-Met-Asp-Phe-NH₂
Human G:2-17-I	Gly-Pro-Trp-Leu-Glu-Glu-Glu-Glu-Glu-Ala-Tyr-Gly-Trp-Met-Asp-Phe-NH₂
Porcine G-17-I	Met (position 5)
Cat G-17-I	Ala (position 8)
Dog G-17-I	Ala (position 8)
Sheep G-17-I	Val (position 5) — Ala (position 9)
Cow	Val (position 5) — Ala (position 9)
Human G-17-II	Tyr (position 12) with SO₃H
Human G-13-I	Leu-Glu-Glu-Glu-Ala-Tyr-Gly-Trp-Met-Asp-Phe-NH₂
Human G-34-I	*Pyr-(14-Amino Acid Residues)-Lys-Lys-Gln-Gly-Pro-Trp-Leu-Glu-Glu-Glu-Glu-Glu-Ala-Tyr-Gly-Trp-Met-Asp-Phe-NH₂
Tetrapeptide	Trp-Met-Asp-Phe-NH₂
Pentagastrin	Boc-β-Ala-Trp-Met Asp-Phe-NH₂
Human G:1-13	*Pyr-Gly-Pro-Trp-Leu-Glu-Glu-Glu-Glu-Glu-Ala-Tyr-Gly
Porcine	Lys-Ala-Pro-Ser-Gly-Arg-Val-Ser-Met-Ile-Lys-Asn-Leu-Gln-Ser-Leu-Asp-NH₂
Cholecystokinin	Pro-Ser-His-Arg-Ile-Ser-Asp-Arg-Asp-Tyr-Met-Gly-Trp-Met-Asp-Phe-NH₂ with SO₃H
CCK Octapeptide	Asp-Tyr-Met-Gly-Trp-Met-Asp-Phe-NH₂ with SO₃H
Caerulein	Asp-Tyr-Thr-Gly-Trp-Met-Asp-Phe-NH₂ with SO₃H

* Pyr = pyroglutamyl
Arabic figures on left refer to number of amino acids in the peptide.
G = gastrin
CCK = cholecystokinin
Caerulein is included since it may be used to test antisera to gastrin. The points of similarity to gastrin may be noted.

fate group.[17] As with other peptide hormones, this heterogeneity in the serum has complicated the measurement and interpretation of immunoreactive gastrin concentrations in the serum. The newer developments are discussed as completely as possible in this chapter. It is realized, of course, that much necessary information is not yet available.

MOLECULAR FORMS OF GASTRIN

In normal subjects and in hypergastrinemic subjects the major forms of immunoreactive gastrin in the circulation have greater apparent molecular weights and are relatively less negatively charged than the heptadecapeptides. Some of these gastrins have been prepared in pure form sufficient to permit analysis of their amino acid composition. Others have been characterized only by their elution patterns on gel filtration. Figure 17-1 indicates an idealized elution pattern on Sephadex G-50 superfine columns which might be obtained from a patient with a gastrin-secreting tumor.

The largest component elutes in the void volume on G-50 and was named "big-big" gastrin by Berson and Yalow.[18] Big-big gastrin is present in relatively low amounts in patients with gastrin-secreting tumors but may comprise a major fraction of normal fasting serum gastrin activity in normal man and dog as determined by RIA.[19] The biological activity of this material is unknown. Similar material purified from a tumor extract was found to have a half-life of approximately 90 minutes in the dog, far greater than the half-life of the other forms of gastrin.[20] Our own studies in the dog suggest that big-big gastrin has relatively more immunochemical than biological activity, since no relationship has been established between basal circulating big-big gastrin and basal acid secretion. This material may be especially abundant in the serum following partial gastric resection.[19] In the dog, stimulation of gastrin release with acetylcholine did not change the concentration of big-big gastrin in the serum (Dockray and Debas,

unpublished observations). Until sufficient quantities of big-big gastrin have been purified from serum or from normal tissues, the biological properties of this material cannot be determined. The presence of big-big gastrin may explain the difficulties encoun-

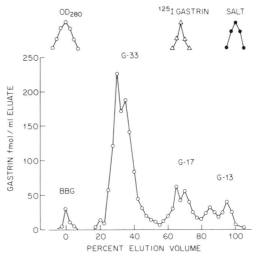

Fig. 17-1. Elution pattern of gastrin immunoreactivity obtained by chromatography of 0.1 ml serum from a patient with Zollinger-Ellison syndrome on a 1 x 100 cm column of Sephadex G-50 superfine gel. Fractions were 1 ml, eluted with 0.02 M veronal buffer, pH 8.6, at a rate of 6 ml per hour. Internal markers included serum protein (identified by measurement of optical density at 280 nm), monoiodinated 125-I gastrin, and sodium chloride (identified by measurement of conductivity). Percent elution volume was measured from the protein peak (0 percent) to the salt peak (100 percent). Gastrin content of each tube of eluate was measured by radioimmunoassay with antibody 1296 and was expressed as fmol/ml with a G-17 standard. This elution pattern is a composite of the results obtained with 2 different patients which were combined to illustrate the different components identified in this system. "Big-big gastrin" was eluted in the void volume, "big gastrin" (G-34) between 30 and 40 percent, "little gastrin" (G-17) between 60 and 70 percent, and "minigastrin" (G-13) between 80 and 100 percent. Component I of Rehfeld is not regularly identified in columns of this size but may be represented by the small shoulder preceding the G-34 peak.

Table 17-2. Molecular Weights and Extinction Coefficients of Gastrin Peptides.

Molecule	Molecular Weight	Extinction coefficient
Human G-34-I	3,839	12,261
Human G-34-II	3,919	10,754
Human G-17-I	2,098	12,261
Human G-17-II	2,178	10,754
Human G:2-17-I	1,987	12,261
Human G-13-I	1,674	6,884
Human G-13-II	1,727	5,377
Porcine G-17-I	2,116	12,261
Porcine G-17-II	2,196	10,754
Porcine G-13-I	1,665	6,884
Porcine G-13-II	1,745	5,377
Porcine CCK	3,918	5,377
Octapeptide CCK	1,143	5,377
Caerulein	1,352	5,377
Tetrapeptide	597	5,377
Pentagastrin	769	5,377

Based on extinction coefficients for Trp = 5,377
Tyr = 1,507
SO_3H-Tyr = nil

tered in preparation of gastrin-free serum, since this material is not removed by dialysis or by charcoal absorption. Its presence in high relative concentrations may also explain some of the difficulties encountered in attempts to correlate basal gastrin with basal acid secretion. No more precise name can be assigned to big-big gastrin until more is known about its chemical nature.

The other gastrin component about which little is known is Component I of Rehfeld. This fraction has been identified only on very long columns of Sephadex G-50 superfine and elutes with an apparent Stokes radius of 2.3.[21] Under more ordinary conditions of gel filtration, Component I is merged into the "big gastrin" peak. It has been speculated that this component is some type of gastrin precursor, but its chemical nature and gastric acid-stimulating capacity have not been determined.

Three other forms of gastrin have been identified in the serum that have been characterized chemically. Each of these forms appears to circulate in sulfated and nonsulfated states. The presence of sulfate does

not appear to affect biological activity on gastric secretion. This is markedly different from the situation with the cholecystokinin peptides in which the sulfate group is essential for optimal activity.[22] Based on the chemical analysis of purified preparations obtained from tumors and from antral extracts by Gregory and Tracy, a tentative nomenclature has been proposed as shown in Table 17-2.

The principal form of gastrin identified in most sera has an apparent molecular weight greater than twice that of the heptadecapeptide. This form was named "big gastrin" by Yalow and Berson. A component with similar characteristics later was named Component II by Rehfeld but appears to be identical. This material has been identified in extracts of normal stomach and intestine[23] and in tumor extracts. Gregory and Tracy purified this material from Z-E tumors and determined that it was composed of 34 amino acids,[24] hence the name G-34. Both sulfated and nonsulfated forms have been identified. Trypsin converts G-34 into 2 major fragments. The C-terminal fragment is identical with heptadecapeptide gastrin (G-17). The N-terminal fragment is a linear peptide which does not contain tryptophan, tyrosine, or phenylalanine. Thus major portions of G-34 and G-17 are identical. The N-terminal peptide of G-34 appears to be linked to the C-terminal G-17 chain through a lysyl-glutaminyl peptide bond.

The difference between the actual calculated molecular weight of G-34 and the earlier estimates, which were approximately twofold higher, can be resolved by noting that G-34 is a linear peptide, whereas estimates of molecular weight assume a globular configuration. The full sequence of the N-terminal hexadecapeptide has not yet been published, but it is known that the amino acid content differs only slightly from the tentative composition published recently by Gregory.[24] G-34 has been identified in extracts of gastric antral mucosa and upper intestinal mucosa from man and other species, in Z-E tumor extracts, and in serum.

However, G-17 usually predominates in tissue extracts from the same persons in whom G-34 predominates in the serum. This discrepancy may be explained in part by the longer half-life of G-34,[25] but it also is possible that G-17 is the form in which gastrin is stored in the granules of G-cells and tumor cells.

G-17 or "little gastrin" is the heptadecapeptide originally isolated from the antrum as "gastrin." It has been well characterized structurally and is available as synthetic human gastrin I.* The biological activities of synthetic human gastrin and of purified natural porcine gastrins I (nonsulfated) and II (sulfated) have been studied in some detail. The only known physiological functions of G-17 in man, as the term is defined by Grossman, are stimulation of gastric acid and pepsin secretion and contraction of antral smooth muscle. However, larger doses, which probably are pharmacological rather than physiological, cause contraction of the gastroesophageal sphincter. In the dog, large doses of gastrin also cause stimulation of pancreatic enzyme secretion, inhibition of salt and water absorption by the intestine, contraction of the gallbladder, and smooth muscle contractions in other areas ·of the gastrointestinal tract.

Another component recently identified in serum has been called "minigastrin."[26] This material appears to be identical with the C-terminal 13 amino acid sequence of G-17 and we have named this substance G-13. Very little is known about the activity of G-13. Preliminary experiments in the dog suggest that it is somewhat less potent than G-17 as a stimulant of gastric acid secretion.[27] Minigastrin also has been identified in extracts of antrum and of Z-E tumors (Gregory and Tracy, personal communication). The possibility that gastrin fragments smaller than G-13 are present in the circulation has not been excluded, but such fragments have not yet been reported. Such

fragments could be of considerable significance, since it is known that the C-terminal tetrapeptide amide possesses considerable acid-stimulating activity.

The usual distribution of gastrin components in normal serum is not well known. Considerably more information is available about serum and plasma specimens from patients with hypergastrinemia due either to Z-E syndrome or to pernicious anemia. In such subjects, the major form of circulating gastrin in the fasting state appears to be G-34, but usually there also is a significant amount of G-17.[28] The relative amount of G-13 is not known but usually is less than that of G-17. Rehfeld has reported that his Component I comprises a significant fraction of Z-E serum gastrin, and he has not identified significant amounts of big-big gastrin.[26] Yalow has not reported Component I but finds big-big gastrin in virtually every plasma sample. She reported that the relative amount of big-big gastrin in Z-E plasma was quite low but that in normal subjects or those with partial gastrectomy this fraction could represent the major form of circulating gastrin.[19] The representation shown in Figure 17-1 might be typical for a patient with Z-E syndrome, although according to Yalow, and in our own experience, the proportion of big-big gastrin is larger in normal fasting subjects and lower in most patients with ZES.

The biological interpretation of the heterogeneity of circulating gastrins has not been established in man. Recent experiments in the dog indicated that it is necessary to increase the circulating gastrin concentration several-fold higher on a molar basis with G-34 to produce the same amount of acid stimulation achieved with G-17.[25] If these observations also are true in man, a "normal" serum gastrin concentration could be associated with a physiologic hypergastrinemia if the circulating gastrin was composed chiefly of G-17. In patients with Z-E syndrome who have gastrin concentrations of several hundred pg/ml to many ng/ml the distinction probably is irrelevant, since con-

---

* Imperial Chemical Industries, Ltd., Cheshire, England.

centrations in this range should produce near maximal stimulation regardless of the predominating molecular form. At the present time, such fine distinctions between circulating forms of gastrin have not proved of great clinical significance, and the radioimmunoassay diagnosis of Z-E syndrome is based on measurement of total immunoreactive gastrin in the serum.

The known structure of gastrins and related peptides is presented in Table 17-1. In Table 17-2 are listed molecular weights and molar extinction coefficients used to determine peptide concentrations in pure solutions.

Preparation of Antibodies

Pure G-17 has proved to be a poor antigen when injected into guinea pigs or rabbits without prior conjugation to a carrier protein. On the other hand, Yalow and Berson were successful in producing satisfactory antibodies in guinea pigs by immunization with partially purified porcine gastrin.[12] Other molecular forms of gastrin such as G-34 currently are not available and antibodies have not yet been produced that are specific for G-34. McGuigan produced antibodies to the C-terminal tetrapeptide amide of gastrin by conjugation to serum protein.[29,30] Such an antibody was reported to have equal immunoreactivity with gastrin and cholecystokinin (CCK), another gastrointestinal hormone with a C-terminal pentapeptide sequence identical with gastrin. Although antibodies produced by immunizing with crude porcine gastrin seem to have a good spectrum of cross-reactivity with the molecular forms of gastrin and minimal cross-reactivity with CCK, this immunization method is less reliable and may depend to a great extent on the exact preparation of crude gastrin for its success. Such antibodies have been commercially available for several years,* although a number of laboratories have experienced difficulty in obtaining satisfactory binding with these antibodies.

It seems reasonable for any laboratory wishing to produce its own antibodies for gastrin radioimmunoassay to begin by immunizing with conjugated gastrin. There have been many variations reported,[31,32] and the one detailed here is presented not because it is best but because it has been successful in our laboratory.

Synthetic human gastrin is purchased either as the whole molecule which has a pyrollidocarboxylic acid residue in the N-terminal position or as the 2:17 hexadecapeptide (ICI, England). It has been advocated that 2:17 be used for conjugation with carbodiimide to bovine serum albumin so that the conjugation takes place through the free amino group. However, since carbodiimide cross-links equally well through acidic side chains and since gastrin has 5 consecutive glutamic acid and one aspartic acid residue, it is unlikely that a high proportion of conjugation occurs through the single amino group of 2:17. The whole 1:17 synthetic human gastrin molecule is easily conjugated and produces suitable antibodies. One consideration in choice of antigen for conjugation is that some rabbits in a group immunized with 1:17 gastrin may develop antibodies with specificity for the N-terminal portion of the gastrin molecule while such specificity cannot be achieved with 2:17 conjugates.[33] Such N-terminal specificity offers no advantage when an antibody with broad reactivity is sought but might be useful in distinguishing between molecular forms. Excellent antibodies have been prepared both in rabbits and in guinea pigs. One practical advantage in use of rabbits is that blood is easier to obtain.

The conjugation procedure we use is as follows: We mix 1 mg synthetic gastrin 1:17 or 2:17 (dissolved in 1 ml 0.05M ammonium bicarbonate), 1.5 mg crystalline bovine serum albumin and 10 mg carbodiimide (ECDI, N-ethyl-N′-(3-dimethylamino propyl)–carbodiimide HCl)* each in 1.5 ml 0.05M sodium phosphate buffer, pH 6.7 and stir for 4 to 6 hours. We then dialyze the

* Wilson Laboratories, Chicago

* K & K Laboratories, Inc., Hollywood, Calif.

mixture for 48 to 72 hours prior to injection. Efficiency of conjugation can be assessed in several ways, the simplest being to measure optical density at 280 nm before and after dialysis. A blank is prepared containing all reagents except gastrin. The molar concentration of gastrin in the original mixture is calculated after subtraction of the blank by application of the molar extinction coefficient, 12,300. The amount conjugated is calculated as the nondialyzable fraction. Minor corrections may be necessary for dilution and for incomplete dialysis, but the exact degree of conjugation is not critical, as long as more than half the gastrin has been bound to albumin. An easy alternative method to monitor conjugation is to include radiolabeled gastrin in the incubation and to measure the change in radioactivity after dialysis. A Sephadex G-50 column can be substituted for the dialysis procedure. The degree of substitution also has been determined by amino acid analysis and the results have agreed with the above methods reasonably well. The chief purpose for monitoring the conjugation procedure is to determine that conjugation has occurred with reasonable yield.

We have found that the multiple intradermal injection technique combined with simultaneous pertussis vaccine immunization in rabbits[34] produces antibodies in at least 3 of 4 animals after the second dose. A dose of conjugated antigen equivalent to 50 to 100 μg unconjugated gastrin per animal is sufficient for each dose. This is given as an emulsion of 1 ml antigen solution plus 1 ml complete Freund's adjuvant in 30 to 40 intradermal sites over the shaved back of the rabbit. This is followed by 0.5 ml intramuscular pertussis vaccine. The rabbits are bled 4 and 6 weeks after the initial immunization, and an identical booster immunization is administered 6 weeks after the first dose. Animals then are tested at weekly intervals for antibody titer. A third dose may be given 4 to 6 months after the first 2. Many other schedules have been proposed and may be equally satisfactory.[31,32] This time schedule

is very similar to the procedure of McGuigan, but it differs in the smaller amount of antigen and the multiple intradermal injections. Useful antiserum often is obtained after the second injection, but the titers may become much higher after the third. Other immunization schedules are not discussed but are covered in the references.[11,12,31,32,35,36,37] Ear lobe bleedings may be done at weekly intervals and each bleeding can produce 10 ml of antiserum.

Evaluation of Titer and Sensitivity

The most reproducible measurements of titer are made by incubation until equilibrium is reached with a fixed amount of monoiodinated gastrin which is known to bind 90 percent or more with excess antibody. Usually incubation for 3 days at 4°C is sufficient to reach equilibrium. The amount of label used is arbitrary. We usually use 1 or 2 fmol*/2 ml incubation volume. Initial titering can be done in tenfold dilutions to find the approximate dilution which binds 50 percent of the label. This point then can be defined more precisely with twofold dilutions. We usually try to work in a B/F range of 1.0 to 1.5 in the absence of added gastrin.

More precise mathematical models of sensitivity are considered in other chapters in this book. The best antibodies produced in rabbits and guinea pigs have had equilibrium constants (K_o) between 10^{11} and 10^{12} l/mol. The working definition of sensitivity in our hands is the concentration of G-17-I, either human or porcine, required to decrease the B/F ratio from 1.0 to 0.5. With the most sensitive antisera this has required between 1 and 5 fmol/ml or 2 to 10 pg/ml. All concentrations are stated in terms of final concentration in the incubation tube.

Specificity is tested in several ways. One test is the determination of immunochemical potency of a number of peptides chemically related to gastrin. A number of these substances are shown in Table 17-1. Other synthetic fragments have been made avail-

---

* fmol = 10^{-15} mol

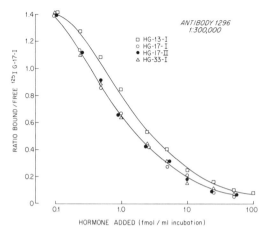

Fig. 17-2. Inhibition curves produced by pure natural human gastrin components known to be present in human serum on binding of labeled HG-17-I with antibody 1296. Sulfated heptadecapeptide gastrin (HG-17-II), nonsulfated heptadecapeptide gastrin (HG-17-I), and nonsulfated "big gastrin" (HG-34-I) produced identical inhibition curves while nonsulfated "minigastrin" (HG-13-I) had an inhibitory potency of approximately 60 percent. All concentrations are expressed in molar terms and were determined from the absorbence at 280 nm of pure solutions.

able on a limited basis. For ordinary measurement of serum gastrin, the antiserum should have good reactivity with all the forms of gastrin known to circulate in human serum. It should have equal reactivity on a molar basis with G-17-I, G-17-II, G-34-I, and G-34-II, which are the major forms of biologically active gastrin known to be present in the human circulation. Cross-reactivity with gastrins from different species is important only when studies are done in these species and then only serve to convert relative values to absolute values. It is important that the cholecystokinin (CCK) peptides not cause significant interference. CCK cross-reactivity of 1 percent or less does not appear to influence gastrin values obtained during physiological studies. Some examples of tests for specificity are shown in Figures 17-2, 17-3, and 17-4. Figure 17-2 illustrates equal immunochemical potency of HG-17-I, HG-17-II, and HG-34-I with one antibody

but less than equal immunopotency of another known circulating form of gastrin, G-13-I. Varying degrees of cross-reactivity with peptides structurally related to gastrin are seen in Figure 17-3. Figures 17-4 *A* and *B* demonstrate that different antibodies differ in reactivity with gastrins from different species and probably distinguish substitutions in position 10 of the G-17 molecule.

Another test of specificity is the demonstration that serum obtained from subjects with normal and with elevated gastrin values can be diluted serially and produce dilution curves that are parallel to the inhibition curves produced with gastrin standards. This demonstration indicates that all immunoreactive components detected in the serum produce the same type of inhibition curve and that nonspecific factors such as salt concentration, protein concentration, and serum enzymes do not produce significant effects in the range of serum concentrations to be assayed. If special conditions are to be used, such as eluates from column chromatography

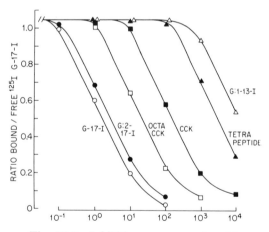

Fig. 17-3. Inhibition curves produced by some peptides structurally related to gastrin on binding of labeled HG-17-I with antibody 1296. G:2-17-I = synthetic C-terminal hexadecapeptide of human gastrin; OctaCCK = synthetic C-terminal octapeptide of cholecystokinin; CCK = porcine cholecystokinin; Tetrapeptide = C-terminal tetrapeptide amide sequence common to gastrin and CCK; G:1-13-I = synthetic N-terminal tridecapeptide of human gastrin.

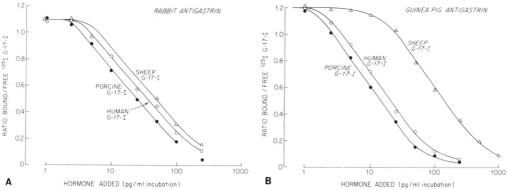

A   HORMONE ADDED (pg/ml incubation)   **B**   HORMONE ADDED (pg/ml incubation)

Fig. 17-4. Demonstration of a specificity directed at the glutamic acid sequence in the midportion of G-17. Natural porcine and synthetic human and sheep heptadecapeptide gastrins were tested with 2 antisera. *A,* The immunochemical potencies in a rabbit antiserum agree very well with the biological potencies determined by bioassay in cats. *B,* The relative potencies of human and porcine are the same but sheep gastrin, which differs from human and porcine gastrins in the 10 and 5 positions, demonstrates much less inhibitory potency in a guinea pig antiserum generated by immunization with crude unconjugated porcine gastrin.

obtained in strong buffers, it should be established that these conditions do not affect immunoreactivity.

Preparation of Labeled Gastrin

One of the major factors influencing the ultimate sensitivity of the gastrin assay is the specific activity of the labeled gastrin. If high-specific activity ^{125}I (15 mCi/μg iodide)* is used for iodination, 1 nmol produces 4.16×10^9 dpm. If 1 mol iodide is substituted per mol gastrin, each nmol labeled gastrin also should produce 4.16×10^9 dpm, and 1 fmol (10^{-15} mol) = $4.16 \times$

---

* Amersham-Searle

Fig. 17-5. Separation of labeled gastrin from unreacted free iodide on a 1 x 20 cm Sephadex G-10 column. Fractions of 1.5 ml were eluted every 3 minutes with 0.05 M ammonium bicarbonate which also served as starting buffer for subsequent ion exchange chromatography. The reaction mixture contained 2.5 mCi 125-I (1.43 nmol, supplied as 100 mCi/ml containing >14 mCi/μg I),* 3 μg natural HG-17-I (1.43 nmol),† 30 μg chloramine T (107 nmol),‡ and 100 μg sodium metabisulfite (526 nmol)§ in a final

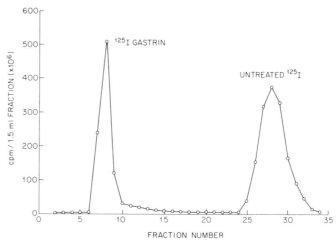

FRACTION NUMBER

volume of 165 μl 0.25 M sodium phosphate buffer, pH 7.4. Reagents were added in the order listed; oxidation with chloramine T was allowed to proceed for 15 seconds before addition of metabisulfite. An aliquot of 40 μl was saved for starch gel electrophoresis and the remainder (120 μl) was applied to the G-10 column. Tubes 7, 8, and 9, which contained approximately 24 percent of radioactivity applied to the column, were pooled for application to AE resin.

---

* Amersham-Searle, Arlington Heights, Ill.   ‡ Eastman-Kodak, Rochester, N.Y.
† Professor R. A. Gregory, Liverpool, England   § Mallinckrodt Chemical Works, St. Louis, Mo.

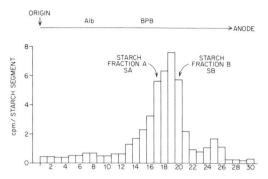

Fig. 17-6. Separation of iodinated gastrin fractions by starch gel electrophoresis. A 25 μl sample of reaction mixture described in Figure 17-5 was applied to a central well on the starch plate. The 2 immediately adjacent wells received the same volumes of bromphenol blue (BPB) dissolved in phosphate buffer and the outermost wells received serum stained with bromphenol blue (Alb). After the wells were sealed with paraffin, vertical electrophoresis was carried out for 5 hours at 200 v (25 mA). The starch was removed from the mold and placed on a sheet of parafilm. The positions of the free bromphenol blue and bromphenol blue-stained protein markers were noted. A longitudinal strip of starch was cut to include the labeled gastrin mixture, then consecutive sections of approximately 0.5 cm were cut from the origin to a point several cm anodal to the BPB marker. Sections were frozen overnight then thawed. Extraction was performed by addition of 1 ml 0.05 M ammonium bicarbonate and application of pressure with a small glass tube. The figure indicates the pattern of radioactivity relative to the positions of the protein and BPB markers. Two fractions were taken for further analysis; SA, near the BPB front, and SB, 3 fractions nearer the anode. In this system unreacted iodide migrates rapidly to the anode and enters the anodal buffer reservoir.

10^3 dpm. Expressed as counts per minute, in a gamma counter with 60 percent efficiency, 1 fmol = 2,500 cpm and 1 pg = 1,200 cpm. In a counter with 80 percent efficiency 1 fmol = 3,300 cpm and 1 pg 1,600 cpm. For monoiodinated gastrin the specific activity of the labeled product equals approximately 900 mCi/mg gastrin.

The chloramine T method has been satisfactory for production of labeled gastrin.[11,12] Conditions of a typical iodination are described in the legend to Figure 17-5. In this instance the proportion of gastrin and iodide was calculated to produce about 1 substitution per molecule. However, purification on Sephadex G-10 revealed less than 30 percent incorporation of label into the gastrin. In some instances the incorporation is higher, but it seldom exceeds 80 percent. It is now possible to repurify label not only to remove unreacted iodide but also to separate unlabeled gastrin from gastrin with single and double substitutions of radioiodine. Such separation can be achieved partially by means of starch gel electrophoresis (see Fig. 17-6). This system separates molecules which differ in size and charge. Gastrin is quite negatively charged at alkaline pH due to the multiple glutamic acid residues and migrates anodally about twice as rapidly as albumin and at a rate similar to that of free bromphenol blue, which is used as a migration marker. Partial separation of labeled and unlabeled gastrins can be achieved by starch gel electrophoresis. The major disadvantages of this method are the relatively small volume which can be applied (40 μl per well), technical difficulty in handling the starch, incomplete recovery, and incomplete separation of products. However, the quality of labeled material obtained from starch is superior to that obtained by gel filtration with Sephadex G-10.

The optimal system for repurification of labeled gastrin in our hands has been chromatography on AE-41 aminoethyl cellulose resin by ion exchange (AE system). This system has been used by Gregory for separation of sulfated and nonsulfated gastrins[38] and was applied to separation of iodinated gastrins by Stadil and Rehfeld.[39] The separation which can be achieved by this system (performed in our laboratory by Dr. G. Dockray) is illustrated in Figure 17-7. The AE system also separates molecules by charge and size and is very efficient for separation of forms of gastrin which differ

Fig. 17-7. Elution diagram demonstrating separation of unlabeled gastrin from singly and doubly iodinated gastrin by chromatograph on AE-41 aminoethyl cellulose. Fractions 7, 8, and 9 from the G-10 eluate illustrated in Figure 17-5 were applied in 0.05 M ammonium bicarbonate to a 1 x 10 column containing AE-41 equilibrated with 0.05 M ammonium bicarbonate. A gradient was established by pumping 0.5 M ammonium bicarbonate into a 125 ml mixing vessel which contained 0.05 M buffer at a rate of 6 ml per hour. The pump, mixing vessel and column were arranged into a continuous system. Fractions of 1 ml were collected in continuous 10 minute intervals and were analyzed for radioactivity. Aliquots from fractions 50 through 60 were tested for gastrin activity by radioimmunoassay. The pattern of radioactivity is indicated by the circles and solid lines while the pattern of nonradioactive immunoreactive gastrin is indicated by triangles and a dashed line.

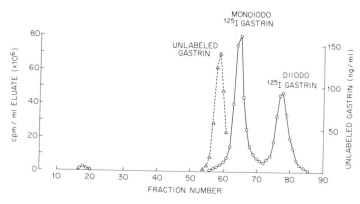

by no more than single substitutions of sulfate or iodide. Unlabeled gastrin is eluted before monoiodinated gastrin, which in turn is separated clearly from doubly iodinated gastrin. In this example the mixture applied to AE was the gastrin peak obtained from Sephadex G-10. It is apparent that the same peak contained labeled and unlabeled gastrin and that the labeled gastrin included both singly and doubly iodinated forms. Calculated recovery in the unlabeled, mono- and diiodo gastrin peaks were 73, 20, and 7 percent.

With some antibodies doubly-labeled gastrin can exhibit a high degree of immunoreactivity (Fig. 17-8). Here doubling amounts of labeled gastrin fractions were incubated with a fixed dilution of rabbit antigastrin. If the number of counts required to produce 50 percent binding is taken as a rough estimate of specific activity (this depends in large measure on the antibody used), it can be seen that fraction 78 from the AE doubly-iodinated peak had the highest activity and was approximately twice as active as the AE-65 monoiodinated peak. The most rapidly migrating starch fraction, S2, was between the mono- and diiodo activity, while the slower moving starch fraction had activity similar to the G-10 peak except that the

maximal binding was greater. In other experiments with this antiserum it was found that the inhibition curves produced by unlabeled and labeled gastrins, both mono- and diiodo, were parallel. It then could be estimated that the following number of counts per 2 ml incubation volume produced a concentration of labeled gastrin of 1 fmol/ml in the incubation:

AE 79	7,000 cpm/2 ml
AE 65	3,500 cpm/2 ml
S2	5,000 cpm/2 ml
S1	1,200 cpm/2 ml
G-10	1,000 cpm/2 ml

It is not uncommon to encounter serum gastrin concentrations as low as 10 fmol/ml (21 pg/ml). It is routine to dilute the serum tenfold in the final incubation mixture. Thus the above counts are the maximum which can be used to produce a concentration of tracer less than the minimal concentration of gastrin which is to be measured. Here there appears to be a definite advantage in using doubly labeled gastrin.

Other parameters of satisfactory label include nonspecific binding (separation by resin in absence of antibody) less than 8 percent, maximal binding with excess antibody greater than 80 percent, and good retention of binding, with nonspecific binding less than

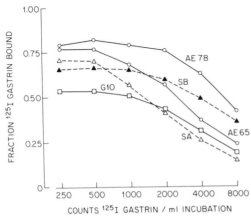

Fig. 17-8. Inhibition curves produced by addition of doubling amounts of labeled gastrin fractions to a series of tubes containing the same concentration of antigastrin in a final incubation volume of 2 ml. Counts added per ml are shown on the abscissa and fraction bound (counts bound/total counts after correction for nonspecific binding) on the ordinate. Fractions were obtained from purification steps illustrated in Figures 17-5, 17-6, and 17-7. Maximal percent binding with tenfold excess antibody is indicated in parentheses. Solid circles = AE 78 (85), the peak tube from the AE eluate doubly iodinated region; open circles = AE 65 (88), the peak tube from the AE eluate singly iodinated region; solid triangles = S2 (66), the more anodally migrating starch fraction; open triangles = S1 (79), the starch fraction taken near the BPB marker; open boxes = G-10 (72), the pool of tubes 7, 8, and 9 from the G-10 column. Counts per ml at which 50 percent radioactivity was bound ranged from 1,000 per ml with the G-10 fraction to 6,500 per ml with the doubly iodinated AE fraction.

10 percent, when stored frozen at −40°C for up to 60 days.

Gastrin Standards. Standard porcine gastrin II (PG-17-II) and synthetic human gastrin I (HG-17-I) are available through the British Medical Research Council.*

These standards were prepared several years ago and may not be as potent as other recent preparations of pure gastrin. Pure

synthetic human gastrin is available† either as the 1:17 or 2:17 sequence. Differences in potency among various vials, which were noted with the synthetic lot prepared several years ago,[12] have not been reported with the newly synthesized material. In the near future, vials containing known amounts of natural human gastrin I and gastrin II, purified from Z-E tumor tissue, will be distributed through the Peptic Ulcer Center at Wadsworth VA Hospital, Los Angeles, California. Presently there is no satisfactory source for pure G-34 (big gastrin) or G-13 (minigastrin). Since G-34 is the predominant form of gastrin in the serum of hypergastrinemic patients with Z-E syndrome, serum from several such patients can be diluted serially to determine parallelism of inhibition between G-34 and the G-17 standard. An estimate of cross-reactivity can be obtained by assaying the G-34 peak from Sephadex G-50 chromatography of a Z-E serum before and after trypsinization. Trypsin converts G-34 to G-17. Conversion should be confirmed by rechromatography on the same column. A G-17 control tube should be exposed to the same conditions of trypsinization because most trypsin preparations contain some chymotrypsin contaminant which may destroy G-17. Trypsin has no effect on G-17.

It is our custom to prepare standards in moderately concentrated solutions in 0.05 M ammonium bicarbonate. These are prepared by dilution from more concentrated solutions of 50 to 100 nmol/ml in which the amount of peptide present has been confirmed by measurement of absorbance at 280 nm and application of the appropriate molar extinction coefficient (Table 17-2). For G-17-I the coefficient is 12,261. If the OD_{280} for G-17-I is multiplied by 81.6 the product equals concentration of gastrin in nmol/ml; when multiplied by 172 the product equals gastrin concentration in µg/ml. Other standards can be prepared to test cross-reactivity of gastrin fragments and related peptides

---

* National Institute for Biological Standards and Control, Holly Hill, Hempstead, London, NW3 6RB, England.

† Imperial Chemical Industries, Cheshire, England.

such as cholecystokinin in assays with different antibodies.

Incubation Conditions. Exact incubation conditions vary with the nature of the antibody and the range of gastrin concentrations in unknown samples to be measured. In order to measure concentrations of less than 1 fmol in the incubation mixture, it is necessary to work under equilibrium conditions with optimal dilutions of antiserum and low concentrations of labeled gastrin. This may require incubation for as long as 5 days at 4°C in a system containing 500 to 1,000 cpm/ml of labeled monoiodogastrin (0.2 – 0.4 fmol). An antibody of very high-binding energy ($K_o \geqq 10^{11}$ l/mol) also is required for such sensitivity. On the other hand, concentration of antibody and labeled gastrin may be increased and incubation time shortened to 24 to 48 hours for measurement of higher concentrations of gastrin. Even shorter incubation times (e.g., 2 hours) have been proposed. We have been unable to achieve equilibrium in this short a time and have been unable to obtain accurate measurements when more than one centrifugation had to be performed. Such a short incubation may be suitable for rapid rough estimates of gastrin activity in a few samples tested with several standards and sera with known gastrin concentration.

Sensitivity of the RIA system to such variables as temperature and salt concentration must be determined empirically. Each new antibody should be evaluated for effects of salt, protein, etc. With some antibodies there is evidence for dissociation of the antigen-antibody complex at higher temperatures, such as those which may be generated in a nonrefrigerated centrifuge after several spins. Exposure to ion exchange resin for prolonged periods also can cause dissociation. With some antibodies it is possible to premix antibody and labeled gastrin and add them together to diluted unknowns and standards. However, we have obtained evidence for some irreversible binding with several antisera treated in this way. Such binding results in standard inhibition curves which

differ, when they are pipetted immediately after label and antibody are mixed, from those prepared after a delay of an hour or more. The standard curve obtained with premixed antibody may be flatter and reveal incomplete inhibition when high concentrations of unlabeled gastrin are added to the tube. Unless these conditions are pretested it is safer to add labeled gastrin, unknown and antibody simultaneously or to add antibody to unknown followed by labeled gastrin.

Antibody can be prediluted at a convenient dilution (e.g., 1:1000 in normal saline) and stored at 4°C. Carrier serum or gamma globulin should be added to prevent adsorption of antibody to glass walls of the container, and usually a preservative such as 0.02 percent thiomersol is added to minimize bacterial overgrowth. Labeled gastrin can be stored in solution. We believe, but have not confirmed with formal tests, that stability is better when the solution is maintained at −40°C or lower as compared with the usual freezer temperature of −20°C.

Standard curves are prepared from standard gastrin solutions. Our own method is to dilute a 10 pmol/ml standard serially to produce solutions containing 1,000, 100, and 10 fmol/ml. Each of these solutions is pipetted in volumes of 200, 100, 50, and 20 μl and the volume in the tube is adjusted to 1 ml before addition of another 1 ml label and antibody. The 200 and 20 μl volumes provide 2 points of overlap to assess the accuracy of dilutions. The final concentration of gastrin in the standard curve thus ranges from 0.1 to 100 fmol/ml (0.21 to 210 pg/ml) as shown in Figure 17-2. There are of course many alternate methods for preparation of standard curves and the range covered depends on the sensitivity of the antibody used. It is our custom to prepare at least 2 standard curves made up with different standard solutions for each large assay. Each tube is pipetted in duplicate. Alternate tubes are pipetted as the first and last tubes in the assay and also are separated first and last as a control for shifts in binding during preparation of a large assay. The standard diluent used in our assays is composed of 0.02 M sodium barbital with 2.5 Gm albumin/l. Other buffers such as phosphate, phosphate-buffered saline, and borate probably are equally suitable.

Serum and unknown samples must be diluted so that they cause B/F values which lie on the sensitive part of the dose-response curve. With our antisera a final dilution of 1:10 to 1:20 in the assay is suitable for normal sera. The normal sera usually contain between 10 and 100 fmol gastrin/ml. Such dilutions are suitable for physiologic studies. When screening for presence of Z-E syndrome, a higher dilution may be more suitable. Serum samples with very high gastrin concentrations and extracts of gastrin-containing tissues often must be diluted over a wider range.

Separation Methods

A number of separation methods have been used successfully for gastrin RIA including double antibody, charcoal, ethanol precipitation, and immuno-absorption.[11,14,15] The method we use is the ion-exchange resin method described by Yalow and Berson.[12] Amberlite resin (IRP 58-M)* is prepared as a suspension of 100 Gm per l 0.02 m veronal buffer, pH 8.6. It is allowed to stand with mild agitation for an hour or two. The resin is allowed to settle for a few minutes and the supernatant fluid, containing fine particles, is poured off and replaced with fresh buffer. Tubes to be separated contain similar concentrations of protein that can be added immediately prior to separation if necessary. The resin is resuspended by swirling of the flask and is then pipetted quickly in volumes of 0.1 to 0.2 ml into a series of reaction tubes. The tubes are agitated quickly then centrifuged for a few minutes in a refrigerated centrifuge until well packed. The supernatant is decanted into a separate tube and both tubes, the resin tube containing free-labeled gastrin and the supernatant con-

---

* Rohm and Haas

taining antibody-bound labeled gastrin, are saved for counting. The separation procedure is performed quickly, since prolonged standing may result in some dissociation of antigen-antibody complexes.

A major source of interference in the resin separation system is heparin present in heparinized plasma. Very lightly heparinized plasma is suitable for assays (e.g., wetting the walls of a syringe with 1,000 units/ml heparin). Heavier heparinization causes interference with the resin separation by competition with gastrin for charged binding sites on the resin. This leads to high values for nonspecific binding in nonantibody-containing control tubes. If control tubes are not included for each patient, inadvertent overheparinization may lead to falsely low values for gastrin determinations.

Counting and Calculations

Counting and calculation do not differ in principle from other radioimmunoassays. We count each pair, bound and free, to a total of 10,000 counts and to express binding as B/F ratio after correction for nonspecfic binding. Usually a separate control tube is run for each new patient from whom serum specimens are obtained and the control value for each patient is used to correct his own B/F values.

Gastrin values are read from the standard curve. Presently there is some disagreement concerning the appropriate units for expression of results. The usual method is to express gastrin values as pg G-17 equivalents/ml and this is perfectly satisfactory for serum samples. An alternate method is to express results as fmol/ml, the rationale for use of molar units being that each serum contains gastrins of more than one molecular weight. The major drawback is that antibodies may not detect each molecular form on an equimolar basis. Sulfated and nonsulfated forms are frequently detected equally, although antibodies with specificities in this region have been reported.[40,41] Many antibodies have some degree of specificity for G-17 as opposed to G-34,[41] although some such as the one shown in Figure 17-2 and those reported by Yalow, appear to react with G-17 and G-34 on an equimolar basis. All antibodies we have tested have failed to react more than 70 percent as well with G-13 as with G-17, the average being around 50 percent. For some purposes molar concentrations are preferable. An example is measurement of gastrin components in a chromatographic eluate in which each component can be identified and its reactivity with the antiserum has been determined previously. Another example is in comparison of relative potency of different standards by preparation of multiple standard curves using pure solutions of known concentrations of pure peptides. However, for routine use the designation pg/ml (HG-17-I equivalents) is still acceptable.

Interpretation of Gastrin Results

Normal gastrin values, obtained in fasting individuals, vary between 20 and 180 pg/ml (HG-17-I equivalents) in our assay with our antibody 1,296 and with pure natural of synthetic human gastrin I as the standard. The median is approximately 50 pg/ml. Values from other laboratories are similar or slightly higher.

In most normal subjects the gastrin value increases 50 to 150 percent after a protein meal, with peak values seen within 15 to 30 minutes. Insulin hypoglycemia also increases serum gastrin values, the response being enhanced by continuous neutralization of the gastric contents. Acidification of the gastric contents to below pH 2.0 prevents gastrin release by all known stimulants. On the other hand alkalinization by itself does not appear to be a significant stimulant of gastrin release unless accompanied by some other chemical or mechanical or nervous stimulant.

Gastrin release by a protein meal is similar in patients with duodenal ulcer and in normals, but the ulcer patients tend to show moderately higher responses (Fig. 17-9). Resection of the gastric antrum removes a major source of gastrin. In man the duodenum also is a source of gastrin which can

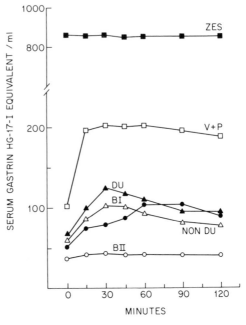

Fig. 17-9. Serum gastrin responses to a protein meal in normal subjects, patients with duodenal ulcer (CU), postoperative DU patients following vagotomy and pyloroplasty (V and P), partial gastrectomy with vagotomy and gastroduodenostomy (BI), or partial gastrectomy with vagotomy and gastrojejunostomy (BII), and patients with Zollinger-Ellison syndrome (ZE).

be released by a protein meal in patients with antral resection and gastroduodenal anastomosis but not in those with gastrojejunal anastomosis (Fig. 17-9).[42] Vagotomy in man increases basal and postprandial gastrin.[42] In patients with Z-E syndrome there is little response to a meal, but the basal gastrin values are elevated.[43]

Some conditions associated with slight to moderate increases in basal and postprandial serum gastrin include gastric ulcer,[44] gastric cancer,[45] and obstructed duodenal ulcer.[46] Moderate to marked elevations in gastrin are found in patients with achlorhydria (absence of gastric acid secretion) who have intact gastric antrum, including patients with pernicious anemia.[47,48] This increase in gastrin is due in part to hyperplasia of gastrin-producing cells and partly to lack of acid inhibition of gastrin release.

The major clinical use of the gastrin assay is for diagnosis of the ZES. This syndrome is caused by a gastrin-secreting tumor, usually originating in the pancreas.[49] Although gastrin was the second hormone discovered,[50] it is only rather recently[4] that a disease entity has been associated with it. Characteristic findings are severe peptic ulcer disease, often accompanied by diarrhea, marked hypersecretion of gastric acid, and hypergastrinemia (7 percent of cases have diarrhea, hypersecretion of gastric acid, hypergastrinemia but no peptic ulcer disease).[53] In many cases the serum gastrin exceeds 800 to 1,000 pg/ml. In the presence of acid hypersecretion such values are virtually diagnostic of ZES. In some patients with ZES the gastrin values fluctuate and may be as low as 200 to 400 pg/ml on some occasions. In these patients stimulation tests may add to the diagnostic confidence. Two methods for stimulating gastrin release from Z-E tumors are by intravenous infusion of calcium gluconate, 5 mg Ca/kg-hr, over a 3-hour period,[51] and by rapid intravenous infusion of secretin, 1 to 2 units/kg.[52] The former stimulant produces a gradual increase in gastrin values which usually reaches a peak after 3 to 4 hours, while the latter produces a rapid release of gastrin to peak values which often are achieved within 5 minutes. Most patients with ZES respond to calcium infusion with an increase in gastrin of more than 50 percent and more than 200 pg/ml. Approximately three-fourths of the patients appear to respond to secretin.

Future of Gastrin Radioimmunoassay

Because of the heterogeneity of gastrins in the circulation, antibodies probably will be developed which will permit identification of individual molecular species. One such antibody, with specificity for the N-terminal portion of G-17 has been described.[33] This antibody was used to identify a previously undetected gastrin fragment in the serum of patients with ZES.[33] When identification of various gastrin components in the serum is made easier by specific antibodies or easier

physical separation methods, it will be possible to explore the role of each component in the physiology of gastric secretion. It also may be possible to identify some forms of ZES in which relatively low concentrations of highly potent gastrins lead to gastric hypersecretion with relatively normal total serum gastrin concentrations.

References

1. Komarov, S. A.: Gastrin. Proc. Soc. Exp. Biol. Med., *38*:514, 1938.
2. Grossman, M. I., Robertson, C. R., and Ivy, A. C.: The proof of a hormonal mechanism for gastric secretion—the humoral transmission of the distension stimulus. Amer. J. Physiol., *153*:1, 1948.
3. Gregory, R. A., and Tracy, H. J.: The constitution and properties of two gastrins extracted from hog antral mucosa. Part I. The isolation of two gastrins from hog antral mucosa. Gut, 5:103, 1964.
4. Walsh, J. H.: Control of gastric secretion. *In* Sleisenger, M. H., and Fordtran, J. S.: Gastrointestinal Disease. chap. 12, pp. 144-162. Philadelphia, W. B. Saunders, 1973.
5. Zollinger, R. M., and Ellison, E. H.: Primary peptic ulcerations of the jejunum associated with islet cell tumors of the pancreas. Ann. Surg., *142*:709, 1955.
6. Grossman, M. I., Tracy, H. J., and Gregory, R. A.: Zollinger-Ellison syndrome in a Bantu woman, with isolation of a gastrin-like substance from the primary and secondary tumors. II. Extraction of gastrin-like activity from tumors. Gastroenterology, *41*:87, 1961.
7. Sircus, W.: Evidence for a gastric secretagogue in the circulation and gastric juice of patients with the Zollinger-Ellison syndrome. Lancet, 2:671, 1964.
8. McGuigan, J. E., and Trudeau, W. L.: Immunochemical measurement of elevated levels of gastrin in the serum of patients with pancreatic tumors of the Zollinger-Ellison variety. N. Eng. J. Med., *278*:1308, 1968.
9. Gregory, H., Hardy, P. M., Jones, D. S., *et al.*: The antral hormone gastrin. Structure of gastrin. Nature, *204*:931, 1964.
10. Morley, J. S.: Gastrin and related peptides. *In* Margoulies, M., and Greenwood, F. C.: Structure-Activity Relationships of Protein and Polypeptide Hormones. vol. 1, pp. 11-17. Amsterdam, Excerpta Medica, 1972.
11. McGuigan, J. E., and Trudeau, W. L.: Studies with antibodies to gastrin: radio-

immunoassay in human serum and physiological studies. Gastroenterology, *58*:139, 1970.

12. Yalow, R. S., and Berson, S. A.: Radioimmunoassay of gastrin. Gastroenterology, *58*:1, 1970.

13. Charters, A. C., Odell, W. D., Davidson, W. D., *et al.*: Development of a radioimmunoassay for gastrin. Arch. Surg., *99*: 361, 1969.

14. Hansky, J., and Cain, M. D.: Radioimmunoassay of gastrin in human serum. Lancet, *2*:1388, 1969.

15. Rehfeld, J. F., and Stadil, F.: Radioimmunoassay for gastrin employing immunosorbent. Scand. J. Clin. Lab. Invest., *31*: 459, 1973.

16. Ganguli, P. C., and Hunter, W. M.: Radioimmunoassay of gastrin in human plasma. J. Physiol., *220*:499, 1972.

17. Yalow, R. S., and Berson, S. A.: Size and charge distinctions between endogenous human plasma gastrin in peripheral blood and heptadecapeptide gastrins. Gastroenterology, *58*:609, 1970.

18. Yalow, R. S., and Berson, S. A.: And now, "big, big" gastrin. Biochem. Biophys. Res. Commun., *48*:391, 1972.

19. Yalow, R. S., and Wu, N.: Additional studies on the nature of big big gastrin. Gastroenterology, *65*:19, 1973.

20. Straus, E., and Yalow, R. S.: Studies on the distribution and degradation of heptadecapeptide, big, and big big gastrins. Gastroenterology, *66*:936, 1974.

21. Rehfeld, J. F.: Three components of gastrin in human serum: Gel filtration studies on the molecular size of immunoreactive serum gastrin. Biochem. Biophys. Acta, *285*:364, 1972.

22. Johnson, L. R., Stening, G. F., and Grossman, M. I.: The effect of sulfation on the gastrointestinal actions of caerulein. Gastroenterology, *58*:208, 1970.

23. Berson, S. A., and Yalow, R. S.: Nature of immunoreactive gastrin extracted from tissues of gastrointestinal tract. Gastroenterology, *60*:215, 1971.

24. Gregory, R. A., and Tracy, H. J.: The isolation of two "big gastrins" from Zollinger-Ellison tumor tissue. Lancet, *2*:797, 1972.

25. Walsh, J. H., Debas, H. T., and Grossman, M. I.: Pure human big gastrin: Immunochemical properties, half life and acid stimulating action in dogs. J. Clin. Invest., In press.

26. Rehfeld, J. F., and Stadil, F.: Gel filtration studies on immunoreactive gastrin in serum from Zollinger-Ellison patients. Gut, *14*: 369, 1973.

27. Debas, H. T., Walsh, J. H., and Grossman, M. I.: Pure natural "minigastrin": biological activity and half-life (abstr.). Gastroenterology, *66*:837, 1974.

28. Yalow, R. S., and Berson, S. A.: Further studies on the nature of immunoreactive gastrin in human plasma. Gastroenterology, *60*:203, 1971.

29. McGuigan, J. E.: Antibodies to the carboxyl-terminal tetrapeptide of gastrin. Gastroenterology, *53*:697, 1968.

30. McGuigan, J. E.: Antibodies to the carboxyl-terminal tetrapeptide amide of gastrin in guinea pigs. J. Lab. Clin. Med., *71*:964, 1967.

31. McGuigan, J. E.: Immunochemical studies with synthetic human gastrin. Gastroenterology, *54*:1005, 1968.

32. Rehfeld, J. F., Stadil, F., and Rubin, B.: Production and evaluation of antibodies for the radioimmunoassay of gastrin. Scand. J. Clin. Lab. Invest., *30*:221, 1972.

33. Dockray, G. J., and Walsh, J. H.: Identification of an N-terminal fragment of heptadecapeptide gastrin in the serum of patients with the Zollinger-Ellison syndrome (ZES) (abstr.). Gastroenterology, *66*:874, 1974.

34. Vaitukitis, J., Robbins, J. B., Nieschlag, E., and Ross, G. T.: A method for producing specific antisera with small doses of immunogen. J. Clin. Endocrin., *33*:988, 1971.

35. Jeffcoate, S. L.: Radioimmunoassay of gastrin: specificity of gastrin antisera. Scand. J. Gastroent., *4*:457, 1969.

36. Stremple, J. F., and Meade, R. C.: Production of antibodies to synthetic human gastrin I and radioimmunoassay of gastrin in serum of patients with the Zollinger-Ellison syndrome. Surgery, *64*:165, 1968.

37. McGuigan, J. E.: Progress report—On antibodies to gastrin: concerning their production, behavioural characteristics, and uses. Gut, *11*:363-367, 1970.

38. Gregory, R. A.: Fractionation on aminoethylcellulose. Chapter 7-1, Gastrin—Preparation, p. 1033. *In* Berson, S. A., and Yalow, R. S. (eds.): Methods in Investigative and Diagnostic Endocrinology: Part III. Peptide Hormones. Amsterdam, North Holland Publishing Co., 1973.

39. Stadil, F., and Rehfeld, J. F.: Preparation of ^{125}I-labelled synthetic human gastrin I for radioimmunoanalysis. Scand. J. Clin. Lab. Invest., *30*:361, 1972.

40. Hansky, J., Soveny, C., and Korman, M. G.: What is immunoreactive gastrin? Studies

with two antisera (abstr.). Gastroenterology, *64*:740, 1973.

41. Walsh, J. H., Trout, H. H. III, Debas, H. T., and Grossman, M. I.: Immunochemical and biological properties of gastrin obtained from different species and of different molecular species of gastrin. Submitted by invitation to Symposium on Recent Advances in Gastrointestinal Hormone Research (Rochester, New York, August 25-26, 1973, William Y. Chey, ed.).

42. Stern, D. H., and Walsh, J. H.: Gastrin release in postoperative ulcer patients: Evidence for release of duodenal gastrin. Gastroenterology, *64*:363, 1973.

43. Berson, S. A., and Yalow, R. S.: Progress in gastroenterology: Radioimmunoassay in gastroenterology. Gastroenterology, *62*: 1061, 1972.

44. Trudeau, W. L., and McGuigan, J. E.: Relations between serum gastrin levels and rates of gastrin hydrochloric acid secretion. N. Eng. J. Med., *284*:408, 1971.

45. McGuigan, J. E., and Trudeau, W. L.: Serum and tissue gastrin concentrations in patients with carcinoma of the stomach. Gastroenterology, *64*:22, 1973.

46. Feurle, G., Ketterer, H., Becker, H. D., *et al.*: Circadian serum gastrin concentrations in control persons and patients with ulcer disease. Scand. J. Gastroenterol., *7*:177, 1972.

47. McGuigan, J. E., and Trudeau, W. L.: Serum gastrin concentrations in pernicious anemia. N. Eng. J. Med., *282*:358, 1970.

48. Berson, S. A., Walsh, J. H., and Yalow, R. S.: Radioimmunoassay of gastrin in human plasma and regulation of gastrin secretion. Nobel Symposium XVI. Frontiers in Gastrointestinal Hormone Research. (pp. 57-66). Andersson, Almquist and Wiksell (eds.), Uppsala, Sweden.

49. Isenberg, J. I., Walsh, J. H., and Grossman, M. I.: Zollinger-Ellison syndrome. Gastroenterology, *65*:140, 1973.

50. Edkins, J. S.: Proc. Royal Soc., *76*:176, 1905.

51. Passaro, E., Basso, N., and Walsh, J. H.: Calcium challenge in the Zollinger-Ellison syndrome. Surgery, *72*:60, 1972.

52. Isenberg, J. I., Walsh, J. H., Passaro, E., *et al.*: Unusual effect of secretin on serum gastrin, serum calcium, and gastric acid secretion in a patient with suspected Zollinger-Ellison syndrome. Gastroenterology, *62*: 626, 1972.

53. Thompson, J. G., Reeder, D. D., and Bunchman, H.: Clinical role of serum gastrin measurements in the Zollinger-Ellison syndrome. Amer. J. Surg., *124*:250, 1972.

18 *Glucagon*

A. M. Lawrence, M.D.

INTRODUCTION

The fiftieth anniversary of the discovery of insulin was celebrated in 1971. Within 2 years of commercial insulin becoming available, the presence of glucagon was suspected but without the fanfare which accompanied the discovery of insulin. Intravenous injection of certain insulin preparations was noted to cause a transient hyperglycemia, the more remarkable when the hormone was injected directly into the portal vein.[1] This phenomenon was initially attributed to some toxic contaminant of insulin. A steadfast group of researchers managed ultimately, through cross-circulation experiments in dogs,[2] and by biochemical characterization and purification,[3,4] to isolate the material and to show its biologic effect. Because it caused release of hepatic glucose, it was called "glucagon" or mobilizer of glucose,[5] and was glycogenolytic, gluconeogenetic, and lipolytic. It stimulates insulin, catecholamine, and growth hormone release. It is available commercially as a porcine glucagon in 1 and 10 mg vials.* Its major therapeutic use is in the treatment of hypoglycemic reactions in insulin-dependent diabetics. Several monographs and reviews are available to those interested in probing this subject in greater depth.[6-9]

Glucagon is a 29-amino acid peptide which is soluble in both acid and alkaline pH. It is secreted from the alpha cell in the islet of Langerhans. Ultrastructural studies suggest that there may be actual membranous links between the glucagon-secreting alpha cell and its neighboring insulin-secreting beta cell. Autonomic innervation of the islet of Langerhans is now an accepted fact.[10] Variations in alpha- and beta-adrenergic reception at the cell membrane undoubtedly modulate secretory events from the alpha cell. Glucagon gains access to the circulation through the pancreaticoduodenal vein and then the portal vein. Lymphatic drainage of glucagon, by which this hormone can gain direct entry into the systemic circulation, probably exists but data is wanting.

As far as is known, the major physiologic role of glucagon is exerted in the liver. Attachment of radiolabeled glucagon to hepatocyte membranes can be demonstrated; that this attachment is specific is concluded from the finding that only added cold glucagon displaces radioactive glucagon from receptor sites on liver cells.[11] Other peptides with immunologic and some biologic similarities to glucagon do enter the circulation. At least 2 have been identified, both of intestinal tract origin, the so-called "entero-glucagons."[12]

There now exists a welter of research articles on glucagon levels in disturbed metabolic events or pathophysiologic states in man. Although the role of glucagon in mammalian physiology clearly gained a surer foothold in the 1960's, its true role in health and disease is still conjectural and subject to speculation. There exists no good animal model of glucagon deficiency analogous to

---

* Glucagon, Eli Lilly & Co.

the classical alloxan or streptozotocin-treated insulin-deficient diabetic animals.

Bioassays of glucagon using liver slices, homogenates or perfusions taught a great deal about the probable physiologic role of glucagon, but distinguishing pharmacologic events from physiologic has and continues to pose interpretive difficulties. Furthermore, innumerable studies in man have had to tally hormonal events on the periphery of the liver. Given the recognized importance of glucagon binding to liver cells for major biologic effects, this feature of glucagon measurement in man clearly introduces problems of analysis. Although the advent in the early 1960's of the very sensitive radioimmuoassay for glucagon, offered a means for enormous data collecting, that has not served as a panacea either. Despite extraordinary sensitivity, these assays are not entirely or strictly specific. Immunologically reactive prohormones and biologically inactive hormone fragments are measured with a given antiserum raised to a pure antigen, as are virtually all radioimmunoassays for peptide hormones. Equating immunologic with biologic activities is still an uncertainty. In the case of glucagon this is particularly true, since more than one molecular species of intestinal origin appear to cross-react with antisera raised to pancreatic glucagon.

This property of antisera should not daunt enthusiasm for the radioimmunoassay, however. Indeed, this feature of the radioimmunoassay helped lead to recognition of the heterogeneity of circulating peptides and to the discovery of precursor or prohormones. These reservations regarding appropriate interpretation of data bearing on glucagon's role in physiology and pathophysiology are largely introduced to caution those who read further, that much of what is now accepted regarding actions of this ubiquitous peptide requires some serious revision with time. A few antisera raised to porcine pancreatic glucagon appear minimally cross-reactive with glucagon-like material of intestinal tract origin, but the majority in use today undoubtedly measure more than one molecular species of glucagon with immunoreactivity.

GLUCAGON ASSAYS
Bioassays

Although the radioimmunoassay offers unparalleled sensitivity and specificity, the presence of cross-reactive peptides and biologically inactive fragments or precursors of the parent peptide make the availability of certain bioassays for glucagon of considerable importance. The greatest problem with such bioassays is relative lack of sensitivity. Most depend on measuring the effect of glucagon upon the handling of hepatic glucose; an occasional bioassay has determined glucagon's effect on lipolysis from chicken fat cells. These assays include study of the effect of intravenous injection of glucagon on blood sugar levels, the effect of glucagon added to liver slices or homogenates, or the effect of glucagon added to a hepatic perfusion system.

Glucagon injected intravenously causes a rise in blood sugar in all mammalian species tested. The cat, being unusually sensitive in this regard, has long been used to test purified insulin preparations for glucagon content after inactivation of the insulin activity.[13] The peak rise in blood sugar which occurs at 10 to 15 minutes is compared to the blood sugar change evoked with standard quantities of crystalline glucagon. In assay by this approach it is important to take cognizance of the fact that innumerable other nonglucagon materials may cause the blood sugar to rise.

Using liver slices and measuring generation of glucose, decrease in glycogen content or activation of phosphorylase, a tenfold increase in bioassay sensitivity can be achieved.[14] Limiting features of these approaches include spontaneous glycogenolysis from slices, lability of glycogenolysis to subtle changes in ionic strength and variability in the capacity of liver slices to inactivate glucagon. Avoidance of certain ions, calcium and magnesium in particular, the addition of insulin to the incubation medium to limit glycogenolysis, and other precautions reduce spontaneous variations in this system. Rabbit liver is preferable to rat liver for these studies. As little as 5 to 10 mμg/ml of glucagon per incubate tube can be measured with these approaches.

Using cat liver particulate fractions, Makman and Sutherland described a technique in which the generation of cyclic AMP was used to estimate the amount of glucagon present.[15] Initially this required a fairly elaborate assay system whereby cyclic AMP generation was deduced from measurement of active phosphorylase. In 1969 Cohen and Bitensky reported a direct measurement for cyclic AMP thereby greatly simplifying the Makman-Sutherland assay. The sensitivity of this assay is of the order of 2 mμg/ml per incubate tube.

Sokol and his associates extensively studied the isolated perfused liver of unfasted rats.[17] In their system measurement of phosphorylase activity, glycogenolysis, gluconeogenesis, or cyclic AMP generation can be studied. Although no more sensitive than the particulate fraction assay, their system does provide a physiologically attractive approach.

Today, however, groups interested in the assay of glucagon in animals and man, by and large lean on some form of radioimmunoassay involving antigen competition for binding sites on a glucagon antiserum. Recently there were attempts aimed at developing a radioligand assay in which radiolabeled glucagon binding to isolated liver cell membranes is quantitatively dissociated by addition of unlabeled hormone.[11] Sensitivity in the immunoassay is for quantities as low as 20 to 40 pg/ml plasma in some laboratories. The useful range in the radioligand assay has not been generally established.

Immunoassays

The first radioimmunoassay for glucagon was reported by Roger Unger in 1961,[18] two years after the now famous technique of radioimmunoassay was described for insulin by Rosalyn Yalow and Solomon Berson.[19] Because raising antibodies to glucagon is particularly difficult, no additional reports using the radioimmunoassay appeared until 1964-65. By then it was appreciated that in order to produce usable antisera against pancreatic glucagon it was necessary to immunize many animals and to repeat immunization schedules for 6 to 18 months or longer. Further, in order to develop usable glucagon antisera it is almost necessary to mix or couple glucagon to albumin, beeswax, and/or complete Freund's adjuvant, and to appreciate that glucagon antisera may have to be used at titers far below that which has worked in the analogous insulin and growth hormone assays.[20] Although many animals develop glucagon antibodies on repeated immunizations, there is a general belief that the guinea pig probably yields more sensitive antisera (i.e., dissociate radiolabeled glucagon faster in the presence of unlabeled hormone). In this assay, as in other types of radioimmunoassay, radioactive glucagon of high specific activity, labeled with either Iodine-131 or Iodine-125, is added to an incubation tube containing buffer, standard amounts of cold glucagon or unknown, and the mixture incubated an additional 24 hours at which time antibody-bound glucagon is separated from nonantibody-bound hormone (see p. 261). The greater the quantity of unlabeled glucagon in the system, the less radioactive glucagon is absorbed to the antiserum. Separation of antibody-bound from free radioactive hormone utilizes the techniques of paper chromatography, albumin-coated dextran (absorbs the free peptide), or precipitation of the glucagon bound to antiserum with a second antiserum directed against the gamma globulin of the animal species from which the glucagon antiserum was originally harvested (the double antibody method).[12] Most glucagon radioimmunoassay work must be conducted in the cold (e.g., at −4°C). Problems associated with the assay have been extensively reviewed by Heding and others.[12] For example, immunoassay of glucagon levels in man requires the addition of a protease inhibitor such as Trasylol*[21] or benzamidine†[22] in order to prevent rapid destruction of endogenous glucagon during handling and storage of serum samples, and of the labeled hormone during incubation in the assay. (See p. 261 for assay procedure used in our laboratory.)

The iodination of peptide hormones for these assays primarily utilizes the remarkably simple method described by Hunter and Greenwood.[23] Using I-131 or I-125 in the presence of the powerful oxidant, Chloramine-T, Tyrosine and Histidine residues are iodinated. The oxidation is brought to a quick halt (before injury to the parent peptide) by the addition of a strong reducing agent such as sodium metabisulfite. The resulting reaction mixture, consisting of labeled hormone, unreacted radioiodine, and damaged fragments—some iodinated, some not —is then subjected to one or more purification steps. Standard techniques utilize the addition of Dowex resin to the mixture. Unreacted radioiodine is adsorbed on the resin and after spinning this down, the supernatant is passed over a small cellulose or Sephadex column and a peak of pure radiolabeled hormone obtained. Hormones labeled to high-specific activity, 200 to 400 mc/mg, are recoverable in this manner.

Sensitivity of the radioimmunoassay requires careful tailoring in each laboratory to each peptide. Each radioimmunoassay is sensitive to temperature, time and pH. Many complete kits are now commercially available for a variety of radioreceptor assays.

There are other iodination modifications for ligand or receptor assay work that should be mentioned. Although radiolabeled products from the Hunter and Greenwood method have worked well in the radioimmunoassay, investigators working with cell and membrane receptors have found the standard chloramine-T oxidation too harsh. This appears to alter significantly the peptide hormone so that binding to receptor sites (e.g., to lymphocytes, peripheral or tissue cultured)

is lessened or even prevented. Accordingly, techniques are now being reported whereby monoiodinated hormone is prepared.[24] In essence this is achieved by adding chloramine-T in a stepwise manner, starting with an amount calculated not to exceed iodination of the hormone by more than 50 percent. After the addition of a one-tenth molar equivalent of the oxidant, the mixture is checked for percent TCA precipitable protein iodination and the further addition of chloramine-T stopped when the desired amount of protein iodination is achieved. An alternative modification is the addition of a large amount of hormone to the radioiodine and one-tenth molar equivalent of chloramine-T, and then the utilization of some method for separating clearly monoiodinated hormone from unlabeled hormone. These latter techniques lean on subtle characteristics of these preparations on ion-exchange columns and must be developed for each hormone. In the last analysis a radiolabel with fewer iodine molecules is obtained. This appears to provide a tracer label which is more readily bound by what are believed to be specific receptor sites on certain cell lines.

Some may find the relatively new iodination procedure of Thorell and Johansson of interest.[25] In this enzymatic procedure lactoperoxidase and hydrogen peroxide are used to oxidize, and the reaction is brought to a stop by the addition of sodium azide. Although receptor assayists believe the hydrogen peroxide procedure to be too harsh, excellent iodinations have been reported, particularly of hormones such as human prolactin, a peptide easily injured by the chloramine-T reaction.

PHYSIOLOGIC REGULATION OF GLUCAGON SECRETION

With the advent of the glucagon radioimmunoassay, progress in understanding the regulation of glucagon secretion has soared. Data has come from in vivo studies in man and animals and from the study of pancreatic slices and isolated islets of Langerhans.

---

* FBA Pharmaceuticals
† Eastman Chemical

Glucagon Release

Glucagon release (Table 18-1) appears to be normally stimulated by a threat of *impending glucopenia* or by frank *hypoglycemia.*[26-28] In dogs below 50 mg/100 ml glucagon is secreted, when intravenous glucose exceeds a blood sugar of 160 mg/100 ml glucagon secretion is suppressed. In man it is possible to show a rise in peripheral blood levels of glucagon with insulin-induced hypoglycemia. Extreme *restriction in carbohydrate* intake results in raised basal levels.[29] Physiologic kinds of *stress,* (e.g., infection, burns, trauma) which call upon rapid substrate mobilization, also seem to be associated with a significant rise in basal glucagon levels. In *starvation* this is most evident during the first week, a period of intense gluconeogenesis.[30,31] Glucagon's role in gluconeogenesis is of considerable importance during starvation, since it can increase hepatic uptake of the important gluconeogenetic amino acid, alanine. Heightened glucagon secretion and accelerated gluconeogenesis are viewed as important for the prevention of fasting hypoglycemia. *Exercise,* too, may act as a stimulus to glucagon release.[32,33] In Unger's study[32] a small rise was seen in 2 human subjects at the moment of collapse. In the study reported by Felig and his associates, 4 subjects showed a significant rise during moderately severe exercise.[33] With our antiserum we have been unable, however, to document a consistent rise in circulating glucagon in exercising normal volunteers.

Ingestion of a *protein meal* or the intravenous infusion of certain amino acids, particularly *arginine* and *alanine,* consistently provokes a significant glucagon rise with a modest hyperglycemia.[34,35] In dogs, and less certainly in man, the protein digestive enzyme *pancreozymin* also stimulates glucagon release.[36] Certain studies suggested that growth hormone and alpha-adrenergic blockers accentuate the alpha cell's response to provocative stimuli such as an arginine infusion.[37,38]

Table 18-1. Conditions Associated with Raised Levels or Enhanced Release of Pancreatic Glucagon.

Hypoglycemia
Carbohydrate restriction
Starvation

Protein meal
Pancreozymin
Glucogenic amino acids

Beta-adrenergic stimuli
Epinephrine
Exercise
Stress

Infection
Burns
Trauma

Recent work indicates that in infection there is a definite rise in the level of blood glucagon,[39] which, it is suggested, meets the body requirements for extra energy during infection, helping to mobilize glucose. This is beneficial to the host even though it is paid for at the cost of a transient diabetic state with negative nitrogen balance. It is possible that this has therapeutic implications, and measures to increase the availability of the various body fuels can be helpful to patients with generalized infection.

Glucagon Suppression

Suppression of pancreatic glucagon secretion is seen during postabsorptive or intravenously-induced hyperglycemia in man.[12,40,41] A *high carbohydrate* isocaloric diet also appears to lower basal levels. Raising circulating levels of *free fatty acids* in dogs is also associated with a decrease in blood glucagon concentration.[42] *Secretin* may also lower glucagon secretion in man, but additional studies are required to settle this point.[43] Beta-adrenergic blockade is associated with dampened glucagon secretion in several studies.[44]

Some of these observations confirm and extend the concept of glucagon as a hormone of fuel needs. Unger furthered this idea by drawing attention to what he believes is an even more important consideration, the "insulin glucagon ratio of biologic equality."[45]

This concept advances the belief that a high ratio promotes nutrient storage, a low ratio represents catabolism or nutrient mobilization. It can be argued that a significant change in the anabolic/catabolic milieu may occur without much absolute change in glucagon titers if the change was primarily an alteration in insulin levels. This question is raised because several recent articles have adopted this approach in order to demonstrate the significance of certain data. Whether or not this represents a meaningful approach to analysis of physiologic data, considering the alpha and beta cell as a single functional unit, nevertheless deserves serious thought.

CLINICAL USES AND PHARMACOLOGIC ACTIONS OF GLUCAGON

Treatment of Hypoglycemia

(Tables 18-2, 18-3, and 18-4)

Glucagon is a well-established remedy for the treatment of insulin-induced hypoglycemia and is uniquely safe and effective. The blood sugar begins to rise within 10 minutes after a subcutaneous injection and the majority of patients are awake and alert within 30 minutes of an administered dose of 1 to 2 mg. Its use in treatment of insulin reactions is associated with a notable drop in professed reactions by children in diabetic camp, pointing up a potential side benefit from its use for this particular problem. It may be of use in the treatment of certain forms of hypoglycemia associated with glycogen storage disease, but it is useless in treating alcohol hypoglycemia and should never be relied upon to treat sulfonylurea-induced hypoglycemia. Hypoglycemia associated with these drugs is often a complicated process and in some patients reflects a serious disturbance in hepatic gluconeogenesis.

Autonomic Nervous System

The administration of pharmacologic doses of glucagon, 0.5 mg or greater intravenously, results in release of norepinephrine and adrenal medullary epinephrine. This nor-

Table 18-2. Therapeutic Uses of Glucagon.

Hypoglycemia
Von Gierkes disease
*Cardiogenic shock
†Hypercalcemia
†Pancreatitis
†Obesity

* Investigational
† Of dubious clinical value.

Table 18-3. Diagnostic Uses of Glucagon.

Glycogen storage disease
Pheochromocytoma
Insulinoma
Growth hormone deficiency
*Medullary carcinoma of the thyroid

* Not established

Table 18-4. Pharmacologic Effects of Glucagon.

System	Effects
Autonomic Nervous System	Release of Catecholamines
Cardiovascular	+Inotropic; chronotropic; ↑ myocardial blood flow
Gastrointestinal	Decreases motility and pancreatic secretions; anorexia
Renal	Increases clearance, sodium, chloride, potassium, and phosphorus
Endocrines	Stimulates release of GH, calcitonin, insulin and catecholamines

mally causes some slight increase in heart rate but little if any alteration in blood pressure. Glucagon, 0.5 to 1 mg administered in similar fashion, however, provokes a hypertensive crisis in some patients with pheochromocytoma.[46,47] A few chromaffin tumors lacking a glucagon specific adenylcyclase do not respond to this signal.[48] Thus, glucagon has an established clinical usefulness as a provocative agent in some patients suspected of harboring a pheochromocytoma. When the diagnosis of pheochromocytoma is difficult, this test is of great diagnostic usefulness. The hazards of provoking severe hypertension must be thoroughly appreciated and suitable precautions, such as the immediate availability of alpha-adrenergic blockers, taken when administering this test. Although no cases have been described, it is likely that a similar hypertensive episode can be provoked in patients taking monoamineoxidase inhibitors. In such cases large amounts of catecholamines stored in neurosecretory vesicles are discharged by glucagon.

Cardiovascular-Renal System

Glucagon has a definite *positive inotropic* effect even in patients who are maximally digitalized. It resembles isoproterenol in most of its cardiovascular effects but does not carry the hazards of dysrhythmias so characteric of isoproterenol administration. Many have studied glucagon's effect on cardiac performance in patients with cardiac disease undergoing catheterization. *Positive inotropic* and *chronotropic* effects and *increased myocardial blood flow* are shown in most but not all patients.[49] Glucagon, accordingly was promoted for use in treatment of cardiogenic shock and severe congestive heart failure.[50] Using doses of 2 to 50 mg over minutes to hours, reports have noted impressive improvement in cardiac performance. Others have seen little or short-lived effects, and the place of glucagon in the therapeutic armamentarium for cardiogenic shock and intractable congestive heart failure is still investigative.[50]

Glucagon is mildly *naturetic*.[51,52,53] This diuretic feature is a transient phenomenon in congestive heart failure patients treated with glucagon. It probably is of very little if any therapeutic benefit under such circumstances.

Gastrointestinal Features

Glucagon almost consistently evokes nausea when doses above 0.5 mg are administered to humans. The severity of nausea and ensuing vomiting seem to be dose related and these side effects seriously limit its long-range therapeutic usefulness.[53] In patients with gastric balloons in place,

glucagon administration causes marked *reduction in gastric contractions* and motility.[54] Similar studies in animals show that this effect is generalized along the entire gastrointestinal tract.[55] In addition to reduction in tonus and motility, it also shows that glucagon administration sharply *decreases pancreatic exocrine secretion*.[56] Pancreozymin, as noted earlier, stimulates glucagon secretion. It has been speculated that the handling of the protein meal incorporates a built-in servomechanism whereby stimulation of glucagon release by pancreozymin acts subsequently to diminish pancreatic secretion after protein digestion has been completed.

Based in part on these effects of glucagon, it has been used in obesity and in acute pancreatitis.[57] Limited trials of glucagon and placebo demonstrated its anorectic quality; multiple daily injections negated its long-term application to the management of obesity, however. The treatment of pancreatitis with glucagon, although of theoretical value, has no adequate application to experimental or clinical material.

Endocrines

In addition to glucagon's effect on the release of stored catecholamines, glucagon in large doses also stimulates release of insulin, growth hormone, calcitonin, and perhaps other peptide hormones.[58-61]

When 1 mg of glucagon is administered subcutaneously or intramuscularly there is a 5 to 15 ng/ml rise in circulating growth hormone in most normal subjects. Pretreatment of a subject with a beta-adrenergic blocker such as a single 40 mg oral dose of propranolol beforehand enhances growth hormone secretory responsiveness and may result in a glucagon-mediated growth hormone rise not seen without propranolol pretreatment.[62] A similar enhancement of growth hormone secretion to provocative stimuli such as glucagon also can be achieved with estrogen pretreatment. The glucagon test, with or without additional priming, is used by some pediatric groups as an outpatient screening procedure for testing growth hormone reserve in children with retarded growth. Advocates of the glucagon-growth hormone testing feel it is simpler and safer as a screening test than other growth hormone provocative stimuli (e.g., arginine infusion, insulin-induced hypoglycemia, or exercise).

Glucagon stimulates insulin release as demonstrated by injecting subhyperglycemic doses of glucagon into animals or man, or by studying insulin release from pancreatic slices or isolated islets of Langerhans in the presence of added glucagon.[58,59] This phenomenon can be put to diagnostic advantage in patients suspected of having an insulin-producing islet cell neoplasm.[59] Whereas glycogenolysis and hyperglycemia overshadow any enhanced insulin secretion in normal subjects, hypoglycemia may be precipitated in the insulinoma patient following administration of the usual 1 mg intravenous bolus of glucagon. A remarkable rise in serum insulin is detectable by radioimmunoassay 5 to 10 minutes after the glucagon injection. A small blood sugar rise followed by a fall into a hypoglycemic range at 45 to 90 minutes is seen in responsive patients. Since insulinoma patients vary greatly in their response to provocative stimuli (e.g., intravenous tolbutamide, oral leucine, glucose or intravenous arginine), the glucagon test can be of diagnostic importance in a given case.

Glucagon infusions have been reported to lower the serum calcium, particularly in patients with hypercalcemia,[63] but there is some evidence that this is secondary to glucagon-stimulated calcitonin release.[61] These observations though interesting are of uncertain clinical usefulness. In acute pancreatitis, glucagon levels rise markedly and may contribute to the hypocalcemia associated with acute pancreatitis.[64]

Finally, glucagon may be diagnostically useful in patients with medullary carcinoma of the thyroid. This neoplasm is of thyroidal C-cell origin, a source of the calcium-lowering peptide calcitonin. This particular neo-plasm appears to be an inherited phenomenon, and immunoassayable calcitonin levels are high in patients with clinically evident disease but may be normal in equivocal or unsuspected cases. Glucagon probably does stimulate secretion of calcitonin. In limited trials the administration of glucagon provoked an abnormal or exaggerated calcitonin rise in patients suspected to be at risk for developing medullary carcinoma of the thyroid.[65] Some time is required to assess the overall usefulness of this diagnostic approach in patients with this syndrome.

Glycogen Storage Disease

Failure of a rise in blood sugar after the administration of a 1 mg intravenous bolus of glucagon suggests that there is some difficulty mobilizing hepatic glucose output, as is the case in certain forms of the glycogen storage diseases.[66] In the variety characterized by glucose 6-phosphatase deficiency, no glucagon associated rise is seen in either the fed or fasted state; whereas in Cori's disease characterized by a deficiency of debrancher enzyme, a normal response is seen after the child is fed. Chronic therapy of certain children with long-acting forms of glucagon has resulted in remarkable diminution of liver size and avoidance of recurring hypoglycemia.

GLUCAGON IN HEALTH AND DISEASE

There now seems little question that glucagon serves an important role in moment-to-moment regulation of blood sugar homeostasis. Whether its total lack results in impaired glucoregulation and recurring hypoglycemia is still debatable. Indeed in all of what follows it is imperative to realize that despite the burgeoning radioimmunoassay data glucagon's pathyphysiologic role in disease states must be regarded as quite speculative and requiring a firmer data base before full acceptance.[67] Nevertheless, several interesting observations have been made to suggest that this hormone is abnormally secreted in several clinical situations (Table 6).

Glucagon Deficiency States (Table 18-5)

Cases of glucagon deficiency have been suspected or documented several times in man. Prior to availability of the radioimmunoassay several infants were seen with *idiopathic hypoglycemia* and in whom light microscopy of the islets disclosed an apparent paucity of alpha cells.[68] Application of the radioimmunoassay to later cases did not support the suspicion of glucagon deficiency in similar patients. Bleicher, however, reported a case of a child characterized by fasting hypoglycemia in whom fasting glucagon levels were virtually unmeasurable and response to infused arginine negligible.[69] Foa and his associates have recently studied two similar cases in adults.[70]

A rare case of advanced *chronic pancreatitis* with fasting hypoglycemia may be encountered. Some studies have demonstrated poor glucagon response to arginine or to insulin-induced hypoglycemia.[69] By and large, however, glucagon levels in patients with pancreatitis are normal or abnormally high.[64]

Many suspect that a tonic relationship exists between function of the anterior pituitary and the islets of Langerhans. Thus, it is not surprising that in some instances of *hypopituitarism* there is a tendency to develop fasting hypoglycemia with associated low basal glucagon levels.[67] This finding has been challenged, however, and additional investigations will be required to settle this issue.

The relationship of glucagon secretion to certain *dyslipidemias* is suspected, but not thoroughly studied at this time. Glucagon possesses lipolytic properties generally masked in the whole organism by the simultaneous secretion of insulin which counteracts potently this effect on lipolysis. Glucagon enhances fatty acid uptake by the liver and may limit hepatic synthesis of very low-density lipoprotein thereby impeding reester-

Table 18-5. Clinical States of Glucagon Deficiency.

Idiopathic glucagon deficiency
Advanced chronic pancreatitis
Hypopituitarism
Beta-adrenergic blockade

ification and transport of free fatty acids from the liver as triglyceride. Reports of the beneficial effect of long-acting zinc glucagon on lowering of elevated triglycerides in certain hyperlipidemic states may be related to such an observation.[72] Based on these kinds of data it has been speculated that a relative glucagon deficiency may exist in the ketosis-resistant hypertriglyceridemic diabetic or in nondiabetic patients with hyperlipoproteinemic states. There is still insufficient data to support or disprove these speculations.

Glucagon deficiency in the extraordinarily brittle or extremely *insulin-sensitive diabetic* has long been suspected. Data to date have shown normal or elevated basal levels of glucagon. Lack of a glucagon rise in response to insulin-induced hypoglycemia has been noted,[73] however, and may explain brittleness as a result of inadequate and tardy hepatic glycogenolysis.

Many drugs almost certainly influence endocrine secretion. Although this area of clinical pharmacology requires intense study, little is yet known of drug influence on glucagon secretion. Long-term *sulfonylurea therapy* may marginally lower glucagon levels in diabetics. Since beta-adrenergic receptor activity clearly enhances alpha-cell secretory responsiveness and points up the importance of the autonomic nervous system to the proper functioning of the islets of Langerhans it is no surprise that *beta-adrenergic blockers* have been associated with increased insulin sensitivity and inadequate glucagon responses (e.g., to hypoglycemia).[44] A similar situation has been noted in a few patients with severe autonomic insufficiency.[75]

Glucagon Excess (Table 18-6)

Glucagon-secreting islet cell tumors, adenomas and adenocarcinomas are now incontrovertibly established as a cause of glucagon excess. Alpha-cytoid tumors were described before, but in 1964 Unger and his associates, utilizing their new radioimmunoassay, reported large quantities of glucagon in a hepatic metastasis of a bronchogenic carcinoma.[76] Whether this particular case represented the ability of hepatic metastases to take up peptides, insulin and glucagon reaching the liver, or indicated synthetic properties of the tumor was not settled conclusively. With expanding interest in the peptide synthetic potential of neoplasms in general, it is possible that in the future under suitable conditions many malignancies can synthesize glucagon; the clinical consequences of such a phenomenon requires careful scrutiny.

The first bona fide case of a glucagon-secreting islet cell tumor was reported by McGavran and his associates in 1966.[77] A 42-year-old woman who sought medical advice for an eczematoid dermopathy was found to have mild diabetes and an enlarged liver. An I-131 rose bengal liver scan demonstrated hepatic lesions, and arteriography of the celiac axis showed a mass in the tail of the pancreas. Glucagon levels in plasma and in pancreatic extracts of the tumor were enormously elevated. Electromicroscopy of the tumor showed cells containing morphologically distinct alpha-cell granules. A few

Table 18-6.
Clinical States of Glucagon Excess or Reduced Insulin/Glucagon Ratio.

Glucagon-secreting tumors

Acute pancreatitis
Stress (burns, trauma, etc.)
Cirrhosis; portal caval shunts

Ketoacidosis
Diabetes mellitus

Pheochromocytoma
Acromegaly
Hyperparathyroidism
Cushing's syndrome
Polyglandular syndrome

additional cases of glucagon-secreting islet cell tumors have since been reported.[78,79] In addition, hyperglucagonemia and diabetes mellitus have been reported in a few patients with islet microadenomatosis or alpha-cell hyperplasia.[80] In the latter case, a patient with chronic pancreatitis and hyperparathyroidism, resection of the pancreas for intractable pain led to diminution in insulin requirement.[81]

Several endocrine disorders such as *acromegaly, pheochromocytoma,* hyperparathyroidism, Cushing's disease and the *multiple endocrine tumor syndrome* have on occasion been associated with higher than normal glucagon levels.[67]

In *acromegaly* basal levels appear normal but glucagon secretion in response to an arginine infusion seems to be particularly exaggerated.[38] Many, but not all, patients with primary *hyperparathyroidism* have raised basal levels;[75,79] a serious study of this population's response to infused arginine has not been carried out, however. Patients with chronic calcific pancreatitis syndrome and primary hyperparathyroidism are more likely to demonstrate hyperglucagonemia because of associated alpha-cell hyperplasia in this syndrome.[80] Raised basal levels of glucagon have been noted sporadically in several patients with *pheochromocytoma*.[67] As in other endocrine disorders, these isolated observations have not been scrutinized in any systematic manner. Whether catecholamines directly stimulate glucagon secretion in man is a question still being debated.[82] Elevated glucagon in patients with pheochromocytoma can also reflect adjustments to impaired glucose tolerance in this syndrome. Epinephrine and norepinephrine interfere with insulin secretion[83] and the ensuing diabetic state is often the basis for extra glucagon secretion, perhaps analogous to that seen in caloric restriction, starvation and in diabetes mellitus.[30,40] No information is available to indicate whether elevated titers of glucagon fell after removal of the chromaffin tumors in the few patients found to have hyperglucagonemia preoperatively.

Others have demonstrated adrenal medullary tissue capable of synthesizing such biologically active peptides as calcitonin, so that there remains the possibility that the pheochromocytoma is the source of hyperglucagonemia in these cases. Glucocorticoid administration results in raised glucagon secretion, and elevated titers are seen in *Cushing's syndrome.*[84] Finally, raised glucagon levels in these seemingly diverse endocrinopathies may simply represent a feature characteristic of the *polyglandular syndrome.* Raised levels of islet hormones, insulin, glucagon, and gastrin in patients and families of patients with this syndrome have been reported.[85] In several, no clinically detectable endocrinopathy was present, in others a single problem such as primary hyperparathyroidism was found. These observations led to speculation that hyperglucagonemia frequently represents an expression of polyadenomatosis. Further speculation in this area recently dealt with the suggestion that all peptide-secreting endocrine cells are of neuroectodermal or neural crest origin, thereby offering a format for explaining a bewildering nexus of associations seen in such endocrine disorders as the MEA (multiple endocrine adenoma) syndrome and the syndrome of ectopic hormone secretion by nonendocrine malignancies.[86,87] Elevated glucagon levels have also been reported in *cirrhosis* and in patients with *portal caval* shunts; this may simply reflect less than normal hepatic extraction in the former situation and direct access of the hormone to the peripheral circulation in the latter case.

GLUCAGON AND DIABETES MELLITUS

Since we are still faced with uncertainties concerning the actual pathogenesis of diabetes in man, it is only natural that any abnormality of alpha-cell function in diabetes will be quickly seized as a potential explanation in these patients. Whether elevated glucagon levels causally contribute to the development of diabetes mellitus or strongly influence metabolic derangements in this disease is another existing controversy. Nevertheless, observations have been made which can incriminate glucagon in diabetes mellitus. Dr. Roger Unger and his associates in Dallas pioneered glucagon research in this area almost from the time they introduced the radioimmunoassay for glucagon in the early 1960's. This group in particular has been extraordinarily interested in the issue of glucagon in diabetes mellitus.[89]

Immunoreactive glucagon levels are markedly elevated in all patients with ketoacidosis.[90] As therapy corrects the gross metabolic disturbances, glucagon levels decline but often remain elevated above normal basal levels. Increasingly it is shown that stress, and in particular stress which theoretically calls for rapid mobilization of endogenous fuels, is associated with remarkable elevation in circulating glucagon levels. Indeed it has been proposed that the insulin-resistance and impaired glucose tolerance seen in such patients is related to excessive glucagon secretion; often there is impaired insulin secretion in these situations as well. To date it has been shown that *hyperglucagonemia,* insulin-resistance, and impaired glucose tolerance are characteristically *seen with severe burns, blunt trauma,*[91,92] *violent exercise,*[32] *pyogenic infection,*[93] and in *psychic stress* (in animals).[93] Studies have suggested, as indicated earlier, that epinephrine may stimulate glucagon release,[82] but confirmation is needed. The point that needs to be settled is whether a general autonomic discharge causes hyperglucagonemia in these stressful circumstances. Until this issue is more adequately studied and defined it is possible that ketoacidosis also reflects another in the list of "stress conditions" associated with hyperglucagonemia in man and animals. The hypothalamo-pituitary-adrenal axis response to stress may also play a role. Glucagon secretion is enhanced in Cushing's syndrome and by the administration of glucocorticoids. Cortisol secreted in response to stress may be partially responsible for the elevated glucagon titers in many of these situations.

Stress hyperglucagonemia notwithstanding, other peculiarities of glucagon secretion may be seen in diabetics. Many, but not all, have truly elevated basal levels even when diabetic control appears adequate.[89]

Some juvenile diabetic patients, particularly those prone to rapid and recurring ketosis, demonstrate continuously elevated basal glucagon levels and markedly exaggerated glucagon response to arginine infusion. Another unusual feature is that hyperglycemic suppression of peripheral glucagon levels is often absent in diabetics.[40,41] Normal subjects show a significant suppression of basal levels following intravenous glucose. Diabetics of all kinds generally fail to suppress,[12,41] and in many a definite early rise is seen during postabsorptive hyperglycemia. Unger proposed the islet of Langerhans as a functional unit or organ that has even greater significance as the molar ratio of insulin to glucagon. He believes that this ratio best reflects the net effect of these 2 potent and opposing peptides on glucose handling by the liver. Despite basal glucagon levels in the normal range, most if not all diabetics show a lower than normal I/G ratio. Such a situation favors catabolism and leads to accelerated glycogenolysis, gluconeogenesis from protein and fat, and lipolysis, phenomena characteristic of the diabetic state. Some argue that relative or absolute glucagon excess in diabetics more accurately reflects intracellular difficulty in metabolism of glucose secondary to insulin deficiency with elevated glucagon levels akin to what obtains in starvation.[95] Indeed, the administration of insulin to animals with experimental diabetes mellitus results in correction of their hyperglucagonemia;[96] infusions of insulin for up to 72 hours in human diabetics failed to alter raised basal glucagon levels nor did it lead to hyperglycemic suppression. Arguably, 72 hours may be insufficient for restoration of normal alpha-cell metabolism after years of relative insulin lack. Extension of such studies in time should help clarify whether abnormalities of glucagon secretion in diabetics are causal or secondary to the diabetic state. A final feature of insulin-dependent diabetics is their apparent inability to generate a glucagon rise in response to insulin-induced hypoglycemia.[73] In diabetes with its attendant and complex metabolic alterations, it may be that the alpha cell is relatively insensitive to major changes in circulating glucose levels.

THE ENTEROINSULAR AXIS

No chapter on glucagon can escape mention of the "other glucagon," and the "enteroinsular axis."[97,98] In 1943 Sutherland and DeDuve noted that extracts of gastric mucosa stimulated a rise in blood sugar;[99] subsequent studies showed that this was secondary to hepatic glucose output and that the mode of action of this material was in essence identical to that of pancreatic glucagon.

In the late 1960's several workers demonstrated that oral glucose provoked a greater insulin rise than intravenous glucose despite comparable blood sugar levels, thus suggesting that a material of enteric origin might be involved.[100] Today it is a reasonably accepted conclusion that secretin, gastrin, pancreozymin, and as yet unidentified peptides of enteric origin stimualte insulin release in a variety of in vitro and in vivo situations. In addition there is peptide material of enteric origin that is bound by many antisera raised to pancreatic glucagon.[97,98,101] These enteroglucagons are yet to be purified; preliminary studies indicate that although they may share certain biologic activities of pancreatic glucagon, they are far less potent. Despite uncertainties as to the exact role of these peptides in priming early insulin release, extensive investigation is ongoing in this area.

Potential clinical significance of the enteroinsular axis has surfaced in several areas (Table 18-7). An early enteric signal to insulin

Table 18-7. Possible Clinical Role of Enteroglucagon.

Promotes early insulin release
Cause of reactive hypoglycemia
Cause of postgastrectomy diabetes mellitus

release explains the remarkably flat glucose tolerance curves of strictly normal subjects. A striking rise in enteroglucagon in patients demonstrating profound reactive hypoglycemia has been reported, suggesting that either excessive immunoreactive glucagon-mediated insulin release or binding of enteric glucagon to liver cells was responsible. In the latter case, binding to receptor sites might prevent pancreatic glucagon from exerting its normal biologic effect on hepatic glycogenolysis. Impaired glucose tolerance or a pseudodiabetes mellitus develops after gastric operations such as gastrectomy or pyloroplasty.[103] Enteric glucagon rises dramatically in these patients when they are subjected to an oral glucose challenge, and this may be responsible for the disordered carbohydrate metabolism observed. Finally, there is the possibility that some deficiency in this enteric signal to early insulin release plays a role in the development of diabetes mellitus a possibility that is being pursued in several laboratories.[105]

A remarkable case of an "enteroglucagon"-secreting renal carcinoma was recently described.[104] A 44-year-old woman presented with edema, mild diabetes mellitus, skin rash, anemia, and severe constipation. Villous hypertrophy of the small bowel with coarse dilated mucosal folds and extraordinarily slow intestinal transit time was shown. Steatorrhea was present as well as mild diabetes. After resection of the tumor all of these abnormalities disappeared. Immunoassay of tumor extracts revealed poor cross-reactivity with antisera more specific for pancreatic glucagon but close cross-reactivity with glucagon antisera known to react well with enteroglucagon fractions.

Clinical Indications for Ordering Blood Glucagon Levels. The radioassay era has clearly revolutionized scientific and clinical data collection and correlative analysis. Radioreceptor assays of various kinds are here to stay in clinical chemistry. In the field of endocrinology these radioreceptor assays already have their clinical application in which insulin, growth hormone, LH, FSH, TSH, and renin are involved. Parathyroid

Table 18-8. Some Clinical Indications for Determining Blood Glucagon.

Idiopathic hypoglycemia in which inadequate glucagon secretion may be responsible

Drug-associated hypoglycemias (e.g., beta-blockers and other drugs, as yet unrecognized, which may prevent adequate glucagon secretion)

Hyperglycemic syndromes in which diabetes mellitus is not believed to be the cause (e.g., suspicion of alpha-cell hyperplasia, glucagonoma, glucagon-secreting islet cell carcinoma, or ectopic production of glucagon from non-islet malignancies)

Ketotic syndromes (other than starvation and diabetes out of control) in which excess glucagon may be responsible

Potential value for screening for prediabetes either by demonstrating raised basal levels and/or demonstrating inadequate suppression of glucagon levels associated with hyperglycemia from intravenous glucose administration

---

hormone, proinsulin, glucagon, gastrin, calcitonin, and secretin determinations are still largely research measurements, but in time the techniques of measurement of these latter hormones may be sufficiently standard that routine clinical application can be carried out.

A variety of clinical circumstances is listed (Table 18-8) wherein the measurement of glucagon could contribute to a diagnostic formulation, and thereby assist a directed therapeutic disposition. At this time, however, glucagon measurements are performed almost solely for clinical investigative purposes, the single exception being measurements of serum from patients with suspect or recognized islet cell adenomas or carcinomas.

NONEQUILIBRIUM DOUBLE ANTIBODY ASSAY FOR SERUM GLUCAGON

Reagents and Materials (Glucagon I-125)

Order from Cambridge Nuclear, 575 Middlesex Turnpike, Bellerica, Mass. 08121, received monthly immediately after production. Keep material frozen until use, then divide into 50 λ (lambda) aliquots. Store frozen. For minimal interassay variance, use freshly provided glucagon I-125 within one week. (Mono-iodinated glucagon not yet commercially available, does not deteriorate as quickly as high-specific activity I-125 glucagon prepared by the Hunter and Greenwood iodination procedure.)

Glucagon Standards

Obtain purified insulin-free porcine glucagon. Prepare stock solution by dissolving glucagon in borate buffer pH 9.6 at a concentration of 1 mg/ml. Prepare further dilutions in veronal albumin buffer, pH 8.6 to a concentration of 1 μg/ml. Store 0.5 ml aliquots frozen in *glass* dram vials with tight-fitting plastic snap-top caps. On day of assay thoroughly thaw and completely mix (vortex) glucagon aliquot (1 μg/ml). Prepare standards in 0.1% gelatin buffer. A useful and simple procedure is to add 10 λ to stock (10,000 pg) to 4 ml of gelatin buffer (2,500 pg/ml) and by serial double diluting prepare 6 standard solutions, ranging from 1,250 pg/ml through 39 pg/ml.

Veronal Buffer (also called barbital buffer) 0.075 M, prepared in batches of 19 l: 292.6 Gm sodium barbital plus 52.44 Gm barbital. Dissolve barbital first by heating in 4 l distilled water until totally dissolved. Add sodium barbital. Dissolve and bring to 19 l volume with distilled water.

Gelatin Buffer 0.1%: Dissolve 400 mg gelatin in 300 ml warmed veronal. Cool. Add 25 ml 0.2 M EDTA, 16 ml 25% human albumin. Bring to 400 ml with veronal.

Veronal Albumin Buffer (contains 2.5 mg human albumin/ml): Prepare by adding 10 ml of 25% human albumin to 1 l veronal buffer.

Glucagon Assay Buffer: 50 ml 0.2 M EDTA, 32 ml 25% human albumin, veronal buffer enough to make 800 ml.

Antibody Buffer: Glucagon assay buffer plus 0.07% normal guinea pig serum (as carrier protein).

Trasylol (Aprotinin): 10,000 KIU (Kallikrein Inactivator Units) distributed by FBA Pharmaceuticals, Division of Baychem Corp., 425 Park Avenue, New York, N.Y. 10022.

Test Tubes: 100 x 10 mm, No. 9446, Arthur Thomas Co., Philadelphia, Pa.

Automatic Gamma Counter

Glucagon Antiserum: Guinea pig glucagon antiserum produced in male guinea pigs by the method of Goldfine.[106] Determine ability of undiluted glucagon antiserum to completely bind tracer quantity of I-125 glucagon (approximately 7,000 counts per minute, 10-20 pg). Dilute such antiserum serially from 1:100 to 1:3000 (initial dilution). Choose dilution in which approximately 30 to 40 percent of radiolabeled glucagon is bound. Set up a standard curve and judge whether sensitivity is adequate for radioimmunoassay. Note 2 to 5 percent dissociation of radioactivity from the glucagon antiserum with addition of 20 to 40 pg/ml.

It is sometimes possible to pool antiserum because it is important to accumulate a sufficient amount to last for research and applied clinical service determinations for many years. In the glucagon immunoassay particularly, different antisera yield significantly different absolute measurements. It is important to start with sufficient antiserum for long-range studies. Utilizing a different antiserum from month to month makes it impossible to compare measurements from normal and diseased subjects.

Second Antibody: Raise in rabbits by immunizing to guinea pig gamma globulin; or purchase anti-guinea-pig-serum rabbit, for radioimmunoassay, 5 ml/vial from Wellcome Research Laboratories, Beckenham, England. Generally used as 1:6 to 1:10 dilution. Determine optimal concentration which completely precipitates I-125 glucagon-glucagon antiserum complex used in assay. Store frozen undiluted. Thaw on day of assay. Dilute appropriate aliquot for assay run in glucagon assay buffer.

Assay Procedure

(Glucagon radioimmunoassay is generally sensitive to temperature and unless determined otherwise carry out all work, after addition of the glucagon antiserum, in a coldroom or in an ice bath.)

Add to test tubes in the following order:

1. 200 λ standards or unknown plasma.*
2. 100 λ glucagon antibody at proper dilution to give 30 to 40 percent initial binding. Prepare antibody dilution in glucagon assay buffer containing 0.07 percent normal guinea pig serum as carrier.

3. Mix tubes on vortex; incubate for 2 to 3 nights at 4° C.

4. Add in coldroom or at ambient temperature keeping sample trays in ice bath:
   200 λ Trasylol (2,000 KIU)
   200 λ glucagon I-125 (6,500-7,500 cpm/200 λ)
   200 λ rabbit or goat antibody to guinea pig gamma globulin at proper dilution (usually 1-6 to 1-10)

5. Mix on vortex.

6. Incubate at 4° C overnight, spin, carefully decant, carefully touch neck of tube to absorbent paper, count precipitate in gamma counter, 10 min per tube.

7. Prepare standard curve and determine unknowns.

---

* All blood drawn for glucagon immunoassay must be drawn into Trasylol, 500 KIU/10 ml. Keep samples refrigerated and spin in a refrigerated centrifuge, remove serum or plasma and store frozen until assay.

References

1. Collip, J. B.: Delayed manifestation of the physiological effects of insulin following administration of certain pancreatic extracts. Amer. J. Physiol., *63*:391, 1923.

2. Foa, P. P., Weinstein, H. R., and Smith, J. A.: Secretion of insulin and of a hyperglycemic substance studied by means of pancreatic femoral cross-circulation experiments. Amer. J. Physiol., *157*:197, 1949.

3. Staub, A., Sinn, L., and Behrens, O. K.: Purification and crystallization of glucagon. J. Biol. Chem., *214*:619, 1955.

4. Bromer, W. W., Sinn, L. G., Staub, A., and Behrens, O. K.: The amino acid sequence of glucagon. J. Amer. Chem. Soc., *78*:3858, 1966.

5. Murlin, J. R., Clough, H. D., Gibbs, C. V. F., and Stokes, A. M.: Aqueous extracts of the pancreas. I. Influence on the carbohydrate metabolism of depancreatized animals. J. Biol. Chem., *56*:253, 1923.

6. Foa, P. P., and Galansino, G.: Glucagon, chemistry, and function in health and disease. Springfield, (Ill.), Charles C Thomas, 1962.

7. Lawrence, A. M.: Glucagon. Ann. Rev. Med., *20*:207, 1969.

8. Lefebvre, P. J., and Unger, R. H.: Glucagon, Molecular Physiology, Clinical and Therapeutic Implications. Oxford, Pergamon Press, 1972.

9. Foa, P. P.: The secretion of glucagon. *In* Freinkel, N., and Steiner, P. (eds.): The Endocrine Pancreas. Handbook of Physiology. Williams & Wilkins, Baltimore, 1972.

10. Munger, B. L.: The histology, cytochemistry and ultrastructure of pancreatic islet A-cells. *In* Lefebvre, P., and Unger, R. (eds.): Glucagon. pp. 7-25. Oxford, Pergamon Press, 1972.

11. Rodbell, M.: Regulation of glucagon at its receptors. *In* Lefebvre, P., and Unger, R. H. (eds.): Glucagon. pp. 61-75. Oxford, Pergamon Press, 1972.

12. Heding, L. G.: Radioimmunological determination of pancreatic and gut glucagon in plasma. Diabetologia, *7*:10, 1971.

13. Staub, A., and Behrens, O. K.: The glucagon content of crystalline insulin preparation. J. Clin. Invest., *33*:1629, 1954.

14. Vuylsteke, C. A., and DeDuve, C.: The assay of glucagon on isolated liver slices. Arch. Int. Pharmacodyn Ther., *111*:437, 1957.

15. Makman, M. H., and Sutherland, E. W., Jr.: Use of liver adenylcyclase for assay of glucagon in human gastrointestinal tract and pancreas. Endocrinology, *75*:127, 1964.

16. Cohen, K. L., and Bitensky, M. W.: Inhibitory effects of alloxan on mammalian adenylcyclase. J. Pharmacol. Exp. Ther., *169*:80, 1969.

17. Sokal, J. E.: Bioassay of glucagon using the isolated perfused rat liver. Endocrinology, *87*:1338, 1970.

18. Unger, R. H., Eisentraut, A. M., McCall, M. S., and Madison, L. L.: Glucagon antibodies and an immunoassay for glucagon. J. Clin. Invest., *40*:1280, 1961.

19. Yalow, R. S., and Berson, S. A.: Immunoassay of endogenous plasma insulin in man. J. Clin. Invest., *39*:1157, 1960.

20. Heding, L.: Immunologic properties of pancreatic glucagon: Antigenicity and antibody characteristics. *In* Lefebvre, P. J., and Unger, R. H. (eds.): Glucagon. Oxford, Pergamon Press, 1972.

21. Eisentraut, A. M., Whissen, N., and Unger, R. H.: Incubation damage in the radioimmunoassay for human plasma glucagon and its prevention with "Trasylol." Amer. J. Med. Sci., *255*:137, 1968.

22. Ensinck, J. W., Shepard, C., Dudl, R. J., and Williams, R. H.: Use of benzamidine

as a proteolytic inhibitor in the radioimmunoassay of glucagon in plasma. J. Clin. Endocr., *35*:463, 1972.

23. Hunter, W. M., and Greenwood, F. C.: A radio-immunoelectrophoretic assay for human growth hormone. Biochem. J., *91*: 43, 1964.

24. Freychet, P., Roth, J., and Neville, D. M., Jr.: Monoiodoinsulin: Demonstration of its biological activity and binding to fat cells and liver membranes. Biochem. Biophys. Res. Commun., *43*:400, 1971.

25. Thorell, J. I., and Johansson, B. G.: Enzymatic iodination of polypeptides with 125-I to high specific activity. Biochim. Biophys. Acta, *251*:363, 1971.

26. Unger, R. H., and Lefebvre, P. J.: Glucagon physiology. *In* Glucagon. Oxford, Pergamon Press, 1972.

27. Ohneda, A., Aguilar-Parada, E., Eisentraut, A. M., and Unger, R. H.: Control of pancreatic glucagon secretion by glucose. Diabetes, *18*:1, 1969.

28. Persson, I., Gyntelberg, F., Heding, L., and Boss-Nielsen, J.: Pancreatic-glucagon-like immunoreactivity after intravenous insulin in normal and chronic pancreatitis patients. Acta Endocrinol., *67*:401, 1971.

29. Muller, W. A., Faloona, G. R., and Unger, R. H.: The influence of the antecedent diet upon glucagon and insulin secretion. N. Eng. J. Med., *285*:1450, 1971.

30. Aguilar-Parada, E., Eisentraut, A. M., and Unger, R. H.: Effects of starvation on plasma pancreatic glucagon in normal man. Diabetes, *18*:717, 1969.

31. Marliss, E. B., Aoki, T. T., Unger, R. H., *et al.*: Glucagon levels and metabolic effects in fasting man. J. Clin. Invest., *49*:2256, 1970.

32. Boettger, I., Schlein, E. M., Faloona, G. R., Knochel, J. P., and Unger, R. H.: The effect of exercise on glucagon secretion. J. Clin. Endocrin., *35*:117, 1972.

33. Felig, P., Wahren, J., Hendler, R., and Ahborg, G.: Plasma glucagon levels in exercising man. N. Eng. J. Med., *287*: 184, 1972.

34. Aguilar-Parada, G., Eisentraut, A. M., and Unger, R. H.: Pancreatic glucagon secretion in normal and diabetic subjects. Amer. J. Med. Sci., *257*:415, 1969.

35. Marreiro Rocha, D., Faloona, G. R., and Unger, R. H.: Glucagon-stimulating activity of 20 amino acids in dogs. J. Clin. Invest., *51*:2346, 1972.

36. Unger, R. H., Ketterer, H., Dupre, J., and Eisentraut, A. M.: The effects of secretin, pancreozymin, and gastrin on insulin and glucagon secretion in anesthetized dogs. J. Clin. Invest., *46*:630, 1967.

37. Eaton, R. P., Conway, M., and Duckmann, M.: Role of alpha-adrenergic blockade on alanine induced hyperglucagonemia. Metabolism, *21*:371, 1972.

38. Goldfine, I. D., Kirsteins, K., and Lawrence, A. M.: Excessive glucagon response to arginine in active acromegaly. Horm. Metab. Res., *4*:97, 1972.

39. Beisel, Wm. R.: A role for glucagon during infection (Editorial). N. Eng. J. Med., *288*:734, 1973.

40. Unger, R. H., Aguilar-Parada, E., Muller, W. A., and Eisentraut, A. M.: Studies of pancreatic alpha-cell function in normal and diabetic subjects. J. Clin. Invest., *49*: 837, 1970.

41. Muller, W. A., Faloona, G. R., Aguilar-Parada, E., and Unger, R. H.: Abnormal alpha-cell function in diabetes mellitus. Response to carbohydrate and protein ingestion. N. Eng. J. Med., *283*:109, 1970.

42. Madison, L. L., Seyffert, W. A., Unger, R. H., and Barker, B.: Effect of plasma free fatty acids on plasma glucagon and serum insulin concentrations. Metabolism, *17*: 301, 1968.

43. Santensanio, F., Faloona, G. R., and Unger, R. H.: Suppressive effect of secretin upon pancreatic alpha cell function. J. Clin. Invest., *51*:1743, 1972.

44. Lawrence, A. M., Hagen, T. C., and Kirsteins, L.: Propranolol hyperglycemia and impaired glucagon secretion. Clin. Res., *20*:770, 1972.

45. Unger, R. H.: The organ of Langerhans in new perspective. Amer. J. Med. Sci., *260*:79, 1970.

46. Lawrence, A. M.: Glucagon provocative test for pheochromocytoma. Ann. Int. Med., *66*:1091, 1967.

47. Lefebvre, P. J., Cession-Fossion, A. M., Luyckx, A. S., Lecomte, J. L., and Cauwenberge, H. S., Van: Interrelationships glucagon-adrenergic system in experimental and clinical conditions. Arch. Int. Pharmacodyn. Ther., *172*:393, 1968.

48. Dexter, R. N., and Allen, D. O.: A glucagon-sensitive adenyl cyclase system in pheochromocytoma. Clin. Res., *18*:601, 1970.

49. Goldschlager, N., Robin, E., Cowan, C. M., Leb, G., and Bing, R. J.: The effect of glucagon on the coronary circulation in man. Circulation, *40*:829, 1969.

50. Parmley, W. W., and Sonnenblick, E. H.: Glucagon: A new agent in cardiac therapy. Amer. J. Cardiol., *27*:298, 1971.

51. Simanis, J., and Goldberg, L. I.: The effects of glucagon on sodium, potassium, and urine excretion in patients in congestive heart failure. Amer. Heart J., *81*:202, 1971.

52. Pullman, T. N., Lavender, A. R., and Aho, I.: Direct effects of glucagon on renal hemodynamics and excretion of inorganic ions. Metabolism, *16*:358, 1967.

53. Galloway, J. A.: The pharmacology and clinical use of glucagon. *In* Unger, R. H., and Lefebvre, P. J. (eds.): Glucagon. p. 299. Oxford, Pergamon Press, 1972.

54. Stunkard, A. J., Van Itallie, T. B., and Reis, B. B.: The mechanism of satiety: Effect of a glucagon on gastric hunger contractions in man. Proc. Soc. Exp. Biol. Med., *89*:258, 1955.

55. Necheles, H., Sporn, J., and Walker, L.: Effect of glucagon on gastrointestinal mobility. Amer. J. Gastroenterol., *45*:34, 1966.

56. Dyck, W. P., Texter, E. C., Jr., Lasater, J. M., and Hightower, N. C., Jr.: Influence of glucagon on pancreatic exocrine secretion in man. Gastroenterology, *58*:532, 1970.

57. Clayton, G. W., and Librick, L.: Therapy of exogenous obesity in childhood and adolescence. Pediatr. Clin. N. Amer., *10*:99, 1963.

58. Samols, E., Marri, G., and Marks, V.: Promotion of insulin secretion by glucagon. Lancet, *2*:415, 1965.

59. Marks, V., and Samols, E.: Glucagon test for insulinoma: A chemical study in 25 cases. J. Clin. Pathol., *21*:346, 1968.

60. Cain, J. P., Williams, G. H., and Dluhy, R. G.: Glucagon stimulation of human growth hormone. J. Clin. Endocrinol., *31*:222, 1970.

61. Avioli, L. V., Birge, S. J., Scott, S., and Shieber, W.: Role of the thyroid gland during glucagon induced hypocalcemia in the dog. Amer. J. Physiol., *216*:939, 1969.

62. Parks, J. S., Amrhein, J. A., Vaidya, V., Moshang, T., Jr., and Bongiovanni, A. M.: Growth hormone responses to propranolol-glucagon stimulation: A comparison with other tests of growth hormone reserve. J. Clin. Endocrinol. Metab., *37*:85, 1973.

63. Paloyan, E., Paloyan, D., and Harper, P. V.: Glucagon-induced hypocalcemia. Metabolism, *16*:35, 1967.

64. Paloyan, E.: Recent developments in the early diagnosis of hyperparathyroidism. Surg. Clin. N. Amer., *47*:61, 1967.

65. Deftos, L. J.: Radioimmunoassay for calcitonin in medullary thyroid carcinoma. JAMA, *226*:403, 1973.

66. Cornblath, M., and Schwartz, R.: Disorders of Carbohydrate Metabolism in Infancy. Philadelphia, W. B. Saunders, 1967.

67. Lawrence, A. M.: Pancreatic alpha-cell function in miscellaneous clinical disorders. *In* Unger, R. H., and Lefebvre, P. J. (eds.): Glucagon. pp. 259-274. Oxford, Pergamon Press, 1972.

68. McQuarrie, I.: Bell, E. T., Zimmermann, B., and Wright, W. S.: Deficiency of alpha cells of pancrease as possible etiologic factor in familial hypoglycemosis. Fed. Proc., *9*:337, 1950.

69. Bleicher, S. J., Spergel, G., Levy, L., and Zarowitz, H.: Glucagon-deficiency hypoglycemia: A new syndrome. Clin. Res., *18*:355, 1970.

70. Foa, P. P.: Personal communication.

71. Aguilar-Parada, E., Eisentraut, A. M., and Unger, R. H.: Pancreatic glucagon secretion in normal and diabetic subjects. Amer. J. Med. Sci., *257*:415, 1969.

72. Paloyan, E., Dumbrys, N., Gallagher, T. F., Rodgers, R. E., and Harper, P. V.: The effect of glucagon on hyperlipemic states. Fed. Proc., *21*:2, 1962.

73. Gerich, J. E., Langlois, M., Noacco, C., *et al.*: Primary alpha-cell defect in juvenile diabetes mellitus: Lack of glucagon response to insulin induced hypoglycemia. Clin. Res., *21*:624, 1973.

74. Foa, P. P.: Personal communication.

75. Lawrence, A. M.: Unpublished observations.

76. Unger, R. H., Lochner, V. J., and Eisentraut, A. M.: Identification of insulin and glucagon in a bronchogenic metastases. J. Clin. Endocrinol., *24*:823, 1964.

77. McGavran, M. H., Unger, R. H., Recant, L., Polk, M. C., Kilo, C., and Lefin, M. E.: A glucagon-secreting alpha-cell carcinoma of the pancreas. N. Eng. J. Med., *274*:1408, 1966.

78. Croughs, R. J. M., Hulsmans, H. A. M., Israel, D. E., Hackeng, W. H. L., and Schopman, W.: Glucagonoma as part of the polyglandular adenoma syndrome. Amer. J. Med., *52*:690, 1972.

79. Leichter, S., Pagliara, A., Pohl, S., and Kipnis, D.: Uncontrolled diabetes mellitus and hyperglucagonemia associated with an islet cell carcinoma. Clin. Res., *21*:886, 1973.

80. Paloyan, E., Lawrence, A. M., Straus, F. H., Paloyan, D., Harper, P. V., and Cummings, D.: Alpha cell hyperplasia in calcific pancreatitis associated with hyperparathyroidism. JAMA, *200*:757, 1967.

81. Paloyan, E., Paloyan, D., and Harper, P. V.: The role of glucagon hypersecretion in the relationship of pancreatitis and hyperparathyroidism. Surgery, *62*:167, 1967.

82. Gerich, J. E., Karam, J. H., and Forsham, P. H.: Stimulation of glucagon secretion by epinephrine in man. J. Clin. Endocrinol. Metab., *37*:479, 1973.

83. Porte, D., Jr., Graber, A. L., and Kuzuya, T.: The effect of epinephrine on immunoreactive insulin levels in man. J. Clin. Invest., *45*:228, 1966.

84. Marco, J., Calle, C., Roman, D., Diaz-Fierros, M., Villanueva, M. C., and Valverde, I.: Hyperglucagonism induced by glucocorticoid treatment in man. N. Eng. J. Med., *288*:128, 1973.

85. Vance, J. E., Stoll, R. W., Kitabchi, A. E., Williams, R. H., and Wood, F. C.: Nesidioblastosis in familial endocrine adenomatosis. JAMA, *207*:1679, 1969.

86. Weichert, R. F.: The neural ectodermal origin of the peptide-secreting endocrine glands. Amer. J. Med., *49*:232, 1970.

87. Lawrence, A. M.: Glucagon and pheochromocytoma. Ann. Int. Med., *73*:852, 1970.

88. Marco, J., Diego, J., Villanueva, M. L., Diaz-Fierros, M., Valverde, I., and Segovia, J. M.: Elevated plasma glucagon levels in cirrhosis of the liver. N. Eng. J. Med., *289*:1107, 1973.

89. Unger, R. H.: Pancreatic alpha cell function in diabetes mellitus. *In* Lefebvre, P. J., and Unger, R. H. (eds.): Glucagon. Oxford, Pergamon Press, 1972.

90. Muller, W. A., Faloona, G. R., and Unger, R. H.: Hyperglucagonemia in diabetic ketoacidosis. Its prevalence and significance. Amer. J. Med., *54*:52, 1973.

91. Lindsey, C. A., Willmore, D. W., and Moylan, J. A.: Glucagon and the insulin: glucagon ratio in burns and trauma. Clin. Res., *20*:802, 1972 (abstr.).

92. Meguid, M. M., Brennan, M. F., Muller, W. A., and Aoki, T. T.: Glucagon and trauma. Lancet, *2*:1145, 1972.

93. Marreiro Rocha, D., Santensanio, F., Faloona, G. R., and Unger, R. H.: Abnormal pancreatic alpha-cell function in bacterial infections. N. Eng. J. Med., *288*:700, 1973.

94. Bloom, S. R.: Glucagon, a stress hormone. Postgrad. Med. J., (In press), 1973.

95. Felig, P.: Glucagon: Physiologic and diabetogenic role. N. Eng. J. Med., *283*:149, 1970.

96. Unger, R. H., Madison, L. L., and Muller, W. A.: Abnormal alpha-cell function in diabetes: response to insulin. Diabetes, *21*:301, 1972.

97. Creutzfeldt, W.: Gastrointestinal hormones and insulin secretion. N. Eng. J. Med., *288*:1238, 1973.

98. Valverde, I., Villanueva, M. L., Lozano, I., Roman, D., Diaz-Fierros, M., and Marco, J.: Chromatographic pattern of human intestinal glucagon-like immunoreactivity (GLI). J. Clin. Endocrinol. Metab., *36*:185, 1973.

99. Sutherland, E. W., and DeDuve, C. V.: Origin and distribution of hyperglycemic-glycogenolytic factor of the pancreas. J. Biol. Chem., *175*:663, 1948.

100. McIntyre, N., Holdworth, C. D., and Turner, D. S.: New interpretation of oral glucose tolerance. Lancet, *2*:20, 1964.

101. Creutzfeldt, W.: Gastrointestinal hormones and insulin secretion. N. Eng. J. Med., *288*:1238, 1973.

102. Rehfeld, J. F., Heding, L. G., and Holst, J. J.: Increased gut glucagon release as pathogenic factor in reactive hypoglycemia. Lancet, *1*:116, 1973.

103. Breuer, R. I., Hamilton, M., III, Hagen, T. C., and Zuckerman, L.: Gastric operations and glucose homeostasis. Gastroenterology, *62*:1109, 1972.

104. Bloom, S. R.: An enteroglucagon tumor. Gut, *13*:520, 1973.

105. Lawrence, A. M., Hagen, T. C., and Kirsteins, L.: Delayed enteroglucagon secretion in prediabetes. Clin. Res., *19*:679, 1971.

106. Goldfine, I. D., and Ryan, W. P. G. P.: Rapid production of glucagon antibodies. Hormone Metab. Res., *2*:47, 1970.

19 Radioisotopic Measurements of Insulin

Thaddeus Prout, M.D.

Studies of insulin have had a unique place in the development of our knowledge of biology. Beginning with Abel's monumental work in the crystallization of insulin at the Johns Hopkins Hospital in 1927,[1] this molecule has been the model on which theories of physicochemical structure have been tested and applied more broadly to many other problems. The work of Sanger and his coworkers,[2] on the amino acid sequence of insulin, and of Hodgkin, and her associates[3] on crystallography, are excellent examples of fundamental research performed on insulin as a model that have had far-reaching consequences in other biologic fields. Clinical endocrinology owes its phenomenal surge of research activity in the past 15 years to the pioneering work on immunoreactive assays of insulin in biologic fluids.

Before discussing the technique and application of insulin measurements, it is important to recall the complex mechanisms likely to be involved in insulin secretion and utilization. These concepts,[4] while not proven, take advantage of recent advances in our knowledge of insulin metabolism.[5,6]

It is likely that the stimuli to produce insulin are initiated by the same metabolites that are now known to bring about insulin release. Although for many years glucose was believed to be the only substance capable of insulin stimulation, there are now a number of known stimulators and inhibitors of insulin secretion (Table 19-1).

The manner in which glucose or other metabolites bring about the secretion of insulin is unknown. It is reasonable to postulate that a sensing device must be present which recognizes the amount of the specific stimulator present and informs the pancreas that insulin is needed. This immediately raises the possibility that a pathologic state could exist wherein a faulty sensing device would fail to inform the pancreas of the need, and insulin would not be secreted despite the presence of normal quantities of insulin in the pancreas. Studies with the sulfonylurea drugs may perhaps be interpreted as bearing on this question. It is clear that insulin can exist within the islet cells quite unaware of the hyperglycemic blood flowing past and that sulfonylurea drugs can bring about the release of this insulin. These drugs may activate a sensing device. It is equally possible that they may activate a releasing mechanism, for we cannot separate these 2 postulated functions. In individuals with adequate pancreatic stores of insulin which are not responsive to elevated levels of glucose, the sulfonylurea drugs bring about a more timely response to the stimuli. There is increasing evidence that there is carbohydrate intolerance that advances with age and again it seems likely that this relative insensitivity comes about through a failure either of the sensing device or of the releasing mechanism. Perhaps other conditions which alter insulin release, such as the glucose intolerance following fasting, may relate to these mechanisms.

Although we can say little about the mechanisms of release of insulin, we are in-

267

Table 19-1. Factors Stimulating or Inhibiting Insulin Secretion.*[5]

Stimulants	Inhibitors
Glucose	2-Deoxyglucose
Mannose	Mannoheptulose
Arginine	Epinephrine
Leucine	Diazoxide
β-Ketoacids	Thiazide diuretics
Secretin	
Pancreozymin	
Glucagon	
cAMP	
Theophylline	
Sulfonylureas	

* Calcium and potassium ions are necessary for the act of secretion; all stimulating substances operate better in the presence of glucose; growth-hormone excess, obesity and glucocorticoids lead to β-cell hypertrophy and hyperplasia; thus, all stimuli have hypernormal effects under these circumstances.

debted to the beautiful studies of Lacy[7] with the electron microscope for an exposition of the migration of the insulin granule across the beta cell to the cell surface. On reaching the cell surface, the envelope of the beta granule appears to coalesce with the surface membrane whereupon the beta granule is discharged into the extracellular space. At this point, unfortunately, the resolution of the electron microscope does not allow further physical view of the discharged granule. After discharge of the previously stored insulin, empty sacs are again seen in the beta

cell; these are frequently surrounded in part by a protein believed to be ribonuclear protein. The ribonuclear protein granules clustered about the sac slowly disappear as the amorphous material fills the empty sac, and it is easy to presume that we have witnessed the synthesis of insulin on a template. The amorphous material in the sac is next seen to condense into a storage form that is typical of the beta granules previously discharged. The discharge of these granules in response to known stimuli, such as glucose and sulfonylurea drugs, adds further to the circumstantial evidence that we are in fact witnessing the synthesis and release of insulin.

It has been shown that the polypeptide synthesized by the pancreas is a single chain with 84-amino acid residues containing 3 disulfide bonds or proinsulin[8] (Fig. 19-1). The 21-amino acid residue of the A-chain is connected to the B-chain containing 31-amino acids[9] (Fig. 19-1) by a connecting peptide of 33-amino acids known as the C-peptide.[8] Soon after the proinsulin leaves the assembly line in the pancreas and before it is stored in the beta granule, it is subjected to enzymatic action by which the C-peptide is removed. Thus, except under conditions of rapid synthesis and release, insulin secreted by the pancreas is largely in the form of the dipeptide molecule consisting of the A- and B-chains. Evidence has now been

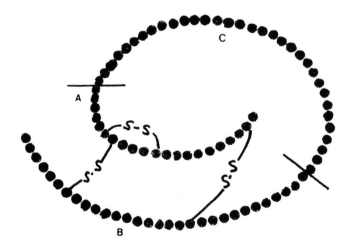

Fig. 19-1. Proinsulin. *A,* The A chain of insulin (21 amino acid residues). *B,* The B chain (30 amino acid residues) containing 3 disulfide bonds (S-S). *C,* The connecting peptide is removed by enzymatic action to produce biologically active insulin. (Adapted from Steiner and Oyer)[8]

Table 19-2. Human Plasma Insulin Sephadex Fractions.

Diagnosis No. of Patients	No. of Samples	Range of Plasma Insulin μU/ml	"Big Insulin" Fraction Percent
Lean, normal 5	9	138-562	5-19
Lean, diabetic 4	8	18-625	0-12
Obese, normal 4	8	65-475	0-6
Obese, diabetic 4	9	65-675	0-14
Myotonic dystrophy 4	8	88-500	3-20
Uremic 1	2	40-65	4-12
Miscellaneous A. Oral glucose stimulation (insulinoma, myxedema, prolonged fasting, postinsulin-hypoglycemia) 4 patients, 5 samples		52-1,000	5-13
B. Intravenous glucagon, glucose, arginine, tolbutamide 5 patients, 6 samples		128-500	5-12
C. Islet cell adenoma, glucagon, tolbutamide 1 patient, 4 samples		70-110	24-55

This study gives no support to the concept that hyperinsulinemia in the problems studied is attributable to "big" insulin. (Goldsmith, S. J., Yalow, R. S., and Berson, S. A.: Diabetes, *18*:834, 1969)[11]

accumulated that "big" insulin and proinsulin are probably identical.[10] The possibility that serum levels of proinsulin might account for the relatively ineffective levels of immunoreactive insulin in states characterized by hyperinsulinism is unsupported (Table 19-2). Between 5 and 15 percent of the insulin secreted in reference to glucose stimulation and separated from human plasma in Sephadex fractions is proinsulin.[11]

The manner and the state in which insulin is transported in blood is not clear, but measurements of insulin or insulin-like activity in the blood have given rise to the concept that there may exist in blood material capable of acting in an insulin-like manner but not demonstrable by immunoassay. The question of "typical" versus "atypical" insulin and of "suppressible" versus "nonsuppressible" insulin has been thoroughly reviewed.[12] We can conveniently consider together the "bound," "complex," "nonsuppressible," and "atypical" insulins and contrast then to insulin that is measured by the immunoassay (Table 19-3). These differ-

Table 19-3. Differences Between "Typical" and "Atypical" Insulin.*

	Typical	Atypical
Assay	Measured immunossay	Measured by fat-pad
Effect of antiserum	Inhibited	Not inhibited
Effect of pancreatectomy	Disappears	Remains
Origin	Pancreas	Unknown
Keto-acidosis	Absent	Present in large quantity
Other unresolved questions	Biologic activity of insulin measured immunologically is not known	Cannot be converted reproducibly to typical form

* Atypical insulin is used here as synonymous with nonsuppressible bound and complexed insulin. See text for discussion.

ences have led many to deny that "atypical" insulin has any real relationship to true pancreatic insulin. Despite these difficulties, it is theoretically possible that some form of insulin may exist that is different from the insulin measured immunologically, but further study of this problem may be necessary.

We can now picture the glucose-insulin regulating mechanism as a feedback system (Table 19-4). A metabolic stimulator, usually glucose, is measured by a sensing device which tells the pancreatic cell to release and to resynthesize insulin in relation to metabolic need. After insulin has arrived in the blood, it is picked up by a specific cell receptor and initiates a cellular response. The cellular response not only serves a metabolic need but also removes from the blood some of the metabolic stimulator that initiated the cycle. As a result of the decrease in the metabolite, no further stimulation for insulin release is given, and the feedback mechanism is satisfied. Various factors can presumably inhibit or potentiate the different steps of this process.

In this framework the diabetes with which we have been most familiar in the past is associated with failure of insulin release from the pancreas. This is most typically exemplified as the pancreatic exhaustion of juvenile diabetes. It is also true of the pancreas that has been destroyed by pancreatitis, hemochromatosis, or removed by the surgeon's knife. It may be seen in cases in which pancreatic exhaustion results from metabolic stresses such as hyperthyroidism, multiple pregnancies, or long-standing obesity. In all cases the pancreas is no longer able to respond to demand and clinical diabetes is seen. In true pancreatic exhaustion the sulfonylureas are, of course, unable to stimulate insulin release.

Also note that a state of functional low insulin output exists when there is either dulling of the sensing device or interference with insulin release; either of these mechanisms impairs the ability of the pancreas to deliver insulin on demand. In these instances, the sulfonylureas release insulin. Epinephrines and the thiazides inhibit release of insulin.

The new concept that must be brought into this scheme is the clinical situation in which metabolic abnormalities of the type seen in diabetes are present in spite of high circulating levels of insulin. A state of im-

Table 19-4. Insulin Stimulation and Response.*

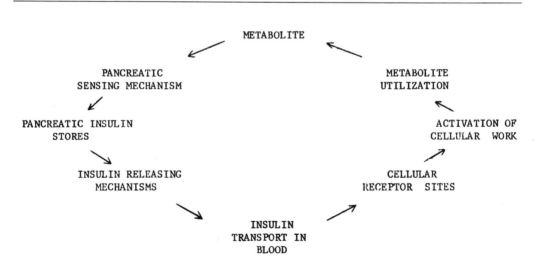

* Each step implies the existence of both stimulator and inhibitor mechanisms.

paired carbohydrate intolerance in association with a high level of plasma insulin can be understood if the insulin present is defective. It is also possible to recognize the clinical syndrome in which normal high levels of insulin compete with antagonists such as growth hormone, acromegaly, or adrenal steroids. A less well-defined impairment of insulin effectiveness is seen in association with obesity in which there is impaired carbohydrate tolerance in the presence of high circulating levels of insulin.[13] In this state it appears likely that the impairment to insulin action is located primarily at the level of cellular response. Roth and coworkers[14] recently developed a method whereby insulin receptors in man can be studied directly in the cultured and circulating lymphocyte. They have found that higher concentrations of unlabeled insulin are necessary to displace insulin labeled with I-125 from the receptor site of obese individuals with insulin resistance as compared with patients of normal weight. This measures indirectly the affinity of the receptor site for insulin and has provided for the first time evidence for a defect in the insulin receptor in certain insulin-resistant states in man.

Although much of the concept presented here is speculative, much has already been verified. The purpose of this global concept of diabetes as a complex metabolic problem is to serve as a reminder that extensive diagnostic interpretation should not be given to single values of insulin taken at variable points in a complex clinical setting even when obtained by a reliable radioimmunoassay.

The radioimmunoassay of insulin has its origins in the early work on the antigenicity of insulin by Tuft,[15] Banting[16] and Lowell[17] as was noted in a previous review.[18] These early studies set the stage for the development by Moloney and Coval[19] for the induction of diabetes by the injection of potent insulin antisera derived from guinea pigs into other laboratory animals. Arquilla and Stavitsky,[20] utilizing agglutination techniques on insulin-coated red blood cells, appear to be the first investigators who actually attempted to apply immunologic techniques to the measurement of insulin. However, an observation by Kalee[21] utilizing paper electrophoresis to separate insulin labeled with I-131 from small samples of sera led to the demonstration in Berson's laboratory of the presence of insulin-binding antibodies in the sera of insulin-treated patients.[22] Subsequently, an immunoassay for insulin in biologic fluids was developed by Berson and Yalow,[23] introducing the era of the radioimmunoassay of physiologic quantities of peptide hormone in biologic fluids by various competitive binding techniques[24] (Table 19-5).

Although the basic methodology both for labeling peptides with radioisotope and for competitive binding has been reviewed elsewhere (Chap. 9), it is worthwhile to point out some of the variations of this procedure that have been applied specifically to the immunoassay of insulin. In the original technique introduced by Berson and Yalow,[23] the insulin I-131 added to serum was found to be proportioned between a fraction bound to insulin-binding antibody and an unbound or free fraction that could be separated by paper electrophoresis. The insulin I-131, added to a mixture of the test serum and a specific titer of insulin-binding globulin, competed for a binding site with any endogenous insulin present. Thus, the free/bound ratio of the insulin I-131 varied directly with the quantity of endogenous insulin present in

Table 19-5. Competitive Binding Radioassay* Peptide Hormones

Insulin	Vasopressin
Growth hormone	Angiotensin
ACTH	Oxytocin
Parathyroid hormone	Bradykinin
Glucagon	Thyroglobulin
TSH	α MSH
HCG	β MSH
FSH	Gastrin
HCS	Calcitonin
Proinsulin	Proinsulin
Secretin	C-peptide
LH	PZ-CCK

* (Odell and Daughaday, p. 7)[24]

the test serum. The essential fact of establishing a reliable method for determining the bound-to-free ratio was the basis of all variations of the assay techniques that followed. Separation of free and bound fractions can be hastened by combining hydrodynamic flow with electrophoretic separation.[25] Other materials including charcoal and cellulose powder have been used to separate these components by adsorption of the free fraction.[26] Hales and Randle[27] incorporated the insulin-binding antibody into a filtration system whereby the bound insulin is separated out and counted on the filter paper while the free insulin passes through into the filtrate.

Morgan and Lazarow altered the procedure significantly by converting the soluble insulin antibody complex into a precipitate by the addition of an antiglobulin antibody.[28] The bound/free ratio is then established by comparison between the precipitated and nonprecipitable radioactivity. Precipitation of insulin-bound globulin with a differential sodium sulfite solution was successfully used by Grodsky and Forsham,[29] but this is perhaps less popular than the Berson and Yalow or Morgan and Lazarow techniques. Acid precipitation of intact protein after destruction of free insulin I-131 by proteolytic enzymes has also been used successfully.[30]

In all of these methods, it must be remembered that all patients who have received intermediate forms of insulin for 6 weeks or longer have developed endogenous antibodies to insulin and special precautions must be taken if an accurate estimate of the circulating insulin in such sera is to be made. Utilizing the double antibody assay of Morgan and Lazarow, endogenous antibodies lead to an interpretation of a circulating insulin value higher than is actually present. This relates to the fact that insulin bound to the human antibody is not precipitated by the rabbit anti-guinea-pig globulin serum used in this assay technique and this fraction appears as free rather than bound under these circumstances. Contrarily, in techniques in which the free insulin is separated from bound insulin by other techniques, the

presence of endogenous antibodies added to the antibodies inherent in the test procedure leads to a high bound fraction and to a lower insulin value than is actually present. It should be pointed out, however, that since endogenous antibodies to insulin stay relatively stable in any of the test conditions utilized, such comparisons in individual patients would clearly and accurately demonstrate any significant change in insulin secretion under certain test conditions.

In general, it may be stated categorically, as noted in the discussion above, that the evidence for so called insulin-like activity, other than that measurable by immunoassay methods, is not sufficiently secure as to challenge successfully the physiologic data available on insulin derived from normal pancreatic cells that are based on the immunoassays. The much greater sensitivity of the immunoassay under physiologic conditions as compared to all methods of bioassay has allowed the immunoassay to stand virtually unchallenged. In one patient, reported with a pancreatic adenoma, however, immunologic identity of the insulin produced was lost at a time when the presence of insulin by bioassay could be readily demonstrated.[31] This report appears to be unique, however, since bioactivity and immunologic identity are expected to be synonymous and hypoglycemia caused by tumors in which no insulin-like material is detectable must have their effect on blood glucose by some means other than the secretion of identifiable insulin.[32] Although the immunoassay of insulin correlates well with physiologic evidence, one must not lose sight of the fact that great care must be taken to alter the insulin compound as little as possible in the labeling procedure if the labeled compounds are to be used as tracer substances for the biologically active hormones. As shown by Izzo and coworkers, excess labeling with radioactive materials leads to major alterations in the behavior of the labeled insulin.[33]

The sensitivity of the various immunologic procedures must be tested in each laboratory but reliable assays to approximately 1

μU/ml of biologic fluid are to be expected and assays in excess of 1,000 μU have been reliably demonstrated in patients with excess insulin production. Thus, by altering the antibody dilution curve, it is quite possible to bring the level of insulin under consideration into the appropriate portion of the assay curve and to improve the reliability of the test (Chap. 9).

With the discovery by Steiner and his co-workers[8] of proinsulin and the C-peptide linkage, studies of insulin in the sera of normal subjects have become more complex. The immunologic half-life of proinsulin in animals is between 15 to 20 minutes or about twice that of insulin. Complexes of the insulin molecules studied after intravenous injection of radioactive insulin are taken up principally by liver, kidney and muscle. Proinsulin, however, is extracted principally by kidneys and it is assumed that this is the major site for its degradation. Most of the physiologic effects of insulin on muscle, adipose tissue and liver can be mimicked by proinsulin, although the potency on a milligram basis is much less than for insulin. No biologic effects have been recognized for the C-peptide preparations, but it is of physiologic importance to note that the levels of C-peptide in serum under a variety of conditions have been found to correspond very closely to those of insulin.[34] This suggests that these 2 compounds are secreted in essentially equal amounts from the beta cell.[35] Proinsulin antibodies exist in some patients treated with commercially available insulin products,[36] but it has been recently shown that measurement of C-peptide can be made in the presence of insulin antibodies in insulin-treated patients, thus making it possible to determine more accurately the presence of beta-cell activity in such individuals.[37,38]

In spite of these apparent difficulties, the immunoassay of insulin in serum can be performed with excellent reliability. Studies have established a range of normality for mean insulin concentrations after overnight fasting in nonobese adults of 15.0 $\pm$ 4.8

μU/ml of plasma with values for obese adults at 36.0 $\pm$ 17.6 μU/ml of plasma but with considerable overlap.[39] Obviously each laboratory must establish its own range of normality for this test.

Following ingestion of 100 Gm of glucose, Rabinowitz and Merimee[40] increased plasma glucose concentrations in normal subjects from 82.9 to 140.9 mg/100 ml declining to 90.3 mg/100 ml in 180 minutes. At the same time, plasma insulin levels rose from 17.2 to 77.3 μU/ml and returned to the basal levels in 4 hours. Following ingestion of 360 to 460 Gm of tenderloin beef, plasma glucose values remained relatively stable and a small but definite rise in plasma insulin was seen in 8 of 9 subjects studied. These increments were usually observed approximately an hour after the ingestion of beef, but were often sustained for several hours (maximal mean increase 15.7 μU/ml). When glucose and insulin were combined in the test procedure, there was a flattening of the glucose tolerance curve relative to that observed after glucose alone but despite this, there was an exaggerated plasma-insulin response. Peak values were about twice those encountered for glucose alone and about 4 times those observed after protein alone (100.5 μU/ml). Similar results were reported by Floyd and coworkers.[41]

Studies by Perley and Kipnis[42] were undertaken to determine the relative insulin response to oral and intravenous glucose in normal and diabetic subjects in which both groups were divided into patients of normal weight and those with obesity. In patients of normal weight, plasma-insulin levels rose to approximately 70 μU/ml 1 hour after oral ingestion of the glucose. In contrast, levels of insulin in obese subjects rose to approximately 240 μU/ml 1 hour after oral ingestion of glucose or approximately 4 times that of the normal subjects. Values of approximately one-third of these were seen in all subjects after glucose by intravenous infusion, thus illustrating the effect of gastrointestinal stimuli such as glucagon and

Table 19-6. Causes of Hypoglycemia.

DECREASED ENTRANCE OF GLUCOSE INTO BLOOD

IMPAIRMENT OF
HEPATIC OUTPUT OF GLUCOSE
1. Hepatic disease
   (a) Acute
   (b) Chronic
2. Alcohol ingestion
3. Enzymatic defects
   (a) Glycogen
   (b) Hereditary fructose intolerance
   (c) Galactosemia
   (d) Other rare conditions
4. Hormone deficiency states
   (a) Adrenal cortical insufficiency
   (b) Glucagon deficiency

IMPAIRMENT OF CALORIC INTAKE
1. Starvation—exercise
2. Malabsorption
3. Deficiency of amino acids

INCREASED REMOVAL OF GLUCOSE FROM BLOOD

ABSOLUTE OVERPRODUCTION
OF INSULIN*
1. Pancreatic origin
   (a) Adenoma, single or multiple
   (b) Carcinoma
2. Infants of diabetic mothers

RELATIVE OVERPRODUCTION
OF INSULIN
1. Sensitivity to insulin
   (a) Stimulated ("functional") hypoglycemia
   (b) Leucine sensitivity
   (c) Idiopathic
2. Abnormal stimulation of insulin
   (a) Alimentary
   (b) Sulfonylureas
   (c) Others

INDUCED HYPOGLYCEMIA
1. Factitious

HYPOGLYCEMIA OF UNDETERMINED ETIOLOGY

EXTRAPANCREATIC TUMORS
1. Fibrosarcoma, mesothelioma

IDIOPATHIC CAUSES

---

* Only a small number of possible causes of hypoglycemia is likely to be associated with excess production of insulin in the fasting state.[53]

secretin on the secretion of insulin under physiologic conditions.[43]

Studies have also been undertaken to maximize insulin secretion[44] and to demonstrate the immediate rise of insulin following the injection of intravenous tolbutamide and glucagon.[45] Evidence for limited insulin reserves of the pancreas has been documented in insulin-dependent patients[46] and in patients with chronic pancreatitis.[47]

Perhaps the most important lesson to be gleaned from these and many other studies of insulin secretion and insulin levels in normal subjects and in patients is the great variation in insulin levels among the individuals studied. These studies make clear the fact that a wide range of values may reflect biologic variations and that individual values in a single patient will always be difficult to interpret. Thus, from the point of view of the practicing physician, a single value for insulin taken at random or even under test conditions is virtually worthless for clinical diagnosis. The same can be said for the use of insulin values in patients with hyperglyceridemia with or without diabetes despite claims to the contrary.[48] Attempts have been made to redefine the mild diabetic state .with correlations of blood glucose and insulin response in the so-called insulogenic index[49]; however, the diagnosis of mild diabetes is based primarily on blood glucose and not on the serum insulin. Studies on the use of insulin in the urine[50] and free insulin in serum[51] have only recently emerged and the clinical usefulness of these tests has not yet been determined. None of these tests are now useful in the regulation of insulin therapy.

The intricacies of the differential diagnosis of hypoglycemia cannot be reviewed here but other reviews are available (Table 19-6).[52,53] Symptomatic hypoglycemia is a much overdiagnosed condition, but fortunately the diagnosis of functional hypoglycemia is quite direct and forthright and is based primarily on the history and provocations of symptoms under test conditions, and is not expected to give rise to abnormal levels of serum insulin. The diagnosis of organic hypoglycemia is based largely on history, the effect of a prolonged fast on blood glucose, and to some degree on the levels of serum insulin during fasting. It is important to emphasize, however, that organic hypoglycemia can occur in patients in whom levels of insulin in the fasting state are well within the normal range for the general population. Fajans and coworkers[54] have reported that approximately one-fifth of the patients with insulinoma on whom serial measurements of circulating insulin were made after overnight fast for up to 7 consecutive days did not display a single elevated level of plasma insulin. On the other hand, attempts to relate insulin levels to blood glucose and to judge the appropriateness of the glucose-insulin ratio can also be misleading. As an example, a level of 20 μg of insulin was found in our laboratory in an infant with ketotic hypoglycemia, having a blood glucose of less than 30. This did not imply hyperinsulinism secondary to a pancreatic tumor, although without other data it might have been so interpreted. The use of tolbutamide, glucagon and leucine as diagnostic tools in the diagnosis of organic hypoglycemia can be useful but both false-negative and false-positive tests are found (Table 19-7).[55] For these reasons, it must be stated categorically that the diagnosis of organic hyperinsulinism is based primarily on demonstrations of continually falling blood glucose and rising or high-serum insulin values during a prolonged fast.

The insulin assay can be very useful and is much less equivocal in the diagnosis of islet cell carcinoma.[56,57] The assay can also be used to demonstrate the therapeutic efficacy of streptozotocin in the treatment of this condition. Following intravenous infusion of streptozotocin, insulin levels climb rapidly to extremely high levels and may be associated with hypoglycemic convulsions even in the presence of rapidly infused hypertonic glucose.[58] In subsequent treatment of metastatic insulin-producing tumors with streptozotocin, a clear demonstration of the efficacy

Table 19-7. Tests for Diagnosis of Organic Hypoglycemia.

1. Prolonged Fast	(30 hours) plasma glucose over 60 mg/100 ml RIA 2-20 μU/ml
2. Tolbutamide Test*	1 Gm Na tolbutamide IV Glucose falls to 70% fasting RIA up to 200 μU/ml
3. Glucagon Test*	1 mg IV RIA up to 150 μU/ml
4. Leucine Test*	200 mg (kg IV in 30 minutes) RIA up to 2 x normal fasting

Limits for normality must be set for each laboratory. False-negative test may be seen in 15 to 30 percent of patients with islet cell adenoma. False-positive test is unlikely to be seen in functional hypoglycemia. Hormone deficiency states and alcoholic hypoglycemia require special care in the use of these tests.

* (Modified from Fajans, S. S.: Excepta Medica, *172*:894, 1967)[54]

of therapy can be made based on the changes of serum levels of insulin. In hyperinsulinism due to benign islet cell tumors, streptozotocin is seldom needed in view of the excellent results which may be obtained by surgery.[59]

Much work remains to be done in determining the clinical significance of the insulin antibodies. Early work in this field has shown that insulin resistance is frequently attributable to the presence of insulin antibodies, but insulin antibodies in vivo may be saturated by daily injections of proper amounts of insulin without increasing antibody production.[60] Additionally, insulin antibodies tend to increase only slightly with duration of insulin therapy but in most patients do not reach clinically significant levels.[60] It has also been shown that insulin derived from a species causes antibody production in homologous species and that the antigenicity of insulin in man is related more to the insulin preparation itself than to the species from which it is derived.[61]

The techniques for study of insulin-binding antibodies may now be based on a simple, standard procedure.[62] Utilizing a similar technique, it has been shown that regular crystalline insulins from both pork and beef are less antigenic than are intermediate insulins from either of these 2 species or indeed than is desalinated intermediate pork insulin.[60,18]

In the patient whose course is illustrated in Figure 19-2, insulin had been stopped 4 years previously because of insulin resistance. Before restarting insulin, antibodies to insulin were of the level seen in all insulin-treated patients which are usually without clinical significance (less than 50 μU/ml). When insulin therapy was started using beef NPH insulin 2 events took place, both of which were predictable. First, the patient responded to insulin during the first week and had normal blood glucose levels for the first time in 4 years. Second, the patient increased antibodies rapidly to over 500 μU/ml and became unresponsive to doses of insulin up to 1,500 units daily. Prednisone therapy did not reverse the resistance to insulin. It was later found that the patient was responsive to crystalline pork insulin. Intermediate pork insulins (NPH, Globin, and Lente) usually lead to antibody production and insulin resistance in such patients. Other studies of the use of insulin antibodies include the demonstration that insulin antibodies may be found in patients suspected of factitious hypoglycemia following surreptitious use of insulin,[63] and that patients with

labile diabetes may lack insulin antibodies which could act as a buffering system between insulin degradation and peripheral use.[64]

New insulins are less contaminated by noninsulin products than were the commercial preparations in use up to this time. Regular commercial insulin which contained 25 U/mg of insulin has been replaced by single peak insulin with 26.3 U/mg which is 99 percent pure and by single component insulin with 28.3 U/mg which is over 99 percent pure.[65] On the basis of this purification it is expected that these insulins will be less antigenic in human subjects,[66] but the proof of this fact and its influence on the development of complications in the diabetic requires further study. In addition to antibodies to exogenous insulin products, a new important finding suggests that autoantibodies may develop following a viral infection of the pancreas and may be of etiologic importance in development of diabetes.[67] Thus far the autoimmune or indeed the viral etiology in the development of diabetes has remained intriguing but difficult to prove. On the basis of these observations, however, it seems likely that future studies relating to the etiology and pathogenesis of diabetes

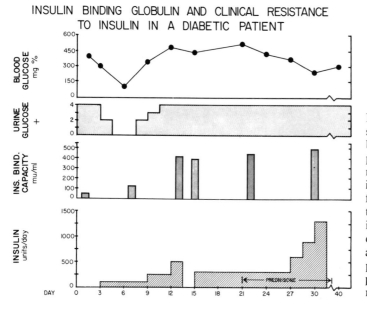

Fig. 19-2. Development of insulin resistance. Insulin antibodies were stimulated in this patient after several years of not receiving insulin. As the insulin-binding antibodies rose from less than 50 to greater than 400 mu/ml the effect of insulin was lost. A Somogyi effect was ruled out on day 13 and 14. Steroids did not improve insulin sensitivity. The patient was later found to be responsive to pork insulin.

will necessarily involve immunologic techniques utilizing the radioimmunoassay.

References

1. Abel, J. J.: Chemistry in relation to biology and medicine with especial reference to insulin and other hormones. Science, *66*:307, 337, 1927.
2. Sanger, F.: Chemistry of insulin. Br. Med. Bull., *16*:183, 1960.
3. Hodgkin, D. C., Blundell, T. L., Phil, D., Cutfield, J. F., Cutfield, S. M., *et al.*: Three-dimensional atomic structure of insulin and its relationship to activity. Diabetes, *21*: 492, 1971.
4. Prout, T. E.: The state of insulin in the blood. Med. College Va. Quart., *2*:14, 1966.
5. Levine, R.: Mechanisms of insulin secretion. N. Eng. J. Med., *283*:522, 1970.
6. Matschinsky, F. M., Landgraf, R., Ellerman, J., and Kotler-Brajtburg, J.: Glucoreceptor mechanisms in islets of Langerhans. Diabetes, *21*:555, 1971.
7. Lacy, P. E.: Electron microscopy of the beta cell of the pancreas. Amer. J. Med., *31*:851, 1961.
8. Steiner, D. F., and Oyer, P. E.: The biosynthesis of insulin and a probable precursor of insulin by a human islet cell adenoma. Proc. Natl. Acad. Sci. USA, *57*: 473, 1967.
9. Prout, T. E.: The chemical structure of insulin in relation to biological activity and to antigenicity. Metabolism, *12*:673, 1963.
10. Sherman, B. M., Gorden, P., Roth, J., and Freychet, P.: Circulating insulin: Proinsulin-like properties of "big" insulin in patients without islet cell tumors. J. Clin. Invest., *50*:849, 1971.
11. Goldsmith, S. J., Yalow, R. S., and Berson, S. A.: Significance of human plasma Sephadex fractions. Diabetes, *18*:834, 1969.
12. Berson, S. A., and Yalow, R. S.: Plasma insulin in diabetes mellitus: Theory and practice. p. 308. (Ed. Ellenberg, M., and Rifkin, H.), New York, McGraw-Hill, 1970.
13. Karam, J. H., Grodsky, G. M., and Forsham, P. H.: Excessive insulin response to glucose in obese subjects as measured by immunochemical assay. Diabetes, *12*:197, 1963.
14. Roth, J., Archer, J., Gavin, J. R., Jr., *et al.*: A defect in the insulin receptor in insulin resistant states in man: Studies in the cultured and circulating lymphocyte. (Abstr.)

p. 76. International Congress Series No. 280. VII Congress of the International Diabetes Federation; Brussels, Belgium; July 15-30, 1973. Excerpta Medica, Amsterdam, 1973.
15. Tuft, L.: Insulin hypersensitiveness; immunologic considerations and case reports. Amer. J. Med. Sci., *176*:707, 1928.
16. Banting, F. G., Franks, W. R., and Gairns, S.: Physiological studies in metrazole shock. VII. Anti-insulin activity of insulin treated patients. Amer. J. Psychiatry, *95*: 562, 1938.
17. Lowell, F. C.: Immunologic studies in insulin resistance. II. The presence of a neutralizing factor in the blood exhibiting characteristics of an antibody. J. Clin. Invest., *23*:233, 1944.
18. Prout, T. E.: The antigenicity of insulin: A review. J. Chron. Dis., *15*:879, 1962.
19. Moloney, P. J., and Coval, M.: Antigenicity of insulin: Diabetes induced by specific antibodies. Biochem. J., *59*:179, 1955.
20. Arquilla, E. R., and Stavitsky, A. B.: Evidence for insulin-directed specificity of rabbit anti-insulin serum. J. Clin. Invest., *35*:467, 1956.
21. Kalee, E.: Uber J-signiertes insulin. I. Mitteilung (Nach weis). Z. Naturforsch., *7b*:661, 1952.
22. Berson, S. A., Yalow, R. S., Bauman, A., *et al.*: Insulin I-131 metabolism in human subjects: Demonstration of insulin binding globulin in the circulation of insulin treated subjects. J. Clin. Invest., *35*:170, 1956.
23. Berson, S. A., and Yalow, R. S.: Quantitative aspects of the reaction between insulin and insulin-binding antibody. J. Clin. Invest., *38*:1996, 1959.
24. Odell, W. D., and Daughaday, W. H. (eds.): Principles of Competitive Protein-binding Assays. p. 7. Philadelphia, J. B. Lippincott, 1971.
25. Grodsky, G. M., Reng, C. T., and Forsham, P. H.: Effect of modification of insulin on specific binding in insulin resistant sera. Arch. Biochem. Biophys., *81*:264, 1959.
26. Herbert, V., Lau, K., Gottlieb, C. W., *et al.*: Coated charcoal immunoassay of insulin. J. Clin. Endocrinol., *25*:1375, 1965.
27. Hales, C. N., and Randle, P. J.: Immunoassay of insulin with insulin-antibody precipitate. Biochem. J., *88*:137, 1963.
28. Morgan, C. R., and Lazarow, A.: Immunoassay of insulin: Two antibody system. Diabetes, *12*:115, 1963.
29. Grodsky, G. M., and Forsham, P. H.: An immunochemical assay of total extractable

insulin in man. J. Clin. Invest., *39*:1070, 1960.

30. Beck, L. U., Zaharko, D. S., Roberts, N., *et al.*: Insulin assay by combined use of I-131 labeled insulin, anti-insulin serum and insulinase. Life Sci., *3*:545, 1964.

31. Boshell, B. R., Kirshenfeld, J. J., and Sateres, P. S.: Extrapancreatic insulin-secreting tumor. N. Eng. J. Med., *270*:338, 1964.

32. Kreisberg, R. A., Hershman, J. M., and Spenny, J. G., *et al.*: Biochemistry of extrapancreatic tumor hypoglycemia. Diabetes, *19*:248, 1970.

33. Izzo, J. L., Roncone, A., Izzo, M. J., *et al.*: Relationship between degree of iodination of insulin and its biological, electrophoretic and immunochemical properties. J. Biol. Chem., *239*:3749, 1964.

34. Oyer, P. E., Cho, S., and Steiner, D. F.: Studies on human proinsulin: Isolation and amino acid sequence of the human pancreatic C-peptide. J. Biol. Chem., *246*: 1375, 1971.

35. Melani, F., Rubenstein, A. H., Oyer, P. E., *et al.*: Identification of proinsulin and C-peptide in human serum by a specific immunoassay. Proc. Natl. Acad. Sci. USA, *67*:148, 1970.

36. Kumar, D., and Miller, L. U.: Proinsulin-specific antibodies in human sera. Diabetes, *22*:361, 1973.

37. Rubenstein, A. H., and Steiner, D. F.: Proinsulin. Ann. Rev. Med., *22*:15, 1971.

38. Block, M. B., Rosenfield, R. L., Malso, M. E., *et al.*: Sequential changes in beta-cell function in insulin-treated diabetic patients assayed by C-peptide immunoreactivity. N. Eng. J. Med., *288*:1144, 1973.

39. Bagdade, J. D., Bierman, E. L., and Porte, D., Jr.: The significance of basal insulin levels in the evaluation of the insulin response to glucose in diabetic and non-diabetic subjects. J. Clin. Invest., *46*:1549, 1967.

40. Rabinowitz, D., Merimee, T. J., Maffezzoli, R., *et al.*: Patterns of hormonal release after glucose, protein and glucose plus protein. Lancet, *2*:454, 1966.

41. Floyd, J. C., Jr., Fajans, S. S., Conn, J. W., *et al.*: Insulin secretion in response to protein ingestion. J. Clin. Invest., *45*:1479, 1966.

42. Perley, M., and Kipnis, D. M.: Plasma insulin response to glucose and tolbutamide of normal weight and obese diabetic and non-diabetic subjects. Diabetes, *15*:867, 1966.

43. Kipnis, D. M.: Nutrient regulations of insulin secretion in human subjects. Diabetes, *21*:606, 1971.

44. Ryan, W. G., Schwartz, T. B., and Nibbe, A. F.: Serum immunoreactive insulin levels during glucose tolerance and intensive islet stimulation. Diabetes, *20*:404, 1971.

45. Yalow, R. S., Block, H., Villazon, M., *et al.*: Comparison of plasma insulin levels following administration of tolbutamide and glucose. Diabetes, *9*:356, 1960.

46. Cremer, G. M., Molnar, G. D., Taylor, W. F., *et al.*: Studies of diabetic instability: II. Tests of insulinogenic reserve with infusions of arginine, glucagon, epinephrine and saline. Metabolism, *20*:1083, 1971.

47. Raptis, S., Rau, R. M., Schroder, K. E., *et al.*: Role of exocrine pancreas in stimulation of insulin secretion by intestinal hormones: III. Insulin response to secretin, pancreozymin and to oral and intravenous glucose in patients suffering from chronic insufficiency of the exocrine pancreas. Diabetologia, *7*:160, 1971.

48. Levy, R. I., and Glueck, C. J.: Hypertriglyceridemia, diabetes mellitus and coronary vessel disease. Arch. Intern. Med., *123*:220, 1969.

49. Seltzer, H. S., and Smith, W. L.: Plasma insulin activity after glucose: An index of insulogenic reserve in normal and diabetic man. Diabetes, *8*:417, 1959.

50. Rubenstein, A. H.: The significance of immunoassayable insulin in urine. JAMA, *209*:254, 1969.

51. Nakagawa, S., Nakayama, H., Sasaki, T., *et al.*: A single method for the determination of serum free insulin in insulin-treated patients. Diabetes, *22*:590, 1973.

52. Freinkel, W.: Hypoglycemic disorders in diabetes mellitus: Diagnosis and treatment. p. 393, vol. III. Amer. Diab. Assoc. Inc., New York, 1971.

53. Prout, T. E.: Hypoglycemia. Diab. Croat., *1*:265, 1972.

54. Fajans, S. S.: Diagnostic tests for functioning pancreatic islet cell tumors. Excerpta Medica, *172*:894, 1967.

55. Seltzer, H. S.: Insights about diabetes and hyperinsulinism gained from the insulin immunoassay. Postgrad. Med., *46*:73, 1969.

56. Gorden, P., Freychet, P., and Nankin, H.: Unique form of circulating insulin in human islet cell carcinoma. J. Clin. Endocrinol., *33*:983, 1971.

57. Lazarus, N. R., Gutman, R. A., Penhos, J. C., *et al.*: Biologically active circulating proinsulin-like materials from islet cell carcinoma patient. Diabetologia, *8*:131, 1972.

58. Taylor, S. G. III, Schwartz, T. B., Zannini, J. J., *et al.*: Streptozotocin therapy for metastatic insulinoma. Arch. Intern. Med., *126*:654, 1970.

59. Streptozotocin for islet-cell carcinoma. Leading article. Lancet, *2*:1063, 1973.

60. Prout, T. E., and Katims, R. B.: The effect of insulin binding serum globulin on insulin requirement. Diabetes, *8*:425, 1959.

61. Lockwood, D. H., and Prout, T. E.: Antigenicity of heterologous and homologous insulin. Metabolism, *14*:530, 1965.

62. Sebriakoua, M., and Little, J. A.: A method for the determination of plasma insulin antibodies and its application in normal and diabetic subjects. Diabetes, *22*:30, 1973.

63. Palumbo, P. J., Molnar, G. D., Taylor, W. F., *et al.*: Insulin antibody binding in diabetes mellitus and factitious hypoglycemia. Mayo Clin. Proc., *44*:725, 1969.

64. Dixon, K., Exon, P. D., and Hughes, H. R.: Insulin antibodies in aetiology of labile diabetes. Lancet, *1*:343, 1972.

65. Root, M. A., Chance, R. E., and Galloway, J. A.: Immunogenicity of insulin. Diabetes, *21*:657, 1971.

66. Galloway, J. A., and Root, M. A.: New forms of insulin. Diabetes, *21*:637, 1971.

67. LeCompte, P. M., and Legg, M. A.: Insulin (lymphocytic infiltration of pancreatic islets) in late-onset diabetes. Diabetes, *21*:762, 1972.

20 Radioimmunoassay of the Calcium-regulating Hormones

CARLOS R. HAMILTON, JR., M.D.

The role of parathyroid hormone in the regulation of calcium metabolism as well as in a variety of clinical disorders has been established since the studies of Fuller Albright and his associates. The inability to measure levels of parathyroid hormone in blood, however, has left many questions unanswered. Until very recently only indirect tests of parathyroid function and clinical judgment were available for the diagnosis of disorders of calcium metabolism. Currently available techniques for the measurement of parathyroid hormone in blood have not replaced these time-proven methods but have greatly contributed to diagnostic precision and an understanding of the nature of parathyroid gland secretion and its regulation in normal and pathologic states.

The discovery of the hypocalcemic peptide, calcitonin and advances in the understanding of vitamin D metabolism have greatly expanded knowledge of calcium homeostasis and metabolic bone diseases. Radioimmunoassays for calcitonin have been developed in several laboratories and have contributed significantly to the diagnosis of medullary carcinoma of the thyroid. New radioligand assays for vitamin D hold promise for additional insights in physiology and clinical medicine.

PARATHYROID HORMONE

The measurement of parathyroid hormone by radioimmunoassay was first accomplished in 1963 by Berson, Yalow, Aurbach and Potts.[1] Unlike assays for most other peptide hormones, widespread application of this technique was delayed by several factors. The initial assay was fraught with technical difficulties and was unable to clearly distinguish normal and hyperparathyroid patients. Preparations of bovine hormone of suitable purity for iodination or for use as standards were scarce and purified human parathyroid hormone was nonexistent.

At the present time, all immunoassays for parathyroid hormone use heterologous antisera (i.e., antibody raised against bovine or porcine hormone). The cross-reactivity of these antisera with purified human hormone has been in the range of only 50 percent of the reactivity with the bovine hormone.[2] Problems of greater significance in the interpretation of results of parathyroid hormone measurement became apparent as assays were developed in other laboratories. Immunoheterogeneity of circulating serum PTH, first identified by Berson and Yalow in 1968,[3] explains discrepancies in results reported by various investigators. Although these discrepancies confused initial PTH assay results, the considerable effort involved in identifying the nature of the heterogeneous immunoreactive PTH peptides has greatly expanded knowledge of the synthesis, secretion and metabolism of the hormone.

Immunoassay Techniques

Assays for parathyroid hormone each using a different antiserum have been reported from several laboratories.[1,3-8] Anti-PTH antibodies have been produced in guinea pigs or in chickens against crude or partially purified preparations of bovine or porcine parathyroid hormone.[1,3-8] Each of these assays utilizes bovine PTH, radioiodinated by standard methods with ^{125}I or ^{131}I, as the labeled hormone. The earlier chromato-electrophoresis separation of free PTH from that bound to antibody has been replaced by methods using silica granules or dextran-coated charcoal.[1,3,5]

Special problems in the immunoassay of PTH require correction factors for the precise calculation and interpretation of results. These factors are required to correct for incubation "damage" of the radiolabeled PTH and to correct for nonspecific inhibition of the hormone-antibody reaction by serum.[5] The term "damaged hormone" is used to refer to the portion of radiolabeled material which behaves as though it were bound to antibody but in fact is not. This material is not removed from the incubation mixture by charcoal absorption and is probably caused by nonspecific binding of labeled material to serum protein. Control tubes with the usual incubation mixture but without anti-PTH antiserum must be assayed and the resultant value for "damage" subtracted from the values of subsequent tubes. This degree of damage is influenced by the amount of protein in the incubation mixture; hence the values derived for varying amounts of standard or unknown serum must be corrected by adding appropriate concentrations of human hypoparathyroid serum. A description of the protocol for such an assay has been described in detail in Arnaud, et al.[5]

The dextran-coated charcoal method of separating bound from free radiolabeled hormone is particularly useful in the assay for PTH, since this method permits calculation of the damage factor and hence for correction of the values. Double-antibody phase separation techniques underestimate this damage and have not been successfully applied to the assay of PTH, since this hormone appears to be more susceptible to damage during radioiodination than most other peptides. Damage appears to increase with the age of the labeled hormone; hence the need for using the material soon after iodination. Repurification of older tag by gel filtration prior to its use in an assay may extend the time between iodinations of the peptide.

An adaptation of the usual method of preparing dextran-coated charcoal was described by Arnaud, et al.[5] A suspension of charcoal and dextran was mixed overnight by magnetic stirring at 4°C. The suspension was then centrifuged and the supernate discarded. The residue was then resuspended in buffer containing human albumin but no dextran. If the dextran-containing buffer was not replaced approximately 20 percent of the radiolabeled PTH remained in the supernate after phase separation.

At the present, there is no widely available preparation of human PTH to standardize the assays in use in various laboratories. Results of hormone concentration in serum, therefore, have been expressed in terms of immunoreactive equivalence with serum from patients with severe hyperparathyroidism (μl equivalents per ml of "unknown" serum) ($\mu lEq/ml$) or with purified preparations of bovine hormone.[9] Theoretical problems in interpretation of assays from different laboratories result when there is potential dissimilarity between the radioiodinated peptide and the hormone standard against which its displacement is being compared. These problems, however, have not prevented the various assay systems from yielding clinically useful results.

The principal discrepancies in results reported from different laboratories involved the ability of the assays to discriminate between normal subjects and those with hyperparathyroidism on the basis of serum concentrations of PTH. Reiss and Canterbury[10] also observed no suppression of serum PTH in patients with parathyroid adenomas dur-

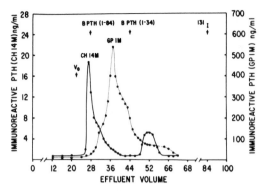

Fig. 20-1. Immunoreactivity of fractions from Bio-Gel P30 gel filtration of serum from a patient with primary hyperparathyroidism. Material reacting with CH 14M antiserum has a molecular weight similar to intact PTH (1-84) while antiserum GP 1M reacts with material of 7,000 MW. (From Arnaud, C. D., et al.: *In* Clinical Aspects of Metabolic Bone Disease. Excerpta Medica, Int. Congress Series, No. 270)

ing calcium infusion while Potts, et al., reported that serum iPTH (immunoreactive PTH) values in such patients were decreased during calcium infusion and increased by EDTA-induced hypocalcemia.[11] Explanations for these disparities have come from work characterizing the immunoheterogeneous forms of circulating PTH.

Metabolism of Parathyroid Hormone

The previously described discrepancies between laboratories using PTH immunoassay methods are explained by immunologic differences between the glandular and circulating hormone. This was first noted by Berson and Yalow[3] from studies comparing the immunoreactivity of extracts of parathyroid glands and plasma from patients with primary hyperparathyroidism or renal insufficiency with different antisera. A species of immunoreactive PTH which differed from glandular hormone was especially prominent in the plasma of patients with renal insufficiency.

Immunologic differences between glandular and serum PTH were also noted by Arnaud, et al.[12] and Sherwood, et al.[13] It was suggested that PTH secreted in vitro was a fragment of the glandular 84-amino

acid peptide and that this fragment was immunologically similar to the predominant form of the hormone in hyperparathyroid serum.[14] These concepts were clarified by the studies of Habener, et al.,[15] using radioimmunoassay and gel filtration of serum from the peripheral circulation and parathyroid effluent blood obtained by venous catheterization. Immunoreactive PTH in serum from the inferior thyroid vein draining a parathyroid adenoma was similar in molecular weight (M.W.) to the 84-amino acid peptide (molecular weight of 9,500) extracted from parathyroid tissue. Most immunoreactive PTH in peripheral blood had a molecular weight of about 7,000. These studies indicate that the 9,500 M.W. glandular hormone is secreated into the circulation and subsequently cleaved into one or more fragments which comprise the predominant form of circulating immunoreactive hormone.

These observations were extended by Arnaud, et al.[15A] who obtained 2 different antisera to PTH which react specifically with the 2 molecular species of human PTH (9,500 M.W.—"glandular" hormone and 7,000 M.W.—"circulating" hormone). Their antiserum CH 14M reacts almost exclusively with material of 9,500 M.W. while antiserum GP 1M reacts with 7,000 M.W. material (Fig. 20-1). The measurement of immunoreactive PTH in serum from hyperparathyroid patients with these 2 antisera revealed marked differences in the values obtained. Patients with chronic renal failure had strikingly elevated PTH values when assayed with antiserum GP 1M, while 40 percent of the PTH values of these patients were within the normal range when measured by antiserum CH 14M (Fig. 20-2). Serum immunoreactive PTH values were normal in only 10 percent of patients with primary hyperparathyroidism when measured with GP 1M, while PTH values were normal in 40 percent of these patients when measured with CH 14M. They concluded from calcium infusion studies that antisera reacting primarily with 9,500 M.W. material most closely reflects the acute secretory status of the parathyroids, while the chronic hyperparathyroid state was most accurately indicated by antisera reacting with 7,000 M.W. material.

The chemical nature of these hormonal fragments has been deduced by the studies of Segre, et al.,[16] which defined the antigenic recognition sites of antibovine PTH antisera by saturating the antisera with selected synthetic fragments of the hormone. These studies indicate that the 7,000 M.W. immunoreactive material lacks a portion of the amino-terminal sequence of intact hormone that is required for biological activity.

Studies of Canterbury, et al.,[17] confirmed that the 7,000 M.W. fraction of serum immunoreactive PTH was biologically inactive as indicated by its lack of effect on renal cortical adenylate cyclase. The 9,500 M.W. material as well as a third fraction with M.W. of 4,500 to 5,000 significantly increased cyclic 3', 5'—AMP accumulation in their bioassay system. The nature of this smaller molecular weight material is unknown but presumably contains the 2-27 sequence of N-terminal amino acids required for biological activity.[18]

These findings have been recently summarized.[19,20] In brief, the parathyroid glands secrete the 9,500 M.W. glandular form of PTH (1-84) which is rapidly cleaved to form a 7,000 M.W. carboxyl-terminal fragment (biologically inert) and smaller amino-terminal fragments which are potentially biologically active. The glandular hormone and N-fragments have short half-lives in serum. Assays which are specific for these N-terminal components of circulating PTH accurately reflect rapid changes in PTH secretion. The C-fragments have longer half-lives in serum and their measurement is a more sensitive indicator of the state of chronic hyperparathyroidism. As would be expected, N-specific assays have been of greatest use in localizing parathyroid adenomas by their ability to recognize the secreted form of the hormone which predominates in the parathyroid effluent blood.

Clinical Applications of PTH Immunoassay

The principal clinical use for measurement of parathyroid hormone in blood is in

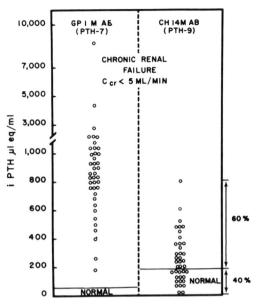

Fig. 20-2. Immunoreactive PTH in serum of patients with end-stage renal failure, measured by antisera GP 1M and CH 14M. The former antisera, measuring material with 7,000 MW more accurately reflects the severe hyperparathyroidism in these patients. (From Arnaud, C. D., et al.: *In* Clinical Aspects of Metabolic Bone Disease, Excerpta Medica Int. Congress Series No. 270)

the differential diagnosis of hypercalcemia. The recognized causes of hypercalcemia (Table 20-1) are often detected by careful

Table 20-1. Causes of Hypercalcemia.

1. Primary hyperparathyroidism—parathyroid adenoma, hyperplasia or carcinoma
2. Nonparathyroid malignancies (carcinomas)
   With bone metastasis
   Without bone metastasis
   With or without ectopic production
   of PTH
3. Other malignancies
   Lymphoma, Hodgkins disease, multiple myeloma, leukemia
4. Other causes
   Sarcoidosis
   Vitamin D intoxication
   Milk-alkali syndrome
   Addison's disease
   Dysproteinemias
   Immobilization (especially with Paget's disease)
   Thiazide diuretics
   Hyperthyroidism

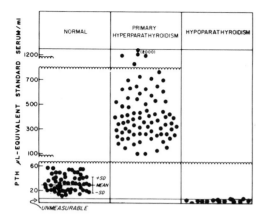

Fig. 20-3. Results of radioimmunoassay of PTH in normal subjects and patients with hyperparathyroidism and with hypoparathyroidism. (From Reiss, E., and Canterbury, J. M.: Amer. J. Med., *50*:680, 1971)

clinical evaluation with the aid of standard laboratory and radiographic studies. The diagnosis of hyperparathyroidism is generally established by the presence of compatible clinical findings and hypercalcemia when other causes of an elevated serum calcium have been reasonably excluded. The wide use of blood chemistry screening tests has identified a group of patients having hypercalcemia which is often only slightly above the normal range and not associated with recognized symptoms.

Measurement of immunoreactive PTH is a useful tool for the diagnosis of hyperparathyroidism in such cases. Serum for PTH measurement should be obtained in the early morning hours, since a consistent diurnal variation in these values has been observed.[5] There is an increase in serum PTH throughout the day and levels at 8 P.M. were twice those at 8 A.M. As described in the previous section, the discrimination between normal and hyperparathyroid serum on the basis of the level of PTH alone depends on the molecular species of the hormonal peptide recognized by different antisera. Reiss, et al.[21] observed complete separation of normal and hyperparathyroid subjects (Fig. 20-3), while Berson and Yalow[9] noted a large overlap of the values in these 2

groups.[9] Antisera reacting with the carboxyl-terminal, 7,000 M.W. fragment of PTH appear to give the best resolution between these groups. When the serum PTH value is compared by discriminate analysis with the serum calcium value, excellent separation of normal subjects from patients with hyperparathyroidism is obtained with all assays currently in use (Fig. 20-4).[5] Patients with hypercalcemia resulting from disorders other than excessive secretion of parathyroid hormone invariably have undetectable immunoreactive PTH in serum.

The most vexing problem to the clinician is the differentiation of cases of primary hyperparathyroidism from those with ectopic production of parathyroid hormone by other malignancies. The association of hypercalcemia and hypophosphatemia with such malignancies as carcinoma of lung, kidney, cervix, ovary, colon, parotid gland and with reticulum cell sarcoma is observed in the absence of demonstrable bone metastasis.

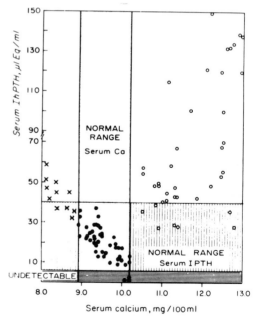

Fig. 20-4. Serum immunoreactive PTH as function of serum calcium in normal subjects (●), hypocalcemic patients (×) and patients with surgically proven primary hyperparathyroidism (○). (From Arnaud, C. D., et al.: J. Clin. Invest., *50*:21, 1971)

The presence of immunoreactive PTH in extracts of such tumors or in the patient's serum has been demonstrated by several laboratories.[9,22,23] Not all patients with hypercalcemia and these malignancies, however, have elevated serum PTH values, and some tumors such as those of breast, usually produce hypercalcemia without detectable immunoreactive PTH. Hence, measurement of serum PTH may not consistently help distinguish primary hyperparathyroidism from ectopic PTH production.

It has been suggested that nonparathyroid malignancies may produce PTH which is immunologically different from normal PTH.[7] Roof, et al., found that the immunoreactivity of serum PTH from patients with malignancies differed from that in primary hyperparathyroidism when measured with other antisera.[7] Riggs, et al. found lower values for serum immunoreactive PTH in patients with malignancies and hypercalcemia than in those with primary hyperparathyroidism.[24] The slopes of dilutional curves of the sera from patients with ectopic hyperparathyroidism differed significantly from dilutional curves of primary hyperparathyroid sera. These observations point to an immunologically distinct PTH in sera of patients with ectopic hyperparathyroidism. It is possible that some malignancies may secrete a disproportionate amount of proparathyroid hormone. Proparathyroid hormone has been identified as having a molecular weight of about 11,500 with an additional 15 to 20 amino acids at the amino-terminal of the PTH molecule.[27,28] Assay methods for measurement of pro-PTH are not yet available but may eventually provide an additional useful diagnostic tool.

The application of PTH assay to serum samples obtained by selective venous catheterization holds great promise for the differentiation of primary and ectopic hyperparathyroid patients. The results of preoperative localization of abnormal parathyroid tissue in a series of 94 patients with primary hyperparathyroidism has been recently reviewed.[25] When blood was obtained from the thyroid veins, significant elevations of the PTH value were observed in 82 percent of patients with parathyroid adenomas and 74 percent of patients with hyperplasia. Detailed studies of the venous drainage of the parathyroid glands[26] permitted differentiation between adenomas and hyperplasia. Of patients with unilateral gradients 98 percent had adenoma and 85 percent with bilateral elevations of PTH in thyroidal veins had hyperplasia.[25] An increased value of PTH in the venous drainage of a suspected mass in the lung, kidney or elsewhere may be the most certain clue to the presence of ectopic PTH production.

Future developments in the radioimmunoassay of PTH may be expected with the recent identification and synthesis of the amino-terminal sequence of human PTH.[29,30] It is likely that antisera reacting specifically with portions of the human hormone will provide more sensitive measurements of parathyroid gland function than currently available techniques.

CALCITONIN

Calcitonin, a hypocalcemic peptide hormone, secreted by thyroid parafollicular cells in mammals and by the ultimobranchial gland in fish, was discovered in 1962 by Copp, et al.[31] Shortly thereafter this hormone was purified, its amino acid sequence established and synthesized. The chemistry and physiology of calcitonin have been recently reviewed.[32,33] The hormone exerts hypocalcemic and hypophosphatemic effects primarily through the inhibition of bone resorption. There is evidence for a physiologic role of calcitonin in the prevention of postprandial hypercalcemia in lower mammals[34] but the significance of this hormone in human physiology has not been determined. Currently available assays are unable to demonstrate convincingly that calcitonin is secreted in normal human subjects. This hormone can often be measured in the blood of patients with medullary carcinoma of the thyroid and is a valuable diagnostic test in such cases.

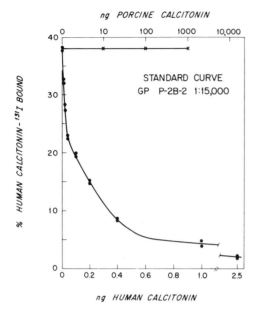

Fig. 20-5. Standard curve for human calcitonin (○) and porcine calcitonin (×) using antihuman calcitonin antiserum. (From Tasjian, A. H., Jr., et al.: N. Eng. J. Med., *283*:891, 1970)

Bioassay methods for measuring calcitonin based on the hypocalcemic effect of this peptide played an important role in the early studies of this hormone.[35] Subsequent bioassay methods have been developed using the inhibition of PTH-stimulated bone resorption in tissue culture by calcitonin.[36] These techniques are relatively laborious and expensive and have been largely replaced by immunoassay methods. They still are applicable in measuring calcitonin in various species, since available immunoassays are rather species-specific.

Immunoassay Techniques

Radioimmunoassay of porcine calcitonin was first reported by Deftos, et al. in 1968.[37] As quantities of human hormone became available assays for its measurement were developed.[38-41] These assays have utilized antiserum produced in guinea pigs or rabbits by injection of calcitonin extracted from human medullary carcinoma of the thyroid or with synthetic human calcitonin. Purified or synthetic hormone has been radioiodin-

ated by standard techniques with specific activities of 250 to 750 $\mu c/\mu g$. Purification of labeled calcitonin has been accomplished by absorption and elution from silica or by gel filtration on Bio-gel P-10[41] or Amberlite CG 400 columns.[38]

Currently used assays have been standardized by the calcitonin preparation MRC Research Standard A supplied by the Medical Research Council. Highly sensitive assays have utilized nonequilibrium reaction conditions and antiserum-bound and -free hormone are separated by dextran-coated charcoal[39-41] or dioxane.[38] These assays have been able to detect as little as 50 to 100 pg calcitonin/ml of human plasma.[41] The lability of calcitonin in blood specimens requires prompt separation and immediate freezing of the plasma sample obtained for immunoassay measurement.

Physiological Studies of Calcitonin Secretion

The initial immunoassay for calcitonin, using antiserum against porcine hormone had some cross-reactivity with calcitonin of other species such as rabbit.[37] There was only slight reactivity of this assay with human calcitonin, inadequate for measurement of hormone in blood. Subsequent studies have shown no significant cross-reactivity between antihuman calcitonin antisera and porcine hormone (Fig. 20-5). Studies using the porcine calcitonin immunoassay demonstrated that the hormone is secreted under basal conditions in both the rabbit and pig. Both calcium and pentagastrin infusion stimulate calcitonin secretion in these species.[34] Munson, et al., suggested that calcitonin is of physiologic significance in these species; the secretion of this hormone protects the animals against transient hypercalcemia and hypercalciuria which would occur during absorption of dietary calcium.[34]

A possible role of calcitonin in normal human physiology has not been fully demonstrated. Initial studies suggested the presence of immunoreactive calcitonin in normal human plasma. Additional studies by Deftos indicated that these low values may occur because of nonspecific interference by human plasma with the immunoassay (Fig. 20-6). His studies have shown the peptide to be undetectable in peripheral plasma and in thyroid venous blood of normal subjects (values less than 100 pg/ml). The presence of calcitonin in peripheral blood of patients with medullary carcinoma of the thyroid has been established. Deftos has also clearly demonstrated that calcitonin may be secreted in patients without this malignancy.[41] He detected calcitonin in the peripheral blood of patients with diseases associated with chronic hypocalcemia. Calcitonin levels were markedly increased after calcium infusion or the administration of pentagastrin. Chronic hypocalcemia may result in increased storage of calcitonin in the c-cells. These studies suggest that calcitonin may indeed be secreted in normal humans but at levels which are undetectable by current immunoassay techniques.

An immunoassay for human calcitonin developed by Samaan, et al., using a double-antibody phase separation technique has been reported to be able to detect calcitonin

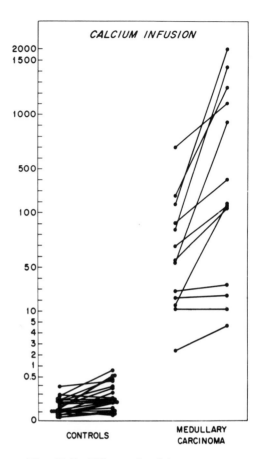

Fig. 20-7. Effects of calcium on serum calcitonin in control subjects and patients with active medullary carcinoma. (From Tasjian, A. H., Jr., et al.: Immunoassay of human calcitonin. N. Eng. J. Med., *283*: 893, 1970)

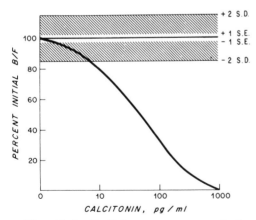

Fig. 20-6. Radioimmunoassay standard curve for human calcitonin. The shaded zone represents the standard deviation around the zero point of the standard curve. Measurements within this area are subject to artifact. (From Deftos, L. J.: assay of calcitonin in man. *In* Clinical Aspects of Metabolic Bone Disease. Excerpta Medica, Int. Congress Series, No. 270)

levels in normals.[42] Their studies included the removal of immunoreactive material by charcoal adsorption in normal serum and serum from patients with medullary carcinoma. Hence the displacement of labeled calcitonin from their antibody was not a result of nonspecific displacement caused by human serum.[41] They were able to detect increased calcitonin concentrations in the serum of neonates by their assay.[42]

Calcitonin and Medullary Carcinoma

The usefulness of calcitonin measurements in the diagnosis of medullary carcinoma of the thyroid gland has been clearly established. The similarity of these tumor cells to the parafollicular cells (c-cells)[43] of the normal thyroid was suggested by Williams, Brown and Doniach.[43] The presence of high concentration of calcitonin in these tumors was soon demonstrated by bioassay[44-46] and by immunoassay.[37,38] Patients with this malignancy were consistently found to have marked increases in plasma calictonin following calcium infusion (Fig. 20-7).[47]

The importance of using this measurement for the detection of occult malignancy in family members of patients with medullary carcinoma has been demonstrated.[48] In some cases the diagnosis can be made in the absence of any abnormality of the thyroid on physical examination or on thyroid scintiscan. These observations have made the measurement of plasma calcitonin an essential screening procedure for families with persons having medullary carcinoma, since this tumor has an autosomal-dominant mode of inheritance. The inhibitory effect of calcitonin on osteoclastic bone resorption has led to investigation of its clinical usefulness in a variety of disorders. This hormone has been found effective in treatment of Paget's disease of bone and in lowering serum calcium in patients with hypercalcemia. It may be particularly useful when severe hypercalcemia is complicated by cardiac or renal failure.

VITAMIN D

Important advances in the understanding of the metabolism of vitamin D and its physiologic actions have been made in the past decade and are the subjects of recent reviews.[49,50] These insights offer promise for understanding the pathophysiology of disorders characterized by apparent resistance to the action of vitamin D and for effective therapy.[51]

Bioassay techniques for measurement of vitamin D have been generally not applicable to the diagnosis of clinical disorders. Techniques for measurement of vitamin D and its metabolies by competitive-binding assays have been recently developed. These assays utilize the specific vitamin D-binding protein from the serum of D-deficient rats or rachitic kidney cytosol and ^{3}H-25-OH vitamin D.[52,53] The measurement requires extraction of the serum sample and chromatography of the lipid extract on silicic acid. Both assay systems which have been reported have cross-reactivity between 25-OH-vitamin D_3 and vitamin D_3 and D_2. Belsey has described an assay using chicken D-binding protein which is insensitive to D_2 or its metabolites.[54]

Haddad and Chyu found plasma 25-hydroxycholecalciferol levels of 27.3 ± 11.8 ng/ml in normal subject, 6.4 ± 2.6 ng/ml in patients with biliary cirrhosis and 64.4 ± 8.7 ng/ml in lifeguards with prolonged sun exposure.[53] Such measurements of vitamin D and its metabolites may help clarify the role of these compounds in the pathophysiology of disorders of calcium homeostasis.

References

1. Berson, S. A., Yalow, R. S., Aurbach, G. D., and Potts, J. T.: Immunoassay of bovine and human parathyroid hormone. Proc. Natl. Acad. Sci. USA, *49*:613, 1963.
2. O'Riordan, J. L. H., Aurbach, G. D., and Potts, J. T.: Immunological reactivity of purified human parathyroid hormone. Proc. Natl. Acad. Sci. USA, *63*:392, 1969.
3. Berson, S. A., and Yalow, R. S.: Immunochemical heterogeneity of parathyroid hormone in plasma. J. Clin. Endocrinol. Metab., *28*:1037, 1968.
4. Tashjian, A. H., Jr., Frantz, A. G., and Lee, J. B.: Pseudohypoparathyroidism: assays of parathyroid hormone and thyrocalcitonin. Proc. Natl. Acad. Sci. USA, *56*:1138, 1966.
5. Arnaud, C. D., Tsao, H. S., and Liddledike, T.: Radioimmunoassay of human parathyroid hormone in serum. J. Clin. Invest., *50*:21, 1971.
6. Reiss, E., and Canterbury, J. M.: Radioimmunoassay for parathyroid hormone in man. Proc. Soc. Exp. Biol. Med., *28*:501, 1968.
7. Roof, B. S., Carpenter, B., Fink, D. J., and Gordan, G. S.: Some thoughts on the nature of ectopic parathyroid hormones. Amer. J. Med., *50*:686, 1971.
8. Blair, A. F., Hawker, C. D., and Utiger, R. D.: Ectopic hyperparathyroidism in a patient with metastatic hypernephroma. Metabolism, *22*:147, 1973.

9. Berson, S. A., and Yalow, R. S.: Parathyroid hormone in plasma in adenomatous hyperparathyroidism, uremia, and bronchogenic carcinoma. Science, *154*:907, 1966.

10. Reiss, E., and Canterbury, J. M.: Primary hyperparathyroidism: application of radioimmunoassay to differentiation of adenomas and hyperplasia and to preoperative localization of hyperfunctioning parathyroid glands. N. Eng. J. Med., *280*:1381, 1969.

11. Potts, J. T., Jr., Murray, T. M., Peacock, M., et al.: Parathyroid hormone sequence, synthesis, immunoassay studies. Amer. J. Med., *50*:639, 1971.

12. Arnaud, C. D., Tsao, H. S., and Oldham, S. B.: Native human parathyroid hormones: an immunochemical investigation. Proc. Natl. Acad. Sci. USA, *67*:415, 1970.

13. Sherwood, L. M., Rodman, J. S., and Lundbery, W. B.: Evidence for a precursor to circulating parathyroid hormone. Proc. Natl. Acad. Sci. USA, *67*:1631, 1970.

14. Arnaud, C. D., Sizemore, G. W., Oldham, S. B., et al.: Human parathyroid hormone: glandular and secreted molecular species. Amer. J. Med., *50*:630, 1971.

15. Habener, J. F., Powell, D., Murray, T. M., et al.: Parathyroid hormone: secretion and metabolism in vivo. Proc. Nat. Acad. Sci. USA, *68*:2986, 1971.

15A. Arnaud, C. D., Goldsmith, R. S., Sizemore, G. W., et al.: Studies on characterization of human parathyroid hormone in hyperparathyroid serum-practical considerations. *In* Frame, B., et al.: Clinical Aspects of Metabolic Bone Disease. Excerpta Medica, Amsterdam, 1973.

16. Segre, G. V., Habener, J. F., Powell, D., et al.: Parathyroid hormone in human plasma-immunochemical characterization and biological implications. J. Clin. Invest., *51*:3163, 1972.

17. Canterbury, J. M., Levey, G. S., and Reiss, E.: Activation of renal cortical adenylate cyclase by circulating immunoreactive parathyroid hormone fragments. J. Clin. Invest., *52*:524, 1973.

18. Potts, J. T., Jr., Habener, J. F., Segre, G. V., et al.: Parathyroid hormone: chemical and immunochemical studies in relation to biosynthesis, secretion and metabolism. *In* Frame, B., et al.: Clinical Aspects of Metabolic Bone Disease, Excerpta Medica, Amsterdam, 1973.

19. Arnaud, C. D.: Immunochemical heterogeneity of circulating parathyroid hormone in man: sequel to an original observation by Berson and Yalow. Mt. Sinai J. Med., *40*:422, 1973.

20. Arnaud, C. D.: Parathyroid hormone: coming of age in clinical medicine. Amer. J. Med., *55*:577, 1973.

21. Reiss, E., and Canterbury, J. M.: Genesis of hyperparathyroidism. Amer. J. Med., *50*:679, 1971.

22. Tashjian, A. H., Levine, L., and Munson, P. L.: Immunochemical identification of parathyroid hormones in non-parathyroid neoplasms associated with hypercalcemia. J. Exp. Med., *119*:467, 1964.

23. Sherwood, L. M., O'Riordan, J. L. H., Aurbach, G. D., and Potts, J. T., Jr.: Production of parathyroid hormone by non-parathyroid tumors. J. Clin. Endocrinol. Metab., *27*:140, 1967.

24. Riggs, B. L., Arnaud, C. D., Reynolds, J. C., and Smith, L. H.: Immunologic differentiation of primary hyperparathyroidism from hyperparathyroidism due to nonparathyroid cancer. J. Clin. Invest., *50*:2079, 1971.

25. Bilezikian, J. P., Doppman, J. L., Shimkin, P. M., et al.: Preoperative localization of abnormal parathyroid tissue. Cummulative experience with venous sampling and arteriography. Amer. J. Med., *55*:505, 1973.

26. Doppman, J. L., and Hammond, W. G.: The anatomic basis of parathyroid venous sampling. Radiology, *95*:603, 1970.

27. Kemper, B., Habener, J. F., Potts, J. T., Jr., and Rich, A.: Proparathyroid hormone: identification of a biosynthetic precursor to parathyroid hormone. Proc. Natl. Acad. Sci. USA, *69*:643, 1972.

28. Habener, J. F., Kemper, B., Potts, J. T., Jr., and Rich, A.: Bovine proparathyroid hormone: structural analysis of radioactive peptides formed by limited cleavage. Endocrinology *92*:219, 1973.

29. Brewer, H. B., Jr., Fairwell, T., Ronan, R., et al.: Human parathyroid hormone: amino-acid sequence of the amino-terminal residues 1-34. Proc. Natl. Acad. Sci. USA, *69*:3585, 1972.

30. Andreatta, R., Hartman, A., Gohl, A., et al.: Synthese der sequenz 1-34 von menschlichen parat-hormon. Helv. Chim. Acta, *56*:410, 1973.

31. Copp, D. H., Cameron, E. C., Cheney, B., et al.: Evidence for calcitonin—a new hormone from the parathyroid that lowers blood calcium. Endocrinology, *70*:638, 1962.

32. Potts, J. T., Jr., and Deftos, L.: Parathyroid hormone, thyocalcitonin, vitamin D and bone mineral metabolism. *In* Bondy, P. K. (ed.): Duncan's Textbook of Diseases of

Metabolism. Philadelphia, W. B. Saunders, 1974.

33. Hirsch, P. F., and Munson, P. L.: Thyro-calcitonin. Physiol. Rev., *49*:548, 1969.

34. Munson, P. L., Gray, T. K., Cooper, C. W., *et al.*: Psychological significance of thyro-calcitonin in mammals. *In* Frame, B., *et al.*: Clinical Aspects of Metabolic Bone Disease. Excerpta Medica, Amsterdam, 1973.

35. Munson, P. L., and Hirsch, P. F.: Discovery and pharmacologic evaluation of thyro-calcitonin. Amer. J. Med., *43*:678, 1967.

36. Raisz, L. G., Au, W. Y. W., Simmons, H., and Mendelstam, P.: Calcitonin in human serum. Detection by tissue culture bioassay in medullary carcinoma of the thyroid and other disorders. Arch. Int. Med., *129*:889, 1972.

37. Deftos, L. J., Lee, M. R., and Potts, J. T., Jr.: A radioimmunossay for thyrocalcitonin. Proc. Natl. Acad. Sci. USA, *60*:293, 1968.

38. Clark, M. B., Byfield, P. H. G., Boyd, G. W., and Foster, G. V.: A radioimmuno-assay for human calcitonin. Lancet, *2*:74, 1969.

39. Tashjian, A. H., Jr., Howard, B. G., Melvin, K. E. W., and Hill, C. S., Jr.: Immunoassay of human calcitonin. N. Eng. J. Med., *283*: 890, 1970.

40. Bell, P. H., Dziokowski, C., and Barge, W. F., Jr.: Plasma calcitonin in man. Lancet, *2*:104, 1970.

41. Deftos, L. J.: Immunoassay for human cal-citonin. I. Method. Metabolism, *20*:1122, 1971.

42. Samaan, N. A., Hill, C. S., Jr., Beceiro, Jr., and Schultz, P. N.: Immunoreactive calci-tonin in medullary carcinoma of the thyroid and in maternal and cord serum. J. Lab. Clin. Med., *81*:671, 1973.

43. Williams, E. D., Brown, C. L., and Doniach, I.: Pathological and clinical findings in series of 67 cases of medullary carcinoma of thyroid. J. Clin. Pathol., *19*:103, 1966.

44. Meyer, J. S., and Abdel-Bari, W.: Granules and thyrocalcitonin activity in medullary carcinoma of thyroid gland. N. Eng. J. Med., *278*:523, 1968.

45. Milhaud, G., Tubiana, M., Parmentier, C., and Coutris, G.: Epithelioma de la thyroide secretant de la thyrocalcitonine. C. R. Acad. Sci. (Paris), *266*:608, 1968.

46. Tashjian, A. H., Jr., and Melvin, K. E. W.: Medullary carcinoma of the thyroid gland. Studies of thyrocalcitonin in plasma and tumor extracts. N. Eng. J. Med., *279*:279, 1968.

47. Tashjian, A. H., Jr., Howland, B. G., Melvin, K. E. W., and Hill, C. S., Jr.: Immuno-assay of human calcitonin. Clinical mea-surement, relation to serum calcium and studies in patients with medullary carci-noma. N. Eng. J. Med., *283*:890, 1970.

48. Melvin, K. E. W., Miller, H. H., and Tash-jian, A. H., Jr.: Very early diagnosis of medullary carcinoma of the thyroid by means of calcitonin assay. N. Eng. J. Med., *285*:1115, 1971.

49. DeLuca, H. F.: The dynamics of vitamin D metabolism: a new component of calcium homeostatis. *In* Frame, B., *et al.*: Clinical Aspects of Metabolic Bone Disease. Ex-cerpta Medica, Amsterdam, 1973.

50. Kodicek, E.: The story of vitamin D from vitamin to hormone. Lancet, *1*:325, 1974.

51. Avioli, L. V.: Vitamin D_3 metabolism in man and its relation to disorders of mineral metabolism. *In* Frame, B., *et al.*: Clinical Aspects of Metabolic Bone Disease. Ex-cerpta Medica, Amsterdam, 1973.

52. Belsey, R., DeLuca, H. F., and Potts, J. T., Jr.: Competitive binding assay for vitamin D and 25 OH vitamin D. J. Clin. Endo-crinol. *22*:554, 1971.

53. Haddad, J. G., and Chyu, K. J.: Competitive protein binding radioassay for 25-hydroxy-cholecalciferol. J. Clin. Endocrinol., *33*: 992, 1971.

54. Belsey, R., Clark, M., DeLuca, H. F., and Potts, J. T. Jr.: A direct assay for 25 OH vitamin D_3. *In* Frame B., *et al.*: Clinical Aspects of Metabolic Bone Disease. Ex-cerpta Medica, Amsterdam, 1973.

21 The Renin-Angiotensin System and Aldosterone

KEVIN CATT, M.D., PH.D., AND JANICE DOUGLAS, M.D.

Abnormalities in the activity of the renin-angiotensin system and the secretion of aldosterone, are frequently encountered in clinical disorders characterized by hypertension and/or disturbances in electrolyte metabolism. Although the renin-angiotensin system is only one of several factors which influence aldosterone secretion in vivo, there is abundant evidence that plasma renin levels and aldosterone secretion usually show a close correlation in the human during normal sodium balance, and during minor degrees of sodium restriction. This association has been observed also during fluctuations accompanying postural change, circadian variations, and short-term secretory changes, and is consistent with the current view that the renin-angiotensin system is a significant regulating factor of aldosterone secretion in man under normal dietary conditions.[1,2,3] However, departures from parity between renin and aldosterone during induced sodium depletion and repletion in animals and man indicate that the actions of other regulatory determinants of aldosterone secretion may predominate under certain circumstances.[4,5,6] The relative influences of ACTH, potassium balance, serum sodium and other possible trophic factors upon aldosterone secretion during sodium depletion have proven to be extremely complex, and are not yet completely elucidated. Despite this complexity, the demonstrated role of the renin-angiotensin system as a major regulator of aldosterone secretion, under normal conditions and in disease states, clearly indicates the need for evaluation of renin secretion during the diagnostic interpretation of disorders of aldosterone secretion. The trophic relationship between angiotensin II and the zona glomerulosa of the adrenal cortex has been demonstrated by the results of numerous experimental observations in animals and man.[7,8] Additional evidence for this interaction has been provided by clinical studies which demonstrate a close association between increased renin secretion and elevated aldosterone production,[9,10] and conversely by the classic demonstration of suppressed renin levels in the presence of autonomous hypersecretion of aldosterone by the adrenal gland.[11,12] For these reasons, and because of their frequently associated diagnostic significance in clinical medicine, it is convenient to consider together the methodologic aspects of procedures for the determination of renin-angiotensin activity and aldosterone secretion.

THE RENIN-ANGIOTENSIN SYSTEM

The renin-angiotensin system consists of a group of interacting renal and plasma proteins leading to the formation of angiotensin II, an octapeptide which exerts potent effects upon smooth muscle, the adrenal cortex, and the nervous system. The "classical" scheme describing this system is illustrated in Figure 21-1. Renin, a proteolytic enzyme released from the cells of the juxtaglomerular apparatus, acts upon renin substrate, a plasma α_2 globulin, to liberate the decapeptide angiotensin I, which is rapidly cleaved to form angiotensin II by converting enzymes present predominantly in lung and to a lesser extent in kidney and plasma. Angiotensin II is rapidly degraded by "angiotensinases" present in plasma and tissues; the half-life of angiotensin II in the circulation is less than 1 minute, and plasma angiotensin II is largely inactivated during a single circulation through tissue-vascular beds. The octapeptide is the most potent pressor agent known, and has long been proposed to play a role in the regulation of normal blood pressure, as well as in the initiation or maintenance of certain forms of hypertension, particularly those associated with renal ischemia. However, although a direct relationship between angiotensin II and elevated blood pressure has been demonstrated in several types of experimental and clinical hypertension of renal origin, precise definition of the role of angiotensin II in hypertension is frequently complicated by the effects of associated changes in body fluid volume and sodium metabolism, which modify the secretion rate and pressor activity of circulating angiotensin II.

The effectiveness with which angiotensin stimulates aldosterone secretion varies markedly in different species, but is well established in man. The influence of angiotensin II on aldosterone production by the glomerulosa cells of the adrenal cortex has been implicated as the cause of excessive aldosterone secretion which occurs in a variety of conditions characterized by increased renin secretion with electrolyte disturbances and sometimes edema, but frequently with normal blood pressure. The sodium retention and body fluid expansion caused by aldosterone normally lead to a decrease in renin release from the kidney, and thus act to reduce angiotensin II formation. Also, plasma angiotensin II exerts a direct negative feedback effect upon the kidney to reduce renin secretion so that rising levels of circulating angiotensin II tend to reduce plasma renin levels under normal physiological conditions. However, most conditions associated with pathologically increased blood angiotensin II and aldosterone levels are characterized by an abnormal rise in renin secretion, and occur under circumstances in which the negative feedback control does not operate effectively.

Actions of angiotensin II upon the nervous system have also been well documented, particularly the potentiation of sensitivity to catecholamines in the autonomic control of peripheral vessels, and the regulation of the CNS-mediated mechanism controlling water intake in response to thirst. However, the major actions of clinical relevance are those concerned with blood pressure regulation and mineralocorticoid secretion, and it is

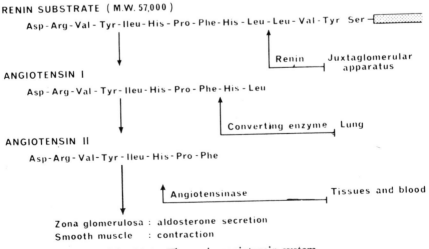

Fig. 21-1. The renin-angiotensin system.

with these aspects that the present description is concerned.

Since angiotensin II is the final product of the reaction between renin and plasma renin substrate, the activity of the renin-angiotensin system is most directly indicated by the level of angiotensin II in the circulation. Determination of angiotensin II in blood or plasma extracts has been performed by radioimmunoassay employing antisera to the octapeptide and radioiodinated angiotensin II as tracer. The circulating levels of angiotensin II in blood are extremely low, with a mean value of about 25 pg/ml. Such assays have shown that blood angiotensin II levels are significantly elevated in a high proportion of patients with renal hypertension and malignant hypertension; a less-marked increase is frequently present in women during oral contraceptive therapy.[13] The technical difficulties in measuring angiotensin II in blood are such that the method has been established in only a few laboratories, and much wider use has been made of the relatively more simple assay procedures for plasma renin. Since angiotensin II levels are generally a direct reflection of the plasma renin activity, measurement of plasma renin has been more commonly employed to evaluate the activity of the renin-angiotensin system. Radioimmunoassay of angiotensin I generated during incubation of plasma at 37°C provides a useful estimate of the plasma renin content, providing a measure of renin activity in terms of the product of the reaction between enzyme and substrate. Such incubations are carried out under conditions designed to protect the generated angiotensin I from degradation or conversion to angiotensin II. The duration of incubation should be chosen to give linear generation of angiotensin I, thus providing a measure of the initial velocity of the reaction between renin and substrate. The relatively large quantities of angiotensin I generated during incubation in vitro, up to several ng/ml of plasma per hour, are readily measured by radioimmunoassay. When the procedure is performed by incubation of plasma alone, the angiotensin I generation

rate represents the plasma renin activity (PRA) (i.e., the product of the action of endogenous renin upon endogenous substrate). Because the concentration of plasma renin substrate (PRS) can also influence the rate of the renin reaction, the PRA is not always directly proportional to the concentration of renin in plasma. For the measurement of plasma renin concentration (PRC), it is necessary to add exogenous renin substrate to the plasma sample in order to reach saturating levels of substrate at which the generation of angiotensin I depends only upon the concentration of renin. An alternative procedure for assay of the PRC depends upon the addition of known quantities of renin to plasma samples to determine by extrapolation the endogenous renin concentration responsible for angiotensin I generation (i.e., the PRA) in the absence of added renin. These procedures are described in more detail below.

Control of Renin Secretion

There is still uncertainty about the relative roles of renin as an intrarenal regulatory factor and as a circulating source of the pressor peptide angiotensin II. However, the implication of the renin-angiotensin system in the pathogenesis of certain forms of hypertension, notably malignant and renovascular hypertension, and in the control of aldosterone secretion and plasma volume homeostasis, indicates that secretion of renin into the circulation leads to important extrarenal effects which contribute to the pathophysiology of several clinical conditions. The numerous factors which influence renin secretion are believed to operate through 2 major intrarenal mechanisms:

1. A baroreceptor in the afferent arterioles which is responsive to changes in tension of the vessel wall, and is modulated by the renal sympathetic nerves.[14,15,16]

2. A sodium-sensitive receptor in the macula densa which responds to alterations in the sodium content of the tubule fluid.[17]

The baroreceptor mechanism appears to be the dominant controlling factor, and accounts for the marked dependence of renin secretion upon the mean renal perfusion pressure and extracellular fluid volume. The effects of hemorrhage and other disturbances of plasma volume upon renin secretion are believed to operate through this mechanism. The role of the macula densa receptor is less well defined, but may be of more importance as an intrarenal regulating mechanism to control the functional activity of each nephron.[18] The macula densa may also operate as an intrarenal cation-sensitive mechanism to provide fine regulation of renin secretion during normal fluctuations of sodium and potassium balance. Renin secretion and plasma renin activity, like aldosterone secretion and plasma aldosterone levels, generally show a close inverse relationship with sodium intake and plasma sodium concentration. The effects of potassium upon renin secretion are similar to those of sodium, with increased plasma renin during potassium depletion and decreased renin levels after potassium loading. However, alterations in potassium balance have opposite actions to those of sodium upon aldosterone secretion, with stimulation following potassium administration and reduction during depletion of potassium.[19,20] Thus, high potassium intake can lead to a reduction in plasma renin activity and a concomitant increase in aldosterone secretion.

Aldosterone Secretion and Metabolism

The major actions of aldosterone are upon ion transport in the distal tubule of the kidney, to increase sodium reabsorption and potassium excretion. Secretion of aldosterone from the glomerulosa layer of the adrenal cortex is predominantly controlled by dietary sodium and potassium under normal circumstances; additional factors, including posture and stress, may operate to modify the rate of aldosterone secretion and metabolism.[21] The manner in which alterations in electrolyte balance influence the glomerulosa cells is quite complex, and includes several well-recognized mechanisms.

1. The renin-angiotensin system, by way of angiotensin II.
2. A direct effect of serum potassium.
3. The direct action of ACTH.
4. Reduced serum sodium concentration.
5. An additional factor which may operate during sodium depletion.

The secretion rate of aldosterone in normal subjects is 75 to 150 μg/day, and the steroid has a plasma half-life of 20 to 30 minutes. Metabolic clearance is rapid, due to lack of a specific plasma-binding protein, and metabolism occurs predominantly in the liver (to tetrahydroaldosterone) and to a lesser extent in the kidney, to the 18-glucuronide of aldosterone. The plasma level of aldosterone is 5 to 15 ng/100 ml, being lowest in samples obtained from supine subjects. Urinary excretion of aldosterone has been most frequently measured by acid hydrolysis of the 18-glucuronide metabolite, the upper level of this "pH 1 fraction" being about 15 μg per day in normal subjects during usual dietary conditions.

Factors Which Influence Renin Secretion

Determinants of Renin Secretion and PRC/PRA in Normal Subjects. In man, the most important factors influencing renin secretion and PRA under normal conditions are:

1. *Posture.* Recumbent PRA levels are usually substantially lower than those measured in the upright position.

2. *Diurnal variation.* In both the recumbent and upright positions, a diurnal variation in PRA has been observed with maximal levels at 11 A.M. to noon followed by a decline over the succeeding several hours.

3. *Sodium balance.* PRA is suppressed by high sodium intake, and is increased during low sodium intake. The action of dietary potassium is similar, though less marked. Knowledge of the prevailing dietary sodium content is essential for the interpretation of plasma renin measurements performed during diagnostic evaluation.

4. *Age, sex and race.* Little is known about the effects of age on renin secretion in

normal subjects, apart from the observation of high PRA levels in the neonatal period. PRA values are generally similar in men and women under comparable dietary conditions. However, a rise in PRA has been observed during the luteal phase of the menstrual cycle, and is attributed to the natriuretic effect of progesterone secreted at this time. During pregnancy, marked elevations of PRS, PRC, and PRA are observed from the first few weeks following conception, and persist until term.[22] Oral contraceptive therapy or other forms of estrogen treatment are accompanied by a marked and consistent increase in PRS, with a variable effect on PRA ranging from normal to increased values, and usually with a significant decrease in renin secretion as reflected by the PRC.[23,24]

No systematic studies on the normal ranges for renin levels in different populations have been performed, and dietary sodium content is probably the major variable to be considered when comparing renin data obtained in different ethnic groups. However, the occurrence of low or suppressed PRA levels has been observed recently in a significant proportion of normotensive black subjects, whereas this appears to be a relatively uncommon finding in normotensive whites.

Alterations of Renin Secretion and PRC/PRA During Disease States and Drug Therapy. Pharmacologic and pathophysiologic effects on renin secretion are seen in a wide variety of circumstances that are mainly associated with changes in blood pressure, sodium balance, or mineralocorticoid secretion.

1. *Increased renin secretion.* Sodium restriction, sodium loss and diuretic administration are potent stimuli to renin secretion. The combination of sodium depletion and reduction of blood pressure is particularly effective, and it is not surprising that some of the highest PRA values are seen in untreated Addison's disease, or postadrenalectomy with inadequate steroid replacement. The long-term effects of chronic diuretic treatment are less certain, and renin levels probably lie in the normal range in many patients in prolonged diuretic therapy for nonedematous states. However, renin levels tend to be higher during continued diuretic treatment for salt and fluid retention, and are frequently elevated during administration of aldosterone antagonists such as spironolactone.

A variety of hypotensive agents, including nitroprusside and diazoxide, are also potent acute stimuli for renin release.

2. *Reduced and suppressed renin secretion.* Low plasma renin levels, which do not rise following the stimulus of sodium restriction and diuretic administration, were first observed as a characteristic of primary aldosteronism and have become established as one of the diagnostic criteria of that condition.[25] In addition, low or suppressed plasma renin has since been recognized to be relatively common in patients with essential hypertension, occurring in 20 to 40 percent of the hypertensive population.[26] Estimates for the incidence of low-renin hypertension have varied considerably according to the racial composition of the hypertensive patient groups studied, being more common in black patients than in whites, and also according to the criteria employed to define the condition of low-renin hypertension. In general, 3 methods of selection have been used.

(a) Subdivision of hypertensive patients into low, normal and high renin groups by comparison of random renin values with those of an appropriate normotensive control group. This is the least satisfactory method.

(b) Subdivision by comparison of plasma renin activity and 24-hour sodium excretion with the normal range for both factors in a normotensive population.

(c) Selection of low-renin patients as those in whom the basal PRA value is below the normal range, and remains low despite the stimulus of low sodium diet and/or diuretic administration. This is the most reliable method for identifying patients with suppressed PRA.

Clinical Implications of Low-Renin Hypertension

The significance of low-renin essential hypertension has not yet been clarified, but appears likely to reside in the relation to volume-dependent factors; definition of the condition may be of value for selection of patients most likely to show a satisfactory blood pressure response to diuretic therapy.

Previously, low-renin hypertension has been proposed to be of major significance as a manifestation of mineralocorticoid excess, caused by steroids other than aldosterone. This line of reasoning, based on the analogy with primary aldosteronism, has led to the recognition that occasional patients with low-renin hypertension excrete an excessive quantity of a weak mineralocorticoid (18 hydroxy DOC) in their urine; in addition, a very small number of patients has been found to exhibit excessive secretion of DOC from the adrenal gland, usually from an adenoma.[27] Apart from these examples, the search for a cryptic mineralocorticoid to explain the relatively high incidence of low-renin hypertension has not been fruitful.

Additional interest in low-renin hypertension has been stimulated by the proposal that such patients may be protected from the vascular complications of hypertension, particularly strokes and myocardial infarction.[28] However, analysis of the incidence of such complications in several series of hypertensive patients has failed to confirm this suggestion, and has shown that the frequency of strokes and heart attacks in patients with uncomplicated essential hypertension bears no relationship to the plasma renin activity.[29,30,31] Therefore, there is no indication to perform PRA measurements for prediction of the likelihood of complications in patients with hypertension. Nevertheless, the detection of low-renin hypertension remains an important diagnostic responsibility of the hypertension clinic, as an adjunct to the diagnosis of mineralocorticoid hyperten-

sion, and as an index of the likelihood that control of blood pressure will be achieved by therapy with diuretics or spironolactone.

Determination of Plasma Renin Parameters—PRA and PRC

All current procedures for renin assay are based upon the enzymatic action of plasma renin upon plasma renin substrate, with measurement of the angiotensin I generated during a period of incubation in vitro under defined conditions.[32-35] Although the principle of such renin assays is quite simple, a degree of confusion has been caused by the influence of 3 major factors.

1. Methods have been developed for measurement of 2 related but different parameters—plasma renin activity (PRA) and plasma renin concentration (PRC).

2. For measurement of both PRA and PRC, different conditions have been employed in various laboratories; there is no standard procedure for either assay.

3. Until recently, no standard preparations of renin or angiotensin I have been available.

For these reasons, it is not possible to provide a description of a single, universally accepted method for renin assay. However, the several variations in assay technique can be grouped into a small number of essentially similar procedures, which will be described with comments upon their individual advantages or deficiencies.

Assay of PRA. All methods are based upon the incubation of plasma samples without addition of exogenous renin or substrate. The generated angiotensin I therefore represents the resultant of the action of circulating renin upon endogenous substrate, and thus provides a useful measure of the effective activity of the prevailing plasma renin concentration. It is important to note that the generation of angiotensin I in vitro during incubation of plasma is influenced by several factors in addition to the major determining action of the endogenous plasma renin concentration.

1. *The conditions of blood sample col-*

Fig. 21-2. Influence of renin substrate concentration upon the generation of angiotensin I by increasing concentrations of human renin. (The standard renin preparation was obtained through the kindness of Dr. E. Haas.)

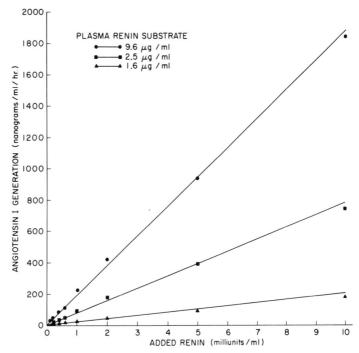

lection. In addition to the effects of sodium intake and drug therapy on prevailing renin levels, more short-term variations relevant to sample collection should also be controlled. The well-known effects of posture and diurnal variation upon renin secretion require that standard conditions for sample collection be employed if valid comparisons are to be made between various sets of renin determinations. Unless recumbent samples are required for particular studies, the most general approach is to collect venous blood samples during the late morning after patients have been up and about for 3 to 4 hours. Blood is taken into chilled tubes containing EDTA to give a final concentration of about 2.5 mM. Heparin has been shown to inhibit the renin reaction at concentrations of 5 U/ml, and should not be employed as an anticoagulant in blood samples taken for renin assay. EDTA has the additional advantage of protecting angiotensin I from conversion and degradation during plasma incubation. Blood samples are immediately placed into ice and transported to the laboratory for separation of

plasma in a refrigerated centrifuge, followed by storage at -15°C or below. Little is recorded about the stability of plasma renin during storage, but no loss of activity is apparent in samples stored at -15°C for up to several months. It is important to note that renin activity is not completely inhibited by low temperature, and that significant generation of angiotensin I can occur in plasma samples kept for several hours at 0 to 4°C. This results in a higher "blank" in the assay system unless plasma samples are pretreated to remove endogenous angiotensin I prior to assay—a step not widely performed and not usually necessary. The true endogenous circulating level of angiotensin I is extremely low (< 50 pg/ml), and does not significantly contribute to the blank of the assay. The "blank" determined in many assay procedures, by measurement of the immunoreactive material present in an aliquot of each plasma sample kept at 4°C for 3 hours, is largely caused by a minor nonspecific interfering effect of plasma in the immunoassay, and by a variable amount of angiotensin I generated during blood collection and plasma preparation. In some methods, addition of a constant proportion of plasma to the assay tubes has been performed to minimize the nonspecific effect of aliquots of incubated plasma in the radioimmunoassay.

2. *The concentration of plasma renin substrate*. Because the circulating concentration of plasma renin substrate is of the same order as the Km of the renin-substrate reaction, variations in plasma renin substrate can significantly influence the rate of angiotensin I generation by a given concentration of plasma renin (Fig. 21-2). The normal range for renin substrate concentration is relatively narrow (1.56 ± 0.35 μg/ml), but significant variations in the rate of the reaction can occur at the extremes of the normal substrate concentration range. In general, effects of substrate concentration upon PRA appear to be negligible at normal substrate levels. However, marked increases in renin substrate occur during pregnancy and oral contraceptive therapy, and significantly enhance the activity of a given concentration of plasma renin. Also, a less striking but significant increase in PRS has been observed in patients with malignant hypertension.[36]

3. *Conditions of incubation*.

(a) The pH of plasma during incubation. There is no agreement concerning the "correct" pH for renin assay; the 2 major alternatives are to incubate at "physiological" pH (7.4) or at the pH optimum of the enzyme-substrate reaction in plasma, which is close to 6.0. Whichever condition is employed, it is essential to ensure that the chosen pH is maintained throughout the period of incubation by addition of an appropriate buffer. The pH of untreated plasma always rises during incubation at 37°C by an average of about one pH unit. Similarly, acidification of plasma to the region of the pH optimum must also be accompanied by addition of buffer to prevent a rise during incubation. The major advantage of incubation at pH 6 is the greater generation of angiotensin I (about twofold) with correspondingly better sensitivity for low-renin plasma samples. However, proponents of the pH 7.4 pro-

cedure, while conceding the need for a buffer to maintain this pH, have shown that generation of immunoreactive angiotensin I is detectable after incubation of nephrectomized human plasma at pH 5.7, presumably due to the action of nonrenal proteolytic enzymes in plasma, whereas no such effect is detectable after incubation at pH 7.4.

(b) The extent of plasma dilution. In general, dilution of plasma during renin assay is avoided because the renin reaction is substrate-dependent at the concentration of renin substrate which exists in plasma under most normal circumstances. A minor dilution caused by pH adjustment and addition of inhibitors cannot be avoided, but has little effect on the rate of the renin reaction in normal plasma if kept below +20 percent of the original plasma volume. A twofold dilution of plasma reduces angiotensin generation by 12 to 20 percent (Fig. 21-3), and more marked effects are seen at higher dilutions. It should be noted that this effect is also amenable to standardization, and that the use of minimally diluted plasma for renin assay is based upon custom rather than on a well-defined scientific requirement.

(c) Efficacy of chemical inhibitors of converting enzyme and "angiotensinase" activity. A variety of agents have been employed to "protect" generated angiotensin I from conversion to angiotensin II (which is not detected by radioimmunoassay for angiotensin I) and from proteolytic degradation during incubation at 37°C. The most universal agent employed to block converting enzyme is EDTA, which is the preferred anticoagulant for blood samples to be subjected to renin assay. It is also an inhibitor of angiotensinase and has been used for this purpose in earlier bioassay procedures in association with acidification, heating or dialysis of plasma to destroy angiotensinase activity. Such physical manipulations are no longer employed, having been replaced by additional chemical inhibitors including diisopropylfluorophosphate (DFP), dimercaprol (BAL), and 2,2′ dipyridyl. Until recently, the most effective single inhibitor was

Fig. 21-3. Effect of a twofold dilution of plasma upon the determination of PRA. Dilution of plasma by addition of an equal volume of 0.5 M sodium acetate buffer pH 6.0 causes a mean decrease of 12 percent in the rate of the renin reaction.

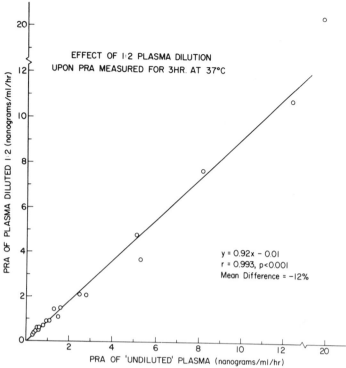

EFFECT OF 1:2 PLASMA DILUTION
UPON PRA MEASURED FOR 3HR. AT 37°C

$y = 0.92x - 0.01$
$r = 0.993, p < 0.001$
Mean Difference = −12%

PRA OF PLASMA DILUTED 1:2 (nanograms/ml/hr)

PRA OF 'UNDILUTED' PLASMA (nanograms/ml/hr)

undoubtedly DFP, which, when present in concentrations of about 7 mM in EDTA-treated plasma provides almost complete protection of angiotensin I from conversion and degradation. DFP has most frequently been employed as an inhibitor in assays performed at pH 5.5 to 6.0, but has also been claimed to be effective at pH 7.4. For incubations performed at pH 7.4, the most frequently employed inhibitors, in addition to EDTA, have been BAL and 8-hydroxy-quinoline. This combination is said to be less effective at lower pH but gives good recovery of angiotensin I generated during incubation at pH 7.4.

Recently, the availability of alternative protease inhibitors of considerably lower toxicity than DFP has increased the convenience and safety of this class of compound for routine assay use. We have found that 5 mM phenylmethyl sulfonylfluoride (PMSF) is somewhat more effective than DFP as a protective agent during renin assay at pH 6.0, and is considerably easier to handle than the volatile and highly toxic

DFP. At present, the combination of EDTA and PMSF appears to be the inhibitory procedure of choice for plasma incubation during renin assay.

(d) Duration of incubation. Most incubations for plasma renin assay are performed for a period of 3 hours. In principle, the shortest practical time should be employed for determination of enzyme activity to provide the best estimate of initial velocity of the reaction, and to minimize substrate consumption and possible inhibitory effects of the reaction products. The sensitivity of most direct radioimmunoassay methods for generated angiotensin I is such that incubation for at least 3 hours are necessary to permit precise determination of the PRA of many low-renin plasma samples. With recent emphasis on the prevalence and possible significance of low-renin hypertension, the need for accurate measurement of angiotensin I generation rates below 1 ng/ml per hour has indicated that more prolonged incubation of plasma, for up to 18 hours, may be required for precise measurement of

PRA in a significant proportion of plasma samples.

Whichever duration is employed for incubation, it is necessary to demonstrate that linear generation of angiotensin I occurs throughout the incubation period, and that recovery of angiotensin I is adequately ensured by the inhibitors added to plasma prior to incubation. With plasma samples of high-renin content, incubation for more than a few hours may be accompanied by a significant decline in reaction rate due to consumption of substrate. Therefore, the most suitable compromise is to employ a standard incubation period of 3 hours, with reassay of low-renin and extremely high-renin samples for appropriately prolonged or abbreviated periods to provide precise estimates at the extremes of the range encountered in clinical assay samples.

4. *Endogenous inhibitors of the renin reaction.* Although the presence of an inhibitor of renal origin has been described in plasma, there is little evidence to show that such factors influence the rate of the renin reaction under the conditions employed for assay of plasma renin activity.

Representative Assay Methods for PRA

Incubation at pH 7.4. Plasma samples are thawed and 1 ml aliquots are kept in an ice bath during addition of the following reagents.

Reagent	Volume Added per ml Plasma (μl)	Final Plasma Concentration (mM)*
2.0 M Tris-HCl buffer pH 7.4	25	50
1.0 M BAL in ethanol	5	5
0.5 M 8-hydroxyquinoline†	10	5
0.5 M Disodium EDTA†	10	>5‡

* These concentrations are given in round figures without correction for the small effect of plasma dilution of +5%.
† These reagents can be made up in a single solution, 0.25 M in each inhibitor, from which 20 μl is added per ml of plasma. Alternatively, reagents

After addition of buffer and inhibitors, an aliquot of the treated plasma (e.g., 250 μl) is transferred into precooled tubes and maintained at 0 to 4°C in an ice bath for 3 hours. The tubes containing the main portion of the plasma samples are incubated at 37°C for 3 hours in a circulating water bath, then transferred back to the ice bath for removal of aliquots into radioimmunoassay tubes. (If necessary, the incubated samples can be immediately frozen and later thawed for radioimmunoassay.) The optimal size of the aliquots taken for assay depend upon the sensitivity of the radioimmunoassay and on the renin activity of the sample. In general, 2 pairs of aliquots (e.g., 10 μl and 25 μl, each in duplicate) should be taken from each incubated plasma sample, and 1 pair of aliquots (e.g., 25 μl, in duplicate) from the plasma sample kept in ice to determine the "4° blank" of each sample.

Incubation at pH 5.5-6.0. The pH-dependency curve for renin activity is relatively flat in this region, and there is little to choose between the variously employed pH levels of 5.5, 5.7 and 6.0. Assays can be performed with the BAL/EDTA inhibitors described above, or with more potent inhibitors such as DFP or PMSF.

1. *Assay of plasma diluted 1:1, with BAL and EDTA.* The procedure for determination of renin parameters by incubation of plasma diluted with an equal volume of 0.5 M sodium acetate buffer, containing disodium EDTA (20 mM), BAL (10 mM) and 8-hydroxyquinoline (5 mM) is illus-

2, 3 and 4 can be replaced by 25 μl of 0.2 M PMSF in isopropanol, to give a final plasma concentration of 5 mM PMSF.
‡ The concentration of EDTA will be greater than 5 mM by the amount of EDTA originally used as anticoagulant. Blood drawn into an EDTA-Vacutainer tube (color code—lavender) to give 1 mg EDTA/ml of blood will give approximately 2.5 mM EDTA in the plasma specimen.

The use of vacutainers containing EDTA as a solution of potassium EDTA permits more rapid dispersion of the anticoagulant in the blood sample, but vacutainers containing disodium EDTA powder are equally satisfactory if adequate mixing is performed.

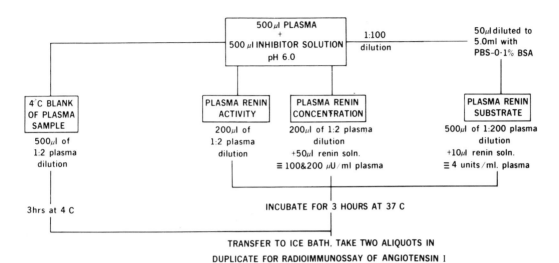

Fig. 21-4. Renin assay procedure for determination of PRA, PRC and PRS in human plasma, by incubation at pH 6.0.

trated in Figure 21-4. Normal values derived for PRA, PRC and PRS by this method are given in Table 21-1.

2. *Assay of undiluted plasma, with PMSF.*

Reagents	Volume Added per ml Plasma (µl)	Final Plasma Concentration (mM)
0.5 M HCl	25	
4.0 M Sodium acetate buffer pH 6.0	40	160
*0.2 M PMSF in isopropanol	25	5

* PMSF provides an effective and safer alternative to DFP, which has previously been used as 20 µl of a 5 percent solution (0.25 M) in isopropanol. In addition, the use of Neomycin sulfate (20 µl of a 10% solution) as a bacteriostatic agent has been recommended during prolonged incubations.

The incubation procedure is performed as for the pH 7.4 procedure described above. Generation of angiotensin I during incubation at pH 6 is usually about twice as great as at pH 7.4, so that correspondingly higher angiotensin levels are present in the aliquots taken for radioimmunoassay. For high-renin samples, it may therefore be necessary to make a dilution of the incubated plasma (e.g., 1:4) before taking aliquots for radioimmunoassay. In addition to the need for dilution to obtain suitable aliquots lying in the optimal portion of the radioimmunoassay standard curve, plasma samples with extremely high-renin content should be subjected to reincubation for shorter time periods (½-1 hr) if it is desired to obtain an accurate estimate of the true PRA (i.e., the

Table 21-1. Normal Values for PRA, PRC and PRS Determined in Blood Donors and Ambulant Males (mean ± SD).

	PRA (ng/ml/hr)	PRC (µ units/ml)	PRS (µg/ml)
Blood donors (Recumbent 1 hr)	(32) 1.66 ± 0.96	(27) 28.5 ± 19.1	(51) 1.56 ± 0.35
Ambulant males	(20) 2.86 ± 2.1	(20) 44.0 ± 31.9	

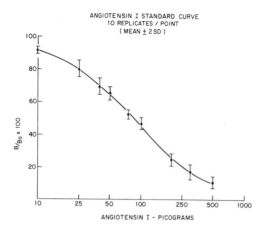

Fig. 21-5. Standard curve for radioimmunoassay of angiotensin I. The within-assay precision of the standard curve is indicated by the vertical bars.

initial velocity determined prior to significant consumption of renin substrate).

Radioimmunoassay of Angiotensin I

The reagents required for radioimmunoassay include a specific, high-affinity antiserum against angiotensin I, a preparation of monoiodinated ^{125}I-labeled angiotensin I, and a suitably pure and accurate standard of angiotensin I. Assays are usually performed by equilibration of antibody with tracer and angiotensin standards or aliquots of incubated plasma, at 4°C for 16 to 24 hours. Separation of antibody-bound and free tracer is most commonly performed by adsorption

of the free peptide to charcoal.[35] Standard curves are usually suitable for measurement of angiotensin I over the range from 5 to 250 pg and show relatively high within-assay precision (Fig. 21-5). The availability of radioimmunoassay kits for angiotensin I has simplified the setting up of such assays in laboratories without ready access to the reagents required for the procedure. Although there is considerable variation in the assay methodology recommended by such kits, this is largely confined to the incubation procedure, and the radioimmunoassay technique is fairly consistent. The antibody and tracer angiotensin I supplied in presently available commercial kits have in our experience been satisfactory. The most important source of potential error lies in the standards supplied in kits, which for reasons of convenience to the consumer are commonly supplied in extremely dilute form (e.g., 10 ng/ml). It has become recognized that angiotensin I, unlike angiotensin II, is relatively unstable during storage at low concentrations. Apart from the intrinsic instability of the peptide, additional problems may arise from the occasional presence of angiotensinase activity in proteins employed as constituents of the diluent solution in which the peptide is stored. This problem could be overcome by provision of standards in lyophilized form, with an appropriate protein carrier or excipient.

1. *Antiserum.* Antisera to angiotensin I

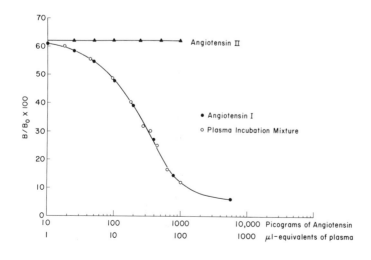

Fig. 21-6. Radioimmunoassay of angiotensin I. The peptide generated during incubation of plasma (O—O) gives a binding-inhibition curve identical to that of the synthetic angiotensin I standards. There is no significant cross-reactivity with angiotensin II (▲—▲).

are prepared by immunization of rabbits with conjugates formed by coupling angiotensin I to a larger and more immunogenic carrier protein. Conjugation to albumin and gamma globulin has been widely performed by the use of water-soluble carbodiimides; more recently, coupling to thyroglobulin with glutaraldehyde has also been shown to provide a highly immunogenic complex suitable for eliciting high-titer antisera in rabbits. Antisera to angiotensin I are usually highly specific, with only a small degree ($< 5\%$) of cross-reaction against angiotensin II (Fig. 21-6). Although the titer of the antiserum is a relatively unimportant factor in determining suitability for radioimmunoassay, high-titer antisera have the advantage of permitting the widespread and/or long-term use of a single well-characterized batch of antibody. The affinity of the antiserum for angiotensin I should be high if adequate sensitivity is to be attained. The maximal attainable sensitivity of a radioimmunoassay is approximately related to the association constant (Ka) of the antiserum by the function: Sensitivity = 0.1/Ka, when sensitivity is defined as the lowest peptide concentration which is significantly distinguished from zero in the assay. Many angiotensin I antisera can be employed at a final dilution in the region of 1:50,000 or higher, and possess affinity constants of the order of 10^{10} M^{-1} (Fig. 21-7).

Apart from the affinity of the antiserum, a further important characteristic is the susceptibility of individual angiotensin antisera to nonspecific interference by plasma added directly to the assay system. This effect varies considerably with different antisera, and can be minimized by selection of antisera which give the lowest reading for blank plasmas (preferably suppressed-renin, nephrectomized-patient or charcoal-stripped normal plasma) which have *not* been incubated at 37°C.

2. *Tracer angiotensin I.* Monoiodinated ^{125}I-labeled angiotensin I tracer of suitable purity and high specific activity (> 500 µc/µg) is available from several commercial sources (e.g., Schwarz-Mann; New England Nuclear). The storage life of such labeled angiotensin I is usually 3 to 5 weeks, and each fresh batch of tracer must be tested for binding to antibody and adsorption to charcoal, before being employed for large-scale assay of angiotensin I generated in plasma samples. It is advisable to subdivide the tracer into small aliquots for storage in the frozen state, to avoid thawing and refreezing of the labeled peptide for each assay.

3. *Angiotensin I standards.* Each laboratory should possess a quantity of standard angiotensin I for use as a reference preparation, or as a source of the diluted angiotensin I solution employed for addition to the radioimmunoassay for construction of the standard curve. For this purpose, a well-characterized commercial preparation of syn-

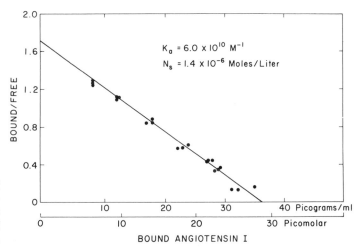

Fig. 21-7. Scatchard plot of antibody-binding data for angiotensin I. The equilibrium association constant (Ka) of the antibody is 6×10^{10} M^{-1}.

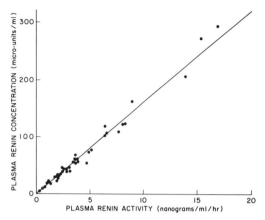

Fig. 21-8. Correlation between PRC (expressed as μ units of Haas human renin per ml plasma) and PRA in plasma samples of normal renin substrate content. When PRS is in the normal range, PRA is linearly related to the PRC.

thetic angiotensin I, of known amino-acid composition and biological activity, is made up as a stock solution, checked by optical density at 275 nm, and stored as frozen or lyophilized aliquots of known concentration. At monthly intervals, aliquots of the stock standard peptide are appropriately diluted to an intermediate standard solution of 10 μg/ml, and this is in turn stored as frozen small aliquots which are used only once to prepare working solutions for the assay standard curve and then discarded. A more convenient alternative is to prepare lyophilized aliquots from an accurately diluted standard solution in ampules each containing an exact quantity (e.g., 10 ng) of the original angiotensin I standard with a suitable quantity of carrier protein (e.g., 1 mg BSA). Whichever method is employed to obtain consistent intra-laboratory quality control, it is also essential to compare the local standard with a suitable reference preparation of national or international acceptance. For this purpose, the only currently available preparation is the angiotensin I standard supplied by the Division of Standards of the Medical Research Council of the United Kingdom. This consists of a synthetic preparation of Ileu[5] angiotensin I in ampules

containing a quantity of peptide which is defined as 9 Units, and is in fact close to 9 μg of angiotensin I. Properly employed, each of those reference ampules provides standards for about 1,000 assays. However, they are more appropriately applied to the calibration of local laboratory standards, for which commercial preparations of synthetic angiotensin I from commercial sources, such as Schwarz-Mann or Beckman, have been most frequently utilized.

Assay of Plasma Renin Concentration (PRC)

Because the renin-substrate reaction follows second-order kinetics at normal levels of plasma substrate, the plasma renin activity does not necessarily provide a proportionate reflection of the circulating concentration of plasma renin. In fact, the normal range for PRS is so relatively narrow that PRA is for all practical purposes a direct reflection of the PRC in plasma of normal nonpregnant subjects (Fig. 21-8). It is only in conditions characterized by elevated plasma renin substrate, notably during pregnancy or oral contraceptive therapy, that the generation rate of angiotensin I becomes a less reliable index of the PRC (Fig. 21-9). Under normal circumstances, the generation rate of angiotensin I per unit of renin concentration is rather constant, and PRA values can be roughly converted to PRC by application of a suitable proportion factor derived from the angiotensin I generation rate of known quantities of standard renin added to normal plasma.

For more precise measurement of PRC, 2 quite different forms of assay have been devised. The simpler methods, originally developed for use with bioassay of generated angiotensin I, employ addition of an excess of heterologous renin substrate from cow or sheep plasma after inactivation of endogenous renin substrate.[37,38] In this way maximal velocity of the renin reaction was attained and depended only upon the concentration of renin present in the plasma samples. Destruction of endogenous human

Fig. 21-9. Influence of wide variations in endogenous renin substrate concentration upon the angiotensin I generated per unit of renin (i.e., PRS is plotted against the ratio PRA/ PRC, after measurement of the 3 parameters in plasma samples from normal, pregnant and contraceptive-treated women). This figure demonstrates that Michaelis-Menten kinetics apply to the renin-substrate reaction in plasma samples containing endogenous concentrations of substrate which occur during pregnancy and oral contraceptive therapy. The Km of the reaction is close to the concentration of substrate in plasma of normal subjects.

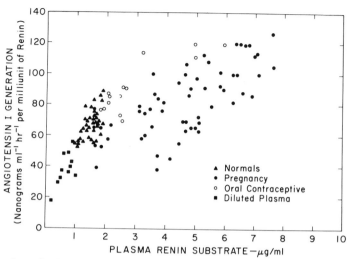

substrate was performed to avoid potential competitive interference during the reaction of renin with the added heterologous substrate. However, a more recent form of PRC assay employed addition of sheep substrate without prior inactivation of endogenous substrate, and was shown to provide a highly sensitive assay for PRC without evidence of competitive interference by the remaining endogenous substrate.[39] In such methods, the PRC is expressed as the maximal velocity of angiotensin I generation (as ng/ml/hr, and can be converted to renin units (e.g., Goldblatt units) by the appropriate factor for angiotensin generation rate per unit of standard renin under the conditions employed for assay.

To overcome the possible effects of factors modifying the renin reaction in individual plasma samples, Haas, et al.,[40] introduced the use of internal calibration of the angiotensin generation rate of each individual plasma sample subjected to PRC, by additional incubations performed in the presence of known concentrations of added standard human renin. Thus, the characteristic angiotensin generation rate per unit of renin is determined and employed to calculate the endogenous renin concentration responsible for the generation rate observed in the absence of added renin. By this method,

renin concentrations in terms of units per milliliter plasma are accurately determined. A modification of this method has been developed in which the renin concentration necessary to account for the PRA is derived by similarly adding standard renin to determine the angiotensin I generation per unit of renin for each plasma sample, with extrapolation to calculate the PRC which corresponds to the PRA of the sample.[34,35]

Assay of Plasma Renin Substrate (PRS)

This assay is relatively rarely required for clinical diagnosis, but is simple enough to perform when the assay method for PRA is an established laboratory procedure. Usually, an excess of homologous renin is added to a small volume of plasma and incubation performed for 2 to 3 hours to permit quantitative conversion of renin substrate into angiotensin I. The usual inhibitors are employed to permit degradation or conversion of the generated angiotensin I, and substrate levels are expressed as μg/ml or as μM, in terms of the angiotensin I formed during incubation. Estimates of the renin substrate content of normal human plasma have varied somewhat, but the mean value is in the region of 1 to 2 μg/ml, rising several-fold during oral contraceptive therapy or pregnancy.[22,23,24]

Assay of Aldosterone in Plasma and Urine

Accurate measurement of aldosterone and its metabolites in plasma and urine previously depended upon relatively elaborate techniques such as double isotope derivative assay, in which labeled derivatives of aldosterone were isolated by multiple chromatographic steps and counted to determine the quantity of steroid present.[41] Extensive losses during purification were corrected by the recovery of a small quantity of labeled aldosterone added prior to extraction from plasma and derivative formation. Such double isotope derivative procedures were extensively employed for physiological and clinical studies of aldosterone secretion and metabolism. They have only recently been replaced by radioimmunoassay methods of equivalent specificity and high sensitivity.

Methods for the determination of aldosterone secretion rate and urinary excretion of aldosterone metabolites have been described in detail[42] and will not be repeated here. Until recently, measurement of the acid-labile glucuronide (pH 1 fraction) or tetrahydro metabolites were mainly employed for clinical diagnosis, and plasma aldosterone assays were performed in only a few laboratories. The upper limit of normal for excretion of the pH 1 fraction is about 15 μg per day, and the normal range for plasma aldosterone is 5 to 20 ng/100 ml.

Development of radioimmunoassays for aldosterone has greatly simplified the measurement of aldosterone in plasma and urine, and has permitted the procedure to be established in laboratories without special expertise in aldosterone methodology. Because the assay of urinary aldosterone excretion provides a useful integrated value of the plasma secretion pattern over a 24-hour period, this measurement continues to be of value in diagnosis, and can most simply be performed by radioimmunoassay after acid hydrolysis of the 18-glucuronide metabolite.[43] However, the present trend is toward determination of the plasma aldosterone concentration, and this is justified by the considerable value of diagnostic tests based upon dynamic changes in plasma aldosterone over short time periods during maneuvers designed to suppress or otherwise evaluate the responsiveness of the peripheral aldosterone level (e.g., upright posture in the distinction between APA* and IHA†). In addition, the plasma assay permits this distinction to be made by selective adrenal venous catheterization, which also enables the location of the lesion to be determined prior to adrenal surgery for APA.[44]

The most readily available antibodies to aldosterone have been produced by immunization of sheep or rabbits with haptenic antigens formed by conjugation of aldosterone-18,21-dihemisuccinate or aldosterone-3-carboxymethyloxime with bovine serum albumin.[45] Like most antisera formed against steroids coupled to protein through existing functional groups, such antisera frequently lack the high immunologic specificity necessary for direct assay of aldosterone in plasma extracts, necessitating the use of at least 1 chromatographic step to permit specific determination of aldosterone in plasma or urine. Although paper chromatography was employed for purification of plasma extracts in the original radioimmunoassays for plasma aldosterone, more recent procedures have utilized partition chromatography on LH-20 columns[46] or thin-layer chromatography.[47] Also, a method for assay of plasma aldosterone has been developed employing antibodies to the oxime of aldosterone-α-lactone; in this procedure, aldosterone is isolated from plasma extracts by cyclohexane-water partition, followed by oxidation to the α-lactone and removal of interfering steroid etienic acids by alkaline washing.[48] In most procedures, the initial extraction step employs methylene chloride (10 vol) for extraction of 2 to 4 ml plasma samples. An alkali-water wash is frequently included before evaporation of the solvent extract under air or nitrogen prior to further purification.

---

* Aldosterone-producing adenoma
† Idiopathic hyperaldosteronism

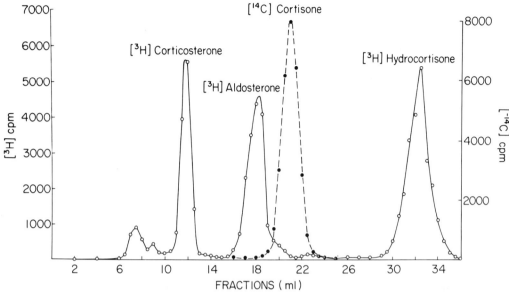

Fig. 21-10. Separation of aldosterone from potentially interfering corticosteroids by column chromatography on Sephadex LH-20. Plasma cortisone is the major source of potential interference in this procedure, and in separations performed by other chromatographic methods.

Methods for Extraction and Purification of Plasma Aldosterone

LH-20 Chromatography. The basic procedure is that described by Ito, *et al.,*[46] in which a methylene chloride extract of plasma is subjected to chromatography on 1 × 60 cm columns of Sephadex LH-20 equilibrated with methylene chloride: methanol 98:2. The order of elution of relevant steroids from such a column is: corticosterone 38 to 46 ml; aldosterone 66 to 72 ml; cortisone 76 to 82 ml; cortisol 118 to 130 ml. Thus, the nearest potentially interfering steroid is cortisone, which is normally present in plasma at concentrations of about 2 μg/ml. The recovery of tritiated aldosterone added as recovery indicator is 56 ± 14 (SD)%. In this method the assay blank is determined largely by the methylene chloride employed for extraction and chromatography, and with purified solvent is less than the limit of sensitivity of the assay (about 6 pg per assay tube). Satisfactory agreement has been demonstrated between this method and a double-isotope derivative technique for assay of plasma aldosterone. The LH-20 columns are washed between uses with 60 ml solvent, and can be used daily for long periods of time without repacking, and with no change in the blank of the assay. The use of smaller columns of LH-20 (0.5 × 20 cm) gives more rapid separation of aldosterone from corticosteroids, with the elution profile shown in Figure 21-10. Once calibrated, the elution position for aldosterone is quite constant, and with minor adjustments for individual columns the recovery of ^{3}H-aldosterone tracer can be improved to the range of 60 to 90 percent. A single technician can process about 60 samples each week by this procedure; as with other techniques, it is convenient to accumulate purified plasma extracts for inclusion in a single radioimmunoassay set up to incubate over the weekend, while recovery aliquots are being counted to accumulate at least 2,000 cpm.

Thin-layer Chromatography. Purification of aldosterone from plasma extracts has been performed by TLC on plates coated with Kieselguhr G, in a solvent system devised to separate aldosterone from other plasma steroids.[47] This method gives a mean recovery of 52 percent, and a blank value (2-10 pg) which is below the sensitivity of the method for aldosterone.

Paper Chromatography. A single paper-chromatography step in the Bush-B5 system has also been utilized prior to radioimmunoassay of plasma aldosterone.[49] Such a method gives satisfactory isolation of aldosterone from other steroids for radioimmunoassay, but is more time-consuming and sometimes more prone to blank problems than the LH-20 and the TLC methods.

Extraction After Oxidation to Aldosterone-α-Lactone. A rapid extraction procedure for use prior to radioimmunoassay with antiserum to aldosterone-α-lactone has employed oxidation of plasma extracts with periodic acid, followed by alkaline washing to separate aldosterone etiolactone from the etienic acids of potentially interfering steroids.[48] This method is sensitive and specific, but the extraction procedure is moderately time-consuming and care must be taken to avoid significant blank values.

Extraction by Aldosterone Antibody. In this method, antiserum to aldosterone is employed for selective isolation of aldosterone from plasma extracts.[50] The procedure is relatively simple and has potential value if abundant and adequately specific antiserum is available. However, the method has not been as thoroughly validated as the alternative procedures described above, and may be less specific than methods which employ chromatography prior to radioimmunoassay. Another version of this approach has utilized an initial extraction with Fuller's earth, to adsorb aldosterone while most of the potentially interfering corticosteroids remain bound to CBG.[51]

Radioimmunoassay of Aldosterone

Although specific antisera suitable for direct assay of aldosterone in simple plasma extracts have been reported,[52] most of the presently available antisera are susceptible to interference by cross-reaction of the high con-

centration of adrenal steroids in plasma. For this reason, assays employing such antisera must be preceded by adequate purification of extracted aldosterone by one of the methods described above. When compared to the elaborate and demanding nature of the double-isotope derivative assay, such purification methods are relatively simple steps to ensure a high degree of specificity in the assay procedure. Certain of the antisera raised against 3-conjugates of aldosterone show relatively low cross-reaction with other steroids, and have been reported to be suitable for direct assay of aldosterone in unpurified extracts of plasma. Even with less specific antisera of the 18,21 hemisuccinate type, the amount of interfering steroid present in methylene chloride extracts of plasma causes only about a twofold increase in the true level of plasma aldosterone, largely due to the cross-reaction of plasma cortisol.

The radioimmunoassay itself is relatively simple to establish, and in most methods employs antiserum against aldosterone-18,21 dihemisuccinate or aldosterone-3-carboxymethyloxime coupled to BSA. An antiserum of the former type[45] is available from the Hormone Distribution Committee of the National Institutes of Health, and can be used for assay at a final concentration of 1 to 2×10^6.

Typically, assays are performed in a phosphate-buffered saline solution containing 1 mg/ml bovine gamma globulin (in addition to the usual role of diluent protein to minimize adsorption artifacts and interference during radioimmunoassay, gamma globulin is an appropriate protein to employ when antiserum is present at high dilution in the assay system). Whichever antiserum is employed, the final dilution is chosen to bind about 50 percent of the added aldosterone tracer.

Tritiated aldosterone of high specific activity (1,2-[3]H: 40-50 Ci/mmole; 1,2,5,6-[3]H: 80 Ci/mmole) is diluted to a convenient concentration (50 μCi/ml) in benzene:ethanol 90:10 and stored at 4°C. Purification of tracer prior to use in the assay by a

Fig. 21-11. Radioimmuno-assay of aldosterone, employing the antiserum (Haning) supplied by the Hormone Distribution Program of the National Institute of Arthritis and Metabolic Diseases, Bethesda, Md. The final dilution of antiserum used in the assay was $1:10^6$, and incubation was performed as described in the text.

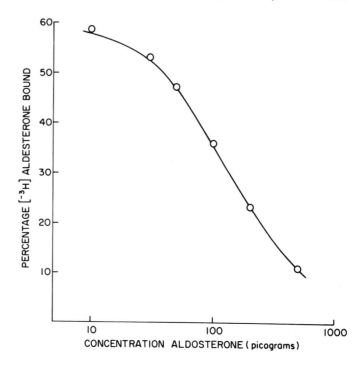

single chromatographic step is sometimes recommended but does not appear to be essential if each fresh batch of tracer is evaluated for binding to antibody and adsorption to charcoal if this adsorbent is used during the separation of antibody-bound and free tracer. An appropriate solution of tracer aldosterone in assay diluent (about 20,000 cpm/ml) is freshly prepared for each assay, and the following reagents are added to 10 × 75 cm glass in polystyrene tubes:

1. Antiserum 1:400,000 in diluent—0.5 ml
2. Aldosterone standards 10-500 pg in diluent—0.1 ml

   or

   aliquots of purified plasma extracts redissolved in diluent—0.1 ml
3. ³H-aldosterone in diluent—0.5 ml

After standing at 4°C for 16 hours (or over the weekend if convenient), separation of bound and free tracer is performed by addition of 0.2 ml of a charcoal suspension containing 5 mg/ml of Norit A in 0.05 percent dextran T70. After mixing, the tubes are stood for 15 to 20 minutes in an ice bath,

then centrifuged at 1,500 g for 15 minutes in a refrigerated centrifuge. The supernatant solutions are decanted into counting vials, followed by the addition of 3 ml dioxane and 10 ml of toluene-based scintillation solution (e.g., Liquifluor* 42 ml/l toluene). After shaking, the radioactivity in each vial is determined by counting in an automatic liquid scintillation spectrometer for sufficient time to accumulate 10,000 cpm.

Other procedures for separation of bound and free tracer include adsorption of free aldosterone to Florisil, and precipitation of the bound tracer by ammonium sulfate or other agents. The charcoal method gives highly precise and reproducible results when used in the manner described, and is somewhat more convenient to perform than the other methods. A typical standard curve for the radioimmunoassay is shown in Figure 21-11. The aldosterone content of plasma samples is most conveniently calculated by computer programs with the facility for simultaneous computation of assay values from the standard curve and corrections for

---

* New England Nuclear

**Table 21-2. Diagnostic Maneuvers to Evaluate Low or High Values
for PRA or Aldosterone.**

	Low Values	*High Values*
Measure PRA after:	Upright posture (3-4 hrs) and acute diuresis (furosemide 120 mg orally) or 10 meq Na diet for 5 days	Overnight recumbency and salt loading (>200 meq Na per day)
Measure aldosterone after:	Salt depletion with constant potassium intake of 80-100 meq/day	High sodium intake (150-200 meq Na^+; 80 meq K^+) for 5 days or until in balance Mineralocorticoid suppression: • DOC acetate 10 mg IM each 12 hrs for 3 days or • Florinef 200 μg by mouth each 8 hrs for 3 days

aliquot factors and individual recovery factors.[53]

Clinical Applications of Renin and Aldosterone Assay

Assays for renin and aldosterone have become particularly useful as adjuncts to the diagnosis of various forms of curable hypertension. As mentioned above, a number of physiologic stimuli, sensed as a decrease in effective blood volume, act through the macula densa and/or baroreceptors of the afferent arterioles to stimulate renin release from the juxtaglomerular cells of the kidney. Factors which acutely stimulate renin release, and in turn aldosterone secretion, include salt depletion, upright posture, hemorrhage and hypotensive drugs or diuretics including diazoxide, hydralazine, nitroprusside and furosemide. Conversely, suppression of plasma renin activity is achieved by recumbency, salt loading, beta-adrenergic blockade (as with propranolol) and mineralocorticoid administration. Changes in serum potassium have a direct effect on aldosterone secretion. Low potassium has an inhibitory effect upon aldosterone secretion, and high potassium directly stimulates the adrenal glomerulosa to cause increased secretion of aldosterone. Therefore, an accurate knowledge of the conditions under which samples for PRA and aldosterone are obtained is essential for appropriate and valid interpretation of the results of plasma assays of these hormones. As with other endocrine diagnostic procedures, more useful information can be derived from the response of PRA and aldosterone to maneuvers designed to suppress or to stimulate renin and aldosterone than from the basal levels of plasma renin activity and aldosterone concentration.

A suggested diagnostic scheme for evaluation of patients with abnormal values for PRA or aldosterone is listed in Table 21-2, with appropriate maneuvers to stimulate or suppress the secretion of renin and aldosterone. The PRA is considered to be suppressed when it remains low despite adequate stimuli with or without preceding sodium restriction (10 mEq diet) for 5 days. Aldosterone secretion is considered to be autonomous if it remains elevated in the face of salt loading and/or administration of mineralocorticoids such as DOCA* or Florinef.†

Since Conn's description of hypertension secondary to excessive aldosterone secretion by an adrenal adenoma,[11] primary aldosteronism has remained the model for mineralocorticoid hypertension, with the cardinal features of

1. High aldosterone secretion which cannot be suppressed by high sodium intake or mineralocorticoid administration.

---

* Trademark, Organon
† Trademark, Squibb

2. Marked suppression of plasma renin levels.

3. Hypokalemia and inappropriate kaliuresis.

There are now 4 recognized forms of primary aldosteronism:

1. Aldosterone producing adenoma (APA).

2. Idiopathic hyperaldosteronism (IHA) associated with bilateral nodular adrenal hyperplasia or normal adrenals.

3. Intermediate hyperaldosteronism with aldosterone levels suppressible by DOCA (20 mg IM each 12 hr for 3 days).

4. Glucocorticoid-remediable hyperaldosteronism, in which excessive aldosterone secretion is suppressible by replacement doses of glucocorticoid.[54]

The distinction between these forms is important, because patients with APA are the only group which responds well to ablative surgery. APA and IHA are the most difficult to distinguish, but the biochemical features of hyperaldosteronism are usually more marked in patients with APA. In particular, plasma renin levels are more extremely suppressed, and aldosterone levels fail to suppress during administration of desoxycorticosterone. It has recently been demonstrated that computer analysis of biochemical characteristics of patients with APA and IHA provided fairly good separation of the 2 groups.[55,56] Also, the plasma aldosterone in normal subjects and patients with IHA increases twofold to fourfold after 4 hours of upright posture, and usually decreases (or increases by < 30%) in patients with APA.[57]

The major clinical situations in which plasma renin assay is of diagnostic value are characterized by

1. Suppression or decrease of renin secretion.

2. Excessive renin secretion.

3. A disparity in renin secretion by the 2 kidneys.

In 2 commonly encountered forms of essential hypertension, plasma renin deter-

Table 21-3. Differential Diagnosis of Primary Aldosteronism

	PRA or PRC	Urinary Aldosterone
Primary aldosteronism	Low	High
Low-renin essential hypertension	Low	Low - Normal
Familial pseudo-aldosteronism	Low	Low
Licorice excess	Low	Low
Excess secretion of other mineralocorticoids:	Low	Low
Congenital adrenal hyperplasia (DOC)		
11β hydroxylase deficiency (DOC)		
17α hydroxylase deficiency (B)		
Adrenal tumor (DOC, B)		
Ectopic ACTH production (DOC)		
Secondary aldosteronism:	High	High
Malignant hypertension		
Renovascular hypertension		
Renin-secreting tumor		

DOC = desoxycorticosterone
B = corticosterone

minations are helpful in identifying patients who will respond to particular forms of drug therapy. One group comprises about 20 to 40 percent of patients with essential hypertension, and is characterized by low PRA (resistant to stimulation), normal- to low-aldosterone secretion, and hypertension which responds to treatment with diuretics and to the mineralocorticoid antagonist spironolactone.[58] The second group is characterized by tachycardia, higher-than-normal PRA, and hypertension which is more readily controlled with propranolol, a beta-adrenergic blocking agent. Other infrequently encountered forms of low-renin hypertension are listed in Table 21-3. Disorders leading to secondary aldosteronism must be considered during the evaluation of patients with high PRA and excessive aldosterone secretion, and can be readily identified on the basis of an adequate history and physical examination. The angiotensin antagonist sar¹-ala⁸-angiotensin II has recently been demonstrated to control the blood pressure of a group of patients with malignant hypertension and secondary aldosteronism, and may prove to be of considerable value as a diagnostic or short-term therapeutic aid in conditions in which elevated plasma renin and excessive angiotensin II formation is suspected to be responsible for the exacerbation of hypertension or the hypersecretion of aldosterone.[59]

The other major diagnostic area in which renin assay is of considerable value is the evaluation of renovascular hypertension, in which the assay is performed as an adjunct to renal arteriography to determine whether a patient is likely to benefit from operative treatment. A supine renin ratio of 1.5:1 or greater between the ischemic and normal kidneys is taken to indicate significant lateralization, in the absence of collateral circulation, to the stenotic kidney. The development of collateral circulation is itself suggestive of significant arterial stenosis, and may be accompanied by a return of the renal venous ratio toward unity. Of a series of 37 patients treated successfully with revascularization for unilateral stenosis,[60] the mean renal venous renin ratio for patients without collaterals was 2.5, whereas patients with demonstrable collaterals showed a mean ratio of 1.8. Recently, renin assay of plasma obtained by segmental catheterization of the renovascular system has been employed to localize small ischemic lesions which were not accompanied by a significant change in the ratio of samples taken from the main renal vein. In the presence of bilateral renal arterial stenosis, renal venous ratios are not helpful in predicting the outcome of renovascular surgical procedures. Whenever feasible, patients should be withdrawn from medications (except guanethidine) for at least 1 month before evaluation, and should be acutely salt-depleted by furosemide administration prior to renal vein catheterization to prevent masking of significant lateralization

by low-renin values.[61] Other maneuvers which have been recommended for acute stimulation of renal venous renin levels include diazoxide, nitroprusside and hydralazine.

An uncommon but dramatic form of surgically correctable hypertension is caused by renin-secreting tumors of the kidney.[62] Findings suggestive of primary aldosteronisms have been initially present in all reported cases but have been subsequently shown to be due to secondary aldosteronism resulting from the unilateral hypersecretion of renin and correspondingly elevated plasma renin levels. Accurate differentiation from renal artery stenosis may be difficult but can be accomplished by adequate renal arteriography and selective venous catheterization.

References

1. Genest, J., De Champlain, J., Veyrat, R., Boucher, R., *et al.*: Role of the renin-angiotensin system in various physiological and pathological states. Hypertension, *13*:97, 1965.
2. Gross, F., Brunner, H., and Ziegler, M.: Renin-angiotensin system, aldosterone and sodium balance. Recent Progr. Horm. Res., *21*:119, 1965.
3. Michelakis, A. M., and Horton, R.: The relationship between plasma renin and aldosterone in normal men. Circ. Res., *26* (suppl. I):185, 1970.
4. Blair-West, J. R., Cain, M. D., Catt, K. J., *et al.*: The mode of control of aldosterone secretion. Fourth International Congress of Nephrology. vol. 2, pp. 33-44. Basel, Karger, 1970.
5. Boyd, G. W., and Peart, W. S.: The relationship between angiotensin and aldosterone. Adv. Metabol. Disord., *5*:77, 1971.
6. Mendelsohn, F. A. O., Johnston, C. I., Doyle, A. E., *et al.*: Renin, angiotensin II and adrenal corticosteroid relationships during sodium deprivation and angiotensin II infusion in normotensive and hypertensive man. Circ. Res., *31*:728, 1972.
7. Davis, J. O.: Renin-angiotensin system in the control of aldosterone secretion. *In* Fisher, J. W. (ed.): Kidney Hormones. pp. 173-205. New York, Academic Press, 1971.
8. Conn, J., Rovner, D., and Cohen, E.: Normal and altered function of the renin-angiotensin aldosterone system in man. Ann. Intern. Med., *63*:266, 1965.

9. Laragh, J. H.: Interrelations between angiotensin, norepinephrine, epinephrine, aldosterone secretion and electrolyte metabolism in man. Circulation, 25:203, 1962.

10. Gowenlock, A., and Wrong, O.: Hyperaldosteronism secondary to renal ischemia. Quart. J. Med., 31:323, 1962.

11. Conn, J. W., Cohen, E. L., and Rovner, D. R.: Suppression of plasma renin activity in primary aldosteronism: Distinguishing primary from secondary aldosteronism in hypertensive disease. JAMA, 190:213, 1964.

12. Fishman, L. M., Kuchel, O., Liddle, G. W., et al.: Incidence of primary aldosteronism in uncomplicated "essential" hypertension. JAMA, 205:85, 1968.

13. Catt, K. J., Cain, M. D., Coghlan, J. P., Zimmet, P. Z., Cran, E., and Best, J. E.: Metabolism and blood levels of angiotensin II in normal subjects, renal disease and essential hypertension. Circ. Res. 26/27 (suppl. II):177, 1970.

14. Tobian, L., Tamboulian, A., and Janacek, J.: Effect of high perfusion pressures on the granulation of juxtaglomerular cells in an isolated kidney. J. Clin. Invest., 38:605, 1959.

15. Skinner, S. L., McCubbin, J. W., and Page, I. H.: Control of renin secretion. Circ. Res., 15:64, 1964.

16. Davis, J. O.: The control of renin release. Amer. J. Med., 55:333, 1973.

17. Vander, A. J.: Control of renin release. Physiol. Rev., 47:359, 1967.

18. Thurau, K., Dahlheim, H., Gruner, A., et al.: Activation of renin in the single juxtaglomerular apparatus by sodium chloride in tubular fluid at the macula densa. Circ. Res., 30/31(suppl. II):182, 1972.

19. Gann, D., Delea, C., Gill, J., et al.: Control of aldosterone secretion by changes of body potassium in normal men. Amer. J. Physiol., 207:104, 1964.

20. Dluhy, R., Axelrod, L., Underwood, R., et al.: Studies on the control of plasma aldosterone concentration in normal men. II. Effect of potassium. J. Clin. Invest., 51:1950, 1972.

21. Horton, R.: Aldosterone: Review of its physiology and diagnostic aspects of primary aldosteronism. Metabolism, 22:1525, 1973.

22. Catt, K. J., Baukal, A. J., and Ashburn, M. J.: The renin-angiotensin system during oral contraceptive therapy and pregnancy. In Fregly, M. J., and Fregly, M. S. (eds.): Oral Contraceptives and Hypertension. pp. 211-222. Gainesville, Dolphin Press, 1974.

23. Skinner, S. L., Lumbers, E. R., and Symonds, E. M.: Alteration by oral contraceptives of normal menstrual changes in plasma renin activity, concentration and substrate. Clin. Sci., 36:67, 1969.

24. Catt, K. J., Cain, M. D., and Menard, J.: Radioimmunoassay studies of the renin-angiotensin system in human hypertension and during estrogen treatment. In Genest, J., and Koiw, E., (eds.): Hypertension, 1972, pp. 591-604. New York, Springer-Verlag, 1972.

25. Conn, J. W.: The evolution of primary aldosteronism 1954-1967. Harvey Lect., 62:257, 1966-67.

26. Dunn, M. J., and Tannen, R. L.: Low-renin hypertension: An editorial review. Kidney International, 5:317, 1974.

27. Melby, J. C., Dali, S. E., and Wilson, T. E.: 18-hydroxy deoxycorticosterone in human hypertension. Circ. Res., 28/29(suppl. II): 143, 1971.

28. Brunner, H. R., Laragh, J. H., Baer, L., et al.: Essential hypertension: Renin and aldosterone, heart attack and stroke. N. Eng. J. Med., 286:441, 1972.

29. Doyle, A. E., Jerums, G., Johnston, C. I., and Louis, W. J.: Plasma renin levels and vascular complications in hypertension. Br. Med. J., 2:206, 1973.

30. Genest, J., Boucher, R., Kuchel, O., and Nowaczynski, W.: Renin in hypertension: How important as a risk factor? Can. Med. Assoc. J., 109:475, 1973.

31. Mroczek, W., Finnerty, F. A., and Catt, K. J.: Lack of association between plasma renin and history of heart attack or stroke in patients with essential hypertension. Lancet, 2:464, 1973.

32. Boyd, G. W., Adamson, A. R., Fitz, A. E., et al.: Radioimmunoassay determination of plasma-renin activity. Lancet, 1:213, 1969.

33. Haber, E., Koernor, T., Page, L. B., et al.: Application of a radioimmunoassay for angiotensin I to the physiologic measurements of plasma renin activity in normal human subjects. J. Clin. Endocrinol. Metab., 29:1349, 1969.

34. Cohen, E. L., Conn, J. W., Lucas, C. P., et al.: Radioimmunoassay for angiotensin I: Measurement of plasma-renin activity, plasma renin concentration, renin substrate concentration and angiotensin I, in normal and hypertensive people. In Genest, J., and Koiw, E., (eds.): Hypertension, 1972, pp. 569-582. New York, Springer-Verlag, 1972.

35. Catt, K. J., Baukal, A. J., and Ashburn, M. J.: Radioimmunoassay determination of plasma renin parameters and circulating

angiotensin II. *In* Fregly, M. J., and Fregly, M. S. (eds.): Oral Contraceptives and Hypertension. pp. 184-210. Gainesville, Dolphin Press, 1974.

36. Gould, A. B., and Green, D.: Kinetics of the human renin and renin substrate reaction. Cardiovas. Res., *5*:86, 1971.

37. Brown, J. J., Davies, D. F., Lever, A. F., *et al.*: The estimation of renin in human plasma. Biochem. J., *93*:594, 1964.

38. Skinner, S. L.: Improved assay methods for renin "concentration" and "activity" in human plasma. Circ. Res., *20*:391, 1967.

39. Stockigt, J. R., Collins, R. D., and Biglieri, E. G.: Determination of plasma renin concentration by angiotensin I immunoassay. circ. Res., *28/29*(suppl. II):175, 1971.

40. Haas, E., Gould, A. B., and Goldblatt, H.: Estimation of endogenous renin in human blood. Lancet, *1*:657, 1968.

41. Kliman, B., and Peterson, R. E.: Double isotope derivative assay of aldosterone in biological fluids. J. Biol. Chem., *235*:1639, 1960.

42. Coghlan, J. P., and Blair-West, J. R.: Aldosterone. *In* Gray, C. H., and Bacharach, A. L., (eds.): Hormones in Blood. pp. 391-488. New York, Academic Press, 1967.

43. Langan, J., Jackson, R., Adlin, E. V., *et al.*: A simple radioimmunoassay for urinary aldosterone. J. Clin. Endocrinol. Metab., *38*:189, 1974.

44. Horton, R., and Finck, E.: Diagnosis and localization in primary aldosteronism. Ann. Intern. Med., *76*:885, 1972.

45. Haning, R., McCracken, J., St. Cyr, M., *et al.*: The evaluation of titer and specificity of aldosterone binding antibodies in hyperimmunized sheep. Steroids, *20*:73, 1972.

46. Ito, T., Woo, J., Haning, R., *et al.*: A radioimmunoassay for aldosterone in human peripheral plasma including a comparison of alternate techniques. J. Clin. Endocrinol. Metab., *34*:106, 1972.

47. St. Cyr, M. J., Sancho, J. M., and Melby, J. C.: Quantitation of plasma aldosterone by radioimmunoassay. Clin. Chem., *18*:1395, 1972.

48. Farmer, R. W., Brown, D. H., Howard, P. Y., *et al.*: A radioimmunoassay for plasma aldosterone without chromatography. J. Clin. Endocrinol. Metab., *36*:460, 1973.

49. Bayard, F., Beitins, I. Z., Kowarski, A., *et al.*: Measurement of plasma aldosterone by radioimmunoassay. J. Clin. Endocrinol. Metab., *31*:1, 1970.

50. Gomez-Sanchez, C., Kem, D. C., and Kaplan, N. M.: A radioimmunoassay for plasma aldosterone by immunologic purification. J. Clin. Endocrinol. Metab., *36*:795, 1973.

51. Martin, B. T., and Nugent, C. A.: A nonchromatographic radioimmunoassay for plasma aldosterone. Steroids, *21*:169, 1973.

52. Africa, B., and Haber, E.: The production and characterization of specific antibodies to aldosterone. Immunochemistry, *8*:479, 1971.

53. Rodbard, D.: Statistical aspects of radioimmunoassay. *In* Daughaday, W., and Odell, W., (eds.): Competitive Protein Binding Assay. pp. 204-259, Philadelphia, J. B. Lippincott, 1971.

54. Biglieri, E. G., Stockigt, J. R., and Schambelan, M.: Adrenal mineralocorticoids causing hypertension. Amer. J. Med., *52*:623, 1972.

55. Ferris, J. B., Brown, J. J., Fraser, A. W., *et al.*: Hypertension with aldosterone excess and low plasma-renin: Preoperative distinction between patients with and without adrenocortical tumor. Lancet, *2*:995, 1970.

56. Biglieri, E. G., Schambelan, M., Slaton, P. E., *et al.*: The intercurrent hypertension of primary aldosteronism. Circ. Res., *26/27* (suppl. I):195, 1970.

57. Ganguly, A., Melada, G. A., Luetscher, J. A., *et al.*: Control of plasma aldosterone in primary aldosteronism: Distinction between adenoma and hyperplasia. J. Clin. Endocrinol. Metab., *37*:765, 1973.

58. Douglas, J. G., Hollifield, J. W., and Liddle, G. W.: Treatment of low-renin essential hypertension. JAMA, *227*:518, 1974.

59. Brunner, H. R., Gavras, H., and Laragh, J. H.: Angiotensin II blockade in man by sar¹-ala⁸-angiotensin II for understanding and treatment of high blood-pressure. Lancet, *2*:1045, 1973.

60. Ernst, C. B., Boakstein, J. J., Montie, J., *et al.*: Renal vein renin ratios and collateral vessels in renovascular hypertension. Arch. Surg., *104*:496, 1972.

61. Strong, C. G., Hunt, J. C., Sheps, S. G., *et al.*: Renal venous renin activity enhancement of sensitivity of lateralization by sodium depletion. Amer. J. Cardiol., *27*:602, 1971.

62. Robertson, P. W., Klidgian, A., Harding, L. K., *et al.*: Hypertension due to a reninsecreting tumor. Amer. J. Med., *43*:963, 1967.

22 *Tumor Antigens*

BENJAMIN ROTHFELD, M.D. AND
STEVEN V. LARSON, M.D.

For many years it has been a dream among medical men to develop a simple blood test which would enable them to screen large numbers of apparently tumor-free individuals to pick up early tumors. It was also hoped that such a test would help detect tumor recurrences before they become detectable with the use of other more complex means. The fact that many different human tumors have tumor-associated antigens has lent encouragement to this hope. Thus tumor-associated antigens have been found in colonic, ovarian, lung, and mammary tumors.[1-4] Such antigens have also been found in association with lymphomata and leukemias.[5,6] The finding that tumor antigens can be released into body fluids raised hopes for a screening test.[7-8] Recently certain developments have given renewed hope for developing such a test. Although such a test is not yet available, by proceeding along lines which have already been developed, it is hoped that it will become possible in time to have a highly efficient tumor-screening test.

BACKGROUND

Before dealing with carcinoembryonic (CEA) antigen, which will form the bulk of the discussion of this chapter, there will be a brief review of other tumor-associated antigens.

An antigen which was originally thought to be associated only with human sarcomas has been found to be widely distributed in patients having other tumors. This antigen is referred to as S_2.[9]

Other authors found an antigen, which they called tumor-associated polypeptide antigen (TPA), to be present in and produced by human cancer cells. Patients with tumor had elevated blood levels of this material.[10] The author felt that TPA had possibilities as a screening test for cancer.

Alpha-fetoprotein is a major protein component in the serum of early rodent and human fetuses.[11] The maximal level in the human fetus is attained around the thirteenth week of intrauterine development. With increasing fetal age these levels decline and the serum albumin concentrations rise so that by the end of the first postnatal week alpha-fetoprotein is no longer demonstrable.[12] Alpha-fetoprotein of human origin is an $alpha_1$-globulin with a molecular weight of 64,000 and a sedimentation constant of 4.5.[13] This substance has been found in association with hepatocellular carcinoma and malignant teratoma and, unfortunately, in persons suffering from acute viral hepatitis.[14,15] With the use of a highly sensitive radioimmunoassay $alpha_1$-fetoprotein has also been found in the plasma of normal controls.[16] Recent work has shown that this substance tends to rise during pregnancy, dropping to normal shortly before term.[17] Extremely high levels may occur before and after fetal death and it has been postulated that an increased release of $alpha_1$-fetoprotein may occur because of fetal distress.[17]

Table 22-1. Human Tumor—Associated Antigens.

Substance	Found In	Drop After Successful Treatment
Carcinoembryonic antigen[1]	See Table 22-2	Yes
alpha$_1$-Fetoprotein (AFP)[7]	Hepatoma (highest values and most frequently) Hepatitis Cirrhosis Metastatic liver cancer Other cancer Normal pregnancy	Yes
alpha$_2$-H-Fetoprotein[14]	Various types of tumors	
beta-S-Fetoprotein[15]	Hepatic tumors Gastric cancer Various types of lymphomas	
Leukemia-associated antigens[6] (LAA)	Leukemias	Not necessarily
Heterophile fetal antigen[16]	Small number patients with leukemia	
Placental alkaline phosphatase[18]	Small percentage patients with various types of tumors	Yes
Fetal sulphoglycoprotein antigen[17] (FSA)	Gastric cancer Benign peptic ulcer	Not necessarily
S$_2$[20]	Many types of tumors	
Tumor-associated polypeptide antigen[21] (TPA)	Many types of tumors	

However the authors were able, in the majority of the cases, to distinguish patients suffering from primary hepatocellular carcinoma from normals in that the alpha$_1$-fetoprotein levels were quite elevated in the carcinoma patients. The test for alphafetoprotein may also be of value in the differential diagnosis of teratoma and seminoma and in following the responses of the former to therapy. It has been noted that patients with raised alpha-fetoprotein levels have more malignant teratomata and also that the majority of alpha-fetoprotein negative malignant teratomatas respond to therapy.[18]

Alpha$_2$H-fetoprotein is found in fetal liver and serum. Although elevated values have been found in various tumors they may also be found in normal individuals.[19]

Another tumor-associated protein is *beta-S-fetoprotein*. This, too, is a protein which normally occurs in fetal serum and has been found in the serum of patients with hepto-carcinoma, cholangiocarcinoma, gastric carcinoma and various types of lymphoma.[20]

There are also *leukemia-associated antigens* which have been found in the serum of as many as one-third of patients with various types of leukemia. Unfortunately these levels do not always decline during remission.[6]

Heterophile fetal antigen has also been found in a relatively small number of patients suffering from leukemia.[21]

Fetal sulphoglycoprotein antigen is another fetal protein which may be found in association with tumors, most commonly with gastric carcinoma. However, its importance is markedly diminished by the fact that it is not uncommonly found with peptic ulcer and additionally that it does not necessarily drop following successful removal of a gastric tumor.[22]

Carcinoplacental alkaline phosphatase is present in maternal serum during the third trimester of pregnancy. It is also found in the serum of a small percentage of patients with a wide variety of neoplasms. It tends to drop with effective therapy of the tumor.[23]

To complete this discussion, Epstein-Barr virus should be mentioned. This is not a tumor-associated antigen but rather an infectious agent. It is most commonly associated with infectious mononucleosis and has been found in 15 of 21 patients with nasopharyngeal carcinoma.[9,24] By contrast antibodies to this virus were found in only 6 of 140 controls. Furthermore, patients with lymphoma of the nasopharynx did not have high titers of this antibody.

The various tumor-associated antigens are summarized in Table 22-1.[24]

A provocative suggestion has been made that these antigens may serve as more than mere markers but actually participate in the pathogenesis of tumor development by disturbing mitotic regulation and facilitating DNA and RNA synthesis.[25]

The most widely used and extensively studied of the various tumor-associated antigens is carcinoembryonic antigen. (CEA) which was first isolated and identified in 1965.[26] This substance was named carcinoembryonic antigen because it was first found in carcinoma of the human colon and was also found to be normally present in the fetal entoderm. This material was first identified in tissue.[27] In 1969 a radioimmunoassay was developed to determine serum levels of CEA.[28] A simpler radioimmunoassay method was subsequently developed which gave similar results but was also positive in non-entodermally-derived tumors and some malignant diseases.[29,30]

Theoretical Background

With the development of more sensitive radioimmunoassay techniques for CEA, this substance has been found even in normal adult tissues.[31] However, it seems that in neoplastic tissue this material is produced in much greater quantity. It has been suggested that CEA is a fetal antigen the production of which is suppressed after birth. Various agents such as viruses, chemical carcinogens, and so on which induce the tumor may at the same time de-press the genome controlling CEA, thereby leading to an increase in its production.[32] An additional explanation for the elevated level of CEA in colonic tumor is that although CEA is produced in normal colonic mucosa it cannot be absorbed through the intact mucosa. As the carcinoma disrupts the normal tissue architecture, cells penetrate the underlying tissue and substances such as CEA enter the vascular system.[33]

As to the location of the antigen in the tumor cell, there are indications that CEA is located on the surface of the tumor cell.[34]

As mentioned above, there have been suggestions that tumor-associated antigens may be intimately involved in the pathogenesis of tumors. One suggestion made was that these antigens may disturb mitotic regulation by facilitating DNA synthesis.[25] Another suggestion based on familial studies was that occurrence of these antigens in family members of individuals with tumors suggested a familial tendency to de-repression which might predispose to malignancy.[9] It should be noted that this study had to do with S_2 antigen rather than with CEA. A suggestion that CEA might be of value in screening tumor-prone persons was made in an article studying the level of CEA in cigarette smokers with no detectable cancer who had a relatively high percentage of positive tests for CEA, as contrasted with nonsmokers.[35] They felt that this association might reflect precancerous changes. The authors suggested that in any study associating CEA with a particular disease the smoking habits be included.

The fact that CEA is not specific for carcinoma but can also be found in normal tissue has been stressed. However, it has been stated that just as the CEA test is not necessarily specific for cancer neither is the Wassermann test for treponema. Despite this the Wassermann test is a very useful laboratory test.[36]

By varying the technique used in studying CEA it was possible to detect tumor antigens specific for digestive tract as well as antigens common to all tumors. It was further possible to detect an antigen present in normal digestive tract tissue.[37] It was suggested that each antigen preparation should be assessed in various ways before it was called CEA.

CHEMISTRY

CEA is a glycoprotein with a molecular weight of 150,000 to 200,000. It migrates as a beta globulin. It is soluble in perchloric acid in concentrations up to 1.0 N. Also, it is soluble in 50 percent saturated ammonium sulfate. It has a sedimentation coefficient of 7 to 8 S. As for its amino acid composition, its major residues are aspartic acid, threonine, serine, glutamic acid, proline, glycine, alanine, leucine, isoleucine, valine. Its minor amino residues are tyrosine, phenylalanine, lysine, histidine, and arginine. Its carbohydrate composition is l-fucose, d-mannose, d-galactose, sialic acid, N-acetyl-d-glucosamine.[38,39]

METHODS

The principle of the radioimmunoassay for CEA is similar to that of other radioimmunoassays discussed throughout this book. That is, labeled CEA is reacted with antibody in the presence of a standard or unlabeled CEA in plasma. The bound CEA is then separated from the free either by precipitation by various salts or by another antibody by means of a double antibody technique. The value of CEA is then read from a curve.

Antisera may be produced by injecting rabbits with extracted tissue from 6- to 7-week human fetuses. The material is suspended in Freund's adjuvant.[40] The most popular method involves developing specific goat anti-CEA serum. This is usually absorbed with an excess of perchloric acid extract of normal spleen in order to absorb antibodies directed against a normal glycoprotein found in serum.[41] This also removes the "nonspecific cross-reacting antigen" of VonKleist, *et al.*[42] If goat antiserum for CEA is used, bound may be separated from free either by using a specific goat antiserum raised from rabbits or by using certain salts as described below.

Blood samples are collected in tubes containing liquid EDTA, centrifuged, and the plasma separated and frozen at $-4°C$. Heparin interferes in some of the assay techniques and care should be taken that heparinized plasma is not used.[37]

With some methods the standard curve produced is nonlinear.[43] Because of this nonlinearity logit transformation is necessary with these techniques in order to linearize the standard curves.[44]

The 2 most widely used methods for determining CEA in the last few years are those of Thomson[28] and Hansen.[45] These 2 methods differ essentially in that Thomson's method involves an ammonium sulfate precipitation to separate bound from free and Hansen's involves a zirconyl phosphate gel to make the separation. Thomson's method is apparently more specific for digestive tract cancer; whereas Hansen's is also positive in patients with nondigestive tract cancer and selected patients without evidence of GI malignancy.[37] Both these methods involve goat antiserum to CEA. They also both use perchloric acid to extract soluble glycoproteins from serum or plasma samples and involve dialysis of the perchloric acid extract. On the whole the dialysis period used for the zirconyl gel assay is shorter than that for the ammonium sulfate assay. A disadvantage of the ammonium sulfate assay when compared to the zirconyl gel is that it is necessary to lyophilize the dialyzed perchloric acid extract. Additionally, it is necessary to incubate the ammonium sulfate assay for one day, the incubation for the zirconyl gel assay being much shorter. An advantage of the zirconyl gel assay, which also has the defect of its virtues, is that it is possible to label CEA with I-125 in the zirconyl gel assay at approximately 10 times the specific activity of that used in the ammonium sulfate assay. However, the use of this high specific activity requires more frequent labeling because of the deterioration of the material, that is, every 1 to 2 weeks rather than the 1 to 2 months required with ammonium sulfate.

All in all, the technical differences between these 2 methods do not appear to cause differing results in the analyses of a patient's sera or plasma.[37]

Currently there is only one assay for CEA which is approved by the FDA. This is the assay developed by Hoffman-LaRoche which uses the zirconyl gel precipitation.

PATHOPHYSIOLOGIC CORRELATIONS

In the past few years it has been determined that CEA levels may be elevated in all malignancies. The exact percentage of elevation in any specific malignancy as well as the level of the titer is related both to the type of malignancy being investigated and the presence or absence of metastases. On the whole the more widespread the tumor, the more elevated the level. However, CEA also has been found to be elevated in a number of nonmalignant disorders and occasionally in apparently normal subjects. The one thing that persons with elevated CEA titers have in common is rapid cellular proliferation with damage to the basement membrane.

Before going into detail on the above statements it is necessary to define the upper limits of normal. Using the most widely accepted method the upper limit of normal is 3.0 ng/cc.[45] The range from 3 to 5 ng/cc is considered a borderline area and values of 5.0 ng/cc and above are considered definitely abnormal.

In Gold's[34] early work he stated that CEA was found only in carcinomas derived from the entoderm of the GI tract. He felt that this antigen was absent from all other tissues and types of carcinoma. This also was the conclusion of Thomson.[28] In fact, they felt that although the anus and pharynx were

part of the GI tract, since they were not entodermally derived, tumors of these tissues did not develop abnormal levels of CEA in the blood. However, more recently, and most likely related to the increased use of the zirconyl-gel precipitation method, CEA has been found in other disorders. Thus using the zirconyl-gel method it was found that 82 percent of patients with malignant tumors of the gastrointestinal tract had positive CEA tests.[43] Additionally, patients with male genitourinary tract cancer had a 30 percent positive rate, female genitourinary 39 percent, localized breast disease 10 percent, disseminated breast disease 60 percent, osteogenic sarcoma 50 percent, neuroblastoma with active disease 100 percent. Abnormally high concentrations of plasma CEA were also found in a number of other types of carcinoma. A substantial incidence of positive CEA tests also has been found in carcinoma of the lung.[46,47,48]

Occurrence of CEA in Benign Conditions. Actually, CEA occurs in normal plasma. The difference with regard to CEA between plasma from normal individuals and those with carcinoma is quantitative rather than qualitative.[49] These workers found that in normal human plasma the average CEA concentration was 1.1 ng/cc of plasma. Various nonmalignant inflammatory diseases, as mentioned above, in their active phase may give rise to elevated CEA titers. These then drop to normal when the disease goes into remission.[50] Here are found diseases such as ulcerative colitis and regional enteritis as well as pulmonary emphysema, cirrhosis of the liver, and pancreatitis.[51,52,53]

As mentioned above, individuals who were heavy smokers frequently had a positive test for CEA in contrast to individuals who were not heavy smokers.[35] Both these groups were apparently free of carcinoma. Other work has indicated that the CEA titer often dropped within 30 to 60 days after cessation of smoking.

One somewhat disturbing finding in some studies involving CEA[43] is a relatively high

Table 22-2. Radioimmunoassay Method.

	Gold				Z-gel		Double Antibody
MALIGNANCIES							
Carcinoma of colon and rectum	97[8]	91[30]	72[55]	64[56]	86[29]	83[57]	69[51]
Other gastrointestinal cancer							
Total	9	70	74	60	84	82	63
Stomach							
Pancreas							
Liver							
Nongastrointestinal cancer							
Total	0	46	55	51	70	39	44
Lung							
Breast							
Reticuloendothelial							
NONMALIGNANCIES							
Gastrointestinal					0		33
Peptic ulcer							
Inflammatory bowel			67	30	30		32
Cirrhosis				48			
Chronic lung disease					11		45
Chronic renal disease		75					
Benign breast lesions							8

Figures are percentage positive

coefficient of variation. In duplicate determinations for 50 samples this was 13.5 percent.

Value of Test

The CEA test has its greatest value in diagnosis of new cases of carcinoma of the colon. In an interesting study the value of the CEA test was compared with the barium enema in diagnosis of new cases of carcinoma of the colon.[54] The authors felt that it was less sensitive than the barium enema in such cases. However, when used in conjunction with conventional radiologic techniques and proctosigmoidoscopy the CEA test increased the accuracy of the operative diagnosis.

All in all this test cannot be used as a screen to detect cancer. It is not an absolute test for malignancy or for a specific type of malignancy. It seems to have a place as an adjunct to the standard methods for detecting cancer.

In persons who have had tumors removed, the CEA test is of value in helping with periodic checks to detect recurrence. By checking the level of CEA in the circulation before and after treatment it may be possible to obtain an early indication of tumor recurrence or the presence of undetected metastases.

It should also be kept in mind that elevations in CEA as discussed above are not pathognomonic of malignancy but not un-

commonly may be related to benign disease.
Some of the results with CEA from the literature are summarized in Table 22-2.

References

1. Gold, P., and Freedman, S. O.: Demonstration of tumor-specific antigens in human colonic carcinoma by immunological tolerance and absorption technique. J. Exp. Med., *121*:439, 1965.
2. Levi, M. M., Keller, S., and Mandl, I.: Antigenicity of a papillary serous cystadenocarcinoma tissue homogenate and its fractions. Amer. J. Obstet. Gynecol., *105*: 856, 1969.
3. Yashi, A., Matsumura, Y., Carpenter, C. M., *et al.*: Immunochemical studies on human lung cancer antigens soluble in 50% saturated ammonium sulfate. J. Natl. Cancer Inst., *40*:663, 1968.
4. Edynak, E. M., Hirshaut, Y., Old, L. J., *et al.*: Antigens of human breast cancer. Proc. Amer. Assoc. Cancer Res., *12*:75, 1971.
5. Smith, R. T., Klein, G., and Klein, E.: Studies of the membrane phenomenon in cultured and biopsy cell lines from the Burkitt lymphoma. *In* Dausset, J., Hamberger, J., Mathe, G. (eds.): Advances in Transplantation. p. 483. Baltimore, Williams & Wilkins, 1967.
6. Harris, R., Viza, D., Topp, R., *et al.*: Detection of human leukemia associated antigens in leukaemic serum and normal embryos. Nature, (Lond.), *233*:556, 1971.
7. Abelev, G. I.: Production of embryonal serum alpha-globulins by hepatomas: review of experimental and clinical data. Cancer Res., *28*:1344, 1968.
8. Thomson, D. M. P., Krupey, J., Freedman, S. O., *et al.*: The radioimmunoassay of circulating carcinoembryonic antigens of the human digestive system. Proc. Natl. Acad. Sci. USA, *64*:161, 1969.
9. Bijay, M., and Yashar, H.: Evidence for fetal antigen in human sarcoma. Science, *181*:440, 1973.
10. Lundstrom, R.: Thirteenth Interscience Conference of Antimicrobial Agents and Chemotherapy, 1973.
11. Kirsh, I., Wise, R., and Oliver, I.: Postalbumin—a fetal specific rat plasma protein. Biochem. J., *102*:763, 1967.
12. Gitlin, D., and Boesman, M.: Serum alpha-fetoprotein. Albumin and alpha-fetoglobulin in the human conceptus. J. Clin. Invest., *45*:1826, 1966.
13. Nishi, S.: Isolation and characterization of a human fetal alpha-globulin from the sera of fetuses and a hepatoma-patient. Cancer Res., *30*:2507, 1970.
14. Kew, M. C., Cos Santos, H. A., and Sherlock, S.: Diagnosis of primary cancer of the liver. Br. Med. J., *4*:408, 1971.
15. Florin-Christenson, A., and Arana, R. N.: Alpha-fetoprotein and anti-alpha-fetoprotein in viral hepatitis. Br. Med. J., *2*:94, 1973.
16. Chayvialle, J. A. T., and Ganouli, T. C.: Radioimmunoassay of alpha$_1$-fetoprotein in human plasma. Lancet, *1*:1355, 1973.
17. Seppälä, M., and Ruoslahti, E.: Radioimmunoassay of maternal serum alpha-fetoprotein during pregnancy and delivery. Amer. J. Obstet. Gynecol., *112*:208, 1972.
18. Abelev, G. I.: Alpha-fetoprotein in ontogenesis and its association with malignant tumors. Adv. Cancer Res., *14*:295, 1971.
19. Buffé, D., Rimbault, C., Lemerle, J., *et al.*: Presence d'u ferroproteine d'origine tissulaire. Fr. J. Cancer, *5*:85, 1970.
20. Wada, T., Anzal, T., Yachi, A., *et al.*: Incidence of three different fetal proteins in sera of patients with primary hepatoma. *In* Peeters, H. (ed.): Protides of the Biological Fluids. p. 22. Oxford, Pergamon Press, 1971.
21. Edynka, E. M., Old, L. J., Vrana, M., *et al.*: A fetal antigen in human tumours detected by an antibody in the serum of cancer patients. Proc. Amer. Assoc. Cancer Res., *11*: 22, 1970.
22. Häkkinen, I., and Viikari, S.: Occurrences of fetal sulphoglycoprotein antigens in the gastric juice of patients with gastric diseases. Ann. Surg., *169*:277, 1969.
23. Fishmann, W. H., Inglis, N. R., Green, S., *et al.*: Immunology and biochemistry of Regan isoenzyme of alkaline phosphatase in human cancer. Nature (Lond.), *219*:697, 1968.
24. Goldmann, J. M., Goodman, M., and Miller, D.: Antibody to Epstein-Barr virus in American patients with carcinoma of the nasopharynx. JAMA, *216*:1618, 1972.
25. Law, L. W.: Studies of tumor antigens and tumor-specific immune mechanisms in experimental systems. Transplant Proc., *2*: 117, 1970.
26. Gold, P., and Freedman, S. O.: Demonstration of tumor-specific antigens in human colonic carcinomata by immunological tolerance and absorption techniques. J. Exp. Med., *121*:439, 1965.
27. Gold, P., and Freedman, S. O.: Specific carcinoembryonic antigens of the human digestive systems. J. Exp. Med., *122*:467, 1965.
28. Thomson, D. M. P., Krupey, J., Freedman,

S. O., *et al.*: The radioimmunoassay of circulating carcinoembryonic antigen of the human digestive system. Proc. Natl. Acad. Sci. USA, *64*:161, 1969.

29. LoGerfo, P., Krupey, J., and Hansen, H. J.: Demonstration of an antigen common to several varieties of neoplasia assay using Zirconyl phosphate gel. N. Eng. J. Med., *285*:138, 1971.

30. Moore, T. L., Kupchik, H. A., and Macon, N.: Carcinoembryonic antigen assay in cancer of the colon and pancreas and other digestive tract disorders. Amer. J. Dig. Dis., *16*:1, 1971.

31. Breborowitz, J., Easty, G. C., and Neville, A. M.: Letter to the editor. Lancet, *2*:1393, 1973.

32. Klavins, J. V., Mesa-Tejaba, R., and Weiss, M.: Human carcinoma antigens crossreacting with antiembryonic antibodies. Nature (New Biol.), *234*:153, 1971.

33. Martin, F., and Martin, M. S.: RIA of CEA in extracts of human colon and stomach. Int. J. Cancer, *9*:641, 1972.

34. Gold, P., Gold, M., and Freedman, S.: Cellular location of carcinoembryonic antigens of the human digestive system. Cancer Res., *28*:1331, 1968.

35. Stevens, D. T., and Mackay, I. R.: Increased carcinoembryonic antigen in heavy cigarette smokers. Lancet, *2*:1238, 1973.

36. Humphrey, L. M.: Discussion of presentation on CEA. Ann. Surg., *176*:563, 1972.

37. Kupchik, H. Z., Hansen, J., Sorokin, J. J., *et al.*: Proceedings of the Second Conference and Workshop on Embryonic and Fetal Antigens in Cancer. p. 264. February, 1972.

38. Krupey, J., Gold, P., and Freedman, S. O.: Physicochemical studies of CEA in the human digestive system. J. Exper. Med., *128*:387, 1968.

39. Krupey, J., Wilson, T., Freedman, S. O., *et al.*: Preparation of purified CEA of the human digestive system from large quantities of tumor tissue. Immunochemistry, *9*: 617, 1972.

40. Klavins, J. F., Mesa-Tejaba, R., and Weiss, M.: Human carcinoma antigens cross reacting with antiembryonic antibodies. Nature (New Biol.), *234*:153, 1971.

41. Mach, J. P., and Pusztasveri, G.: Demonstration of a partial identity between CEA and another glycoprotein. Immunochemistry, *9*:1031, 1972.

42. VonKleist, L. S., Chavanel, G., and Burton, P.: Identification of an antigen from normal human tissue that cross-reacts with CEA. Proc. Natl. Acad. Sci. USA, *69*:2492, 1972.

43. Chu, T. N., and Reynoso, G.: Evaluation of a new radioimmunoassay method for carcinoembryonic antigen in plasma with use of zirconyl phosphate gel. Clin. Chem., *18*: 918, 1972.

44. Rodbard, D., Reyford, T. L., and Cooper, J. A., *et al.*: Statistical quality control of radioimmunoassay. J. Clin. Endocrinol. Metabol., *28*:1412, 1968.

45. Hansen, M. J., Lance, K. P., and Krupey, J.: Demonstration of an ion sensitive antigenic site on carcinoembryonic antigen using Zirconyl phosphate. Clin. Res., *19*: 143, 1971.

46. LoGerfo, P., Krupey, J., and Hansen, H. J.: Demonstration of an antigen common to several varieties of neoplasia. N. Eng. J. Med., *288*:138, 1971.

47. Zamcheck, N., Moore, T., Dhar, T., *et al.*: Immunological diagnoses and prognosis in human digestive tract cancer. N. Eng. J. Med., *286*:83, 1972.

48. LoGerfo, P., Herter, F. P., Braun, J., *et al.*: Tumor associated antigen with pulmonary neoplasma. Ann. Surg., *175*:495, 1972.

49. Chu, T. N., Reynoso, G., and Hansen, H. J.: Demonstration of carcinoembryonic antigen in normal human plasma. Nature, *238*:152, 1972.

50. Rule, A., Strauss, E., Vandevoorde, J., *et al.*: Tumor associated antigen and inflammatory bowel disease. N. Eng. J. Med., *287*:24, 1972.

51. Laurence, D. J., Steven, U., Bettleheim, R., *et al.*: Role of CEA in diagnoses of cancer. Br. Med. J., *3*:605, 1972.

52. Khoo, S. K., and Mackay, E. V.: CEA in cancer—sequential studies. Aust. N.Z. J. Obst. Gynaecol., *26*:475, 1973.

53. Khoo, S. K., Mackay, I. R., *et al.*: CEA in serum in diseases of the liver and pancreas. J. Clin. Pathol., *26*:470, 1973.

54. McCartney, W. H., Hoffer, P., and Paloyan, D.: The role of a CEA test as an adjunct to the diagnosis of colo-rectal carcinoma. Scientific Exhibit Society of Nuclear Medicine, June 1973.

55. Le Bel, J. S., Deodhar, S. D., and Brown, C. H.: Newer concepts of cancer of the colon and rectum. Dis. Colon Rectum, *15*: 111, 1972.

56. Joint National Cancer Institute: American Cancer Society investigation of CEA in patient with cancer of the colon. Can. Med. Assoc. J., *107*:25, 1972.

57. Reynoso, C., Chu, T. M., Holyoke, D., *et al.*: CEA in patients with different cancers. JAMA, *220*:361, 1972.

23 *Fat Absorption*

JOSEPH L. RABINOWITZ, PH.D. AND
RALPH M. MYERSON, M.D.

INTRODUCTION

Definition. The term "fat" is one of the most ambiguous terms currently in use in chemistry and medicine. A loose definition includes all substances that are insoluble in water but soluble in the so-called lipid solvents such as ether, chloroform and acetone. They all have a high caloric content and low density. In the past, the term "fat" was reserved for those lipids that were solid at room temperature, while the term "oil" was utilized for lipids that remained fluid at room temperature. These definitions are now obsolete.

From a biological standpoint it is reasonable to limit the definition of lipids to those compounds that can be metabolized' by an organism. This would exclude certain mineral oils, waxes, gasoline and other materials from consideration. Lipids thus included have in common long acyl (fatty acid)-chains that can be metabolized by an organism to yield energy. Figures 23-1 *A* and *B* depict respectively the chemical structure of compounds soluble in lipid solvents that are not metabolized by humans and those that are capable of being metabolized.

If the above biologically oriented definition is accepted, the useful lipids can be classified into the following groups:

1. Fatty acids.
2. Glycerol esters (glycerides of fatty acids).
3. Phospholipids (glycerol esters containing phosphoric acid and another functional group).
4. Cerebrosides (lipids containing a carbohydrate molecule in addition to a fatty acid).
5. Sulfolipids (containing fatty acids, carbohydrates and a sulfate residue).
6. Sphingomyelins (containing a fatty acid, phosphoric acid, choline and the nitrogenous base, sphingosine).

These compounds differ not only in their chemical structure, but in solubility and other physical properties. From a clinical and practical point of view, however, once ingested, all of the mentioned lipid categories are rapidly saponified and broken down to their component fatty acids. The nonlipid moieties (e.g., glycerol, choline) are digested, absorbed, and metabolized by processes and through pathways that are not relevant to this discussion.

DIGESTION AND ABSORPTION OF FAT

The gastrointestinal digestion and absorption of fat is a complex, multifaceted process which depends on a number of factors for its integrity and normal function. It is beyond the scope or purpose of this chapter to review in depth the many interdependent physicochemical and biochemical reactions which take part in fat absorption and are potentially vulnerable to disruption by a wide spectrum of pathologic processes. However, in order to assess the value and limitations of radioisotopic techniques in the

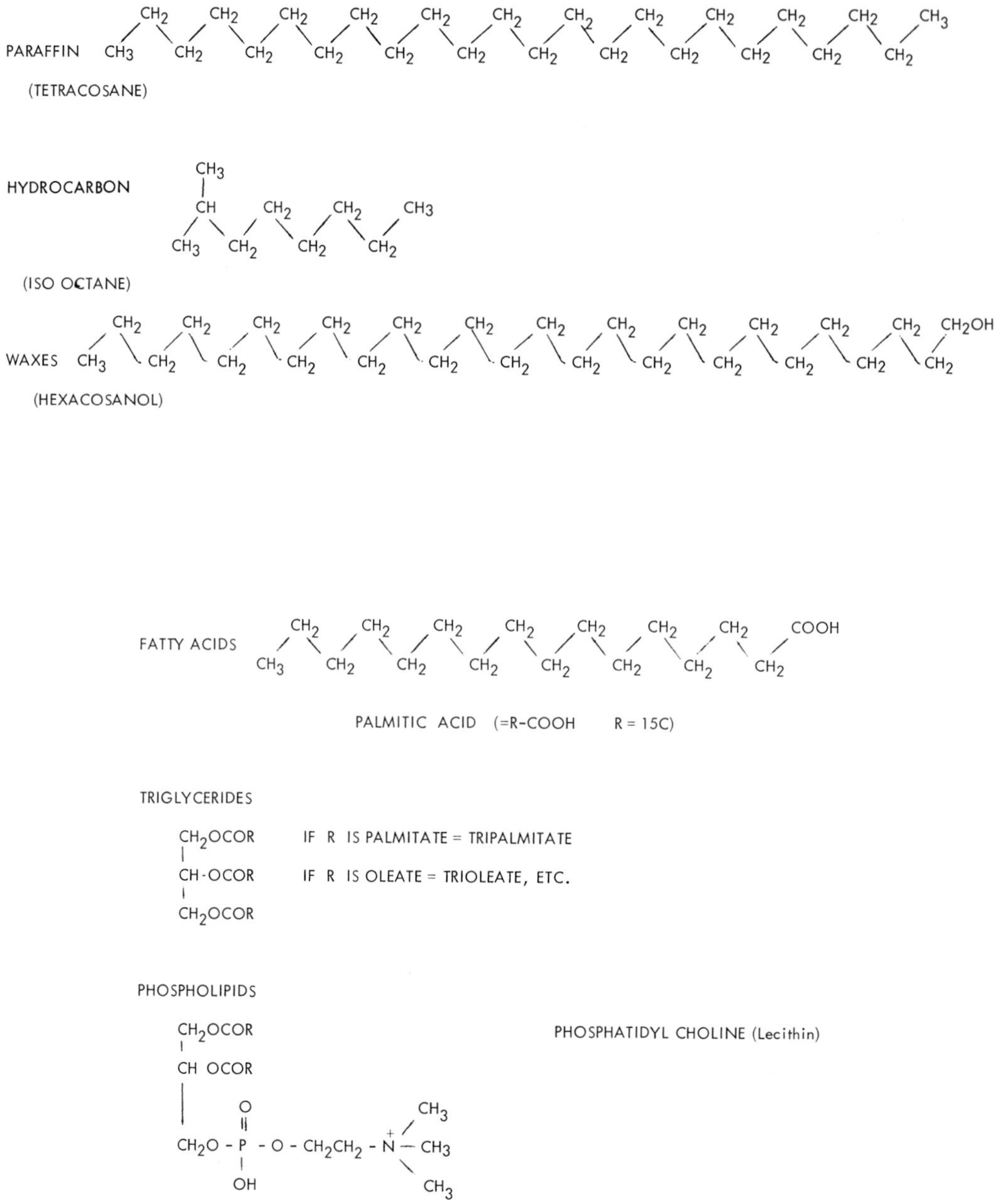

Fig. 23-1. *Top,* Chemical configuration of some lipids not utilizable by humans. *Bottom,* Chemical configuration of lipids most commonly utilized by humans.

diagnosis and investigation of fat malabsorption, a review of the overall process of fat digestion and absorption seems to be indicated.

It is important to recognize that significant differences exist in the digestion and absorption of various ingested lipids due to differences in the solubilities of the liberated fatty

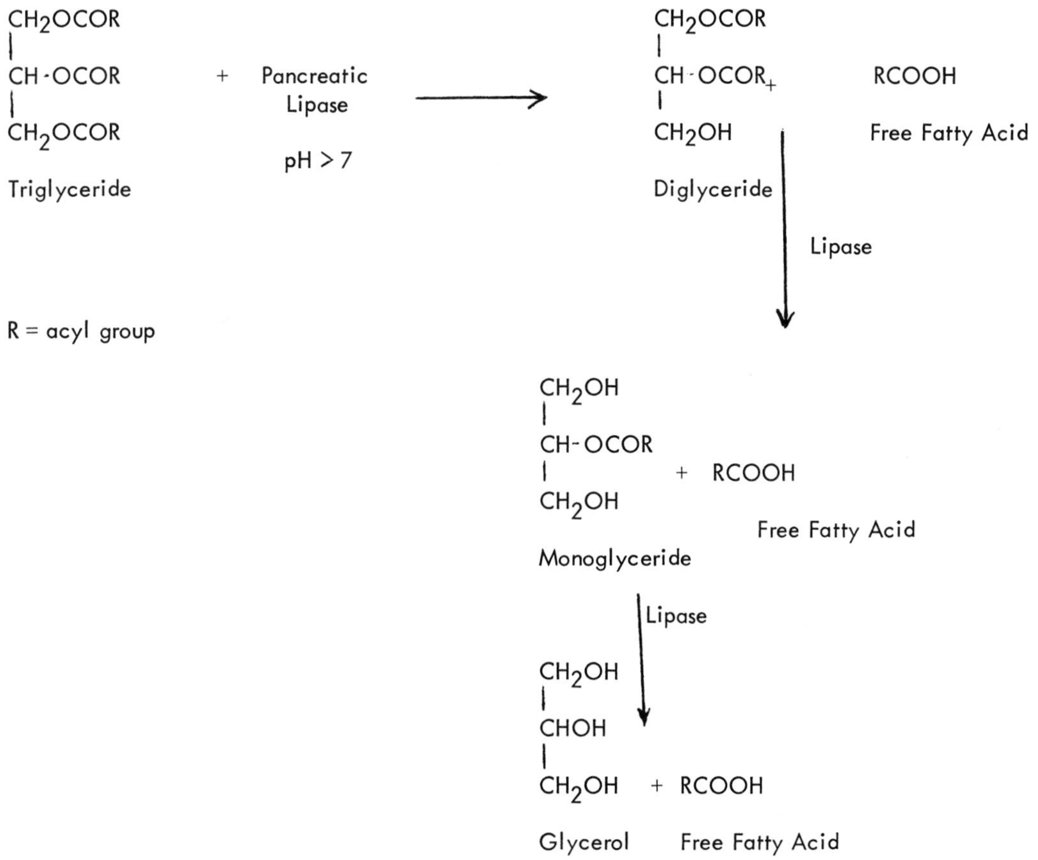

CH$_2$OCOR
|
CH·OCOR   +   Pancreatic   CH$_2$OCOR
| Lipase |
CH$_2$OCOR   CH·OCOR$_+$ RCOOH
                         pH > 7 |
Triglyceride   CH$_2$OH   Free Fatty Acid

                                              Diglyceride

R = acyl group

                                                           Lipase

CH$_2$OH
|
CH-OCOR
| + RCOOH
CH$_2$OH
                          Free Fatty Acid
Monoglyceride

              Lipase

CH$_2$OH
|
CHOH
|
CH$_2$OH   + RCOOH

Glycerol   Free Fatty Acid

Fig. 23-2. Action of pancreatic lipase on triglycerides.

acids. Fatty acids have a distinct solubility that depends on the fatty acid (acyl)-chain length. Basically, the short-chain fatty acids up to 6 carbons are soluble in water and readily cross membranes. The medium-chain fatty acids, 8 to 12 carbons in length, are partially soluble in lipid solvents as well as in water. This has given them unusual physicochemical properties which have prompted their use in various clinical syndromes.

The long-chain (16-24 carbon length) fatty acids are soluble only in lipid or organic solvents. These long-chain fatty acids include palmitic, oleic and stearic acid that are in large part esterified to glycerol to form triglycerides. Inasmuch as the vast majority of the 60 to 100 Gm of fat included in the average daily American diet consist of triglycerides, this discussion will emphasize this group of lipids.

Intraluminal Digestive Phase

An intraluminal digestive phase is usually considered the first step leading toward the absorption of fat. This phase occurs within the lumen of the intestine and consists of 2 parts.

1. *The lipolysis of triglycerides into fatty acids and monoglycerides by the action of pancreatic lipase.* Figure 23-2 depicts the chemical sequence occurring as a result of the action of pancreatic lipase on ingested triglycerides. This reaction depends on the integrity of the pancreas in the enzymatic synthesis and release of lipase. Inadequate

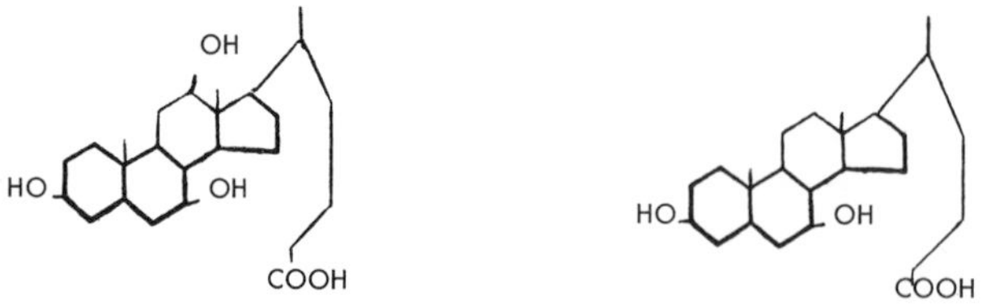

CHOLIC ACID
(3,7,12-Trihydroxycholanic acid)

A

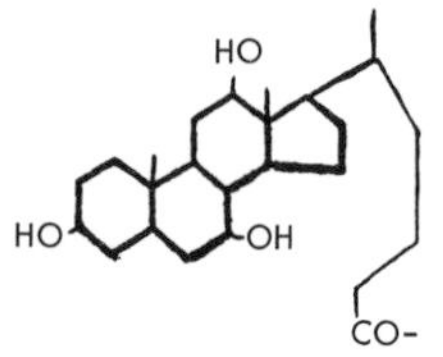

CHENODEOXYCHOLANIC ACID
(3,7-Dihydroxycholanic acid)

= R (CHOLYL-)

R - NHCH$_2$COOH   GLYCOCHOLIC ACID
(Cholylglycine)

R - NHCH$_2$CH$_2$SO$_3$H   TAUROCHOLIC ACID
(Cholyltaurine)

B

Fig. 23-3. *A*, Primary bile acids. *B*, Conjugated forms of cholic acid.

mixing of food with pancreatic lipase, such as may occur following gastrectomy, may interfere with lipolysis because of inadequate contact between the lipid and lipase. There is also evidence that an abnormally low pH of the intestinal contents, such as occurs in the Zollinger-Ellison syndrome, may interfere with the function of pancreatic lipase.

2. *The incorporation of the fatty acid with bile salts into aggregates called micelles.* The complete or partial hydrolysis of triglycerides into fatty acids and monoglycerides results in a change in the solubility pattern of the mixture. It becomes amphiphilic, accepting both water and lipid, and thus permits the formation of micelles with the detergent-like bile salts.

When the mixed micelle composed of fatty acid, monoglycerides and bile salts reaches the microvillus of the intestinal epithelial cell, it splits into its components. This is followed by passage of the mono-glycerides and fatty acid across the membranes of the microvillus. The bile salts, now freed of the micelle, are probably reused and eventually are almost completely reabsorbed in the terminal ileum by a process of active transport.

Abnormalities of Intraluminal Digestive Phase. A number of processes may interfere with the intraluminal phase. In the presence of extrahepatic biliary obstruction, inadequate amounts of bile may reach the intestine, jeopardizing micelle formation. A similar phenomenon may occur in chronic intrahepatic cholestatic processes, particularly biliary cirrhosis. Bile salt deficiency may result from severe disease of the terminal ileum, or from resection or bypass of the terminal ileum. Under these circumstances, the normally highly effective mechanism for bile salt reabsorption is lost and excess bile salts are lost in the feces. The enterohepatic circulation of bile salts is thus disrupted.

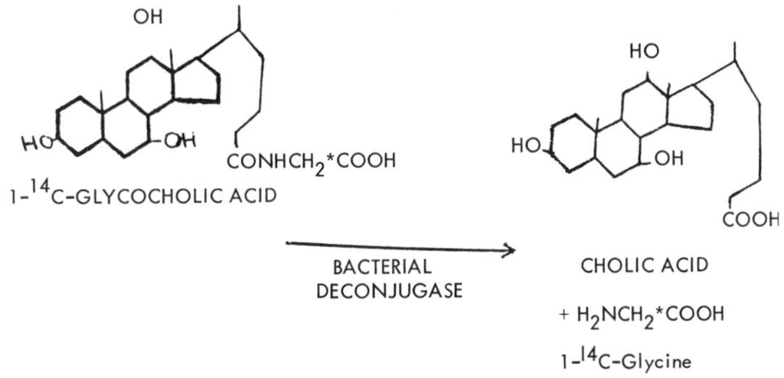

Fig. 23-4. Bacterial deconjugation of 1-^{14}C-glycocholic acid.

OH

HO

HO

HO

OH

OH

CONHCH$_2$*COOH

1-^{14}C-GLYCOCHOLIC ACID

COOH

BACTERIAL
DECONJUGASE

CHOLIC ACID

+ H$_2$NCH$_2$*COOH

1-^{14}C-Glycine

Although increased synthesis by the liver is able to compensate to some degree for bile salt loss, this is an inadequate mechanism in severe bile salt loss, and malabsorption is the consequence.

Optimal bile salt function depends on conjugation of the primary bile acids, cholic and chenodeoxycholic acid, with glycine or taurine. This important conjugating function is performed by the liver and results in the formation of the 4 primary bile salts (i.e., the glycine and taurine conjugates of cholic and chenodeoxycholic acids). Figures 23-3 *A* and *B* depict the chemical structure of the primary bile acids and their conjugated forms.

Certain bacteria, predominantly anaerobes, have the enzymatic capability of deconjugating bile salts, that is, splitting the amino acid moiety from its bile acid base. Deconjugated bile salts have a much reduced detergent activity. Bile salt deconjugation occurs in the colon secondary to deconjugase enzymatic action of the normal anaerobic inhabitants of the large bowel (Fig. 23-4).

Since, however, the reabsorptive ability of the terminal ileum allows only a small fraction of bile salts ($\sim$5%) to reach the colon, large bowel deconjugation is of little or no clinical consequence. In certain circumstances, however, overgrowth of the normally relatively sterile small intestine by anaerobes may result in bile-salt deconjugation that has a significant effect on micellar formation and fat absorption. Clinically, this is most frequently seen in the stagnant loop syndromes, especially that following Billroth II gas-

trectomy in which there may be anaerobic overgrowth of the afferent loop. Figure 23-5 depicts the anatomical situation following Billroth II gastrectomy which may lead to the "afferent loop" syndrome. A similar phenomenon may occur in diverticulosis of the small intestine and in severe motor disorders of the small bowel such as scleroderma.

Intramural Phase of Absorption

Intraluminal digestion is followed by an intramural phase of fat absorption. This phase commences with transport of fatty acids and monoglycerides across the mucosal cell membrane. Once within the mucosal cell, the digestive process is reversed, and fatty acids and monoglycerides are rapidly

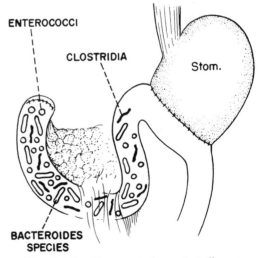

Fig. 23-5. Representation of "afferent loop" syndrome following Billroth II gastrectomy and gastrojejunostomy.

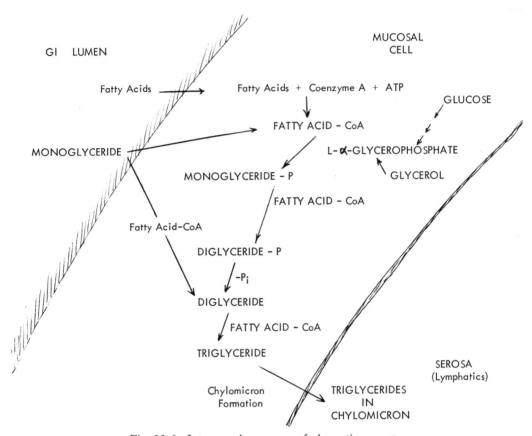

Fig. 23-6. Intramural sequence of absorptive events.

reassembled into triglycerides. Figure 23-6 depicts the intramural sequence of absorptive events.

Abnormalities of Intramural Phase. A host of disorders involving the mucosal absorbing cell may result in malabsorption of fat. The impairment may not be structural, as is the case in a-beta lipoproteinemia. In most cases, however, fat malabsorption is associated with inflammation, infiltration, villous atrophy or neoplasm. Included in this group of disorders are such entities as gluten enteropathy, tropical sprue, regional enteritis, lymphoma and amyloidosis.

Following intracellular reesterification, triglycerides leave the basal or lateral wall of the cell coated with beta-lipoproteins, pass through the lamina propria and enter the lymphatic vessels. This coated triglyceride is known as a chylomicron (Fig. 23-7).

Submucosal disorders such as Whipple's disease, scleroderma and intestinal lymphangiectasia may interfere with this phase of fat absorption. Medium-chain triglycerides are absorbed through the venous drainage of the bowel, thereby entering the portal circulation.

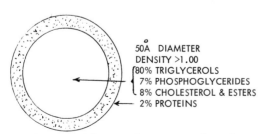

50Å DIAMETER
DENSITY >1.00
80% TRIGLYCEROLS
7% PHOSPHOGLYCERIDES
8% CHOLESTEROL & ESTERS
2% PROTEINS

Fig. 23-7. Diagramatic representation of a chylomicron.

In addition to the entities mentioned above, there are a number of disorders producing malabsorption in which the mechanism is not clear or in which multiple defects play a role (e.g., diabetes mellitus, carcinoid syndrome, mast cell disease, parasitic infestations, drug-induced malabsorption, endocrinopathies and hypogammaglobulinemias).

This cursory overview of fat digestion and absorption makes it apparent that a variety of mechanisms may be responsible for fat malabsorption. Although all have steatorrhea in common, the definition of the responsible defect requires a coordinated work-up including a carefully conducted clinical history and physical examination, appropriate roentgenographic studies, studies of pancreatic function, small bowel biopsy and the utilization of appropriate laboratory tests measuring various parameters of absorption. The latter include d-xylose excretion, serum carotene levels and the use of the Schilling test both with and without intrinsic factor.

RADIOISOTOPES IN FAT ABSORPTION

The use of isotopes in the study of fat absorption was introduced in the late 1940's.

Fats labeled with ^{131}I and with ^{14}C have been utilized for this purpose.

[131]I-Labeled Fats

Because of the restrictions (AEC) on the use of ^{14}C labeled materials in humans, Rutenberg, Seligman and Fine[1] in 1949 suggested that fats labeled with ^{131}I are more practical for chronic in vivo studies. They administered ^{131}I-labeled soy bean oil to dogs and measured specific activity in the blood following metabolism of the fat. Their attempts to separate inorganic ^{131}I from lipid-bound ^{131}I were unsuccessful.

In the same year Thannhauser and Stanley[2,3] reported the use of a similar technique in humans. ^{131}I-labeled triolein was administered to normal individuals and to patients with idiopathic hyperlipemia, and differences in the resultant specific activity of the sera were noted. This work was received with enthusiasm, and subsequently a number of studies appeared in the literature reporting the value of this procedure in the investigation of patients with fat malabsorption.[4-8] The main value of these studies was

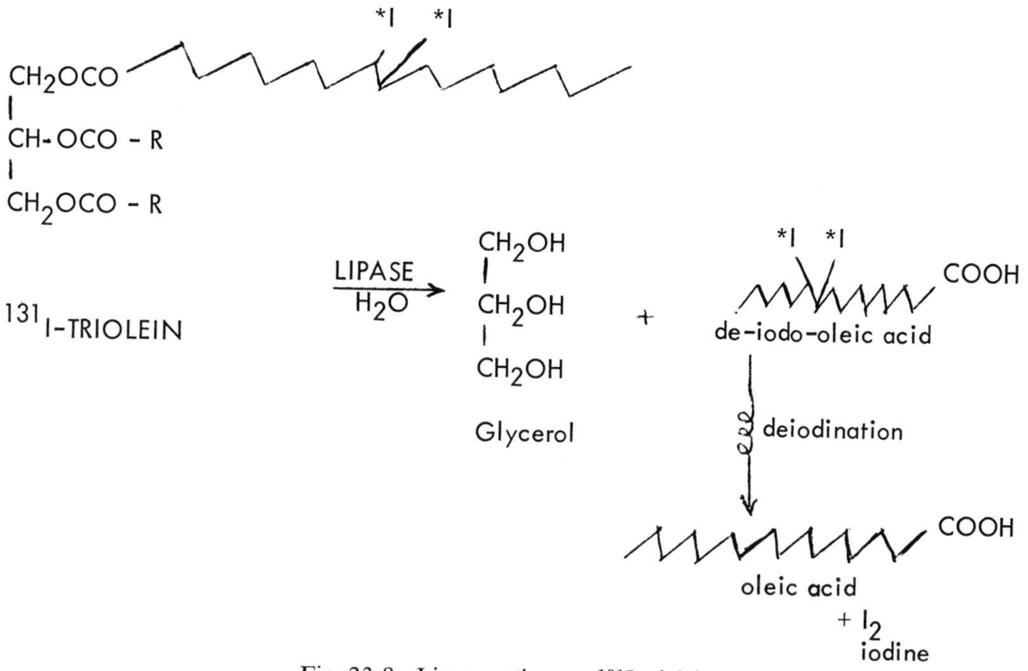

Fig. 23-8. Lipase action on ^{131}I-triolein.

thought to be their ability to differentiate between steatorrhea due to pancreatic insufficiency and that due to other causes. It was felt that this differentation could be made by comparing serum specific activity following administration of ^{131}I-triolein and ^{131}I-oleic acid. Thus, in pancreatic insufficiency and a deficiency of pancreatic lipase, levels of ^{131}I in the serum would be lower following administration of ^{131}I-triolein than after ^{131}I-oleic acid. The theory was that pancreatic lipase was necessary for the hydrolysis of triolein, and in its absence a discrepancy in serum-specific activity would result between ^{131}I-triolein and ^{131}I-oleic acid administration. Figure 23-8 depicts the action of pancreatic lipase on ^{131}I-triolein.

Prior to the study it is standard procedure to give the patient an oral dose of 10 drops of Lugol's solution for 2 days to block the thyroid and thus lower iodine removal from the sample. The fasting subject is given 25 to 35 μCi of ^{131}I-trioleate in a capsule. Shortly after this, a "cold" fat meal is given to the patient (1 ml of fat meal/kg of weight). Lipomul* is a fat emulsion that may be used for this purpose; it consists of a mixture of 67 percent vegetable oils and "Tween-80" as emulsifier. Two hours after the administration of the dose, blood samples are taken in heparinized tubes (5 ml). This is repeated several times at 2-hour intervals. Additional samples are taken 12 and 24 hours later. The exact time of blood withdrawal is recorded. The patient remains fasting for 3 hours after administration of the dose. For additional accuracy total stools may be collected for two 24-hour intervals. The counting of the specimens is reported as percentage of the dose given to the patient. For this purpose it is advisable to have a dose similar to the one given to the patient for control radioassay. The radioactive countings are corrected for estimated total blood volume of the patient and for radioactive decay. Pancreatic function is considered normal if the plasma-lipid radioactivity remains above 8 to 10 percent of

the given dose for a 6-hour period. If the plasma-lipid radioactive level drops below 6 to 8 percent, fat malabsorption due to pancreatic insufficiency should be considered.

The validity of these techniques soon became open to question. When the radioactivity results were correlated with chemical fat balance studies, it became apparent that the ^{131}I-labeled fat absorption test results were often misleading.[9-15] Normal levels of whole blood radioactivity have been reported in a significant number of patients with fat malabsorption.[9,12,15] Measurements of fecal radioactivity correlate somewhat better than blood levels, but their accuracy is still quite poor, especially when steatorrhea is mild or moderate.[14,16] It has also been demonstrated that impurities exist in ^{131}I-triolein, and it is likely that they contribute to the inaccuracies of the test. Thus, a relatively small amount of the ^{131}I label is on triglycerides, the remainder being on nontriglyceride fractions such as monoglycerides, diglycerides and monohydric alcohol esters.[17,18,19]

The process of iodinization of triolein may actually produce an abnormal fat molecule depending on how many double bonds of the triolein are iodinated. A chemically abnormal triglyceride can behave abnormally in any or all phases of fat digestion and absorption (i.e., intraluminal lipolysis, micellar formation, transport across the microvillus membrane) or in its distribution throughout the body. It has also been demonstrated that deiodination may follow the oral ingestion of radioiodinated triolein.[20-23] It is also important to emphasize that changes in gastric emptying may result in variable levels of blood radioactivity.[24]

In an effort to demonstrate the influence that ^{131}I-triolein impurities might have on its use in evaluating fat malabsorption, Tuna and his associates[18] manufactured radiochemically pure ^{131}I-triolein. When this was administered to a small number of patients with steatorrhea, the blood radioactivity was abnormal, whereas results had been normal when commercial ^{131}I had been used. Leinbach and his coworkers[25] recently repeated these studies utilizing 98 percent pure radio-

---

* Trademark, Upjohn.

iodinated triolein in a group of 44 subjects, including 15 normals, 10 with gastrointestinal disease but without fat malabsorption, and 19 with steatorrhea of various etiologies. Whole blood, plasma, plasma lipid, urine, and fecal radioactivity were measured after ingestion of the labeled test material. All of the normal persons had normal levels of blood radioactivity and normal fecal radioactivity. Of the patients with steatorrhea, 11 percent had normal blood radioactivity, but in only 4 percent was there normal fecal radioactivity. Sixteen of the 19 patients with steatorrhea had both excessive fecal radioactivity and low levels of whole blood radioactivity. The authors concluded that radiochemical purification of radioiodinated triolein improves the accuracy of this test of fat absorption.

Until these results are confirmed, the many serious problems inherent in the ^{131}I-triolein test have essentially removed it from our diagnostic armamentarium.

[14]C-Labeled Fats

[14]C-labeled fats were used to study in vivo absorption of fats in animals in 1948 and 1949.[26-27] In the early 1950's ^{14}C-labeled fats were utilized to study normal fat absorption and the differences in pathways and rates of absorption of fatty acids of differing chain lengths.[28,31] The popularity of radioiodinated fats in studying human fat malabsorption overshadowed the use of ^{14}C-labeled fats. With, however, the disillusionment over the use of ^{131}I-triolein, attention was redirected to the ^{14}C-labeled preparations. Van Handel and Zelversmit[32] indeed demonstrated that in animals, ^{14}C-labeled fat gave data of greater reliability than the corresponding ^{131}I-labeled materials in the measurement of fat absorption. Rothfeld and Rabinowitz[33] found that ^{14}C-labeled fat was superior to ^{131}I-labeled fat in evaluating neomycin-induced steatorrhea in humans.

Because of the relatively long half-life of ^{14}C, it was felt that such studies would be of greatest value when there was rapid elimination of the radiolabel from the host. Animal experiments had indicated that the measurement of [14]CO_2 activity in the breath following the oral or intravenous administration of ^{14}C-labeled fatty acids, afforded a means of studying the overall oxidation of fatty acids to CO_2.[27,34-36]

In 1962 Schwabe and his coworkers[37] reported the use in humans of ^{14}C-glyceryl trioctanate labeled with ^{14}C in the carboxyl position. The preparation was administered orally and radioactive carbon measured in the expired air. The results in a group of normal persons were compared to those in a group of 21 patients with a variety of malabsorptive syndromes. Although as a group there was a significant increase in breath-specific activity in the controls, considerable overlap existed with the malabsorbers and the test was unreliable in individual instances. In addition, measurement of the total breath [14]CO_2 is cumbersome and difficult. In 1966 Uthgenanant reported the use of a similar technique.[38]

In 1966 Abt and Von Schuching[39] described a modification of the breath-analysis technique that proved to be simpler, faster and more accurate. In view of the fact that in the fasting and resting person CO_2 production remains approximately constant, these investigators employed periodic rather than continuous sampling. Using a known quantity of an alkaline-trapping solution into which the patient expired, the specific activity of expired CO_2 could be calculated. ^{14}C-tripalmitin or ^{14}C-triolein was administered to normal controls and to patients with various malabsorptive states and arteriosclerotic cardiovascular disease. Significant differences between normals and malabsorbers were noted. In the latter, the heights of the curves of expired radioactivity were definitely lower, less distinct, and more prolonged than those of normal individuals. Abt and Von Schuching[39] also found that in all individuals tested, the specific radioactivity of exhaled [14]CO_2 following ingestion of ^{14}C-triolein was more than double that following the ingestion of ^{14}C-tripalmitin. The peaks of [14]CO_2 excretion from both radioactive fats occurred at identical intervals in each individual.

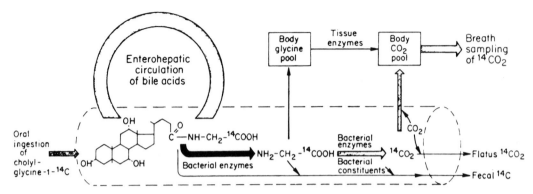

Fig. 23-9. Fate of ^{14}C after labeling endogenous cholylglycine pool with ^{14}C-G.C.A.

Using similar techniques employing ^{14}C-tripalmitate administered orally, Kaihara and Wagner[40] and Antar and his coworkers[41] reported good correlation between the specific activity of CO_2 in the expired air and other measurements of fat absorption such as serum carotene levels and determinations of fecal fat. Antar et al.[40] found that ^{14}C sodium octanoate was absorbed normally and rapidly even in the presence of advanced bowel wall dysfunction and grossly impaired ^{14}C-tripalmitate absorption.

The favorable reports of these investigators and the advantages of technical simplicity, as well as avoidance of the need to collect feces or blood indicate the need for further exploration of this technique in the study of fat malabsorption syndromes.

Detection of Bile Salt Deconjugation by Measurement of the Specific Activity of ^{14}CO$_2$ in Expired Air

Nonisotopic procedures currently available to detect bile salt deconjugation are technically difficult and are not routinely performed in clinical practice. To definitely establish the occurrence of bile salt deconjugation in the presence of a stagnant loop syndrome, for example, one requires intubation of the blind loop, culture of its contents under strictly anaerobic conditions, and in vitro chromatographic testing of the cultured organisms' ability to deconjugate bile salts.

In 1970 Hofmann and his associates[42] reported that when glycine-1-^{14}C-cholate was administered orally to patients who had

undergone ileal resection, the excretion of ^{14}CO$_2$ in expired air was increased when compared to normals. Subsequent reports have confirmed the fact that breath analysis appears to provide a simple, rapid, and effective screening technique for the detection of increased bile salt deconjugation.[43-45] It thus may provide a valuable diagnostic supplement in the study of the patient with steatorrhea.

The principle of the technique relies on the fact that in the presence of a normally efficient enterohepatic circulation, and in the absence of significant deconjugation, the administered radioactive bile salt recirculates in its conjugated form in the enterohepatic circulation. A small amount of bile salt is normally passed into the colon where deconjugation occurs as a result of enzymatic action by the normal anaerobic bacterial flora residing in the large bowel.

Under circumstances in which excessive bacterial deconjugation of bile salts occurs, the amino acid moiety is split from the bile acid and enters the general metabolic pool. Ultimately it emerges as CO_2 in the breath. If radioactive bile salts are administered in the presence of excess deconjugation, there is an increase in the specific activity of the ^{14}CO$_2$ in the expired air (Fig. 23-9).

Generally speaking, excess deconjugation occurs in 2 clinical situations: (1) when there is small intestinal overgrowth by bacteria, especially anaerobic deconjugators, and (2) when there is interference with the normally efficient reabsorption of bile salts by the ileum. The former situation occurs in the so-called stasis or stagnant loop syndromes, such as occurs in the afferent loop syndrome following Billroth II gastric resections (see Fig. 23-5), in small bowel diverticulosis, and in certain disorders interfering with motility of the small bowel such as scleroderma. Ileal malabsorption of bile salts occurs in severe disease of the ileum or under circumstances in which an ileal bypass or resection has been performed.

The authors have utilized this technique in a number of normal controls, and in patients with cirrhosis of the liver, steatorrhea unrelated to abnormalities in bile salt metabolism, stasis syndromes of the small bowel, ileal resection or bypass and in a miscellaneous group of disorders (Table 23-1).

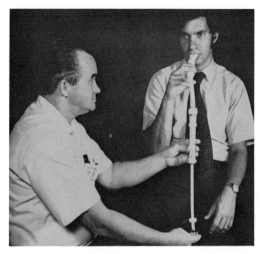

Fig. 23-10. Collection of expired air preparatory to determination of $^{14}CO_2$ specific activity.

Table 23-1—Diagnosis and Test Results

Group	Fecal Fat Gm/24 hrs	Total $^{14}CO_2$ Breath excretion/6 hrs (% administered dose)
1. **Normal controls** (10)	5 Gm	0.4-2.8
2. **Cirrhosis of the liver** (7)	5 Gm (5)	0.6-2.8
	5-10 Gm (2)	0.4, 1.6
3. **Steatorrhea unrelated to abnormality of bile-salt metabolism** (5)		
Chronic pancreatitis	50.8 Gm	2.7
Chronic pancreatitis	32 Gm	3.1
Chronic pancreatitis	34 Gm	1.6
Idiopathic	32.5 Gm	2.6
Idiopathic	23.5 Gm	3.0
4. **Ileal resection or bypass**		
Ileal resection	30-40 Gm	31.6
Ileal resection	26 Gm	19.0
Ileal resection	30 Gm	37.0
Gastrocolic fistula	38.6 Gm	30.7
Postsurgical correction	5.0 Gm	4.8
5. **Bacterial overgrowth syndromes with steatorrhea**		
Billroth II gastrectomy	14 Gm	16.2
Billroth II gastrectomy	22 Gm	29.0
Billroth II gastrectomy	18 Gm	21.0
Scleroderma	20 Gm	12.0
6. **Miscellaneous disorders without steatorrhea**		
Regional enteritis (2)		2.6, 2.7
Scleroderma (3)		0.6, 0.6, 1.2
Billroth II gastrectomy (4)		0.4, 0.6, 0.6, 1.0
Acute pancreatitis (1)		0.6

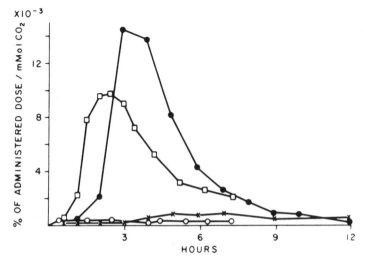

Fig. 23-11. Typical breath analysis curves after administration of 1-^{14}C-glycocholate.

Methods. Fasting subjects received orally 5 μCi of 1-^{14}C-glycocholic acid* dissolved in 1-2 ml ethanol in a glass of orange juice. The purity of the ^{14}C-1-cholylglycine was over 98 percent as determined by the method of Sjovall.[47] Breath samples were taken as a baseline and then every 30 minutes for a period of 6 hours. Exhaled air was desiccated by passage over anhydrous calcium chloride and collected in 2.5 ml of a CO_2-trapping solution (Fig. 23-10). This solution was prepared with 790 ml 1 M hyamine (p-diisobutylcresoxyethoxy-ethyl)-dimethylbenzylammonium chloride,† 1,700 ml of methanol, 20 ml of 1 percent phenolphthalein in methanol, and 1 ml glycerol.

Disappearance of the red color of the phenolphthalein solution is indicative of complete titration of the hyamine, indicating its conversion to hyamine carbonate; 13 ml of liquid scintillation phosphor solution (5.5 Gm PPO [2,5-diphenyloxazole] plus 300 mg POPOP [1,4-bis-2 (5-phenyloxazolyl) benzene] in 1 l toluene) are added to the hyamine-trapping solution and radioassay performed using the Packard Tri-Carb Spectrometer No. 3375, with pulse-height discrimination for [14]C. Counting was for a period long

enough to insure a maximal error of ±2 percent. The specific activity of the [14]CO_2 was calculated in the following manner: to 2.5 ml of a 0.3 M solution of hyamine (containing the phenolphthalein) 0.1 N hydrochloric acid was added until the pink color disappeared (=0.75 M; Fig. 23-11).

Standardization was accomplished by assaying the oral dose of 5 μCi of 1-^{14}C glycocholic acid for its radioactive content in disintegrations per minute (dpm). Since 1 μmol of [14]CO_2 may be generated from 1 μmol of 1-^{14}C glycocholic acid, we divided the obtained radioactivity of the [14]CO_2 in dpm by the total radioactivity administered to the patient. Thus a percentage of the original dose was obtained at each time interval. In many cases the patients contributed duplicate and triplicate breath specimens. These samples differed among themselves by less than 3 percent of their total radioactivity. All calculations were determined as a mole ratio of the original dose of 1-^{14}C-cholylglycine given.

Regular graph paper was utilized to plot results. The percent dose per μmole [14]CO_2 was plotted against time. The area under the 6-hour curve was measured and expressed as percentage of administered dose.

In some patients intestinal intubation and aspiration were performed and anaerobic and

---

* New England Nuclear, Boston, Mass.
† Rohm and Haas, Inc., Philadelphia

aerobic cultures taken using techniques previously described.[48] Following bacteria identification and colony counting, the organisms were tested for their ability to deconjugate bile salts utilizing a technique of thin-layer chromatography.[49,50]

Results. Table 23-1 lists the results of breath analysis in the various groups studied.

Normals. Ten men, 36 to 68 years of age, with no evidence of steatorrhea or gastrointestinal abnormalities were studied. All excreted less than 4 percent of the administered dose as $^{14}CO_2$ over a 6-hour period. This compares favorably with the findings of Fromm and Hofmann,[43] and Sherr and his coworkers.[44]

Cirrhotics. Normal values were obtained in 7 male patients, 44 to 59 years of age, with Laennec's cirrhosis, including 3 with modest steatorrhea (5-10 Gm of fecal fat/24 hours).

Steatorrhea unassociated with an abnormality of bile-salt metabolism. Three patients with chronic pancreatitis with fecal fat values of 32 to 60 Gm per 24 hours had normal breath analyses; 2 with idiopathic steatorrhea had normal values. In one of these patients with a Billroth II anastomosis, an afferent loop syndrome was suspected. The validity of the negative breath analysis was confirmed when intubation and culture of the afferent loop contents revealed insignificant bacterial counts, and no bile salt deconjugation could be demonstrated after thin-layer chromatography was used to identify the original bile salt.

Stasis syndrome associated with steatorrhea. Four patients were studied in whom small bowel bacterial overgrowth and steatorrhea were attributed to stagnant loops or stasis; 3 had an afferent loop syndrome following Billroth II resections and 1 had stasis and bacterial overgrowth secondary to scleroderma of the small bowel. All had significant amounts of steatorrhea, and there were marked increases in $^{14}CO_2$ specific activity in the breath indicating excessive bile salt deconjugation. The patient with scleroderma

had jejunal intubation, and the contents were studied for the presence of aerobic and anaerobic bacteria. There were 10^8 nonhemolytic *Escherichia Coli,* 10^8 B hemolytic *E. Coli* and 10^6 *Bacteroides melaninogenicus.* Dioxycholate was identified in the jejunal fluid utilizing thin-layer chromatography.

Ileal resection and bypass. Three patients were studied in whom ileal resection or ileal bypass had been performed because of regional ileitis. Steatorrhea was present in all. Administration of glycine-1-^{14}C-cholate was followed by the appearance of high levels of specific activity in the breath.

One patient was studied with a gastrocolic fistula following peptic ulcer surgery. Fecal fat content averaged 38.6 Gm/24 hours and there was a marked increase in $^{14}CO_2$ in the breath. Culture of the patient's stomach and stool revealed significant quantities of *Bacteroides.* Following surgical correction of his fistula, both fecal fat values and breath analyses returned to normal levels.

A group of 10 patients with a variety of gastrointestinal disorders unassociated with steatorrhea was studied. Included were 2 patients with regional ileitis, 3 with scleroderma, 4 with Billroth II gastrectomies without manifest afferent loop syndrome and 1 with acute pancreatitis. In all, breath analysis was normal. In one of the patients with a Billroth II procedure, cultures of the afferent loop revealed no bacterial growth and no evidence of bile salt deconjugation.

These findings as well as those of other investigators indicate that determination of breath $^{14}CO_2$ specific activity following the oral administration of a tracer dose of glycine-1-^{14}C-cholate is a rapid, simple and safe method for the detection of increased deconjugation of bile salts. No false-positives were detected.

Breath-specific activity rises to significant levels quite rapidly in positive cases and peak values are obtained in 2 to 3 hours. Though a 6-hour period was employed for monitoring breath-specific activity, it seems likely

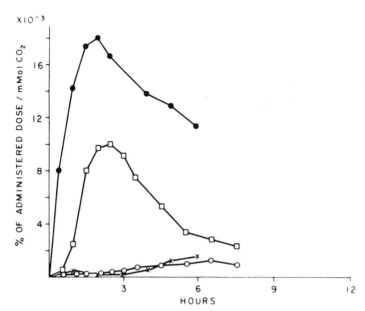

Fig. 23-12. Effect of treatment on $^{14}CO_2$ excretion after oral glycine-1-^{14}C-cholate administration in two patients with bacterial-overgrowth syndromes.

that a single analysis 2 to 3 hours following administration of the tracer dose of bile salts would suffice. Figure 23-12 represents typical breath-analysis curves following the oral administration of labeled glycocholate to 2 individuals before and after treatment.

A positive breath test does not indicate the site of bile salt deconjugation, but in most instances the clinical and roentgenographic findings establish the diagnosis.

Refsum's Disease

Heredopathia atactica polyneuritiformis, usually referred to as Refsum's disease, is an inborn error in metabolism in which phytanic acid (3,7,11,15 - tetramethylhexadecanoic acid) accumulates in many of the body tissues. The clinical picture has been well presented and reviewed recently by Steinberg and his associates.[51] The metabolic pathways of phytanic acid have been elucidated and recently reported by Avigan.[52] The inability of patients with Refsum's disease to utilize phytanic acid or its precursors, phytol, etc. rests in the enzymatic incapacity of formation of α-hydroxyphytanic acid, a necessary step for the oxidation of fatty acids. The presence of this defect permits the evaluation of this disease by a simple radioactive

breath-assay test, or remaining plasma radioactivity.

Patients suspected of having this disease are given 5 μCi of 1-^{14}C or U-^{14}C-phytanic acid intravenously. The oxidative half-life of this compound as shown by plasma levels in normal individuals is less than 1 day. In contrast to this value, patients with Refsum's disease show plasma-lipid radioactivity with a biological half-life of approximately 35 days.

Blood samples are taken at daily intervals, and the plasma assayed for ^{14}C-phytanic acid content by use of a tri-carb liquid scintillation spectrometer. Breath assays may be performed in the same manner as for intestinal bacterial invasion. Refsum's disease patients show only trace quantities of $^{14}CO_2$ in their breath even after 4 or 5 hours; control patients have 5 to 10 percent of the total injected radioactivity in the expired air in the first hour after injection (Fig. 23-13).

The sera of patients with Refsum's disease always show a high content of radioactivity. This level of activity remains approximately constant for 20 or 30 days after the ^{14}C-phytanic acid injection. The lipid is bound to the serum protein and slowly deposits itself through different organs and tissues. In

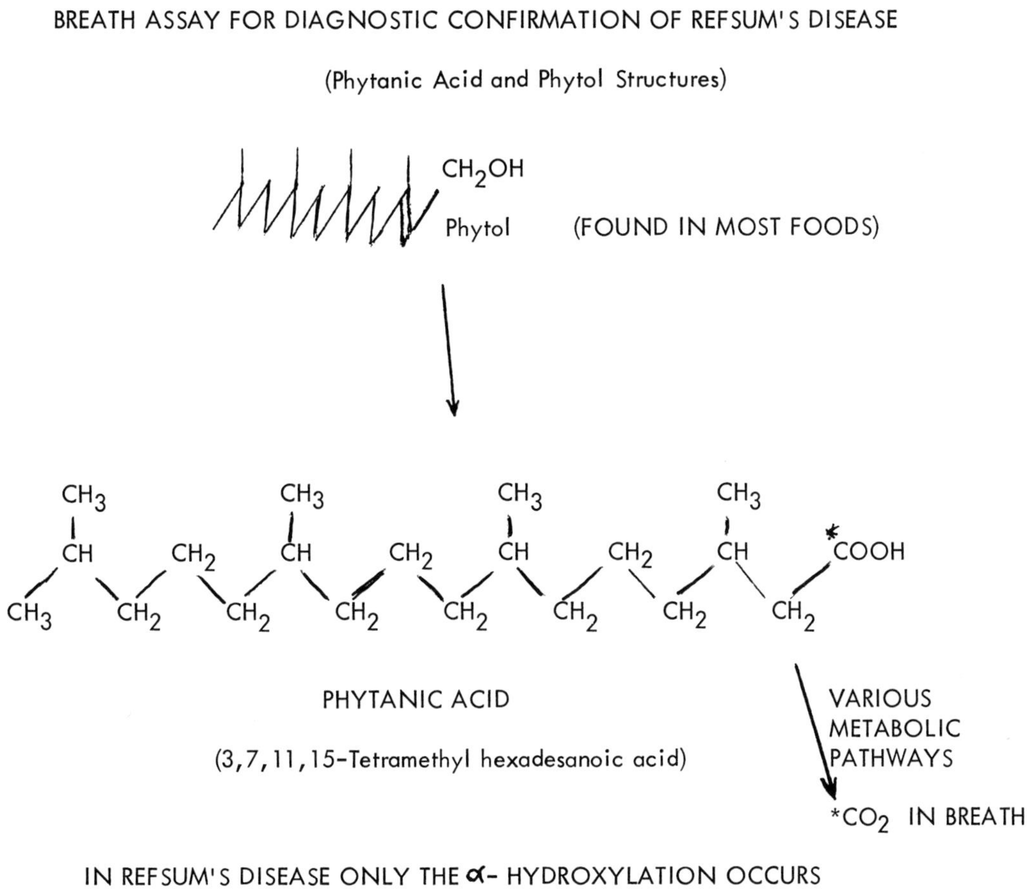

BREATH ASSAY FOR DIAGNOSTIC CONFIRMATION OF REFSUM'S DISEASE

(Phytanic Acid and Phytol Structures)

Fig. 23-13. Breath assay for diagnostic confirmation of Refsum's disease.

a control individual most of the radioactivity injected disappears from the serum protein by the end of 6 to 7 days.

The test is simple to perform and phytanic acid labeled is commercially available from various suppliers.

Research Applications

As pointed out by Hofmann and Thomas,[53] at the present time the Atomic Energy Commission's current list of "recognized medical uses of radioisotopes" does not include a single test using ^{14}C. However, the breath test for measuring bacterial deconjugation of bile acids may soon qualify as the first routine clinical procedure using ^{14}C.

As has been mentioned, $^{14}CO_2$ breath analysis has been utilized as a research tool in the elucidation of lipid metabolism and in the determination of biological half-lives. Thus, breath assay of $^{14}CO_2$ has been determined after the intravenous injection of ^{14}C-palmitate or 26-^{14}C-cholesterol, and from the data obtained, the biological half-life of these substances determined.

Of potential clinical significance has been the use of this technique to study the effect of various drugs on lipid metabolism. Thus, thyroid and its analogs have been studied for their influence on increasing rates of lipid metabolism. Evidence has been accumulated that indicates that dextrothyroxin is effective in increasing the rate of oxidation of fatty acids and cholesterol without appreciable effects on general metabolism.[54,55]

Recently, Edmond and Popjak[56,57] presented evidence that certain fatty acids may be derived through shunt pathways from mevalonate. When these investigators injected 2-^{14}C-mevalonate into rats, extensive labeling was detected in certain fatty acids obtained from the brain, spinal cord and skin. This was a previously unrecognized pathway of fatty acid formation and is an example of an important experimental use for carbon-labeled substances.

References

1. Rutenburg, A. M., Seligman, A. M., and Fine, J.: Studies with radioactive iodized fat. I. Preparation of radioactive fat with observations on the absorption of fat following subcutaneous and intraperitoneal injection in dogs. J. Clin. Invest., *28*:1105, 1949.

2. Thannhauser, S. J., and Stanley, M. M.: Serum fat curves following oral administration of I[131]-labeled neutral fat to normal subjects and those with idiopathic hyperlipemia. Trans. Assoc. Amer. Physicians, *62*:245, 1949.

3. Stanley, M. M., and Thannhauser, S. J.: The absorption and disposition of orally administered I[131]-labeled neutral fat in man. J. Lab. Clin. Med., *34*:1634, 1949.

4. Shingleton, W. W., Wells, M. H., Baylin, G. J., *et al.*: The use of radioactive-labeled protein and fat in the evaluation of pancreatic disorders. Surgery, *38*:134, 1955.

5. Ruffin, J. M., Shingleton, W. W., Baylin, G. J., *et al.*: I[131]-labeled fat in the study of intestinal absorption. N. Eng. J. Med., *255*:594, 1956.

6. Chears, W. C., Jr., McCraw, B. H., Tyor, M. P., *et al.*: The I[131] labeled triolein absorption test: Reproducibility and factors affecting blood levels. South. Med. J., *51*:433, 1958.

7. Likoff, W., Berkowitz, D., Woldow, A., *et al.*: Radioactive fat absorption patterns. Their significance in coronary artery atherosclerosis. Circulation, *18*:1118, 1958.

8. Bonnet, J. D., Hightower, N. C., Jr., and Rodarte, J. R.: Correlation of blood and fecal radioactivity after oral administration of I[131]-labeled triolein. JAMA, *181*:35, 1962.

9. Grossman, M. I., and Jordan, P. H., Jr.: The radio-iodinated triolein test for steatorrhea. Gastroenterology, *34*:892, 1958.

10. Lubran, M., and Pearson, J. D.: A screening test for steatorrhea using ^{131}I-labelled triolein. J. Clin. Pathol., *11*:165, 1958.

11. Jones, R. V.: Estimation of faecal fat. Br. Med. J., *2*:1236, 1960.

12. Pimparker, B. D., Tulsky, E. G., Kalser, M. H., *et al.*: Correlation of radioactive and chemical faecal fat in different malabsorption syndromes. Br. Med. J., *2*:894, 1960.

13. Berkowitz, D., Croll, M. N., and Shapiro, B.: Evaluation of radioisotopic triolein techniques in the detection of steatorrhea. Gastroenterology, *42*:572, 1962.

14. Moertel, C. G., Scudamore, H. H., Wollaeger, E. E., *et al.*: Limitations of the I[131]-labeled triolein tests in the diagnosis of steatorrhea. Gastroenterology, *42*:16, 1962.

15. Wormsley, K. G.: Use of labelled triolein, vitamin A, and D-xylose in the diagnosis of malabsorption. Gut, *4*:261, 1963.

16. Rufin, F., Blahd, W. H., Nordyke, R. A., *et al.*: Reliability of I[131]-triolein test in the detection of steatorrhea. Gastroenterology, *41*:220, 1961.

17. Lakshminarayana, G., Kruger, F. A., Cornwell, D. G., *et al.*: Chromatographic studies on the composition of commercial samples of triolein-I[131] and oleic acid-I[131], and the distribution of the label in human serum lipids following oral administration of these lipids. Arch. Biochem. Biophys., *88*:318, 1960.

18. Tuna, N., Mangold, H. K., and Mosser, D. G.: Re-evaluation of the I[131]-triolein absorption test; Analysis and purification of commercial radio-iodinated triolein and clinical studies with pure preparations. J. Lab. Clin. Med., *61*:620, 1963.

19. Kennedy, J. A., and Kinloch, J. D.: The impurity of radio-iodinated triolein. J. Clin. Pathol., *17*:160, 1964.

20. Beres, P., Wenger, J., and Kirsner, J. B.: The use of I[131] triolein in the study of absorptive disorders in man. Gastroenterology, *32*:1, 1957.

21. Turner, D. A.: The absorption, transport, and deposition of fat. Amer. J. Dig. Dis., *3*:594, 1958.

22. Berkowitz, D., Sklaroff, D., Woldow, A., *et al.*: Blood absorptive patterns of isotopically-labeled fat and fatty acid. Ann. Intern. Med., *50*:247, 1959.

23. Sie, H. G., Valkema, A. J., and Loomeijer, F. J.: Re-evaluation of radio-iodinated triolein as a test fat in fat absorption studies. J. Lab. Clin. Med., *70*:121, 1967.

24. Baylin, G. J., Sanders, A. P., Isley, J. K., *et al.*: I[131] blood levels correlated with gas-

tric emptying determined radiographically. II. Fat test meal. Proc. Soc. Exp. Biol. Med. 89:54, 1955.

25. Leinbach, G. E., Saunders, D. R., and Nelp, W. B.: Radiotriolein revisited: a study of the ^{131}I-triolein absorption test using radiochemically pure triolein in man. J. Nucl. Med., 13:252, 1972.

26. Geyer, R. P., Chipman, J., and Stare, F. J.: Oxidation in vivo of emulsified radioactive trilaurin administered intravenously. J. Biol. Chem., 176:1469, 1948.

27. Lerner, S. R., Chaikoff, I. L., Entenman, C., et al.: The fate of C^{14}-labeled palmitic acid administered intravenously as a tripalmitin emulsion. Proc. Soc. Exp. Biol. Med., 70: 384, 1949.

28. Bloom, B., Chaikoff, I. L., Reinhardt, W. O., et al.: The quantitative significance of the lymphatic pathway in transport of absorbed fatty acids. J. Biol. Chem., 184:1, 1950.

29. Bloom, B., Chaikoff, I. L., and Reinhardt, W. O.: Intestinal lymph as pathway for transport of absorbed fatty acids of different chain lengths. Amer. J. Physiol., 166: 451, 1951.

30. Bergstrom, S., Borgstrom, B., and Rottenberg, M.: Intestinal absorption and distribution of fatty acids and glycerides in the rat. Metabolism of lipids 3. Acta Physiol. Scand., 25:120, 1952.

31. Bergstrom, S., Blomstrand, R., and Borgstrom, B.: Route of absorption and distribution of oleic acid and triolein in the rat. Biochem. J., 58:600, 1954.

32. Van Handel, E., and Zilversmith, D. B.: Limitation of radio-iodine as a label for fat. J. Lab. Clin. Med., 52:831, 1958.

33. Rothfeld, B., and Rabinowitz, J. L.: Comparison of measurement of fat absorption using I^{131}- and C^{14}-labeled fats. Amer. J. Dig. Dis., 9:263, 1964.

34. Weinman, E. O., Chaikoff, I. L., Dauben, W. G., et al.: Relative rates of conversion of the various carbon atoms of palmitic acid to carbon dioxide by the intact rat. J. Biol. Chem., 184:735, 1950.

35. Lossow, W. J., and Chaikoff, I. L.: Carbohydrate sparing of fatty acid oxidation. I. The relation of fatty acid chain length to the degree of sparing. II. The mechanism by which carbohydrate spares the oxidation of palmitic acid. Arch. Biochem. Biophys., 57:23, 1955.

36. Bragdon, J. H.: $^{14}CO_2$ excretion after the intravenous administration of labeled chylomicrons in the rat. Arch. Biochem. Biophys., 75:528, 1958.

37. Schwabe, A. D., Cozzetto, F. J., Bennett, L. R., et al.: Estimation of fat absorption by monitoring of expired radioactive carbon dioxide after feeding a radioactive fat. Gastroenterology, 42:285, 1962.

38. Uthgenannt, H.: Resorptionsstudien mit dem $^{14}CO_2$-Exhalationsmessgerat FHT-50. Nucl. Med., 5:298, 1966.

39. Abt, A. F., and Schuching, S. L., von: Fat utilization test in disorders of fat metabolism. Bull. Johns Hopkins Hosp., 119:316, 1966.

40. Kaihara, S., and Wagner, H. N., Jr.: Measurement of intestinal fat absorption with carbon-14 labeled tracers. J. Lab. Clin. Med., 71:400, 1968.

41. Antar, M. A., Spencer, R. P., Hersh, T., et al.: Specific activity of expired $^{14}CO_2$ after administration of 1-^{14}C-sodium palmitate and 1-^{14}C-sodium octanoate in malabsorption and in normal controls. J. Nucl. Med., 10:(abstr.)385, 1969.

42. Hofmann, A. F., Thomas, P. J., Smith, L. H., et al.: Pathogenesis of secondary hyperoxalura in patients with ileal resection and diarrhea. Gastroenterology, 58:(abstr.)960, 1970.

43. Fromm, H., and Hofmann, A. F.: Breath test for altered bile-acid metabolism. Lancet, 2:621, 1971.

44. Sherr, H. P., Sasaki, Y., Newman, A., et al.: Detection of bacterial deconjugation of bile salts by a convenient breath-analysis technique. N. Eng. J. Med., 285:656, 1971.

45. Parkin, D. M., Cussons, D. J., Rooney, P., et al.: Evaluation of the "breath test" in the detection of bacterial colonisation of the upper gastrointestinal tract. Lancet, 2:777, 1972.

46. Myerson, R. M., Levison, M. E., and Rabinowitz, J. L.: Detection of deconjugation of bile salts by measurement of the specific activity of $^{14}CO_2$ in expired air. Amer. J. Med. Sci., 267:35, 1974.

47. Sjovall, J.: Quantitative determination of bile acids in human bile. Acta Chem. Scand., 10:1051, 1956.

48. Levison, M. E., and Kaye, D.: Fecal flora in man: Effect of cathartic. J. Infect. Dis., 119:591, 1969.

49. Tabaqchali, S., and Booth, C. C.: Jejunal bacteriology and bile-salt metabolism in patients with intestinal malabsorption. Lancet, 2:12, 1966.

50. Parkin, D. M., McClelland, D. B. L., O'Moore, R. R., et al.: Intestinal bacterial flora and bile salt studies in hypogammaglobulinaemia. Gut, 13:182, 1972.

51. Steinberg, D., Vroom, F. Q., Engel, W. K., *et al.*: Refsum's disease—a recently characterized lipidosis involving the nervous system. Ann. Intern. Med., *66*:365, 1967.

52. Avigan, J., Steinberg, D., Gutman, A., *et al.*: Alpha-decarboxylation, an important pathway for degradation of phytanic acid in animals. Biochem. Biophys. Res. Commun., *24*:838, 1966.

53. Hofmann, A. F., and Thomas, P. J.: Bile acid breath test. Ann. Intern. Med. (ed. note), *79*:743, 1973.

54. Rabinowitz, J. L., Rodman, T., and Myerson, R. M.: Effect of dextrothyroxine on metabolism of C^{14}-labeled cholesterol and tripalmitin. JAMA, *183*:758, 1963.

55. Rabinowitz, J. L., Rodman, T., and Smolinsky, T. L.: The effect of dextrothyroxine on the disappearance from the blood of C^{14}-labeled cholesterol. A preliminary report. Angiology, *13*:81, 1962.

56. Popjak, G., and Edmond, J.: The Transmethylglutaconate shunt of intermediates of sterol biosynthesis. Circulation, *44*: (abstr.)272, 1973.

57. Edmond, J., and Popjak, G.: Transfer of carbon atoms from mevalonate to n-fatty acids. Circulation, *48*:(suppl. IV)243, 1973.

24 *Protein-Losing Enteropathy*

MALCOLM M. STANLEY, M.D. AND
GERARD CERNIAK, M.D.

The methods by which, using radioactive isotopes, protein-losing enteropathy (PLE) can be diagnosed and its course evaluated is the main emphasis of this chapter. Most of our discussion is devoted to the technic of these laboratory procedures and interpretation of results of their use. Clinical aspects are considered very briefly, since they have been thoroughly reviewed in several detailed monographs,[1-7] the most recent of which was published in 1966. However, some new clinical developments have been reported since this last review.

HYPOPROTEINEMIA

Since nearly all patients with severe PLE have hypoproteinemia, we shall briefly consider the various etiologies of this manifestation. In the large majority of such patients the causal factors can be readily identified from the results of studies which have long been available (Table 24-1). One large group comprises those in whom the rate of protein synthesis is diminished as a consequence of liver disease or of reduced availability of substrate amino acids resulting from starvation, qualitative dietary inadequacy, or intestinal malabsorption.

A second group includes patients who have abnormally large losses of protein in the urine, from the skin (e.g., burns, pemphigus, chronic ulcerations, dermatitis, etc.),

and from miscellaneous sources (e.g., draining sinuses, fistulas). Although plasma is lost when bleeding from the gastrointestinal tract occurs, no one prior to the era of modern studies could prove that, in the absence of frank hemorrhage, lesions of the gut were responsible for significant losses of plasma proteins. Thus, prior to 1957 this source of protein loss was not recognized and a few patients could not be fitted into any of the other categories at that time.

In the third group, the hypercatabolic states, the common feature is an abnormally high metabolic rate. Examples most frequently seen are those consequent to chronic infections and to widespread cancer.

The mixed category is also large and varied. For example, in the alcoholic cirrhotic, protein synthesis may be acutely and chronically suppressed from the effects of alcohol and inadequate diet upon hepatocellular function. Cirrhosis may lead to PLE. These patients may also develop pancreatitis followed by pancreatic insufficiency and maldigestion.

CURRENT CONCEPTS OF PROTEIN-LOSING ENTEROPATHY
Events in Development

In these few patients in the absence of an apparent etiology the abnormality was designated as "idiopathic" hypoproteinemia. In 1950 Kinsell, et al.[8] found an abnormally rapid rate of loss of isotopically labeled proteins from the intravascular compartment in

Wherever *I appears in this chapter it refers to radioactive iodine, either ^{125}I or ^{131}I; *I-PVP is polyvinylpyrrolidone labeled with radioactive iodine.

Table 24-1. Causes of Hypoproteinemia.

DEFECTS IN SYNTHESIS
IMPAIRED CELLULAR FUNCTION
Liver disease (most common)
Administration of immunosuppressive agents,
    alcohol abuse
Limited to a single protein
    Various rare diseases,
    Analbuminemia, Wilson's disease,
    Agammaglobulinemia

SUBSTRATE INADEQUACY
Starvation
Low-protein diet, adequate in calories
Intestinal malabsorption; maldigestion
    (pancreatic insufficiency)
Competition for nutrients by parasites and
    proliferating bacteria in upper gut

INCREASED EXTERNAL LOSSES
Urine
    Nephrotic syndrome
Skin
    Burns,
    Pemphigus
Miscellaneous
    Draining sinuses,
    Abscesses
Gut
    Protein-losing enteropathy

TRUE HYPERCATABOLIC STATES
Thyrotoxicosis
Infections, Other febrile states
Malignancies
    Lymphomas,
    Leukemias especially
Cushing's disease, ACTH and adrenal cortical
    steroid administration

MIXED
Liver disease and dietary deficiency
Alcohol and dietary deficiency
Malabsorption plus PLE
    Sprue,
    Crohn's disease of small intestine

such patients. By 1957 these findings had been confirmed by improved methods using ¹³¹I-albumin and the syndrome was then called "hypercatabolic" hypoproteinemia.[9] The paper of Schwartz and Thomsen has a good review of the earlier literature on the subject. In 1957, Citrin, Sterling and Halsted[10] found, in a patient with so-called "giant hypertrophy of the gastric mucosa" and hypoproteinemia, an increased turnover

rate of intravenously administered *I-albumin and recovered enough labeled albumin from the stomach lumen to account for this exaggerated rate of loss from the plasma. The total nitrogen and *I excretion rates in the stools were normal in this patient. In the same year Steinfeld, Davidson and Gordon[11] studied patients with ulcerative colitis and regional enteritis and also found abnormally rapid rates of *I-albumin turnover. Very large quantities of the injected *I were excreted in the stools; both albumin and gamma globulin were identified immunochemically in the succus entericus of a patient with regional enteritis. Thus, these pioneering studies disclosed a previously undemonstrated route by which protein could be lost from the body. In 1959 Gordon[12] described the use of *I-PVP. After IV injection of this labeled macromolecular polymer he accurately inferred that excessive protein was lost from the gut by detection of abnormally large quantities of the label in the stools. This finding was immediately confirmed[13] and provided the impetus for a remarkable extension of the scope of such investigations. During the ensuing years, development of better methods has enabled many investigators to study a large number of such patients.

Present Views

Excessive loss of protein through the gut occurs in many diseases. Most of the organic disorders localized in the gastrointestinal tract, and a few generalized processes involving the gut, anatomically or functionally, at some time during their evolution have protein loss as a common feature. In all of these disorders there is nonselective ("bulk") transfer of protein into the gastrointestinal lumen.[14] Although the immediate source of this protein is the extravascular, extracellular pool, if the loss is so large that the capacity for compensation is exceeded, depletion of all related protein pools follows as manifested by decreased concentrations of intravascular (plasma) proteins. Except for α_2 macroglobulin and fibrinogen, there is a generalized reduction in the concentrations of the plasma proteins. If the site of abnormal loss is the colon or distal ileum the stools contain increased quantities of nitrogen, some of which may be in the form of whole protein or that which has been partially degraded by fecal microorganisms. If the protein loss is from the upper gut, complete digestion and absorption usually occur, and the rate of nitrogen excretion in the feces is normal. The fact that the rapid rate of protein loss from the body is reflected by a similar increase in removal rate of appropriately labeled proteins or other macromolecular indicators introduced into the blood stream is often of great diagnostic value. However, if demonstration of excessive protein loss is to be direct and unequivocal (measured in the stool) either this indicator or its label must have the unique property of being nonabsorbable.

The clinical picture is that of the primary disease plus the manifestations of protein depletion in the more severe cases. If the inciting disease is relatively silent, the latter features may be dominant and the patient may present only with edema and fluid accumulations in the serous cavities. The mechanisms by which the gut loses abnormal quantities of protein are incompletely understood. In one group the common feature is leakage of fluid high in protein from lymphatics dilated presumably because of increased intraluminal pressure. In a second large group inflammation and ulceration are present. In some cases both mechanisms may be operative and in a sizeable fraction the mechanisms have not been defined.

NORMAL LOSSES OF BODY PROTEINS INTO THE GUT

In addition to that ingested as food, large quantities of protein enter the gut lumen every day. Nasset[15] estimated that the endogenous fraction is greater than 100 Gm daily. This fraction consists largely of digestive secretions with a smaller component of shed cells and a relatively insignificant contribution from protein circulating outside the gut. Thus, the normal daily plasma loss through the gut is at most equivalent to the proteins contained in 20 to 35 ml of plasma; this is approximately 10 percent of the total quantity catabolized.[16,17] Results of a study by a different method[18] indicate that the size of the cellular contribution is smaller than that from extracellular sources.

RADIO-IODINATED HUMAN SERUM ALBUMIN (RIHSA) IN DIAGNOSIS OF OBSCURE HYPOPROTEINEMIA

The RIHSA test is of considerable diagnostic value in screening the majority of patients in whom the presence of PLE is suspected. With a few exceptions estimation of rate of albumin degradation using RIHSA should precede the more difficult fecal excretion tests. In many instances in which the problem is to detect excessive enteric protein loss in an uncomplicated clinical setting, the results of the RIHSA study when considered in relation to the other available data enables an inferential diagnosis of PLE, or allows the exclusion of this entity. It is often unnecessary to perform the studies involving stool collection.

TECHNIC OF RIHSA TEST

Administration of stable iodide, either as NaI or KI, 20 mg is begun 1 hour prior to the test and continued in the same dosage 3 times daily with meals until completion. An accurately known quantity (approximately 20 μc) of an acceptable, sterile, nonpyrogenic RIHSA preparation is injected intravenously without spillage into the tissues. Accurately timed venous blood specimens are drawn without stasis at 10 minutes after injection and daily thereafter for 14 days. Concentrations of radioiodine are estimated in aliquots of plasma, compared with appropriate standards and expressed as fractions of injected radioactivity. Results are graphed as a concentration-time plot on semilog paper. The data obtained after 7 to 10 days, when the plasma disappearance curve has reached its final slope, are most useful for estimating the rate of turnover of this protein

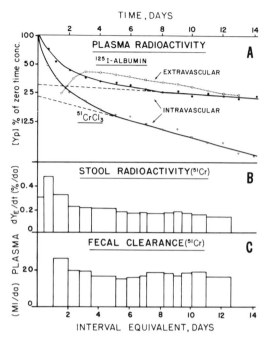

TIME, DAYS

Fig. 24-1. Results of a study using ^{51}CrCl$_3$ and ^{125}I-albumin administered IV simultaneously in a normal person. *A,* The plasma decay curves are graphed as percentages of zero time concentrations. The ^{51}Cr curve attains its final slope more rapidly and this slope is steeper. Comparative T-1/2's for these curves are 7 vs 22 days. The theoretical *extravascular* *I-albumin concentrations are depicted as open circles.[19,20] *B,* Daily rates of fecal excretion of ^{51}Cr for various "interval equivalents" are shown; each bar represents one stool. The width of each bar is proportional to the interval equivalent of the stool, estimated using Cr$_2$O$_3$, and the area is proportional to the total amount of radioactivity in the stool. *C,* The excretion rates have been correlated with plasma activities and the fecal clearances for each stool calculated as ml plasma per day.[21] We recommend that pooled stools, days 5 through 9, rather than individual stools as shown, be used for clearance studies.

in normal persons (Fig. 24-1). However, information from the earlier specimens is also valuable, and may be essential for interpretation in those patients in whom the slope is very steep. Usually a straight line curve is visually fitted to the plot of the appropriate points. A somewhat more precise fit of the

curve to the data is obtained by use of the least squares method. The half-time, T-1/2, is then estimated as the interval between any 2 convenient points on the line, the magnitude of the second of which is one-half that of the first. From a special form of the first order equation, the plasma disappearance rate, k_p is calculated as $k_p = -0.693/T-1/2$. From the quantity (total CPM or DPM) of RIHSA injected, *I, and the concentration of this in the 10-minute specimen, $[*I_P]_{10}$, the plasma volume, V_P, is calculated as $V_P = *I/[*I_P]_{10}$. The intravascular mass of this protein, A_P, is estimated from the equation $A_P = V_P [A_P]$, where $[A_P]$ is plasma-stable albumin concentration.

Interpretation of Results

Normal Values. A knowledge of *normal* values including means and expected variances—standard deviations—is required for interpretation. Assuming a "normal" distribution of results, an abnormal result can then be defined with any desired degree of precision. In the average large hospital laboratory information about mean values and variations to be expected is not available from local experience with a prospective study of a sizeable group of healthy subjects. In any event, the results might be applicable only to the specific preparations used. Hence, one must be satisfied with quotation of results from the literature and assurance that local experience is in agreement with these. This is usually satisfactory; such widespread reproducibility is possible as a consequence of excellent quality control in RIHSA preparation, use of standardized equipment and of adequate standards. For RIHSA prepared by the method of MacFarlane,[22] typical normal plasma disappearance rates (k_p) are 0.032 to 0.05 percent per day; the corresponding T-1/2's range from 14 to 22 days. The normal lower limit of this T-1/2 is 12 days.

Abnormally Rapid Disappearance Rate. This indicates either *true hypercatabolism* or *increased external losses.* Obviously these could also occur in combination. Those instances in which rate of degradation of the protein is likely to be truly increased include hyperthyroidism, infections and any disease in which fever is present, especially the leukemias and lymphomas and other widespread malignancies, inflammatory diseases, Cushing's syndrome and during administration of ACTH or corticosteroids in large doses.[23] Protein is commonly *lost* through the kidneys, the gut and the skin. In most instances in which an explanation for hypoproteinemia is sought, a source from the kidneys or skin is readily detected or excluded. In the absence of any of the hypercatabolic states or evident external sources of loss, the existence of PLE can reasonably be inferred and the source in a subtle gut disease sought by appropriate diagnostic studies. Thus, although an abnormally rapid plasma disappearance rate does not *in itself* allow direct differentiation between PLE and a hypercatabolic disorder, if other easily available data are taken into account this can almost invariably be accurately categorized. In the presence of a known gastrointestinal disease of uncertain activity, detection and quantification of PLE by this method is at least as accurate as with clearance tests. Also, a *normal result* allows exclusion of PLE with as much certainty as that from the more specific but less accurate tests which depend upon collection of stools. Hence, this screening procedure is a very valuable one. One reason for our favorable assessment of the usefulness of this test is the widespread availability of excellent quality labeled-albumin preparations from commercial sources. With present equipment the technic is relatively simple, so that acceptable results are feasible even when large numbers of tests are performed by technicians with average training. A large experience has accumulated. Radiochemical purity of each new lot should be determined by the manufacturer; a certificate with these data should accompany each shipment. However, a defective albumin is occasionally received and good preparations may be denatured as a consequence of bacterial con-

tamination or storage under adverse conditions. Use of denatured albumin in itself leads to an abnormally rapid plasma disappearance rate. Adequacy of a preparation, about which (from its cloudy appearance or other reason) there is doubt, can be verified by culture and radiochemical analysis of fractions obtained by means of polyacrylamide gel electrophoresis or column chromatography with Sephadex or Bio-gel. However, it is preferable to discard such dubious specimens. Because of its longer shelf-life we prefer ^{125}I as a label to ^{131}I. Despite its longer physical half-life (60 days), ^{125}I presents no greater radiation hazard to the patient than ^{131}I. This is in part attributable to lack of beta emission by ^{125}I.[24]

Several assumptions and other practical problems should also be discussed. Basic to such studies is the assumption of a *steady state,* that is that rates of synthesis and total degradation, including external losses of the protein, are equal and do not change during the period of investigation. The labeled products of iodalbumin catabolism are present in the plasma and excreted in the urine mainly as iodide but these also include iodotyrosyl residues. The requirement that *these metabolic products not be reused in vivo in albumin synthesis* seems to be adequately fulfilled. These labeled residues are not separated from the radioiodinated albumin in the plasma before estimating ($*I_P$), plasma concentration of radioiodine; hence this estimate is of the sum of these fractions. Administration of relatively large amounts of stable iodide inhibits accumulation of radioiodide by the thyroid and accelerates excretion in the urine normally. The nonalbumin radioiodine fraction is normally a small portion of the total and is relatively constant throughout the study, so that the error in estimating plasma disappearance rate attributable to presence of this nonprotein-bound *I is insignificant. However, in presence of *renal failure* and abnormally slow iodide excretion, radioiodide may comprise a much larger than normal fraction of total radioactivity. In this situation, especially if there is also truly acceleration of plasma-albumin disappearance rate, there may be substantial error if the nonprotein-bound fraction is not taken into account. It is desirable to have an estimate of adequacy of renal function, at least by such simple means as serum BUN and creatinine concentrations and creatinine clearance, before beginning this study. If manifestations of an authenticated *iodide hypersensitivity* are more than trivial the test is contraindicated. The ^{127}I administered to block thyroid uptake of $*I$, but not the $*I$ itself, is responsible for any iodide hypersensitivity. The mass of the $*I$ is so minute that it has no effect as a drug except that attributable to the radiation.

DIRECT DEMONSTRATION OF LOSS OF MACROMOLECULES THROUGH THE GUT

Properties of Substances Used

Understanding of PLE has improved considerably during nearly 2 decades since its existence was established with certainty. This was possible almost solely because of development and application of methods using radioactive isotopes for directly demonstrating enteric protein loss. Although several procedures allow quantification of this loss none is ideal. Requirements for an ideal label for this purpose have been listed[16] as follows:

1. The radioactive label should not alter the survival or distribution of the protein, nor should the label be eluted from the protein. If this requirement is fulfilled, the labeled protein can be used to quantitate simultaneously the rates of intestinal protein loss, endogenous catabolism and, in the steady state, protein synthesis.

2. There should be no absorption of the label from the intestinal tract; otherwise the extent of the gastrointestinal protein loss will be underestimated.

3. There should be no loss of label into the gastrointestinal tract in any form other than as the intact labeled protein. Excretion of unbound label results in overestimation of the gastrointestinal protein loss.

4. The label should be easy to detect and quantitate in the stools; it should be safe for the subject and should be excreted only minimally in the urine because of possible urinary contamination of the stool.

5. To this list might well have been added: The isotope should have a long enough half-life so that its widespread use would be convenient, feasible and not prohibitively expensive.

Competitive Clearance. Of the labeled indicators to be discussed, $*I$-PVP (polyvinylpyrrolidone labeled with radioiodine), ^{59}Fe-ID (dextran complexed with radioiron) and ^{51}Cr (from ^{51}Cr-albumin or $^{51}CrCl_3$) are removed from the plasma mainly by the reticuloendothelial system (RES). Considerable but smaller fractions of all except ^{59}Fe-ID are excreted in the urine. Normally a very small portion is lost into the gut. Severe dysfunction of the RES or kidneys results in more sustained, higher plasma-label concentrations and a greater excretion in the stools. If this were detected by the semiquantitative stool tests alone this increase over the normal in fecal excretion would be interpreted as indicative of the presence of PLE. On the contrary, increased loss in the urine (nephrotic syndrome), increased uptake by a hyperphagic RES, or dilution in an abnormally large EC fluid volume, reduce fecal excretion. The more precise clearance tests take into consideration the concentrations of label in plasma and are not in error. It should be kept in mind in interpreting results of semiquantitative stool excretion tests that alteration of function of the principal organs of metabolism of these indicators may influence the size of the fraction excreted in the feces. However, this is not a problem with an ideal indicator.

QUANTITATIVE ESTIMATION OF ENTERIC PROTEIN LOSS

Enteric Clearance, C_{gi}.[21,25-29]

In the clearance method, concentrations of label in plasma are related to quantities of label in the stools and expressed as the volume of plasma containing the quantity excreted per unit time. Enteric clearance is specifically defined as follows:

$$C_{gi} = \frac{dY_E(t)/dt}{[Y_P](t)}. \qquad (1)$$

Y = labeled substance cleared

$dY_E(t)/dt$ = rate of entry into the gut

[Y_P] = concentration of the label in plasma at moment of clearance

As studies of gut clearance are carried out over several (usually 4-6) days, and as the results are best expressed as ml plasma (or fraction of IV volume) per day, an integral expression is more appropriate.

$$\frac{\text{Label in Stools}}{\text{Plasma Label Concentration}}$$

$$C_{gi} = \frac{\int_{T_1}^{T_2} Y_E(t) \cdot dt}{\int_{T_1}^{T_2} [Y_P](t) \cdot dt}, \qquad (2)$$

$T_2 - T_1$ is the interval during which clearance is estimated.

To estimate clearance of macromolecules through the gut the following steps are essential.

1. After intravenous injection of an appropriate labeled substance, estimate concentrations of this indicator in sequential, accurately timed specimens of plasma.

2. Collect stools containing the "cleared" indicator during an appropriate interval and estimate the quantity of label. This stool collection must be complete, and the interval during which the food, from which these residues were derived, was eaten ("interval equivalent"—IE) must be known.

3. Match the calendar dates of the interval during which the collected food residues flowed past the area of gut that was the source of the "cleared" indicator to the same interval on the plasma indicator time-concentration plot.

4. After transformation of the 2 sets of raw data, calculate C_{gi} from equation (2).

Data from Indicator in Stools (Numerator)

In the above sequence, problems concerning collection and processing of stools and application of the derived data are difficult to solve.

Traditional Method. Administer by mouth a marker that can be identified in stools, such as carmine red or charcoal, before breakfast on both the first and fifth days of the test. Inject intravenously labeled plasma indicator immediately after breakfast and draw blood specimens at 10 minutes and daily thereafter for the duration of the study. Determine plasma radioactivity concentrations as for the *I-albumin study. Begin the stool collection with the stool in which the colored marker first appears and continue until the first stool containing the second marker is voided; discard this last stool. The interval equivalent (IE) is assumed to be that period separating administration of markers. The calendar interval during which intestinal contents are in contact with the site of entry into the gut of plasma indicator is commonly estimated by assuming that the bolus passed this location 24 hours prior to being voided as a stool.[16,17,30] Bring the stool pool to an appropriate consistency by homogenizing[31] after adding water and stabilizer, such as methyl cellulose, and a convenient aliquot is analyzed for radioactivity.

An alternative method, which reduces handling and eliminates aliquoting of stools, is to collect the entire pool in a suitable standard container from which gamma emissions are quantified directly by means of an appropriate detector system. Add water to a standard volume briefly stir the contents until grossly dispersed. Compensate for nonuniform distribution of stool radioactivity within the container by using an appropriate geometric relation between specimen and detector.

Faults of the traditional method. The outstanding defect of this procedure is uncertainty concerning the interval equivalent. Inability to verify objectively completeness of stool collections adds to this insecurity. If studies are performed while the patient is hospitalized in a metabolic ward, probability for loss is reduced but not eliminated. When the test is carried out under other conditions the likelihood that stools will be lost is great. Use of qualitative indicators such as carmine red or charcoal only slightly improves precision of results of such stool studies. The interval between clearance of labeled indicator into the gut and voiding of this material in stools is highly variable from person to person and depends upon location (stomach vs. colon) of clearance sites. Also, plasma and stool radioactivity concentrations are matched during a period when both, but especially the former, are rapidly changing. These inadequacies and others have led to development of a more precise alternative method.

Steady-state Inert-marker Method.[21,32] Administer an inert nonabsorbable marker, chromium sesquioxide, Cr_2O_3, in accurately weighed quantities by mouth at a constant daily rate. After 3 to 4 days of administration a steady state is attained in which concentrations of this indicator in dried stools are constant and fecal excretion rate is equal to rate of intake. During the period when this steady state is maintained the IE of either a single stool or a fecal pool is precisely defined by the inert-marker content relative to rate of intake. Thus, with a Cr_2O_3 intake rate of 1.50 Gm per day, if a "5-day" accumulation of stools contained 5.25 Gm, the true IE ("stool time") would be 3½ (5.25/1.50 = 3.5) days.

Technic. Begin administration of Cr_2O_3 with a loading dose of 1.500 Gm at breakfast on day 1 and continue in dosage of 0.500 with each meal, 1.500 Gm per day, throughout the study. Within a few minutes after the first dose of Cr_2O_3, give $^{51}CrCl_3$ IV. Draw blood speciments at 10 minutes and daily for 10 days and determine plasma radioactivity concentrations as for the *I-albumin study. Administer brilliant blue[33] on day 5 before breakfast and collect all stools, beginning with the first blue stool, for the following 5 days. Record times of voiding of the first and last stools. Stop Cr_2O_3 administration at the end of the fifth day following appearance of blue marker in stools. Estimate the ^{51}Cr and Cr_2O_3 contents of the pool. (See

Blood Volume, Chapter 5.) Since the pool must be homogenously mixed in order to estimate the Cr_2O_3 content from a representative aliquot, measure ^{51}Cr in the same aliquot or a similar one rather than in the whole collection as described above. Estimation of IE varies somewhat in relation to location of clearance site. If protein loss is from stomach, small bowel or site unknown, calculate the IE from the Cr_2O_3 content of the stool pool divided by intake rate. This interval will extend from the fifth day after injection of ^{51}Cr. If the site of protein loss is in the colon, a better estimator is the calendar interval between times of passage of first and last stools in the pool. This assumes that: (1) The stool bolus sweeps along with it all of the exuded protein; (2) intestinal flow is not obstructed; (3) and no stools are lost. Compare the interval equivalent (calculated as above) with the calendar interval and use the briefer period. Usually if ulcerative colitis is the etiology of protein loss, intervals measured by these 2 methods are quite similar.

Deficiencies of the inert-marker method. This requires more time for completion than the traditional procedure. However, if the recommendation[34] that all clearances be done during the flattest portion of the plasma-indicator curve is followed, the 2 methods are of the same duration. Administration of marker and analysis of this indicator in stools are additional necessary steps in the more precise method. Evidently loss of stools is not detected, but "lost" stools are not spuriously included in the collection. Only analysis of marker in stools collected for the entire period of administration of Cr_2O_3 enables detection of "lost" stools. This additional labor can be justified when the procedure is part of a research project, but may not be indicated under other circumstances.

Shortcomings of both methods. Most plasma indicators are excreted in urine as well as stools. Mixing of these excreta, unavoidable in some patients, especially children, is difficult to detect and increases spuriously the clearance rate.

Estimation of magnitude of numerator. In equation 2 this is the total quantity of indicator isotope in the stool pool. It is corrected for differences in counting geometry so as to be directly comparable to the indicator isotope concentrations in plasma.

Data from Plasma Indicator Concentrations (Denominator)

Relationship of Plasma Indicator Concentrations to Entry of Indicator into the Gut. The concept of clearance is simple, but is somewhat changed by the inference that the immediate source of the excreted label may be a part of the extravascular fluid in which the specific activity (SA) of the label (*I-albumin) is different from that in the plasma. Also the relationship between the specific activities in the intravascular and extravascular compartments is variable with time and depends upon the phase of the plasma-decay curve and the sites of origin and degradation of the labeled compound. For albumin these sites are considered to be in the intravascular compartment, or in specialized cellular compartments in rapid equilibrium with it.[19] Soon after injection of labeled albumin the SA is higher in the intravascular space, but after the first 2 to 3 days equilibration with the general extravascular compartment occurs; thereafter SA in the generalized extravascular fluid remains higher as the compound is metabolized and the label excreted from the intravascular compartment (see Fig. 24-1).[19,20] These considerations may also apply to [51]Cr. Thus in those studies in which excretion of the label has been determined in individual stools, the fecal excretion rate rises to a peak sometime during the 2 to 3 days after IV injection of the labeled compound, after which there is a rapid, then gradual, decrease in the rate, so that it generally parallels concentrations of label in plasma. During the first few days after IV injection the slope of the plasma-decay curve is relatively steep; the integral mean (or the

integral) of the SA's or concentrations can be most accurately estimated after resolution of this composite curve into its several component exponentials.[19,28,35] As a consequence of the uncertainties in intravascular-extravascular specific activity relationships, and of difficulties in calculations and in interpretations during the equilibration phase, Beeken and Harwood[34] urged that clearance studies be done only during the period following that of equilibration. We concur.

From the preceding paragraphs 2 sources of error are evident in: (1) Estimation of the duration of the IE for the stool collection; and (2) matching of the calendar interval during which this collection passed the area of entry of protein into the gut with the calendar interval of the plasma-decay curve. The magnitudes of both errors are minimized if the study is done during the flattest, least steep portion of this curve (see Fig. 24-1).

Estimation of magnitude of denominator. From the stool data we have an estimate of the duration of the IE and have also estimated the calendar dates of this interval so that it can now be located on the plasma time-concentration curve. This curve has been already defined and its slope calculated as described before. The plasma concentration of label at the beginning of the study interval and at the end can now be read from the curve or calculated. If the study has been done during the final phase of the plasma-decay curve when the slope is monoexponential, the integral label concentration for the study interval is

$$\int_{T_1}^{T_2} [Y_P] (T)\, dt = 1/k\, ([Y_P]_{T_1} - [Y_P]_{T_2})$$

For example, in the study shown in Figure 24-1, the T-1/2 for $[Y_P]$ [51]Cr after the fourth day is 7 days; $k = 0.10$ per day, and $1/k = 10$. If the 7 stools, beginning with IE 5.2 and ending with IE 10.1, are pooled the total IE is 4.9 days. The $[Y_P]_{T_1}$ at 5.2 days is 0.139 and $[Y_P]_{T_2}$ at 10.1 days is 0.085. The integral over 4.9 days is $10(0.139 - 0.085) = 0.54$.

These are expressed as multiples of the 10-minute (=100%) concentration; the absolute concentrations in CPM can be readily estimated from these values.

If the study has been performed during the early phase of the plasma-decay curve before equilibration has occurred, and during the period when the concentration of the label is changing rapidly and this curve is multiexponential, estimation of the integral or mean integral of the plasma-label concentration is more difficult. The former may be measured in several ways. A time-honored method is to plot the curve on rectilinear (not logarithmic) graph paper and measure with a planimeter the area under the curve for the interval. A similar result can be obtained by accurately weighing the cutout area and comparing this to the weight of a similar sheet of known area. Finally, by "curve peeling" the curve may be resolved into its 3 or more component exponentials and the integral for each curve determined during the study interval as described above; the sum of the integrals of these component curves is the desired integral of the composite curve. Several authors have published detailed directions for performance of this last calculation.[19,28,35] As indicated previously, when the study is carried out during this early phase of the plasma-decay curve even slight mismatching of the data for plasma and stools results in relatively large error.

Calculation of C_{gi}

After the values in equation 2 for the numerator (total indicator isotope in the stool pool) and for the denominator (integral plasma isotope concentration) during the same interval equivalent are known, C_{gi} is calculated by substituting in this equation. In the example cited, if the stool pool (IE 4.9 days) isotope content was 12,600 CPM (corrected for counting geometry so as to be directly comparable to [Y_P]) and the integral of [Y_P] over the same interval was 636 CPM per ml, $C_{gi} = 12,600/636 = 19.8$ ml plasma per day. For normal persons C_{gi} varies only

slightly when quite different macromolecules are employed as the test material. Normal values are from 2 up to 35 to 40 ml per day.

SEMIQUANTITATIVE DETECTION OF EXCESSIVE ENTERIC PROTEIN LOSS

Common features of all of these empiric procedures are intravenous administration of a known quantity of a labeled macromolecule; over the following 4 to 5 day interval the stools are collected between orally administered markers and the quantity of excreted label estimated as a fraction of the injected dose. Although there are theoretical objections to the collection of stools for this purpose during the rapidly changing preequilibration phase of the plasma-decay curve, this period has invariably been used. Indeed, the rate of loss from the intravascular compartment is so rapid for some of the nonprotein-labeled materials, such as *I-PVP and ^{59}FeID, that this is the only procedure possible. The properties of an ideal indicator or labeled compound have been previously discussed. Subjects without gastrointestinal disease and with normal plasmaprotein concentrations and *I-albumin plasma-decay curves have usually excreted 1.0 to 1.5 percent or less of the injected label during the 4 to 5 days. In early investigations, perhaps because of choice of patients with severe disease, those with PLE excreted so much more of such indicators as *I-PVP and ^{51}Cr-albumin than the controls that the value of these labeled substances was promptly established with small series.

This may be an acceptable alternative procedure to the more difficult clearance test. The likelihood that kidney or RES disease would change competitive clearance and lead to a false outcome from this fecal excretion test has been mentioned before. Variations in results with repeated tests in the same persons under the same conditions are not known. The results are not obtained in terms of meaningful functions such as rate of protein loss. Hence, the term "semiquantitative" is considered appropriate. Currently the best widely available indicator is ^{51}Cr, and $^{51}CrCl_3$ is the preferable compound. (Further details are discussed in the following section devoted to this isotope.)

USE OF VARIOUS INDICATORS FOR ESTIMATING ENTERIC PROTEIN LOSS

^{51}Cr-Albumin, $^{51}Cr^{+++}$[36,37]

The use of ^{51}Cr for studies of this type is feasible because of the physical half-life of 26.5 days and its gamma emission. It is readily quantified, either alone or mixed with ^{125}I, in blood, urine or stools. Because the principal photo-peaks of ^{51}Cr (0.323 MeV) and ^{131}I (0.364 MeV) are close together, quantitative analysis of the components of this mixture is less precise. $^{51}Cr^{+++}$ readily binds to various proteins. Of the plasma proteins it has the greatest affinity for transferrin, but it also complexes loosely with albumin. Transferrin has a greater affinity for Fe than for Cr; thus Fe displaces Cr from this protein in vitro and if it is Fe-saturated no Cr is bound.

After administration by mouth, either as cationic ^{51}Cr or as ^{51}Cr-albumin, virtually 100 percent of the dose is recovered in the stools. After IV injection of either form, only a small fraction is excreted normally in the stools; the major portion is eventually excreted in the urine. The plasma-decay curve is multiexponential with relatively steep slopes during the first 3 to 5 days following IV injection of either material. After about the fourth day the curve becomes monoexponential with a T-1/2 of 6 to 12 days.[17,28,38] Rubini and Sheehy,[36] using $^{51}CrCl_3$, found a T-1/2 of 11 to 16 days in this slowest component in their presumably normal subjects. Although the plasma T-1/2 of iodinated albumin is much longer than that of ^{51}Cr-albumin, the biologic half-life in the body of the latter is several times that of *I-albumin. Thus the slope of the body disappearance curve of *I-albumin parallels that of the plasma, while these ^{51}Cr-decay curves diverge markedly.[39] Much of this difference is accounted for by the prolonged

sequestration of a large fraction of the injected Cr in the liver and spleen. The form in which it is taken up by these organs, whether as colloidal $Cr(OH)_3$ into the RE system or bound to red blood cells[36] in the spleen, is not known. For some years after these differences in the metabolism of ^{51}Cr- and *I-albumins were noted, it was assumed that denaturation of the Cr compound was responsible, as denatured RIHSA exhibited this same shortening of the plasma T-1/2. However, this behavior in plasma is more likely to be the consequence of elution of the ^{51}Cr from albumin and binding to other proteins, especially transferrin, the average normal plasma half-life of which is 8.8 days.[40] Binding to transferrin, either primarily or secondarily, depending upon whether the ^{51}Cr was administered as Cr^{+++} or as ^{51}Cr-albumin, is greater if the ^{51}Cr is of high SA, so that this transport protein is not saturated. Most investigators have found that these ^{51}Cr-labeled indicators behave similarly after IV injection.[17,24,28,41,42]

Normally fecal clearances of both materials range from 2 to 40 ml plasma per day. During the first 4 days after injection normally up to 1.5 percent of the dose is excreted in the stools. Earlier results indicated an upper limit of about one-half this value. This difference can easily be the consequence of variations in individual stool excretion patterns resulting in markedly different interval equivalents for the stools excreted during this calendar interval. When patients with PLE are studied by either fecal excretion method, using either ^{51}Cr preparation, there is excellent separation from the normal group. Likewise, these patients have an abnormally short T-1/2 of the plasma-decay curve. In view of the diagnostic precision that is achieved with use of either substance, these are the preparations of choice for study of enteric protein loss. Actually, they are the only available indicators suitable for estimation of enteric protein loss. The dose range described in the literature is 5 to 20 uC.

Since $^{51}CrCl_3$ is well defined chemically,

more readily available, more easily prepared for parenteral administration, and its longer shelf-life is limited only by the physical half-life of the isotope,[43] it is preferable to ^{51}Cr-albumin. As the initial distribution of ^{51}CrCl$_3$ after IV injection is in a somewhat larger volume than that of *I-albumin, plasma volume cannot be estimated with this preparation of the isotope. Another disadvantage is adsorption of the high SA isotope to glassware, sometimes resulting in loss of as much as 20 percent during injection. This loss is minimized by maintaining pH of the solution at or below 4 and by use of plastic or siliconized glass syringes. Exact knowledge of the quantity injected is essential if fecal excretion over 4 to 5 days is to be estimated as the fraction of the activity administered; so that this loss must be quantified and taken into account. Precision of results of *fecal clearance* studies does not depend upon administration of an exactly known amount of radioactivity. It is only necessary that enough be injected to achieve the objective of the study and that this quantity does not excessively irradiate the patient. Indeed the quantity administered, within the above limits, need not be known; so that loss of an unknown amount of radioactivity during injection does not matter. After injection the subject is "internally standardized," that is the activity in plasma, urine and stools originates from the same source. Activity in body fluids and stools is easily quantified for estimating plasma-decay curves and fecal clearances by comparing the radioactivity of these specimens to that of appropriate arbitrary standards of convenient counting rates and making allowances for differences in geometry. The chief disadvantage of ^{51}Cr-indicators is the long biological half-life consequent to sequestration of isotope in liver and spleen. The isotope is mainly excreted in urine; even slight contamination of stools with urine significantly but spuriously increases fecal clearance. This is also a fault of other indicators except ^{59}Fe-ID. After ^{51}Cr-albumin administration, ^{51}Cr is eluted from albumin and bound predominantly by trans-ferrin. Label elution does not result in apparent difference in plasma-decay pattern from that of ^{51}CrCl$_3$.

^{67}Cu Ceruloplasmin (^{67}Cu-Cp)[16]

Ceruloplasmin (CP) is a plasma protein of 160,000 molecular weight and contains 8 atoms of copper/molecule. Normal plasma concentration is 20 to 35 mg/dl; approximately 70 percent of the body pool of CP is within the intravascular space in man and dog. The physical half-life of ^{67}Cu is 61.8 hours; that of the readily available ^{64}Cu is 12.8 hours. ^{67}Cu-CP is prepared from the cyclotron-produced isotope by in vitro exchange from ^{67}CuNO$_3$. There is significant exchange of the label in vivo, and metabolism of such labeled preparations is normal in man and dog.

Excretion in the stool after oral administration of ^{67}Cu-CP was as follows: 8 patients, 70 to 99 percent (mean 88); 4 dogs, 82 to 100 percent (mean 92); 6 rats, 95 to 100 percent (mean 98). Thus, the copper moiety of ^{67}Cu-CP is poorly absorbed from the gut. However, to minimize absorption of ^{67}Cu by dilution in a relatively large intestinal Cu pool, 10 mg CuSO$_4$ was administered 3 times daily by mouth to patients undergoing clearance studies. A small fraction of the Cu from the daily turnover of CP is excreted in the bile. In 4 dogs from 0.01 to 0.3 percent (mean 0.13) of the circulating radioactivity appeared in the urine per day; no data were given for man.

After intravenous administration of 100 mg of CP labeled with 20 μc ^{67}Cu to 4 control subjects the plasma half-life was from 5.5 to 6.6 (mean 6.1) days. 1.9 to 3.9 percent (mean 2.9) of the plasma pool was cleared into the gut daily; this accounted for a maximum of only 11 to 27 percent of the total catabolism of CP. In 4 patients with intestinal lymphangiectasia, the plasma survival half-time of ^{67}Cu-CP ranged from 2.3 to 3.6 days (mean 3.1), and from 15 to 40 percent (mean 26) of the intravascular volume was cleared through the intestine daily. In these patients approximately 75 percent of CP-catabolism was due to intestinal loss, and in contrast to normal subjects this loss was a major factor in metabolism of this protein. In the experience of these authors hypoceruloplasminemia was a part of generalized hypoproteinemia; in 14 patients with excessive gastrointestinal protein loss the concentration was 16.4 ± 5 mg/dl, whereas in 185 control subjects this was 30.7 ± 3.5 (p < 0.01).

From this excellent but limited study use of [67]Cu-CP enables quantitative estimation of enteric protein loss. Patients with PLE were clearly separated from normals. In addition, loss through the gut normally was a minor factor in the catabolism of this protein. Fecal clearances in normals were about twice those found by other methods in other studies. Indeed, results of fecal clearances estimated from the multicompartmental analysis also done were about one-half those cited above. The excretion of [67]Cu in the bile in various forms may account for the difference. We conclude that [67]Cu-CP fulfills most of the requirements for an ideal substance by which protein transfer into the gut can be quantified. However, the difficulty and expense in production of [67]Cu and its short physical half-life (61.8 hrs) preclude its widespread use in clinical studies.

[59]Fe-Dextran (^{59}Fe-ID)[44,45]

This is an iron-dextran complex; the preparations used by these investigators had an average molecular weight of 180,000 (range 50,000-250,000) and contained no free iron. After slow intravenous injection of a dilute solution, the plasma-disappearance curves are described as "monoexponential," with a T-1/2 of 10 to 20 hours until 2 to 5 percent remain in the plasma. The short half-life of the complex in the plasma reflects rapid uptake by the reticuloendothelial system, from which the iron is slowly released. In the absence of proteinuria insignificant quantities of ^{59}Fe are excreted in the urine following intravenous injection. After oral administration in 7 subjects without PLE

from 51 to 105 percent of the dose was recovered in the stools; in 4 subjects it was less than 80 percent. It is not clear whether the incomplete recoveries in stools were wholly attributable to loss of stools or in part to intestinal absorption. Since there was some evidence for the latter, it seems fair to characterize the complex as "partially absorbable," perhaps "poorly absorbable." Although ^{59}Fe-ID is not a protein, the molecular weights approximate those of the chief plasma proteins and it is not appreciably excreted in the urine. These properties led to studies in PLE because they might be uniquely valuable in direct demonstrations of bulk plasma loss from the gut in children and others who have difficulty in separating feces from urine.

The results showed that subjects without PLE excreted 0 to 0.8 percent of the injected dose in 4-day stool collections started immediately after administration of the labeled complex. During this same interval, daily fecal isotope clearance was 0 to 0.8 percent of plasma volume or 0 to 26 ml plasma, approximately the same as that of [51]Cr. In patients with PLE the results of both measurements were invariably abnormally high, so that the patients were clearly separated from the normal group. Correlation with ^{131}I-albumin degradation rate was excellent, but was no better than that of ^{51}Cr-albumin studied in fewer patients.

It is difficult to compare fecal clearances of ^{59}Fe-ID with those of ^{51}Cr because of the necessity of performing the former studies during the period of rapid disappearance of the indicator from the plasma. Again, this emphasizes the problem of interpretation of results of clearance studies carried out before the indicator has equilibrated between the intravascular and extravascular compartments. Because of the short half-life of the labeled complex in the plasma, ^{59}Fe-ID must enter the gut as a brief pulse, unless, as has been suggested,[45] a portion is stored in the intestinal mucosal cells from which it is released after a delay. Conversely, ^{51}Cr, which has a much slower plasma disappearance rate, must normally have a more sustained pattern of fecal excretion. It is likely to be fortuitous that the same fraction of both of these indicators is excreted in the stools of normal controls during the 4 days following injection. Thus, if the collection period were shortened, relatively more ^{59}Fe-ID would be excreted; and if the stool collection were of longer duration, more ^{51}Cr than ^{59}Fe-ID would appear in the feces. No values for clearances of these 2 substances by the same normals have been published, although the ranges and means are quite similar. In patients with PLE in whom ^{59}Fe-ID and ^{51}Cr-albumin were directly compared concurrently the fecal excretions and clearances of the latter were greater. The authors opined that "bulk loss" was *underestimated* by the ^{59}Fe-ID method. Interestingly, with one exception the T-1/2 of plasma-disappearance curves of patients with PLE were no shorter than those of controls, despite fecal excretions of up to 15 percent of the dose in the patients.

In summary, with the use of ^{59}Fe-ID the authors readily confirmed directly the diagnosis of PLE, but this indicator was no better than ^{51}Cr for this purpose. ^{59}Fe-ID was not excreted in the urine, so that in such studies in patients (especially children) who cannot separate feces from urine this complex might be useful; otherwise, it seems to offer no advantage.

^{95}Nb-labeled Albumin[46]

^{95}Niobium has a peak energy level of its gamma emission of about 760 KeV and a half-life of 35 days. ^{95}Nb-albumin was prepared by "electrolytic labeling" of albumin with ^{95}Nb. Although details of preparation and purification are lacking, a stable product with an acceptably small proportion of denatured protein was apparently obtained only with considerable difficulty. Data concerning intestinal absorption are not available. Urinary excretion of ^{95}Nb after intravenous administration was "low compared to that of ^{131}I (or ^{125}I) in studies with radioiodine-labeled albumin," but again details are not given.

After intravenous administration the plasma-disappearance curves of the best preparations of ^{95}Nb-albumin were nearly identical to those of simultaneously injected ^{131}I-albumin. Subjects without protein loss excreted 0.1 to 7.0 percent (mean 2.0% ± 1.8 S.D.) of injected dose in the stools in 6 days. Fecal clearance was from 0.3 to 2.2 percent (mean 1.2 ± 0.6 S.D.) of the IV pool per day, or 0 to 60 ml plasma per day (mean 29). In patients with PLE fecal excretions and clearances were abnormally high. In those who were comparatively studied with ^{51}Cr-albumin or ^{59}Fe-ID the results were all abnormal.

The ^{95}Nb-albumin prepared by these investigators was suitable for detection of PLE. Their goal, the production of a substance with which both gastrointestinal protein loss and metabolic turnover of albumin can be measured, seems to have been nearly reached. Further data are awaited with interest. A possible disadvantage of this material is that the high energy of ^{95}Nb, combined with its 35-day half-life would give an unacceptably high radiation dose.

COMBINED METHODS

Simultaneous Studies of Enteric Protein Loss and Albumin Catabolism: ^{51}Cr-Albumin and ^{125}I-Albumin.[39] When patients with PLE are studied with either ^{51}CrCl$_3$ or ^{51}Cr-albumin an abnormally short plasma T-1/2 is found. In this respect the behavior of these labeled indicators resembles that of *I-albumin. In a study using ^{51}Cr, the steepness of the slope of the plasma disappearance curve adds to the evidence obtained from stool studies about the magnitude of enteric protein loss. Stool studies are laborious; for example, in patients with PLE, follow-up studies to determine effects of therapy would be more easily accomplished with a method in which plasma specimens alone were used. But even when ^{51}Cr plasma-decay curves are obtained sequentially in the same patient, in the absence of results from a reference study with which they can be correlated, there may be some doubt about their validity. In view of the uncertainty and conflicting evidence concerning exactly what is being measured in the ^{51}Cr plasma-decay curve, some investigators will wish to obtain simultaneous data about albumin turnover. Such a combined study employing ^{51}Cr (preferably ^{51}CrCl$_3$) and ^{125}I-albumin can be easily done. Thus enteric protein loss could be estimated with ^{51}Cr and data obtained simultaneously about the plasma disappearance rates of both isotopes. In follow-up studies using ^{125}I-albumin alone it might be inferred that changes in enteric losses paralleled the changes in albumin "catabolism." Evidence validating this logical assumption has not been published however.

To Obtain Data About the Site of Enteric Protein Loss: ^{59}Fe-ID (or ^{51}Cr) and *I-Albumin.[47] In patients with PLE, of the *I-albumin entering the gut, that fraction which is voided in the stool varies with the site of entry. If this site is in the stomach virtually none of the label appears in the stool, but if the loss is into the left colon the feces contain nearly 100 percent of the exudate. The site of protein loss can perhaps be approximately inferred from this information alone, but the precision of this deduction can be improved by use of either ^{51}CrCl$_3$ or ^{59}Fe-ID administered together with *I-albumin. The preferred combination is ^{51}CrCl$_3$ and ^{125}I-; fecal clearance of both isotopes is estimated for 4 to 5 days after intravenous injection. The ratio of fecal clearance of *I to that of either ^{51}Cr or ^{59}Fe is less than 0.30 in diseases of the upper gut and intestinal lymphangiectasia, greater than 0.90 in inflammatory diseases of colon, and intermediate in Crohn's disease of the ileum. It is assumed that the *I-albumin entering the upper gut is normally digested and absorbed. If pancreatic insufficiency or malabsorption secondary to intestinal resection or other lesion were present the ratio might be falsely increased. Certainly ^{51}Cr would be more reliable to use than ^{59}Fe-ID; these were not compared in the same patients to determine whether the ratios might be different.

METHODS NOW CHIEFLY OF HISTORICAL INTEREST

*I-PVP.[12]

*I-PVP occupies a unique position in the development of present concepts of PLE, since use of this preparation first enabled direct demonstration of enteric "protein" loss from all parts of the gut. It was incorporated into a feasible, reproducible method that was of great value throughout the world in diagnosis of this syndrome. Hence, it is briefly discussed, although it has been superseded by better indicators. PVP is a synthetic polymer used in various cosmetic preparations and formerly as a plasma expander. The iodinated preparations used by Gordon had a wide range of molecular weights, averaging about 40,000. After oral administration of *I-PVP absorption varied greatly, from 10 to 60 percent with different preparations. After IV administration it was rapidly cleared from plasma with a T-1/2 of 0.3 to 3.0 days. Normal persons excreted 1.5 percent or less in 4-day stool collections begun immediately after injection, and those with PLE were invariably well delineated from these by their much greater fecal excretion rates. Although it was widely employed for these properties on an empiric basis, it was unsuitable for use in clearance studies and preparation of a uniform, stably-labeled product was technically difficult. During the past decade the method has gradually fallen into disuse and *I-PVP is now no longer easily obtainable.

Amberlite Resin by Mouth plus *I-Albumin IV.[48-51]

Amberlite resin IRA-400 (Cl) is an anion-exchange resin with a considerable affinity for halogens, particularly iodide. Administration of the resin in doses of 5 Gm every 2 hours by mouth enabled subjects without gastrointestinal disease to excrete in their stools as much as 80 percent of the *I of an orally administered dose of *I-albumin. It was hypothesized that the *I digested from intravenously administered *I-albumin after the latter had entered the gut would be bound by the resin. Hence, its use was advocated in the diagnosis of PLE. However, it was soon learned that fecal excretion of parenterally administered *I-*iodide* was also markedly increased by this agent. Then it seemed probable that the *I in the stool following oral administration of *I-albumin originated from *I-peptides that were digested and absorbed, catabolized and finally secreted as iodide through the salivary glands and gastric mucosa back into the gut. *I (as iodide) from catabolism of IV administered *I-albumin normally enters the gut as above but is also normally nearly completely reabsorbed. The presence of the resin would greatly inhibit this reabsorption. Thus, the label appearing in the stool would have been lost into the gut in a form other than as intact protein. This would lead to overestimation of the magnitude of the loss. Also the *I-resin bond was not firm; as much as 30 percent was split off during passage through the gut. As a consequence of these inadequacies this method was used for only a short time.

CHOICE OF A METHOD

Although we have discussed a number of indicators and isotopes the choice is really quite restricted for most users: either *I-albumin (^{125}I or ^{131}I) or ^{51}Cr (CrCl$_3$ or -albumin). For the reasons given ^{125}I-*albumin* is the labeled indicator of choice for study of albumin degradation and ^{51}CrCl$_3$ that for fecal excretion studies. Use of *I-albumin is advocated as a screening test. Results from this will, in conjunction with other readily available information, enable one to solve this aspect of most relatively simple clinical problems. A normal test result is conclusive. If it is necessary to know beyond doubt that increased "catabolism" is accounted for by enteric protein loss, then one of the fecal excretion studies with ^{51}CrCl$_3$ is indicated. An example of need for this is as a part of the description

of a disease or case report in which PLE is first found to be a part of the picture. Although the semiquantitative type is less laborious, result of the clearance study is less likely to be in error and it produces much more information for a very little increase in work over that involved in the semiquantitative test. We recommend doing the clearance study whenever possible. Quantitative information can be obtained only from clearance studies. A good example[30] is the correlation of the severity of the PLE with extent of involvement in Crohn's disease; in some patients mild enteric protein loss was accompanied by normal serum albumin concentrations ("compensated"). In complex situations in which there are multiple etiologies of hypoproteinemia, to obtain the maximal amount of data, *I-albumin plasma turnover studies may be advantageously combined with ^{51}Cr fecal clearances. In instances in which decreased synthesis is combined with increased enteric protein loss interpretation may be very difficult. Finally, comparative studies have confirmed the adequacy and reliability of ^{51}Cr-clearances in diagnosis of PLE. Thus, correlations of results with use of ^{51}Cr-albumin, *I-albumin and transferrin in PLE are excellent.[17,52]

DISEASES CHARACTERIZED BY PLE

Table 24-2 (p. 357) includes the names of some diseases and other variables associated with PLE, with reference numbers indicating some of the more significant of the clinical findings. Those disorders for which no references are listed are documented in Waldmann's extensive 1966 review.[7]

The desirability of devoting a considerable effort to detection and quantification of PLE, a ubiquitous manifestation of gut disease, should be justified. How can the patient and his physician benefit from results of these studies? In patients whose major symptomatic abnormalities are consequent to protein loss and related phenomena, objective confirmation of the presence of PLE may lead eventually to diagnosis of important

Table 24-2. Diseases and Other Variables Characterized by PLE

Acute transient GI protein loss[53,54]
Agammaglobulinemia and hypogamma-
　　globulinemia
Amyloidosis, primary[17]
Angioneurotic edema
Bezoar[55,56]
Blind loops[57]
Cirrhosis, hepatic[58,59,60]
Diverticulosis of jejunum

Drug poisoning, other noxious agents
　　Arsenic[61]
　　Aspirin[62]
　　Ampicillin[63]
　　Laxatives[64]
　　Methotrexate[17]
　　Nitrogen mustard (experimental)
　　Sulfhydryl reagents (experimental)[65]
　　Fistula, gastrocolic
　　Fistula, thoracic duct—small bowel
　　Gastrectomy, post-
　　Graft versus host reaction[66]
　　Growth hormone[67]

Heart Disease: Decompensated Cardiac States
　　Congestive heart failure[68]
　　Constrictive pericarditis[69,70,71]
　　Familial myocardopathy
　　Interatrial septal defect
　　Lymphopericardium[72]
　　Thrombosis of inferior vena cava
　　Hernia, incarc. ing. (ileum), postoperative[73]
　　Herpetiformis, dermatitis[74,75]
　　Icthyosis[76]

Inflammations, nonspecific
　　Crohn's disease (regional enteritis, granu-
　　　　lomatous enterocolitis, etc.)[77,78]
　　Eosinophilic gastroenteritis[79,80]
　　Gastritis, atrophic[81]
　　Gastritis, hypertrophic, giant (including
　　　　Menetrier's syndrome)[81,82,83]
　　Granuloma, nonspecific, of bowel
　　Jejunal stenosis
　　Pancreatitis, chronic[17]
　　Retroperitoneal fibrosis[84]
　　Ulcerative colitis, idiopathic[78]
　　Ulcerative jejunoileitis[85]

Inflammations, specific
　Infections
　　"Acute gastrointestinal infection"
　　Capillariasis[86]
　　Histoplasmosis[87]
　　Hookworm infection
　　Infectious mononucleosis[88]
　　Schistosomal polyps[89]
　　Shigella dysentery[17]
　　Tuberculosis, chr. GI
　　Whipple's disease[90]
　Allergic gastroenteropathy,[91,92,93]
　　allergic gastritis
Kwashiorkor
Lupus erythematosus[17,94]

Lymphatic obstruction
　　Lymphangiectasis[95]; colon,[96]
　　　　small bowel[90,97,98,99,100]
　　Thoracic duct ligation, dogs[101]
　Mastocytosis[45]
　Megacolon, congenital (Hirschsprung's)

Neoplasms, benign
　　Hemangioma, small intestine[102]
　　Lymphangioma of mesentery[103]
　　Polyp of stomach
　　Polyposis, diffuse gastrointestinal[104,105,106]
　　Mesenchymoma (benign) of mesentery[107]

Neoplasms, malignant
　　Carcinoma esophagus, stomach, colon
　　Carcinoid syndrome[17]
　　Lymphosarcoma of bowel
　　Melanomatosis, generalized[17]
　Nephrotic syndrome[52,108,109]
　Pancreas, cystic fibrosis[17]
　Purpura, anaphylactoid[110]
　Radiation[17,69,70,112]
　Scleroderma[17]
　Sjogren syndrome[17]
　Sjogren-Larsson syndrome[76]
　Sprue, nontropical (gluten-induced, celiac)
　Sprue, tropical
　Treatment[99,112,113]
　Tube, retained intestinal [114]
　Tuberous sclerosis with angiomatous
　　malformation of small bowel
　Ulcers, multiple gastric, with Menetrier's
　　syndrome

---

unsuspected diseases such as Menetrier's syndrome, lymphangiectasia or constrictive pericarditis. Available therapy may be quite specific and effective, but also laborious, expensive and, with gastrectomy, attended by appreciable risk. Hence, an accurate, objective, quantitative basis for initiation of treatment and of evaluating its efficacy is desirable. Quantification of gut protein loss in instances of known disease may lead to modification of therapy such as restriction of dietary long-chain fats in patients with various forms of lymphatic obstruction, addition of protein supplements to the diet, or increasing dosage of steroids in patients with inflammatory bowel disease. Indeed this may be one of the best means of evaluating the extent and activity of Crohn's disease.[30] In patients whose PLE is consequent to loss of lymph into the gut, concomitant deprivation of lymphocytes leads to alterations in immunity that are of considerable general significance. Deficiencies in tissue-immune responses are manifested as increased tolerance to foreign tissue grafts, loss of reactivity to common skin-test antigens and perhaps no decrease in resistance to certain infections. The syndrome was originally described in lymphangiectasia, but after specific search was also found in patients with constrictive pericarditis and congestive heart failure. Thus these studies have benefited many patients directly, and have considerably increased understanding of various related disease mechanisms.

References

1. Jarnum, S.: Protein-losing Gastroenteropathy. Oxford, Blackwell, 1963.
2. Jeffries, G. H., Holman, H., and Sleisenger, M. H.: Plasma proteins and the gastrointestinal tract. N. Eng. J. Med., *266*:652, 1962.
3. Kalser, M. H.: Protein-losing gastroenteropathies. *In* Bockus, H. L.: Gastroenterology, ed. 2, vol. II, pp. 510-529. Philadelphia, W. B. Saunders, 1964.
4. Munro, H. N.: The Role of the Gastrointestinal Tract in Protein Metabolism. Oxford, Blackwell, 1964.
5. O'Meallie, L. P.: Protein-losing gastroenteropathy. Amer. J. Med. Sci., *245*:109, 1963.
6. Schwartz, M., and Vesin, P.: Plasma Proteins and Gastrointestinal Tract in Health and Disease. Baltimore, Williams & Wilkins, 1963.
7. Waldmann, T. A.: Protein-losing enteropathy (Progress in Gastroenterology). Gastroenterology, *50*:422, 1966.
8. Kinsell, L. W., Margen, S., Tarver, H., *et al.*: Studies in methionine metabolism. III. The fate of intravenously administered S[35]-labeled-methionine in normal adult males, in patients with chronic hepatic disease, "idiopathic" hypoproteinemia and Cushing's syndrome. J. Clin. Invest., *29*: 238, 1950.
9. Schwartz, M., and Thomsen, B.: Idiopathic or hypercatabolic hypoproteinemia. Case examined by I[131]-labelled albumin. Br. Med. J., *1*:14, 1957.
10. Citrin, Y., Sterling, K., and Halsted, J.: The mechanism of hypoproteinemia associated with giant hypertrophy of the gastric mucosa. N. Eng. J. Med., *257*:906, 1957.
11. Steinfeld, J. L., Davidson, J. D., and Gordon, R. S., Jr.: A mechanism for hypoalbuminemia in patients with ulcerative colitis and regional enteritis. J. Clin. Invest., *36*:931, 1957.
12. Gordon, R. S., Jr.: Exudative enteropathy: Abnormal permeability of gastrointestinal tract demonstrable with labelled polyvinylpyrrolidone. Lancet, *1*:325, 1959.
13. Schwartz, M., and Jarnum, S.: Gastrointestinal protein loss in idiopathic (hypercatabolic) hypoproteinaemia. Lancet, *1*: 327, 1959.
14. Jarnum, S., and Jensen, K. B.: Plasma protein turnover (albumin, transferrin, IGG, IGM) in Menetrier's disease (giant hypertrophic gastritis): Evidence of nonselective protein loss. Gut, *13*:128, 1972.
15. Nasset, E. S.: Role of the digestive system in protein metabolism. Fed. Proc., *24*:953, 1965.
16. Waldmann, T. A., Morell, A. G., Wochner, R. D., *et al.*: Measurement of gastrointestinal protein loss using ceruloplasmin labeled with [67]Copper. J. Clin. Invest., *46*:10, 1967.
17. Waldmann, T. A., Wochner, R. D., and Strober, W.: The role of the gastrointestinal tract in plasma protein metabolism. Studies with ^{51}Cr-albumin. Amer. J. Med., *46*:275, 1969.
18. DaCosta, L. R., Croft, D. N., and Creamer, B.: Protein loss and cell loss from the small-intestinal mucosa. Gut, *12*: 179, 1971.
19. Matthews, C. M. E.: The theory of tracer experiments with ^{131}I-labelled plasma proteins. Phys. Med. Biol., *2*:36, 1957.
20. Reeve, E. B., and Bailey, H. R.: Mathematical models describing the distribution of I[131]-albumin in man. J. Lab. Clin. Med., *60*:923, 1962.
21. Stanley, M. M.: Plasma protein clearance by the gut. A method of studying the

exudative gastroenteropathies. Amer. J. Dig. Dis., *10*:993, 1965.

22. McFarlane, A. S.: Efficient trace-labeling of proteins with iodine. Nature, *182*:53, 1958.

23. Flick, A. L., and Steinfeld, J. L.: The effect of fever and corticotropin on the in vivo degradation of albumin in man as measured with iodinated human serum albumin. Amer. J. Med. Sci., *236*:65, 1958.

24. Rootwelt, K.: Direct intravenous injection of [51]chromic chloride compared with ^{125}I-polyvinylpyrrolidone and ^{131}I-albumin in the detection of gastrointestinal protein loss. Scand. J. Clin. Lab. Invest., *18*:405, 1966.

25. Beeken, W. L.: Clearance of circulating radiochromated albumin and erythrocytes by the gastrointestinal tract of normal subjects. Gastroenterology, *52*:34, 1967.

26. Stanley, M.: Estimation of rates of fecal excretion and of clearance of plasma albumin by the gut. Fed. Proc., *23*:512, 1964.

27. Stanley, M. M., and Cheng, S. H.: Clearance by the gut of plasma albumin. Gastroenterology, *44*:854, 1963.

28. Van Tongeren, J. H. M., Reichert, W. J., and Kamphuys, T. M.: Demonstration of protein-losing gastroenteropathy. The quantitative estimation of gastrointestinal protein loss, using ^{51}Cr-labeled plasma proteins. Clin. Chim. Acta, *14*:42, 1966.

29. Waldmann, T. A., and Wochner, R. D.: The use of ^{51}Cr-labeled albumin in the study of protein-losing enteropathy. Protides Biol. Fluids, *11*:224, 1963.

30. Beeken, W. L., Busch, H. J., and Sylwester, D. L.: Intestinal protein loss in Crohn's disease. Gastroenterology, *62*:207, 1972.

31. Jover, A., and Gordon, R. S., Jr.: Procedure for quantitative analysis of feces with special reference to fecal fatty acids. J. Lab. Clin. Med., *59*:878, 1962.

32. Stanley, M. M., and Nemchausky, B.: Fecal C^{14}-bile acid secretion in normal subjects and patients with steroid-wasting syndromes secondary to ileal dysfunction. J. Lab. Clin. Med., *70*:627, 1967.

33. Lutwak, L., and Burton, B. T.: Fecal dye markers in metabolic balance studies. Amer. J. Clin. Nutrition, *14*:109, 1964.

34. Beeken, W. L., and Harwood, J. F.: Measurements of gastrointestinal protein loss. Gastroenterology, *60*:987, 1971.

35. Nosslin, B.: In Andersen, S. B.: Metabolism of Human Gamma Globulin (γ_{ss}-globulin). Appendixes A-G, pp. 103-120. Philadelphia, F. A. Davis, 1964.

36. Rubini, M. E., Sheehy, T. W., and Johnson, C. R.: Exudative enteropathy. I. A comparative study of $Cr^{51}Cl$ and $I^{131}PVP$. J. Lab. Clin. Med., *58*:892, 1961.

37. Waldmann, T. A.: Gastrointestinal protein loss demonstrated by ^{51}Cr-labelled albumin. Lancet, *21*:121, 1961.

38. Mabry, C. C., Greenlaw, R. H., and DeVore, W. D.: Measurement of gastrointestinal loss of plasma albumin: a clinical and laboratory evaluation of [51]chromium labeled albumin. J. Nucl. Med., *6*:93, 1965.

39. Kerr, R. M., Dubois, J. J., and Holt, P. R.: Use of [125]I- and ^{51}Cr-labeled albumin for the measurement of gastrointestinal and total albumin catabolism. J. Clin. Invest., *46*:2064, 1967.

40. Awai, M., and Brown, E. B.: Studies of the metabolism of I^{131}-labeled human transferrin. J. Lab. Clin. Med., *61*:363, 1963.

41. Van Tongeren, J. H. M., Majoor, C. L. H., and Kamphuys, T. M.: Demonstration of protein-losing gastroenteropathy. The disappearance rate of ^{51}Cr from plasma and the binding of ^{51}Cr to different serum proteins. Clin. Chim. Acta, *14*:31, 1966.

42. Peterson, M. L.: Transferrin-chomium: A "physiological" index of gastrointestinal loss of serum proteins. Gastroenterology, *52*:1113, 1967.

43. Tengström, B.: Critical evaluation of ^{51}Cr-labelled serum albumin in the study of gastrointestinal protein loss. Scand. J. Clin. Lab. Invest., *17*:299, 1965.

44. Andersen, S. B., and Jarnum, S. J.: Gastrointestinal protein loss measured with ^{59}Fe-labelled iron-dextran. Lancet, *1*:1060, 1966.

45. Jarnum, S., Westergaard, H. O., Yssing, M,. et al.: Quantitation of gastrointestinal protein loss by means of Fe^{59}-labeled dextran. Gastroenterology, *55*:229, 1968.

46. Jeejeebhoy, K. N., Jarnum, S., Singh, B., et al.: [95]Nb-labelled albumin for the study of gastrointestinal albumin loss. Scand. J. Gastroenterol., *3*:449, 1968.

47. Westergaard, H. O., Jarnum, S., Jensen, H., et al.: Topographic diagnosis of gastrointestinal protein loss. Digestion, *1*:341, 1968.

48. Freeman, T., and Gordon, A. H.: The measurement of albumin leak into the gastrointestinal tract using I^{131}-albumin and ion exchange resin by mouth. Gut, *5*:155, 1964.

49. Hoedt-Rassmussen, K., Kemp, E., Moller-Petersen, B., et al.: The measurement of

gastrointestinal protein loss by ^{131}I-labelled protein and resin. Gut, 5:158, 1964.

50. Jeejeebhoy, K. N., and Coghill, N. F.: Measurement of gastrointestinal protein loss by new method. Gut, 2:123, 1961.

51. Jones, J. H., and Morgan, D. B.: Measurement of plasma-protein loss into gastrointestinal tract using I[131]-labelled proteins and oral amberlite resin. Lancet, 1:626, 1963.

52. Jensen, H.: Transferrin metabolism in the nephrotic syndrome and protein-losing gastroenteropathy. Scand. J. Clin. Lab. Invest., 21:293, 1968.

53. Herskovic, T., Spiro, H. M., and Gryboski, J. D.: Acute transient gastrointestinal protein loss. Pediatrics, 41:818, 1968.

54. Mahmoud, J., and McKechnie, J.: Acute transient protein-losing gastroenteropathy in an adult. Amer. J. Gastroenterol., 57:416, 1972.

55. Hossenbocus, A., and Colin-Jones, D. G.: Trichobezoar, gastric polyposis, protein-losing gastroenteropathy and steatorrhea. Gut, 14:730, 1973.

56. Valberg, L. S., McCorriston, J. R., and Partington, M. W.: Bezoar: An unusual cause of protein-losing gastroenteropathy. Can. Med. Assoc. J., 94:388, 1966.

57. Nygaard, K., and Rootwelt, K.: Intestinal protein loss in rats with blind segments on the small bowel. Gastroenterology, 54:52, 1968.

58. Davcev, P., Vanovski, B., Sestakov, D., et al.: Protein-losing enteropathy in patients with liver cirrhosis. Digestion, 2:17, 1969.

59. Marinkovic, M., Miocka, O., and Kallai, L.: Fecal excretion of polyvinylpyrrolidone [131]-I in liver cirrhosis. Digestion, 2:172, 1969.

60. Takada, A., Kobayashi, K., and Takeuchi, J.: Gastroenteric clearance of albumin in liver cirrhosis; relative protein-losing gastroenteropathy. Digestion, 3:154, 1970.

61. Kobayashi, A., and Obe, Y.: Protein-losing enteropathy associated with arsenic poisoning. Amer. J. Dis. Child., 121:515, 1971.

62. Beeken, W. L.: Effect of salicylates on gastrointestinal protein loss in normal subjects. Gastroenterology, 53:894, 1967.

63. Stanley, M.: Protein-losing enteropathy following use of ampicillin in treatment of urinary tract infection. Previously unreported case.

64. Heizer, W. D., Warshaw, A. L., Waldmann, T. A., et al.: Protein-losing gastroenteropathy and malabsorption associated

with factitious diarrhea. Ann. Intern. Med., 68:839, 1968.

65. Davenport, H. W.: Protein-losing gastropathy produced by sulfhydryl reagents. Gastroenterology, 60:870, 1971.

66. Cornelius, E. A.: Protein-losing enteropathy in the graft-versus-host reaction. Transplantation, 9:247, 1970.

67. Pimstone, B., Bank, S., and Buchanan-Lee, B.: Growth hormone in protein-losing enteropathy. Lancet, 2:1246, 1968.

68. Strober, W., Cohen, L. S., Waldmann, T. A., et al.: Tricuspid regurgitation. A newly recognized cause of protein-losing enteropathy, lymphocytopenia and immunologic deficiency. Amer. J. Med., 44:842, 1968.

69. Brohet, C., Rousseau, M., Chalante, C., et al.: Postradiotherapeutic constrictive pericarditis with exudative enteropathy. Acta Cardiol. (Brux), 27:736, 1972.

70. Palmer, H. M., Cocking, J. B., and Emmanuel, I. G.: Irradiation-induced constrictive pericarditis in intestinal lymphangiectasis. Br. Med J., 4:783, 1970.

71. Wilkinson, P., Pinto, B., and Senior, J. R.: Reversible protein-losing enteropathy with intestinal lymphangiectasis secondary to chronic constrictive pericarditis. N. Eng. J. Med., 273:1178, 1965.

72. Offerijns, F. G. J., van der Veen, K. J., Durrer, D., et al.: Lymphopericardium with hypoproteinemia, intestinal loss of protein, and congenital defects of the lymphatic system. Circulation, 39:116, 1969.

73. Lonnum, I.: Protein loss in the small intestine following operation for incarcerated inguinal hernia. Acta Chir. Scand., 131:81, 1966.

74. Gjone, E., and Oyri, A.: Protein-losing enteropathy in dermatitis herpetiformis. Scand. J. Gastroenterol., 5:13, 1970.

75. Van Tongeren, J. H. M., van der Staak, W. J. B. M., and Schillings, P. H. M.: Small-bowel changes in dermatitis herpetiformis. Lancet, 1:218, 1967.

76. Hooft, C., Kriekemans, J., van Acker, E., et al.: Sjögren-Larsson syndrome with exudative enteropathy. Influence of medium-chain triglycerides on the symptomatology. Helv. Paediatr. Acta, 5:447, 1967.

77. Bendixen, G., Jarnum, S., Soltoft, J., et al.: IgG and albumin turnover in Crohn's disease. Scand. J. Gastroenterol., 3:481, 1968.

78. Steinfeld, J. L., Davidson, J. D., Gordon, R. S. Jr., et al.: The mechanism of hypoproteinemia in patients with regional en-

teritis and ulcerative colitis. Amer. J. Med., *29*:405, 1960.

79. Gregg, J. A., and Luna, L.: Eosinophilic gastroenteritis. Report of a case with protein-losing enteropathy. Amer. J. Gastroenterol., 59:41, 1973.

80. Kaplan, S., Goldstein, F., and Kowlessar, O. D.: Eosinophilic gastroenteritis: report of a case with malabsorption and protein-losing enteropathy. Gastroenterology, 58: 540, 1970.

81. Frank, B. W., and Kern, F., Jr.: Menetrier's disease. Spontaneous metamorphosis of giant hypertrophy of the gastric mucosa to atrophic gastritis. Gastroenterology, *53*:953, 1967.

82. Brook, A. M., Isenberg, J., and Goldstein, H.: Giant thickening of the gastric mucosa with acid hypersecretion and protein-losing gastropathy. Gastroenterology, 58: 73, 1970.

83. Roberts, H. J.: Giant rugal hypertrophy of stomach with protein loss and response to drug therapy. Gut, *11*:980, 1970.

84. Chew, C. K., Jarzylo, S. V., and Valberg, L. S.: Idiopathic retroperitoneal fibrosis with protein-losing enteropathy and duodenal obstruction successfully treated with corticosteroids. Can. Med. Assoc. J., 95: 1183, 1966.

85. Corlin, R. F., and Pops, M. A.: Nongranulomatous ulcerative jejunoileitis with hypogammaglobulinemia. Clinical remission after treatment with globulin. Gastroenterology, *62*:473, 1972.

86. Whalen, G. E., Rosenberg, E. B., Strickland, G. T., et al.: Intestinal capillariasis. A new disease in man. Lancet, *1*:13, 1969.

87. Bank, S., Trey, C., Gans, I., Marks, I. N., and Groll, A.: Histoplasmosis of the small bowel with "giant" intestinal villi and secondary protein-losing enteropathy. Amer. J. Med., *39*:492, 1965.

88. Corbus, H. F.: Protein-losing enteropathy in infectious mononucleosis. Calif. Med., *109*:378, 1968.

89. Lehman, J. S., Jr., Farid, Z., Bassily, S., et al.: Intestinal protein loss in schistosomal polyposis of the colon. Gastroenterology, *59*:433, 1970.

90. Dobbins, W. O.: Diseases associated with protein losing enteropathy. South. Med. J., *60*:1077, 1967.

91. Greenberger, N. J., Tennenbaum, J. I., and Ruppert, R. D.: Protein-losing enteropathy associated with gastrointestinal allergy. Amer. J. Med., *43*:777, 1967.

92. Huntley, C. C., Bowers, G. W., and Vann, R. L.: Allergic protein-losing gastroenter-

opathy: Report of an unusual case. South. Med. J., *63*:917, 1970.

93. Lebenthal, E., Laor, J., Lewitus, Z., et al.: Gastrointestinal protein loss in allergy to cow's milk beta-lactoglobulin. Isr. J. Med. Sci., *6*:506, 1970.

94. Pachas, W. N., Linscheer, W. G., and Pinals, R. S.: Protein-losing enteropathy in systemic lupus erythematosus. Amer. J. Gastroenterol., *55*:162, 1971.

95. Strober, W., Wochner, R. D., Carbone, P. P., et al.: Intestinal lymphangiectasia: a protein-losing enteropathy with hypogammaglobulinemia, lymphocytopenia and impaired homograft rejection. J. Clin. Invest., *46*:1643, 1967.

96. Griffen, W. O., Jr., Belin, R. P., Furman, R. W., et al.: Colonic lymphangiectasia: Report of two cases. Dis. Colon Rectum, *15*:49, 1972.

97. French, A. B.: Protein-losing gastroenteropathies. Amer. J. Dig. Dis., *16*:661, 1971.

98. McGuigan, J. B.: Studies of the immunologic defects associated with intestinal lymphangiectasia with some observations on the dietary control of chylous ascites. Ann. Intern. Med., *68*:398, 1968.

99. Mistilis, S. P., and Skyring, A. P.: Intestinal lymphangiectasia: Therapeutic effect of lymph venous anastomosis. Amer. J. Med., *40*:634, 1966.

100. Ross, J. D., Reid, K. D., Ambujakshan, V. P., et al.: Recurrent pleural effusion, protein-losing enteropathy, malabsorption, and mosaic warts associated with generalized lymphatic hypoplasia. Thorax, *26*: 119, 1971.

101. Marshall, W. H., Jr., Neyazaki, T., and Abrams, H. L.: Abnormal protein loss after thoracic duct ligation in dogs. N. Eng. J. Med., *273*:1092, 1965.

102. Jackson, A. E., and Peterson, C.: Hemangioma of the small intestine causing protein-losing enteropathy. Ann. Intern. Med., *66*:1190, 1967.

103. Leonidas, J. C., Kopel, F. B., and Danese, C. A.: Mesenteric cyst associated with protein loss in the gastrointestinal tract. Study with lymphangiography. Amer. J. Roentgenol. Radium Ther. Nucl. Med., *112*:150, 1971.

104. Jarnum, S., and Jensen, H.: Diffuse gastrointestinal polyposis with ectodermal changes: a case with severe malabsorption and enteric loss of plasma proteins and electrolytes. Gastroenterology, *50*:107, 1966.

105. Orimo, H., Fujita, T., Yoshikawa, M., *et al.*: Gastrointestinal polyposis with protein-losing enteropathy, abnormal skin pigmentation and loss of hair and nails (Cronkhite-Canada syndrome). Amer. J. Med., *47*:445, 1969.

106. Takahata, J., Okubo, K., Komeda, T., *et al.*: Generalized gastrointestinal polyposis associated with ectodermal changes and protein-losing enteropathy with a dramatic response to prednisone. Digestion, *5*:153, 1972.

107. Rosati, L. A., and Oberman, H. A.: Protein losing enteropathy and gastrointestinal hemorrhage associated with a benign mesenchymoma in mesentery. Arch. Intern. Med., *122*:50, 1968.

108. DeSousa, J. S., Guerreiro, O., Cunha, A., *et al.*: Association of nephrotic syndrome with intestinal lymphangiectasia. Arch. Dis. Child., *43*:245, 1968.

109. Yssing, M., Jensen, H., and Jarnum, S.: Albumin metabolism and gastrointestinal protein loss in children with nephrotic syndrome. Acta Paediat. Scand., *58*:109, 1969.

110. Jones, N. F., Creamer, B., and Gimlette, T. M. D.: Hypoproteinemia in anaphylactoid purpura. Br. Med. J., *2*:1166, 1966.

111. Vatistas, S., and Hornsey, S.: Radiation-induced protein loss into the gastrointestinal tract. Br. J. Radiol., *39*:547, 1966.

112. Wagner, A.: Treatment of PLE due to idiopathic intestinal lymphangiectasia by parenteral nutrition. Digestion, *2*:167, 1969.

113. Yssing, M., Jensen, H., and Jarnum, S.: Dietary treatment of protein-losing enteropathy. Acta Paediatr. Scand., *56*:173, 1967.

114. Gruhl, V. R., Weis, H. J., Bailey, J. J., *et al.*: Protein-losing enteropathy caused by a retained intestinal tube. Gastroenterology, *58*:217, 1970.

25 *Australia Antigen*

JONATHAN P. MILLER, PH.D. AND
LACY R. OVERBY, PH.D.

Historical Background

In 1961, Allison and Blumberg[1] observed the presence of precipitating antibodies in the sera of persons who had received multiple blood transfusions. During the course of further studies, they discovered an unusual antigen when a panel of sera were tested against the serum of 2 patients with hemophilia, who had received multiple transfusions. One of the serum samples in the panel reacted and contained an antigenic factor which was named "Australia antigen" because the source of this reactive serum was an Australian aborigine.[2]

In 1967, Krugman's group reported the identification of 2 types of viral hepatitis each with distinctive attributes.[3] One type, MS-1, resembled classical infectious hepatitis, had an incubation period of 30 to 38 days, a relatively short period of abnormal levels of serum transaminase, abnormal thymol turbidity values, and infected patients were quite contagious. The other type, MS-2, resembled serum hepatitis with a longer incubation period of 41 to 108 days. MS-2 infection was characterized by a longer period of elevated transaminase activity, relatively normal thymol turbidity values, and patients infected were only moderately contagious.[4] The correlation of the previously described Australia antigen with long-incubation period hepatitis was established by both Blumberg's group[5] and Prince[6] in 1968.

Several synonyms for Australia antigen have appeared in various reports including SH antigen,[6] hepatitis antigen,[7] hepatitis associated antigen,[8] Australia/SH antigen,[9] and MS-2.[4] Currently the preferred designation is hepatitis B virus associated antigen (HB_sAg).

Properties

Using electron microscopy, Almeida, *et al.,*[9] showed that antigen in serum consisted of 2 main forms, an irregularly sized sphere ranging from 16 to 25 nm, and a tubular form having a diameter of 20 nm but with variable lengths up to several nm. More recently, Almeida, *et al.,*[10] observed typical virus-like particles of 27 nm diameter in liver homogenates of 2 patients who died in the acute stage of serum hepatitis. This same particle was examined most thoroughly by Shao-nan Huang who noted that it has a diameter between 23 and 27 nm. It was discovered in the nuclei of hepatocytes from liver transplant patients who contracted hepatitis.[11]

Dane, *et al.,*[12] observed another particle about 45 nm in diameter. It is composed of an outer coat that reacts with antibody specific for HB_sAg and an inner core about 27 nm in diameter. The current designation for the core is HB_cAg. The "Dane particle" has been found in blood serums and in the cytoplasm of infected hepatocytes.

Immune antigen, antibody complexes formed with specific antisera, have been found to contain all 3 particle types.[13,14] The emerging opinion is that the viral core (HB_cAg) is the Huang particle, containing nucleic acid, which replicates in the hepatocyte nucleus thereby causing the tissue damage associated with hepatitis B. Perhaps the transmissible form of the virus is the Dane particle consisting of the Huang particle (HB$_C$Ag) sheathed in the HB$_S$Ag coat. In some instances, there may be an excess production of coat giving rise to a large quantity of circulating HB$_S$Ag.

The 25 nm particles have a buoyant density of 1.20 gm/cm³ in cesium chloride and are sensitive to ether, and are heat stable for 1 hour at 56°C.

There is, as yet, no consistent demonstration that highly purified preparations of HB$_S$Ag contain nucleic acid, although Jozwiak, *et al.,*[15] reported recovery of RNA from a hepatitis B antigen preparation. The finding of a primed DNA polymerase associated with the Dane particle core[16] suggests that the infectious agent is a DNA-type virus.

LeBouvier[17] demonstrated that HB$_S$Ag is made up of at least 3 antigenic determinants (*a, d,* and *y*). Determinant *a* is common to all HB$_S$Ag particles and the *d* and *y* seem to be mutually exclusive. Hepatitis B antigen is usually subtyped as *ad* or *ay* by AGD methods. Further classification of the determinants has been provided by Bancroft, *et al.,*[18] with the discovery of 2 other mutually exclusive determinants, *w* and *r*. Thus, 4 distinct particle types exist: *adw, adr, ayw,* and *ayr*. Subtype evaluation has been useful in epidemiological studies and Feinman, *et al.,*[19] demonstrated that the subtype of chronic HB$_S$Ag carriers appears to be more related to their country of origin than to their country of residence. An evaluation of 63 persons indicated that *adw* carriers were born in Canada, China, Germany and the West Indies. Most of those originating from Mediterranean countries carried the subtype *ayw* and all *adr* carriers studied were from China.

Transmission

The ability of blood or plasma, containing hepatitis B antigen, to cause posttransfusion hepatitis in man has been well-documented.[20]

Indeed, Schoenfield[21] has shown that even when the plasma has been diluted up to 10,000 times it can produce clinical hepatitis.

Although transfusion is the most commonly implicated source of hepatitis B antigen infection, it is by no means unique. Giles, *et al.,*[3,22] found that the antigen can be infectious when given orally. Other sources of transmission include inadequately sterilized needles, particularly among drug addicts,[23,24,25] kissing, menstrual discharge, contaminated toothbrushes, dental instruments, infected scratches, and accidental pricks from handling infected patients.[26] Urine has also been implicated as a possible source of infection[27] as has sexual transmission.[28] The possibility of infection from airborne contaminated blood within a hemodialysis unit was proposed by Almeida, *et al.*[29]

In further studies on subtypes of HB$_S$Ag, LeBouvier, *et al.,*[30] established that the *ad* and *ay* subtypes are mutually exclusive and that during transmission these subtypes "breed true." Drug addicts most commonly carry the *ay* subtype, whereas *ad* is predominant in asymptomatic carriers. The relationships of subtypes to disease are not clear. Two reports suggest that more cases of acute hepatitis are due to *ay,* although acute disease is more severe in patients with ad subtype HB$_S$Ag.[31,32]

Viral hepatitis has been seen in chimpanzees and the effects are comparable to those observed in humans.[33,34] Krushak[35] and Hillis[36] cited evidence that the disease can be transmitted from chimpanzees to humans. Hirschman, *et al.,*[37] observed the presence of HB$_S$Ag in healthy chimpanzees and Maynard, *et al.,*[38] demonstrated anti-HB$_S$Ag in 55 percent of these animals using RIA techniques. These latter authors also demonstrated immunological identity between human and chimpanzee HB$_S$Ag and antibody. Further studies[39] showed that 2 other susceptible chimpanzees developed transient antigenemia and an antibody response following inoculation with dilutions of human plasma containing HB$_S$Ag.

Using a solid phase RIA method, London, et al.,[40] were able to demonstrate the presence of HB$_S$Ag after 5 serial passages in juvenile rhesus monkeys, the first of which was inoculated with HB$_S$Ag-positive serum obtained from a patient with chronic hepatitis.

Seroconversion, usually regarded as a sign of subclinical infection, occurred in all animals examined. In a similar study, Prince[41] found that HB$_S$Ag can be detected in an experimentally infected chimpanzee, followed by seroconversion and elevated SGPT levels, clear signs of clinical infection. The data indicate that the nonhuman primate is a desirable model for the study of hepatitis B virus infection.

It is not uncommon for the antigen to be observed in the blood early in the disease before the development of overt clinical symptoms. Typically, there may be a peak of hepatitis B antigenemia, the antigen disappearing within a few days or weeks after first detection. Following infection, antigenemia may be detectable within days or, in some cases, weeks. Chronic carriers of HB$_S$Ag also exist and such chronic hepatitis has been observed in a high incidence of patients with Down's syndrome.[42] The carrier state is also undoubtedly associated with other diseases in which there is impaired cellular immunity, such as lepromatous leprosy and chronic renal failure.[43]

Methodology

Since the hepatitis B antigen cannot be grown in tissue culture, and there are no suitable laboratory animal models exhibiting infectivity, the detection of the antigen usually depends upon some form of immunological or biophysical test. The types of tests that have been applied to the detection of hepatitis B antigen are listed in Table 25-1.

Immunodiffusion (AGD, ID). The simplest of the techniques for the detection of hepatitis B antigen is immunodiffusion. Conventionally, it is run in agarose gels, and

Table 25-1. Test Methods for the Detection of Hepatitis B Antigen.

Test Method	Typical Abbreviations
Immunodiffusion or Agar-gel Diffusion	ID, AGD
Complement Fixation	CF
Electron Microscopy	EM
Immune Electron Microscopy	IEM
Hemagglutination	HA
Passive Hemagglutination	PHA
Hemagglutination Inhibition	HAI
Reversed Passive Hemagglutination	RPHA
Immunoelectro-osmophoresis	CIEP, IEOP, CEP
Latex Agglutination	LA, LPA
Radioimmunoassay	RIA

a visually observable precipitin line is formed between the antigen and antibody.[6]

The 2 major disadvantages of this technique are that it is relatively insensitive and it is a slow test to perform. Depending upon the concentration of hepatitis B antigen in the unknown sample, it may require 1 to 3 days to complete the test. A major advantage of immunodiffusion is the ease of confirming and classifying antigens with known standards, allowing positive identification.

Complement Fixation (CF). Typically, the complement fixation test is 10 to 50 times more sensitive than immunodiffusion for the detection of hepatitis B antigen. Microtiter techniques widely used include those of Shulman and Barker,[44] and Taylor.[45]

There are several disadvantages to the CF procedure not the least of which is that it is technically very demanding. In addition, strongly positive sera often exhibit a prozone (negative result) so that screening must be arranged to include a range of dilutions.

Electron Microscopy (EM). Use of the electron microscope provides a nonserological method for detecting hepatitis B antigen. Ultracentrifugation is typically used as a preparative procedure and Almeida, et al.,[9] have described a simple negative staining technique.

Disadvantages are obvious in that this technique requires expensive and elaborate equipment as well as personnel who are well-trained in the identification and morphological characterization of the hepatitis B antigen. While the method can obviously be very sensitive, it may require the careful observation of many fields of view to identify characteristic particles in a low titer sample.

Immune Electron Microscopy (IEM). For samples which contain low concentrations of antigen, the addition of specific antiserum to the test serum causes clumping of the hepatitis B particles, thus making identification easier and more specific. Kelen, *et al.,*[46] described a modification of this technique.

Hemagglutination (HA). Hepatitis B antigen itself has not been found to agglutinate red cells. Red cells, however, can be sensitized by coating them with antigen (PHA) or with antibody (RPHA). The hemagglutination methods are especially useful for identifying nonreactive (negative) serum samples rapidly.

Hemagglutination Inhibition. HAI was first reported by Vyas, *et al.,*[47] using cells sensitized with HB_SAg. The sensitized cells will agglutinate in the presence of antibody. Inhibition of the agglutination by a known amount of antibody in the presence of test sera is used as a measure of HB_SAg. The method is less sensitive than radioimmunoassay, but generally is more sensitive than CEP.

Reversed Passive Hemagglutination. RPHA uses red cells sensitized with antibody and gives a direct test for antigen.[48-53] The sensitivity of this method is about 100 times that of complement fixation and the method itself requires typical serological techniques. The increased sensitivity is manifested in increased detection of positive units in donor populations. Disadvantages include the subjectivity of reading results and the tendency to yield a significant number of reactive serum samples on initial

screening. With appropriate confirmatory procedures, however, all reactive sera can be verified conveniently for the presence of HB_SAg.

Immunoelectro-osmophoresis (IEOP, CIEP, CEP). These are rapid methods for the detection of HBAg which are widely used screening tests. The methods are based on the principle that HB_SAg, at a chosen pH, has an electrophoretic mobility similar to that of α_2-globulin, and moves in the same direction as the current. The antibody, at the chosen pH, moves in the opposite direction because of "endosmosis," thus forcing the antigen and antibody together where they react to form a precipitin line. This phenomenon was first observed by Alter and Blumberg[54] and first applied successfully as a detection technique by Bedarida, *et al.*[55] Since that time, a number of modifications have been described by Pesendorfer, *et al.,*[56] Gocke and Howe,[57] Prince and Burke,[58] and others.

Advantages of this method include rapidity and simplicity. Disadvantages include only a modest increase in sensitivity, 2 to 10 times more sensitive than immunodiffusion, and lack of objectivity. False-positives are observed but are not common. False-negatives, however, occur with relative frequency because of poor visual interpretation of the precipitin line.

Latex Agglutination (LPA). Leach and Ruck[59] reported on a detection system in which latex particles are coated with antibody and are then mixed with the test sample. Agglutination of the latex particles indicates a positive reaction to HBAg. Sensitivity of this method is reported to approach that of complement fixation. Fritz and Rivers[60] evaluated a latex method and reported that sensitivity was slightly more than CF. These studies indicated comparable results with LPA, CF, and RIA on selected test panels.

Latex agglutination is a rapid reaction, but poor specificity has been reported to be a major disadvantage.

Radioimmunoassay (RIA). Since radioimmunoassay is directly applicable to the subject of this book, *In Vitro Nuclear Medicine,* this test methodology is reviewed in depth.

Radioimmunoassay

Radioimmunoassay (RIA) techniques are generally useful for the detection of very low antigen concentrations and the need for more sensitive detection systems for HB_sAg has been considered for several years.

Competitive (Indirect) Techniques. Most reported techniques are based upon the classic "competitive" procedure in which radiolabeled antigen competes with unlabeled antigen for a limited amount of antibody.[61-65] This procedure was first used experimentally to measure hepatitis B antigen by Walsh, *et al.,* in 1970.[61]

The principle of the radioimmune competitive assay system is illustrated in Figure 25-1. Using this test methodology, a small amount of labeled antigen is mixed with the unlabeled antigen in the test sera, and this mixture is then allowed to compete for a fixed amount of antibody. After a suitable incubation period, both labeled and unlabeled antigen have complexed with the antibody present. Separation of the complex from noncomplexed material is accomplished by a variety of techniques including electrophoresis, double antibody precipitation, and solid phase antibody. After separation, the level of radioactivity is determined in the antigen:antibody complex.

The principle of competition indicates that the higher the concentration of unlabeled antigen in the test sera, the lower the amount

RADIOIMMUNE ASSAY
Isotope Dilution (Indirect)

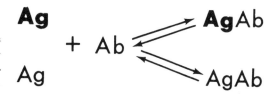

Fig. 25-1. Radioimmune assay isotope dilution (indirect).

of radioactivity in the antigen:antibody complex. Various synonyms for this procedure are competitive radioimmunoassay, isotope dilution radioimmunoassay, and indirect radioimmunoassay.

The solid phase, indirect method is presented in Figure 25-2. In the first step, a mixture of labeled and unlabeled antigen is added to a plastic tube to the interior surface of which antibody has been fixed. After a suitable incubation time, as illustrated in the second step, both labeled and unlabeled antigens will be complexed with the antibody bound to the surface of the tube. The relative amounts of labeled and unlabeled antigen bound depend upon the original ratio which was present in the test sample. The unreacted materials are then washed from the tube and it is assayed for radioactivity. The amount of unlabeled antigen, originally present in the sample, can be estimated by the decrease in count rate from a similar sample which contained no unlabeled antigen.

RADIOIMMUNE ASSAY
Solid Phase (Indirect)

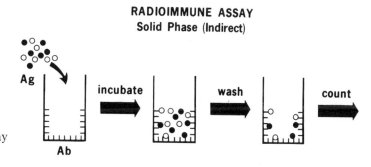

Fig. 25-2. Radioimmune assay solid phase (indirect).

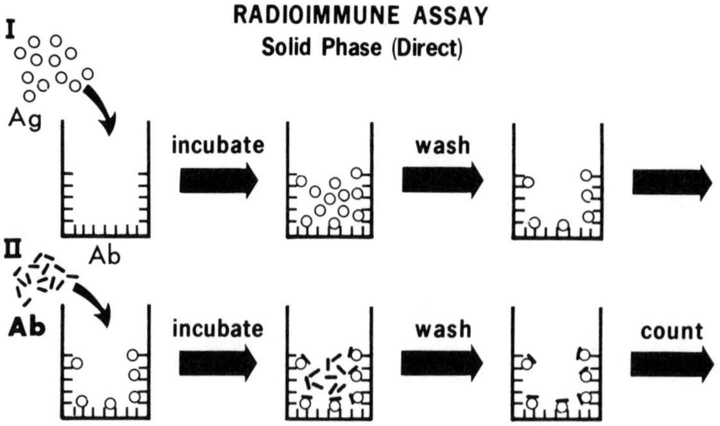

RADIOIMMUNE ASSAY
Solid Phase (Direct)

Fig. 25-3. Radioimmune assay solid phase (direct).

Direct Technique. In 1972, Ling and Overby[66] reported on a 2-step radioimmune technique for the detection of hepatitis B antigen (Fig. 25-3).

1. An unknown amount of antigen is again added to a plastic tube in which specific antibody to HB$_s$Ag has been fixed to the surface.

2. After a suitable incubation time, the tube is washed to remove noncomplexed material and a large excess of specific antibody, labeled with ^{125}I, is added to the tube.

After a suitable incubation period, a number of iodine-labeled antibody molecules re-

act with available determinants on the previously "fixed" HB$_s$Ag creating an antibody: antigen:labeled antibody "sandwich." The tube is then washed to remove unreacted labeled antibody and is finally assayed for radioactivity.

It is obvious, with this technique, that the level of radioactivity in the finally washed tube is directly related to the amount of antigen initially present in the test sample.

A sensitivity comparison of the direct versus the indirect techniques, as well as other techniques, is illustrated in Table 25-2. In this study a sample of purified HB$_s$Ag

Table 25-2. Relative Sensitivity of Five Immunologic Methods for Detecting HB Antigen.

HB$_s$Ag Conc. μg/ml	RIA (Direct) cpm	RIA (Indirect) cpm	CF 1/Dilution	CIEP	AGD
80	10,961+	261+	64	+	+
40	12,208+	370+	32	+	+
20	10,482+	401+	32	+	+
10	10,447+	558+	16	+	+
5	11,253+	656+	4	+	—
2.5	11,291+	1,193+	2	—	—
1.25	11,169+	2,640+	—	—	—
0.6	10,765+	3,455+	—	—	—
0.3	10,080+	5,640+	—	—	—
0.15	8,082+	5,672+	—	—	—
0.075	4,536+	8,833—	—	—	—
0.04	3,198+	7,761—	—	—	—
0.02	1,302+	6,493—	—	—	—
0.01	833+	9,737—	—	—	—
0.005	496—	7,927—	—	—	—
Negative control mean	456—	9,059—	—	—	—

(Ling, and Overby)[66]

was serially diluted and end-point detectability ascertained using the direct and indirect RIA techniques, CF, CIEP and AGD.

In this study, the direct radioimmunoassay was able to detect as little as 0.01 μg/ml of HB_SAg as compared to 0.15 μg/ml for indirect, 2.5 μg/ml for CF, 5.0 μg/ml for CIEP and 10 μg/ml for AGD. The direct technique was thus 1,000 times more sensitive than AGD, 500 times more sensitive than CIEP, 250 times more sensitive than CF and about 15 times more sensitive than the indirect technique.

There are several practical advantages of the solid phase, direct radioimmune assay over those based on competition of unlabeled antigen with labeled antigen in a single reaction. First, in the solid phase, direct method, concentration of antigen and time and temperature of the reaction can be varied in the first step to optimize the kinetics of the antigen-antibody interaction. Second, a high concentration and large excess of ^{125}I-labeled antibody may be used in the second step. This excess favors an increased amount of radioactivity being fixed with increased sensitivity of detection. A third advantage of the direct technique is that antigen can be detected even in the presence of a limited amount of antibody. The simultaneous presence of both antigen and antibody in blood is a frequent occurrence.

Table 25-3 summarizes the results of a study designed to quantify the ability of the direct, solid-phase technique to detect HB_SAg in the presence of antibody. In this study a specific quantity of purified HB_SAg was mixed with an increasing amount of antiserum. Each sample was then tested. The results indicate that there must be an excess of anti-HB_SAg before negative results are attained. The Ab test (Fig. 25-3) is also a direct, solid-phase technique, developed in these laboratories. This technique uses a reverse procedure in which HB_SAg is fixed to the solid phase, anti-HB_SAg in the test sera is complexed to the antigen, and finally ^{125}I-labeled HB_SAg is added to create an antigen: antibody:labeled antigen "sand-

Table 25-3. Test Evaluation of Antigen-Antibody Mixtures.

Ab/Ag Ratio	Ag Test (cpm)	Ab Test (cpm)
0	8,390+	350−
0.5	7,892+	324−
1	9,712+	1,107+
2	7,357+	2,724+
4	2,236+	3,546+
8	484−	6,325+
16	362−	6,053+
32	425−	12,650+
64	405−	11,144+
128	468−	12,740+

(Ling, and Overby)[66]

wich." Results illustrated in Table 25-3 demonstrate that the antibody was easily detected in the presence of antigen as evidenced by increasing count rate.

The direct, solid phase radioimmunoassay procedure, previously described, is presently marketed under the trade name of Ausria-125.* At the time of this writing, an improved version of this test (Ausria II) is the only commercially available, federally approved, RIA system used in the United States. This system has been adopted by the American Red Cross and is widely used as a screening technique for the detection of HB_SAg in donor blood.

Performance Factors

In the development of any test procedure for the detection of HBAg, there are several key questions which must be answered.

1. **Sensitivity.** What is the sensitivity of the method for the detection of HBAg in test sera?

In considering the evaluation of sensitivity of a given test method for the detection of HB_SAg, one must be cognizant of the heterogeneity of this antigen. Ling, *et al.*,[67] and Ginsberg, *et al.*,[68] have reported on the use of the direct, solid phase radioimmune assay

---

* Trademark, Abbott Laboratories, North Chicago, Ill.

Table 25-4. Comparative Sensitivity.

Purified Ag Subtype	Minimal Detectable Dilution			
	Direct RIA	CF	CEP	AGD
ad	1:2,048	1:16	1:4	1:8
ay	1:512	1:4	1:8	1:2
	Relative Sensitivity			
ad	1	1/125	1/250	1/512
ay	1	1/125	1/64	1/256

system for the sensitive detection of *ad* and *ay* subtypes of HB_sAg.

Table 25-4 summarizes the results obtained on purified *ad* and *ay* subtypes using direct RIA, CF, CEP, and AGD methods. This study indicates that the direct RIA is 125 times more sensitive than CF for both subtypes, 64 times more sensitive than CEP for *ay* and 250 times more sensitive than CEP for *ad*. Sensitivity is 250 to 500 times more than AGD for both subtypes.

2. **Specificity.** What is the incidence of false-negatives? What is the incidence of false-positives? Are all serotypes detected with equal specificity?

Initial studies on the direct, solid-phase RIA procedure indicated a high degree of specificity. Hermodsson,[69] Ling and Overby,[66] Matsuda, *et al.,*[70] and Prince, *et al.,*[71] reported that preincubation of samples known to contain HB_sAg with specific antiserum neutralized the positive results. Conversely, preincubation with normal human serum,[71] or with highly diluted antiserum[66,69] did not cause neutralization. Additional specificity

data was provided by Toyoshima, *et al.,*[72] who showed that a number of suspect materials such as fetal calf, mouse, guinea pig, ox and horse sera, Newcastle disease virus, crude and purified influenza virus, trypsin, and insulin did not yield false-positive results.

Sgouris[73] made a preliminary report on false-positive results found in subjects who had been sensitized to guinea pigs and in 1973, Prince, *et al.,*[74] published data indicating that only 21 percent of the positives detected could be confirmed directly by neutralization with specific antiserum; 42 percent were judged to be nonspecific false-positives in that they were neutralized with normal guinea pig serum; and 37 percent of the positives were judged to be equivocal in that they could not be clearly neutralized.

Prince's initial screening results on 5,089 volunteer donor bloods indicated 10 times as many positives detected with the direct, solid-phase system as with CEP. With 21 percent of these judged to be confirmed positives, the solid-phase system detected 2.1 times as many confirmed positives as did CEP.

As a result of these findings, the ^{125}I-labeled antibody formula was modified to contain additional 0.2 percent normal human serum, and 20 percent of normal guinea pig serum. The addition of the latter was capable of greatly reducing the incidence of false-positive results caused by cross-reacting substances in the test sera.

Results, obtained on the plasmas of 5,344 consecutive commercial donors from the west coast are summarized in Table 25-5.

Table 25-5. Specificity Evaluation on 5,344 Donor Sera.

Test	Number Positive		Percent Confirmed	Number per 1,000 Units	
	Detected	Confirmed		False-Positives	False-Negatives
Direct RIA					
Premodification	57	34	59.6	4.3	0
Postmodification	42	34	81.0	1.5	0
Human labeled Ab	34	34	100.0	0	0
CEP	23	23	100.0	0	2.1

Table 25-6. Detectability: Direct Solid-Phase RIA Versus CEP.

Panel Identity	Test Method	No. Units	Confirmed Positives	Percent Positive
Implicated samples	RIA	398	125	31.4
	CEP	398	88	22.1
Commercial donor sera	RIA	6,360	35	0.55
	CEP	6,360	25	0.39
Overall	RIA	6,758	160	23.7
	CEP	6,758	113	16.7

These samples were tested both premodification, prior to addition of 20 percent normal guinea pig serum plus 0.2 percent normal human serum, and also postmodification. The data show a confirmability of 59.6 percent premodification, and 81.0 percent postmodification. Also included in these data is a summary of results obtained using labeled human antibody, instead of guinea pig antibody. This latter modification essentially eliminates potential nonspecificity problems, and overall confirmability of detected positive is 100 percent.

The system using heterologous antibodies (solid phase, guinea pig and labeled human) has now been widely used as a replacement (Ausria II) for the original guinea pig antibodies. There have been no reports of false-positive results. Nevertheless the confirmatory test reagent and procedure is provided to verify the confirmability of positive samples identified. This confirmatory procedure consists of a neutralization test in which 10 percent specfic human antiserum to HB_sAg is mixed with the labeled antibody in the second step of the direct, solid-phase RIA method.[66] In this procedure, a sample is considered confirmed when the count rate is reduced by more than 50 percent with the human antiserum as compared to a normal human serum control.

3. **Detectability.** With a given sensitivity, what is the detectability of the method in finding HB_sAg-positive sera in the population?

Barker[75] estimated that 20 to 25 percent of potentially infectious donors are capable of being detected by ID, CEP, and CF techniques. With a step-function increase in sensitivity, one would expect to detect significantly more positive units in population screening than with other existing methods for the detection of hepatitis B antigen. It is obvious that detectability in a given population is more directly related to the nature of the population than to the sensitivity of the method. Consider the following examples.

(a) An extremely "clean" population which had never been exposed to the hepatitis B antigen.

(b) An extremely "dirty" population which had been repeatedly exposed to the antigen and all individuals had high titer antigenemia.

In these hypothetical cases, one would expect to find 100 percent correlation between a very sensitive test method and an insensitive test method (i.e., 100% negative by both methods in the "clean" population and 100% positive by both methods in the "dirty" population). For this reason, one must be very careful in making inferences as to relative detectability of methods in blood-donor populations if the data is based upon small numbers of units tested.

Table 25-6 summarizes data obtained in our laboratories on 2 distinct populations:

(a) Implicated donor sera where the unit tested was suspect in a specific incident of posttransfusion hepatitis.

(b) Sera obtained from commercial donors from the west coast.

Each implicated serum is not expected to be positive since, in most cases, multiple

Table 25-7. Duration of Positivity.

Investigator	No. Patients	Weeks Ausria-Positive
		(Beyond CEP Detectability)
Johnsson[77]	20	2.6*
Alter[78]		
Chronic hepatitis	2	9-18
Acute hepatitis	4	0
Acute hepatitis	4	1.5-10
		(Prior to CEP Detectability)
Taylor[76]	2	4

* Based on 10 patients (50%) becoming negative by either CEP or Ausria

units are transfused. All positives recorded in Table 25-6 were confirmed to be specific by neutralization with human antiserum specific to hepatitis B antigen. In both populations the RIA detectability was greater and, overall, the CEP method missed a total of 47 confirmed positives in a population of 6,758.

Indications of detectability can also be observed by assessing how long hepatitis B antigen can be detected in the plasma of a patient following infection. Data presented in Table 25-7 summarize the results reported by several investigators.[76,77,78] Typically, the RIA procedure was able to detect hepatitis B antigen from 2 to 10 weeks longer than CEP. Alter[78] reported results from 8 patients but found increased detectability beyond CEP, in only 4 of these. Taylor[76] reported that the direct, solid phase procedure detected the presence of antigen in 2 patients prior to the time that the antigen was detected by CEP. Johnsson[77] evaluated this phenomenon in 20 patients by determining the ratio of positive to negative patient results. On the average, 50 percent of the patients became negative 2.6 weeks sooner with CEP than with the direct, solid-phase RIA technique.

4. **Repeatability.** What is the repeatability of the method on a given sample?

What is the incidence of detection of non-repeatable false-positives?

The direct, solid-phase RIA method is designed to use as a single analysis screening method. Single positive results should be repeated to verify that the results are not caused by possible errors in technique such as inadequate washing of the tube. This parameter can be assessed by determining the number of test results which agree with replicate determinations on the same sample. Results obtained in 3 separate studies, 17,934 individual determinations, demonstrated 105 determinations which did not agree, with respect to positivity or negativity, before repeat testing was carried out. Overall duplicate agreement in these studies was 99.4 percent.

5. **Objectivity.** What is the accuracy of the test method in obtaining true results when run on coded samples by different laboratories?

One of the most significant advantages of an RIA method, as used in a routine screening situation, is that results are based on the analysis of specific numbers instead of visual interpretation such as is necessary with CEP, CF, and AGD. This objectivity can be illustrated by running blind studies on known panels. Panel evaluations tend to be biased because the presence of both positive and negative units is expected, and also because side-by-side intercomparison of test data is possible.

Results obtained on the NIH Serum Panel Number 2, in 6 different laboratories, are summarized in Table 25-8. This panel, of 61 units, consisted of 35 easily identified positives, 6 low-dilution positives not routinely detectable even by very sensitive methods, and 20 negative samples. None of the laboratories involved was 100 percent accurate in that the low dilution positives were not routinely detected.

The overall incidence of false-positives results by RIA, without repeat testing, was 5/366 (1.3%) while the false-positive incidence by CEP was 0. The overall incidence of false-negative results by RIA was 35/366

Table 25-8. Objectivity, Solid-Phase RIA vs. CEP.

Number	Identity	Method	Laboratory (No. Detected)					
			1	*2*	*3*	*4*	*5*	*6*
35	Positives	RIA	34	32	35	35	34	35
6	Low-dilution positives		0	4	0	0	0	0
20	Negatives		26	22	25	26	27	26
	False-positives		1	3	1	0	0	0
	False-negatives		6	4	6	6	7	6
35	Positives	CEP	13	29	29	30	25	
6	Low-dilution positives		0	0	0	1	0	
20	Negatives		48	32	32	30	36	
	False-positives		0	0	0	0	0	
	False-negatives		29	12	12	9	13	
Accuracy								
	Number correct:	RIA	54	56	55	55	54	55
		CEP	33	49	49	51	45	
	Percent correct:	RIA	88.5	91.8	90.1	90.1	88.5	90.1
		CEP	54.1	80.4	80.4	83.6	73.7	

(9.6%) compared to 75/305 (24.6%) by CEP. Thirty-two of 35 samples missed by RIA and 29 of 75 samples missed by CEP were low-dilution positives. The objectivity aspect of these results is further emphasized when consideration is given to the fact that these laboratories had been running CEP for some time and had very little experience with the RIA technique at the time this study was done.

6. **Infectivity.** What is the significance of detecting low levels of HB$_S$Ag in terms of such infected units transmitting clinical or subclinical hepatitis?

In 1970, Barker, *et al.*,[20] demonstrated the presence of hepatitis B antigen in plasma pool samples which had been stored lyophilized since the early 1950's. By correlating the results of their tests with the records of earlier studies, they found that clinical hepatitis had been successfully transmitted by a 1:10,000 dilution of plasma having a CF titer of 1:10. These studies unequivocally demonstrate that very low levels of hepatitis B antigen can cause clinical hepatitis.

The sensitivity and detectability of direct, solid-phase RIA has been previously described. There is little doubt that the more sensitive RIA method is capable of detecting more of the low-titer samples positive for hepatitis B antigen. The potential infectivity of these units is being actively investigated but results to date are incomplete.

Using electron microscopy techniques, Zuckerman's group[79,80] demonstrated the presence of the various particles associated with hepatitis B antigen in samples positive by RIA but negative by other methods. In fact, specificity and sensitivity of the method was confirmed by the evaluation of 2 serum samples which were RIA-positive but negative by AGD, CEP, CF, and IEM. After concentration of these 2 samples, the presence of the hepatitis B antigen could be identified using IEM techniques. Ginsberg, *et al.,*[81] found 25 percent of the specimens collected during the first week of jaundice from 211 patients with hepatitis were positive by RIA techniques versus 12 percent by CEP, 11 percent by CF, 9 percent by HAI, and 4 percent by AGD.

Alter, *et al.,*[82] reported that seroconversion or an anamnestic antibody response occurred in at least 2 patients given blood found to be RIA-positive but AGD, CEP, CF, and HAI-negative. Similarly, Gust[83] identified a serum sample which was negative by all methods previously tested but was RIA-positive. The donor has now been firmly implicated in transmitting hepatitis to at least 3 recipients.

During an evaluation of sera from 211 recipients developing hepatitis in New Jersey, Goldfield, *et al.,*[84] concluded that the use of the direct, solid-phase RIA system would prevent up to 29 percent of all cases of transfusion-associated hepatitis and up to 45 percent of the cases associated with hepatitis B virus infection.

Taswell[85] studied 92 implicated donors involved in blood transfusion to 103 recipients. AGD detected 32 percent of the suspect carriers as positive. When these sera were retested, 9 additional positive samples were detected by RIA.

A specific case of hepatitis transmission was identified by Taylor, *et al.*[76] Blood from a group of 31 apparently healthy donors was given to a patient undergoing cardiac surgery, who subsequently developed hepatitis B antigen positive posttransfusion hepatitis. All of the donor samples were negative by AGD, IEOP, and CF but 1 sample was positive by the direct, solid-phase RIA method (SPRIA).

Prince, *et al.,*[74] made a careful follow-up of transfusions of blood containing both specific RIA reactants, identified by confirmatory neutralization studies, and nonspecific or equivocal RIA-reacting substances. The transfusion of blood containing specific reactants resulted in serologic evidence of HB_SAg infection in 13 or 15 patients followed. Transfusion of nonspecific

RIA reactants resulted in serologic evidence of infection in only one of 18 patients.

Hollinger, *et al.,*[86] reported on a prospective study carried out in 139 presumably susceptible recipients. Units identified as positive by solid-phase RIA were not confirmed by neutralization. Each of the 139 recipients received RIA-positive blood which was negative by CEP. Evaluation of posttransfusion serologic responses indicated that exposure to HB_SAg occurred in 31.6 percent of the recipients of RIA-positive blood, whereas only 6.7 percent of the recipients of RIA-negative blood responded. No hepatitis B occurred in 9 subjects who received RIA-positive blood alone. This study is at variance with that of Giorgini, *et al.,*[87] who found RIA-positive blood to be associated with type B hepatitis in 5 recipients.

Gocke and Kachani[88] evaluated the direct, solid-phase RIA with respect to the ability to detect infectious HB_SAg donors who had been missed by CEP. An assessment of 18 recipients indicated that RIA had the potential for preventing 5 (28%) additional cases of HB_SAg-positive hepatitis. Eighty-nine serum specimens were also tested from 75 patients in the acute phase of hepatitis; 14 additional RIA-positive, CEP-negative, sera were identified.

New Developments in HBAg Testing

Some of the more recent innovations in test methodology for HBAg have been briefly discussed previously. Research on hepatitis B antigen is rapidly moving ahead and continual improvement in test methods is certain. An indication of the rapidly changing technology base can be gained by reviewing developments within the last 2 years (Table 25-9).

The more pertinent details of these particular test systems were:

Ausria-125 (Premodification). With this test system, the test serum sample is added to a tube which was coated with guinea pig antibody to HB_SAg. After incubating overnight at room temperature, the tube is

Table 25-9. Recent Developments in Test Methodology for Hepatitis B Antigen

Method	Form	Incubation Conditions	Reagents	Trade Name	Introduction Date
RIA	Coated tube	First step: Overnight Second step: 90 minutes at room temperature	Solid Phase: Guinea pig Ab Labeled Ab: Guinea pig in calf serum	Ausria-125 (Pre-modification)	August, 1972
RIA	Coated tube	Same as above	Solid Phase: Guinea pig Ab Labeled Ab: Guinea pig plus 0.2% normal human serum and 20% normal guinea pig serum	Ausria-125 (Post-modification)	June, ·1973
RIA	Coated tube	First step: 2 hours Second step: 1 hour at 45° C	Same	Ausria-125 (Ausria-45)	November, 1973
RIA	Coated bead	Same	Solid phase: Guinea pig Ab Labeled Ab: Human plus 0.2% normal human serum and 20% normal guinea pig serum	Ausria II-125	April, 1974
HA	Agglutination test	2 hours at room temperature	Human erythrocytes sensitized with guinea pig Ab	Auscell	April, 1974

washed and guinea pig antibody, labeled with ^{125}I, is added to the tube. After incubating for 90 minutes at room temperature, the tube is washed and counts per minute (cpm) determined in a suitable scintillation detector. Positivity is based upon the ratio of cpm of the test serum to the cpm of the negative-control serum provided. A sample is judged to be negative for hepatitis B antigen if this ratio is less than 2.1.

Ausria-125 (Postmodification). As previously discussed, Prince, *et al.,*[74] reported data which indicated a low degree of specificity of the test system as a result of nonspecific cross-reacting substances in the human test sera. As a result of these findings, the ^{125}I-labeled antibody solution was modified to contain an additional 0.2 per cent of normal human serum and 20 per cent of normal guinea pig serum. These additions are capable of significantly improving the specificity of the test system. The technique involved in running the test is the same as described above.

Ausria-125 (Ausria-45). Taswell[89] presented evidence that incubation at elevated temperature was capable of decreasing the incidence of nonspecificity resulting from cross-reactions. Studies in our laboratories verified these findings and data indicated that optimal sensitivity and specificity can be attained by incubation at 45°C. At this temperature, the first incubation is carried out for 2 hours (with test sera) and the second incubation for 1 hour (with labeled antibody).

Ausria II-125. If there are nonspecific substances in human sera which cross-react with guinea pig antibody, they can be minimized or eliminated by using a heterologous system (i.e., solid-phase object coated with guinea pig antibody combined with the use of ^{125}I-labeled human antibody to HB$_S$Ag).

The Ausria II-125 system utilizes a bead which is coated with guinea pig antibody to HB$_S$Ag. The bead is covered with the test serum and the first incubation is carried out at 45°C for 2 hours. After washing the bead, ^{125}I-labeled human antibody is added and the sample is again incubated at 45°C for 1 hour. After washing, the bead is transferred to a separate tube in order to determine cpm. A sample positive for HB$_S$Ag is defined as one with a cpm ratio to the negative control serum repeatedly greater than 2.1.

Auscell. This hemagglutination test is based on the agglutination of red cells sensitized with anti-HB$_S$Ag. The cells used are specially prepared, stabilized, lyophilized human erythrocytes. In the presence of sufficient HB$_S$Ag, the sensitized cells form a complex leading to an altered visible settling pattern.

All test specimens are diluted 1:8 prior to testing and samples are added to the sensitized erythrocytes. The reactants are then uniformly mixed by rotation and allowed to incubate at room temperature for 2 hours. The test mixtures are then visually observed for indications of agglutination. The test is so designed as to rapidly identify nonreactive samples. All reactive samples must, however, be confirmed for the presence of HB$_S$Ag by carrying out serial dilution titrations and comparing final results with standard control cells.

Table 25-10 summarizes overall results obtained in 2 different studies on blood samples obtained from 5,344 commercial donors (plasma) on the west coast and 9,682 mixed commercial and volunteer donors (sera) from the southeastern portion of the United States. All methods were capable of detecting approximately 40 to 50 per cent more positive units than CEP in this population. Most of the persons tested had been routinely screened by RIA and CEP for many months prior to these studies. These data show that Ausria, postmodification, detected 1.2 false-positive units per 1,000 units tested in this population. The other methods did not detect any false-positives in this population. Although the CEP method was highly specific, it missed 32 true positives in this population with an overall false-negative incidence of 2.1/1,000.

The relative ability of tests to detect the presence of hepatitis B antigen must obviously be related to the sensitivity of the test system for the antigen. The sensitivity of some of the recent hepatitis test systems is summarized in Table 25-11. The most sensitive of the test systems is Auria II-125 utilizing a coated bead and human antibody. Typically, Ausria II, run at 45°C is about 4 to 8 times as sensitive as Ausria-125, which is run at room temperature. The true significance of relative test sensitivity in detecting HB$_S$Ag in various populations must eventually await the accumulation of significant statistics. It appears obvious that the nature of the population screened is an important factor in controlling the relative number of positive units detected. For example, one might expect to find significantly more positive units in a highly implicated population with a more sensitive test method. Conversely, the difference in detectability between sensitive and insensitive methods is expected to be lowest in a low-exposure group. Volunteer donors typically have less exposure to hepatitis B antigen, and it has been well established that posttransfusion hepatitis is more common following the administration of commercial blood.[90,91]

The Value of Hepatitis Testing

Alter has reported[92] that transfusion viral hepatitis is responsible for an estimated 30,000 cases of serious, overt illness and

Table 25-10. Detection and Confirmation Results on 15,026 Blood Donor Samples.

Method	RIA	RIA*	RIA	HA	CEP
Trade Name:	Ausria (Post-modification)	Ausria 45°	Ausria II	Auscell	
Positives detected	111	(34)*	97	89	65
Negatives detected	14,915	(5,310)*	14,929	14,937	14,961
Confirmed positives	93	(34)*	97	89	65
False-positives	18	(0)*	0	0	0
False-negatives	4	(0)*	0	8	32
Confirmed positive/1,000	6.2	6.4	6.4	5.9	4.3
False-negatives/1,000	0.3	0	0	0.5	2.1
False-positives/1,000	1.2	0	0	0	0
Ratio confirmed positives: CEP	1.44	1.49	1.49	1.37	1.0

* Only 5,344/15,026 units tested by Ausria 45°

1,000 to 3,000 deaths annually in the United States. For each case of overt disease, there are at least 5 cases of subclinical hepatitis and the actual incidence of post-transfusion hepatitis probably exceeds 150,000 cases a year. In the United States the task force on a National Blood Policy estimated that hospitalization of overt post-transfusion hepatitis costs the nation 86 million dollars a year.[93]

The medical literature is replete with instances of outbreaks of hepatitis B in renal dialysis and kidney transplant units of the hospital. It would appear to be prudent that both staff and patients in renal and dialysis units be routinely screened for the presence of HB_SAg by sensitive test methods. Obviously, positive findings will dictate hygienic measures. The blood bank has primary responsibility for testing the quality of transfusion blood and the American National Red Cross system has implemented the use of the direct, solid-phase RIA test system. In addition to the routine clearance of transfusion blood, some hospitals have initiated the routine testing of incoming patients for HB_SAg.

It is evident that hepatitis B antigen is an important factor in the diagnosis and prognosis of many cases of liver disease. The antigen has been found in two-thirds of the patients with chronic, persistent hepatitis, and commonly in several forms of cirrhosis. Diagnosis of liver disorders can be puzzling and a sensitive hepatitis B antigen test can provide valuable additional data in conjunction with the usual laboratory tests to establish liver profile. Vogel, et al.,[94] and Sherlock, et al.,[95] reported that a substantial proportion of patients with hepatoma are also HB_SAg-positive. Japanese investigators[96] es-

Table 25-11. Sensitivity Comparison of Test Methods for the Detection of HBAg.

Method	Minimal Detectable Concentration of Purified HBAg ($\mu g/ml$)	
	Subtype ad	Subtype ay
Ausria II	0.0025	0.0025
Ausria-125	0.01	0.02
Auscell	0.02	0.04
CEP	2.56	2.56
	Relative Sensitivity	
Ausria II	1,000*	1,000*
Ausria-125	250	125
Auscell	125	62.5
CEP	1	1

* Arbitrary assignment of 1,000 to Ausria II

timated that patients with circulating HB_SAg are 8 times as susceptible to hepatoma as are those in whom antigen is not detected. In numerous chronic hepatitis cases, the HB_SAg has been detected in a high proportion of the family of the patient.

There is a continued research interest in methods for the detection of anti-HB_SAg that is generally focused on (a) epidemiologic factors associated with transmission of HB_SAg hepatitis, (b) efficacy of the administration of human serum gamma globulin for the prevention of hepatitis B, and (c) evaluation of the recovery and prognosis of infected recipients. Persons under 20 years of age have been shown to have an anti-HB_SAg prevalence significantly less than older persons,[97] and the prevalence of antibody in residents of Harlem was approximately 3 times that of residents in a high socio-economic area.[98] Using a solid-phase radio-immunoassay method developed in these laboratories, Ginsberg, Conrad, *et al.*,[99] showed that the incidence of anti-HB_SAg in military recruits was about 5 per cent, about 14 per cent in older soldiers, and about 25 per cent in soldiers with a year of military service in Korea. These authors were not able to correlate antibody titer in lots of standard human serum gamma globulin versus protection against icteric serum hepatitis. The question of whether anti-HB_SAg affords some protection against hepatitis development is yet to be resolved. Lander, Alter, and Purcell[100] used a double antibody RIA method for determining the frequency of antibody and found an incidence of 14.4 per cent in voluntary blood donors, 22.6 per cent in commercial donors, 14.8 per cent in blood bank personnel, 11.4 per cent in laboratory personnel and 82.6 per cent in persons given multiple transfusions. Reed, *et al.*,[101] studied the infusion of anti-HB_SAg in patients with active chronic hepatitis. The previously described solid-phase RIA method was capable of detecting antibody in one patient up to 93 days post-infusion and in all of 6 patients infused. In only one of the 6 patients was antibody titer

high enough to be detected by immuno-diffusion. The value of routine screening of blood donations for anti-HB_SAg is not established, although some have advanced the proposal that the presence of antibody mandates the biological presence of HB_SAg. Perhaps the most meaningful results from anti-HB_SAg studies will be related to clinical use in monitoring the course and prognosis of established hepatitis.

Safety Precautions

As previously indicated, hepatitis B can be transmitted by several means other than blood transfusion. Precautionary procedures and personnel surveillance programs should be instituted where exposure to the antigen is possible. Schmidt and Lennette[102] have reviewed proper precautions for performing tests. Good practices in handling HB_SAg-containing materials are generally very similar to those dictated by the use and handling of radioactive materials.

Personnel who should be considered for surveillance include clinical chemistry technicians, blood bank technicians, blood product handlers, patients and staff of renal dialysis units, animal handlers for primate colonies, food handlers, surgeons, and paramedical personnel, dentists, dental assistants, autopsy and morgue staff, and surgical patients. London and colleagues[103] carefully investigated an epidemic in renal dialysis units and developed specific preventive measures. Precautions for handling human blood should include care with specimens and specimen collection, use of gloves and hoods, isolation of contaminated equipment, no eating, drinking, or smoking in laboratories, routine decontamination procedures, and careful disposal of contaminated materials.

Other Hepatitis Causative Agents

It is clear that the presence of HB_SAg accounts for only a portion of those blood units capable of causing hepatitis following transfusion.

Hepatitis A. The preferred nomenclature for the agent associated with infectious hepatitis is hepatitis A. Clinical disease is characterized by a relatively short incubation period with no evidence for association with HB_SAg. Sherlock[104] reported that hepatitis A is usually carried in feces and that epidemics often arise following contamination of food and water supplies. Epidemics have been related to contaminated water used to wash dairy equipment and to ingestion of raw clams and oysters from polluted water. The disease is usually mild compared to that caused by transmission of HB_SAg.

It has generally been accepted that hepatitis A and hepatitis B are caused by different and distinct entities. Some epidemiologic studies and similarities in clinical symptomology followng transfusion of HB_SAg-positive and HB_SAg-negative blood[105] have promulgated the concept that the infectious agents may be either closely related or perhaps identical.[106] Recent studies in marmosets[107] have shown encouraging results as to the possibility of finding a suitable animal model for transmitting hepatitis A. This finding will provide the needed biological system, other than man, needed to accelerate the characterization of the hepatitis A agent.

The recent finding of virus-like particles in fecal extracts by IEM using convalescent serum from hepatitis A patients for complexing appears to be a major breakthrough in characterizing the infectious agent.[108] If confirmed, these studies also should help establish the nature of the agents associated with transfusion-related hepatitis, and not identified as hepatitis B.

Hepatitis C. Prince[109] postulated a third major subclass of hepatitis, type C, in addition to hepatitis A and B. Prince's hypothesis for a type C hepatitis virus is based upon: (a) relatively low-detection incidence of infective units even with the best available screening techniques, (b) abnormal precipitin lines when using agar gel diffusion and (c) specific antigen density bands obtained by gradient centrifugation studies.

Dane Core Antigen. The previously de-scribed Dane particle contains a central core, and Almeida[110] obtained evidence indicating that the core antigen (HB_CAg) may be distinctly different from the surrounding surface antigen (HB_SAg). Convalescing serum antibody reacted with the inner core component but not the outer coat to yield aggregates similar to those seen in the liver of patients with serum hepatitis.

Detection systems for the Dane core and core antibody, now available, should provide the means for clarifying the role of the Dane particle. The presence of a DNA polymerase associated with these particles suggests a major role in the infectious process.

References

1. Allison, A. C., and Blumberg, B. S.: An isoprecipitation reaction distinguishing human serum protein types. Lancet, *1*:634, 1961.
2. Blumberg, B. S.: Polymorphisms of serum proteins in the development of isoprecipitins in transfused patients. Bull. N.Y. Acad. Med., *40*:377, 1964.
3. Krugman, S., Giles, J. P., and Hammond, J.: Infectious hepatitis: evidence for two distinctive clinical epidemiological, and immunological types of infection. JAMA, *200*:365, 1967.
4. Krugman, J., and Giles, J. P.: Viral hepatitis: new light on an old disease. JAMA, *212*:1019, 1970.
5. Sutnick, A. I., London, W. T., Gerstley, B. J. J., Cronlund, M. M., and Blumberg, B. S.: Anicteric hepatitis associated with Australia antigen. JAMA, *205*:670, 1968.
6. Prince, A. M.: An antigen detected in the blood during the incubation period of serum hepatitis. Proc. Nat. Acad. Sci. USA, *60*:814, 1968.
7. Gocke, D. J., and Kavey, N. B.: Hepatitis antigen. Lancet, *1*:1055, 1969.
8. Kim, C. Y., and Tilles, J. G.: Immunologic electrophoretic heterogeneity of hepatitis-associated antigen. J. Infect. Dis., *123*:618, 1971.
9. Almeida, J. D., Zuckerman, A. J., Taylor, P. E., and Waterson, A. P.: Immune electron microscopy of the Australia-SH (serum hepatitis) antigen. Microbios, *2*: 117, 1969.
10. Almeida, J. D., Waterson, A. P., Trawell, J. M., and Neale, G.: The finding of virus-like particles in two Australia-antigen-

positive human livers. Microbios, 6:145, 1970.

11. Huang, S.: Hepatitis associated antigen hepatitis. Amer. J. Path., 64:483, 1971.

12. Dane, D. S., Cameron, C. H., and Briggs, M.: Virus-like particles in serum of patients with Australia-antigen-associated hepatitis. Lancet, 1:695, 1970.

13. Cossart, Y. E.: Australia antigen and hepatitis: a review. J. Clin. Path., 24:394, 1971.

14. Jokelainen, P. T., Krohn, K., Prince, A. M., and Finlayson, N. D. C.: Electron microscope observations on virus-like particles associated with SH antigen. J. Virol., 6:685, 1970.

15. Jozwiak, W., Koscielak, K., Madalinski, K., Brzosko, W. J., et al.: R.N.A. of Australia antigen. Nature New Biol., 229:92, 1971.

16. Kaplan, P. M., Greenman, R. L., Gerin, J. L., Purcell, R. H., and Robinson, W. S.: DNA polymerase associated with human hepatitis B antigen. J. Virol., 12:995, 1973.

17. LeBouvier, G. L.: The heterogeneity of Australia antigen. J. Infect. Dis., 123:671, 1971.

18. Bancroft, W. H., Mundon, F. K., and Russell, P. K.: Detection of additional antigenic determinants of hepatitis B antigen. J. Immunol., 109:842, 1972.

19. Feinman, S. V., Berris, B., Sinclair, J. C., Alter, H. J., et al.: Relation of hepatitis-B-antigen subtypes in symptom-free carriers to geographical origin and liver abnormalities. Lancet, 1:867, 1973.

20. Barker, L. F., Shulman, N. R., Murray, R., Hirschman, R. J., et al.: Transmission of serum hepatitis. JAMA, 211:1509, 1970.

21. Schoenfield, L. J.: New aspects of hepatitis. Okla. State Med. Assoc. J., 64:336, 1971.

22. Giles, J. P., McCollum, R. W., Berndtson, L. W., Jr., and Krugman, S.: Viral hepatitis: relation of Australia/SH antigen to the Willowbrook MS-2 strain. N. Eng. J. Med., 281:119, 1969.

23. Fenner, F., and White, D. O.: Medical Virology. ch. 23, pp. 361-362. New York, Academic Press, 1970.

24. Nordenfelt, E., Kaijand, K., and Ursing, B.: Presence and persistence of Australia antigen among drug addicts. Vox. Sang., 19:371, 1970.

25. Sullman, S. F., and Zuckerman, A. J.: Viral hepatitis in drug addicts. Postgrad. Med. J., 47:473, 1971.

26. Sherlock, S.: Progress Report. Long-incubating (virus B, HAA-associated) hepatitis. Gut, 13:297, 1972.

27. Heathcote, E. J. L., Tsianides, A., and Sherlock, S.: Australia antigen in the urine of patients with acute Australia-antigen positive hepatitis and their household contacts. Gut, 13:852, 1972.

28. Editorial: Cherchez l'Homme? JAMA, 225:1645, 1973.

29. Almeida, J. D., Kulatilake, A. E., Mackey, D. H., et al.: Possible airborne spread of serum-hepatitis virus within a haemodialysis unit. Lancet, 2:849, 1971.

30. LeBouvier, G. L., McCollum, R. W., Hierholzer, W. J., Jr., Irwin, G. R., et al.: Subtypes of Australia antigen and hepatitis-B virus. JAMA, 222:928, 1972.

31. Nielsen, J. O., LeBouvier, G. L., and The Copenhagen Hepatitis Acute Program: Subtypes of Australia antigen among paients and healthy carriers in Copenhagen. N. Eng. J. Med., 288:1257, 1973.

32. Editorial: Subtypes of Australia antigen. Br. Med. J., 1:127, 1973.

33. Hillis, W. D.: Viral hepatitis associated with sub-human primates. Transfusion, 3:445, 1963.

34. Atchley, F. O., and Kimbrough, R. D.: Experimental study of infectious hepatitis in chimpanzees. Lab. Invest., 15:1520, 1966.

35. Krushak, D. H.: Application of preventative health measures to curtail chimpanzee-associated infectious hepatitis in handlers. Lab. Anim. Sci., 20:52, 1970.

36. Hillis, W. D.: An outbreak of infectious hepatitis among chimpanzee handlers at a United States Air Force Base. Amer. J. Hygiene, 73:316, 1961.

37. Hirschman, R. J., Shulman, N. R., Barker, L. F., and Smith, K. O.: Virus-like particles in sera of patients with infectious and serum hepatitis. JAMA, 208:1667, 1969.

38. Maynard, J. E., Hartwell, W. V., and Berquist, K. R.: Hepatitis-associated antigen in chimpanzees. J. Infect. Dis., 123:660, 1971.

39. Maynard, J. E., Berquist, K. R., and Krushak, D. H.: Experimental infection of chimpanzees with the virus of hepatitis B. Nature, 237:514, 1972.

40. London, W. T., Alter, H. J., Lander, J., and Purcell, R. H.: Serial transmission of rhesus monkeys of an agent related to hepatitis associated antigen. J. Infect. Dis., 125:382, 1972.

41. Prince, A. M.: Infection of chimpanzees with hepatitis B virus. *In* Vyas, G. N.,

Perkins, H. A., and Schmid, R.: Hepatitis and Blood Transfusion. New York, Grune & Stratton, 1972.

42. Sutnick, A. I., London, W. T., Gerstley, B. J., *et al.*: Anicteric hepatitis associated with Australia antigen. Occurrence in patients with Down's syndrome. JAMA, *205*:670, 1968.

43. Editorial: Australia antigen—the pace quickens. Lancet, *1*:85, 1973.

44. Shulman, N. R., and Barker, L. F.: Virus antigen, antibody and the antigen-antibody complexes in hepatitis measured by complement fixation. Science, *165*:204, 1969.

45. Taylor, P. E.: Viral hepatitis and tests for the Australia (hepatitis-associated) antigen and antibody. IV. Complement fixation tests. Bull. WHO, *42*:966, 1970.

46. Kelen, A. E., Hathaway, A. E., and McLeod, D. A.: Rapid detection of Australia/SH antigen and antibody by a simple and sensitive technique of immuno-electronmicroscopy. Can. J. Microbiol., *17*:993, 1971.

47. Vyas, G. N., and Shulman, N. R.: Hemagglutination assay for antigen and antibody associated with viral hepatitis. Science, *170*:332, 1970.

48. Cook, R. J.: Reversed passive haemagglutination systems for the estimation of tetanus toxins and antitoxins. Immunology, *8*:74, 1965.

49. Cook, R. J.: Titration of *Clostridium oedematiens* antitoxin by reversed passive haemagglutination. Immunology, *9*:249, 1965.

50. Cua-Lim, F., Richter, M., and Rose, B.: The reversed BDB technique. Allergy, *34*:142, 1963.

51. Juji, R., and Yokochi, T.: Haemagglutination technique with erythrocyte coated with specific antibody for detection of Australia antigen. Japan J. Exp. Med., *39*:615, 1969.

52. Nyerges, G.: Reversed passive haemagglutination inhibition method for the estimation of Antivaccinia antibodies. Immunology, *17*:333, 1969.

53. Hirata, A. A., Emerick, A. J., and Boley, W. F.: Hepatitis B virus antigen detected by reversed passive hemagglutination. Proc. Soc. Exp. Biol. Med., *143*:761, 1973.

54. Alter, H. J., and Blumberg, B. S.: Further studies on a "new" human isoprecipitin system (Australia antigen). Blood, *127*:297, 1966.

55. Bedarida, G., Trinchieri, G., and Carbonara, A. O.: The detection of Australia antigen and anti-Au antibodies, by a rapid procedure combining electrophoresis and immunoprecipitation. Haematologica, *54*:551, 1969.

56. Pesendorfer, F., Krassnitsky, O., and Welwalka, F. G.: Viral hepatitis and tests for the Australia (hepatitis-associated) antigen and antibody. V. immunoelectrophoretic methods. Bull. WHO, *42*:974, 1970.

57. Gocke, D. J., and Howe, C.: Rapid detection of Australia antigen by counter-immunoelectrophoresis. J. Immunol., *104*:1031, 1970.

58. Prince, A. M., and Burke, K.: Serum hepatitis antigen (SH): rapid detection by high voltage immunoelectroosmophoresis. Science, *169*:593, 1970.

59. Leach, J. M., and Ruck, B. J.: Detection of hepatitis associated antigen by the latex agglutination test. Br. Med. J., *4*:597, 1971.

60. Fritz, R. B., and River, S. L.: Hepatitis-associated antigen: detection of antibody-sensitized latex particles. J. Immunol., *108*:108, 1972.

61. Walsh, J. H., Yalow, R., and Berson, S. A.: Detection of Australia antigen and antibody by means of radioimmunoassay techniques. J. Infect. Dis., *121*:550, 1970.

62. Aach, R. D., Grisham, J. W., and Parker, C. W.: Detection of Australia antigen by radioimmunoassay. Proc. Natl. Acad. Sci., *68*:1056, 1971.

63. Hollinger, F. B., Vorndam, V., and Dreesman, G. R.: Assay of Australia antigen and antibody employing double-antibody and solid-phase radioimmunoassay techniques and comparison with the passive hemagglutination methods. J. Immunol., *107*:1099, 1971.

64. Coller, J. A., Millman, I., Halbherr, T. C., and Blumberg, B. S.: Radioimmunoprecipitation assay for Australia antigen, antibody, and antigen-antibody complexes. Proc. Soc. Exp. Biol. Med., *138*:249, 1971.

65. Purcell, R. H.: Viral hepatitis and tests for the Australia (hepatitis-associated) antigen and antibody. VII. Radioimmunoassay Techniques. Bull. WHO, *42*:978, 1970.

66. Ling, C. M., and Overby, L. R.: Prevalence of hepatitis B virus antigen as revealed by direct radioimmune assay with ^{125}I-antibody. J. Immunol., *109*:834, 1972.

67. Ling, C. M., Irace, H., Decker, R., and Overby, L. R.: Hepatitis B virus antigen: validation and immunologic characterization of low titer serums with ^{125}I-antibody. Science, *180*:203, 1973.

68. Ginsberg, A. L., Bancroft, W. H., and Conrad, M. E.: Simplified and sensitive

detection of subtypes of Australia antigen (HBAg) using a solid-phase radioimmune assay. J. Lab. Clin. Med., *80*:291, 1972.

69. Hermodsson, S.: Studies with the Ausria test for detection of Au-antigen. Personal communication, November 15, 1972.

70. Matsuda, S., Tada, K., Shirachi, R., and Ishida, N.: Australia antigen in amniotic fluid. Lancet, *1*:1117, 1972.

71. Prince, A. M., Metselaar, D., Kalfuko, G. W., Mukwaya, L. G., *et al.*: Hepatitis B antigen in wild-caught mosquitoes in Africa. Lancet, *2*:247, 1972.

72. Toyoshima, S., Seto, Y., and Inagaki, M.: Specificity of a solid phase radioimmunoassay of Australia antigen. Personal communication, Dec., 1972.

73. Sgouris, J. R.: Limitations of the radioimmunoassay for hepatitis B antigen. N. Eng. J. Med., *288*:160, 1973.

74. Prince, A. M., Brotman, B., Jass, D., and Ikram, H.: The specificity of the direct solid-phase radioimmunoassay for detection of hepatitis B antigen. Lancet, *1*:1346, 1973.

75. Barker, L. F.: Comparative sensitivity of procedures for hepatitis-associated antigen detection. XXIVth Scientific Meeting of the Blood Research Institute, p. 457, 1971.

76. Taylor, P. E., and Kelen, A. E.: Studies of hepatitis B antigenaemia by solid-phase radioimmunoassay. Can. J. Public Health, *64*:67, 1973.

77. Johnsson, T.: Personal communication. Nov., 1972.

78. Alter, H. J.: Evaluation of solid phase radioimmunoassay for hepatitis B antigen: experience of the N.I.H. Clinical Center Blood Bank. *In* Symposium on Hepatitis B Antigen Testing by Radioimmunoassay. Catonsville, Maryland, Mar., 1973.

79. Bowes, A., Preece, J., and Zuckerman, A. J.: Solid-phase radioimmunoassay for hepatitis B antigen. Personal communication, Aug., 1972.

80. Zuckerman, A. J., Earl, P. M., Bowes, A., *et al.*: Detection rate of hepatitis B antigen in serum. Personal communication, Sept., 1972.

81. Ginsberg, A. L., Conrad, M. E., Bancroft, W. H., Ling, C. M., *et al.*: Prevention of endemic HAA-positive hepatitis with gamma globulin. Use of a simple radioimmune assay to detect HAA. N. Eng. J. Med., *286*:562, 1972.

82. Alter, H. J., Holland, P. V., Purcell, R. H., Lander, J. J., *et al.*: Post-transfusion hepatitis after exclusion of commercial and hepatitis-B antigen positive donors. Ann. Intern. Med., *77*:691, 1972.

83. Gust, I.: Personal communication, Oct., 1972.

84. Goldfield, M., Bill, J., Black, H., Pizzuti, W., and Srihongse, S.: Hepatitis associated with the transfusion of HBAg-negative blood. *In* Vyas, G. N., Perkins, H. A., and Schmid, R.: Hepatitis and Blood Transfusion. New York, Grune & Stratton, 1972.

85. Taswell, H. F.: Incidence of HBAg in blood donors: an overview. *In* Vyas, G. N., Perkins, H. A., and Schmid, R.: Hepatitis and Blood Transfusion. New York, Grune & Stratton, 1972.

86. Hollinger, F. B., Aach, R. D., Gitnick, G. L., Roche, J. K., and Melnick, J. L.: Limitations of solid-phase radioimmunoassay for HBAg in reducing frequency of post-transfusion hepatitis. N. Eng. J. Med., *289*:385, 1973.

87. Giorgini, G. L., Hollinger, F. B., Laduc, I., *et al.*: Radioimmunoassay detection of hepatitis type B antigen: a prospective study in blood donors and recipients. JAMA, *222*:1514, 1972.

88. Gocke, D. J., and Kachani, Z. F.: Solid-phase radioimmunoassay for hepatitis B antigen. JAMA, *224*:1425, 1973.

89. Taswell, H. F., Nicholson, L., Cochran, M., and Tauxe, W. N.: A rapid, safe method for the detection of hepatitis B antigen by radioimmunoassay. 26th Annual Meeting Amer. Assn. Blood Banks, Miami, Florida, (abstr.), p. 80, Nov., 1973.

90. Holland, P. V., Alter, H. J., Purcell, R. H., Walsh, J. H., *et al.*: The infectivity of blood containing the Australia antigen. *In* Prier, J. E., and Friedman, H.: Australia Antigen, Baltimore, University Park Press, 1973.

91. Allen, J. G.: Commercially obtained blood and serum hepatitis. Surg. Gynecol. Obstet., *131*:277, 1970.

92. Alter, H. J.: The hepatitis-associated antigen (Australia antigen). Amer. Fam. Physician, *3*:72, 1971.

93. Report of Task Force, Chaired by Dr. Ian Mitchell, U.S. Department of Health, Education, and Welfare, National Blood Policy, July, 1973.

94. Vogel, C. L., Anthony, P. P., Mody, N., and Barker, L. F.: Hepatitis associated antigen in Ugandan patients with hepatocellular carcinoma. Lancet, *2*:621, 1970.

95. Sherlock, S., Fox, R. A., Niazi, S. P., and Scheuer, R. J.: Chronic liver disease and

primary liver cell cancer with hepatitis associated (Australia) antigen in serum. Lancet, *1*:1243, 1970.

96. Nichioka, K., Hirayama, T., Sekine, T., Okochi, K., *et al.*: Australia antigen and hepatocellular carcinoma. GANN Monograph on Cancer Research, *14*:167, 1973.

97. Lander, J. J., Holland, P. V., Alter, J. H., *et al.*: Antibody to hepatitis-associated antigen. Frequency and pattern of response as detected by radioimmunoprecipitation. JAMA, *220*:1079, 1972.

98. Cherubin, C. E., Lander, J. J., Purcell, R. H., *et al.*: Acquisition of antibody to hepatitis B antigen in three socioeconomically different medical populations. Lancet, *2*: 149, 1972.

99. Ginsberg, A. L., Conrad, M. E., Bancroft, W. H., Ling, C. M., and Overby, L. R.: Antibody to Australia antigen: detection with a simple radioimmune assay, incidence in military populations, and role in the prevention of hepatitis B with gamma globulin. J. Lab. Clin. Med., *82*:317, 1973.

100. Lander, J. J., Alter, H. J., and Purcell, R. H.: Frequency of antibody to hepatitis-associated antigen as measured by a new radioimmunoassay technique. J. Immunol., *106*:1166, 1971.

101. Reed, W. D., Eddleston, A. L. W. F., Cullens, H., Williams, R., *et al.*: Infusion of hepatitis-B antibody in antigen-positive active chronic hepatitis. Lancet, *2*:1347, 1973.

102. Schmidt, N. J., and Lennette, E. H.: Safety precautions for performing tests for hepatitis-associated "Australia" antigen and antibodies. Amer. J. Clin. Pathol., *57*: 526, 1972.

103. London, W. T., Figlia, M., Sutnick, A., *et al.*: An epidemic of hepatitis in a chronic-hemodialysis unit. Australia antigen and difference in host response. N. Eng. J. Med., *281*:571, 1969.

104. Sherlock, S.: Acute virus hepatitis: Clinical and pathological aspects. Amer. J. Med. Technol., *38*:333, 1972.

105. Sutnick, A. I., Senior, J. R., Goeser, E., and Millman, I.: Similarity of hepatitis following transfusion of Australia-antigen positive and negative blood. Lancet, *2*: 461, 1973.

106. Editorial: What about type A hepatitis? Lancet, *2*:1007, 1973.

107. Deinhardt, F., Wolfe, L., Junge, U., and Holmes, A. W.: Viral hepatitis in non-human primates. Can. Med. Assoc. J., *106*:468, 1972.

108. Feinstone, S. M., Kapikian, A. Z., and Purcell, R. H.: Hepatitis A: Detection by immune electron microscopy of a virus-like antigen associated with acute illness. Science, *182*:1026, 1973.

109. Special Report: Another hepatitis virus? Med. World News, p. 441, June 25, 1971.

110. Almeida, J. P., Rubenstein, D., and Stott, E. J.: New antigen-antibody system in Australia antigen positive hepatitis. Lancet, *2*:1225, 1971.

26 Bacteriologic Cultures and Sensitivities

Frank H. DeLand, M.D.

HISTORY

Methodologies currently used in microbiology are essentially those that were developed during the "golden era" of technical advancements in bacteriology, from 1870 to 1885. The isolation and identification of bacteria and determining their sensitivity to antibiotics and chemotherapeutic drugs encompass multiple manual procedures. Since the interpretation of the results from these procedures is subjective, demanding experience and judgment, well-trained personnel are essential. The combination of manual methodology and skilled technical personnel inevitably results in a time-consuming, expensive discipline. Experience and medical practice have repeatedly demonstrated that bacteriologic investigation of patients is significantly underutilized because results of bacteriologic tests are so frequently not known until after the fact (i.e., the patient has been treated empirically and often has been already discharged from the hospital or the physician's care before the results are available). Since bacteriologic investigations are expensive, physicians are frequently reluctant to utilize bacteriology more fully. The factors of time and expense have inhibited the optimal use of this discipline to the detriment of the patient.

The application of methodologies which eliminates subjective interpretations and manual operations has tremendous impact on the utilization of the discipline. Clinical chemistry is an excellent example of this approach to laboratory medicine. As the result of eliminating manual procedures and subjective interpretations by means of automated procedures, clinical chemistry has assumed a more important role in diagnostic and preventive medicine because it is so economical. Besides the scientific implications of applying to bacteriology new methodologies that are more sensitive, specific, and rapid there are certain economical and public health factors to be considered. The time required for treatment may be effectively reduced, and offer a financial saving to the patient, a more optimal use of hospital beds, and a shorter hospital stay. The impact of more rapid bacteriologic methodologies should change the role of treatment in outpatient clinics and partially eliminate the subsequent hospital admissions.

In the past 20 years explosive developments in diagnostic and therapeutic medical procedures would have placed an insurmountable burden on medical personnel had not many innovations been applied. Of all the services affected by increased utilization, laboratory medicine experienced the greatest increase in work load. New diagnostic methods and procedural automation have enabled laboratories to meet the tremendous demand upon their services and simultaneously to decrease unit cost very effectively. However, in bacteriology application of automated or semi-automated methods has not kept pace with application in other areas in the clinical laboratory. Kinney and Melville noted that "automation has made the least inroads in this field (microbiology) so far, except for the area of serologic reactions where continuous flow techniques offer considerable promise."[1]

In 1956 Levin, et al.[2] reported one of the first applications of radionuclides for the clinical detection of microorganisms. Their procedure was a rapid presumptive test for coliform organisms in drinking water. By means of a Geiger counter, they measured the release of $^{14}CO_2$ from the bacterial metabolism of ^{14}C-l-lactose. By this method it was possible to detect metabolism of lactose by coliform organisms (10^9 concentration per ml of *Escherichia coli*) in less than 1 hour. Roberts, *et al.* found that when ^{14}C-formate was metabolized by *Escherichia coli,* 86 per cent of the carbon-14 was recovered as $^{14}CO_2$, 12 per cent was incorporated into the bacteria and 2 per cent remained in the culture media.[3] Levin, *et al.*

reported that the ^{14}C-formate substrate method for the detection of coliform was adequate for detecting bacterial concentrations in the range of 10^1 to 10^2 organisms/ml.[4]

The application of the radionuclides for the detection of microorganisms was investigated by means of liquid scintillation counting by DeLand and Wagner in 1968.[5] When bacteria were incubated (37°C) in a glucose-free thioglycolate medium with carbon-14 uniformly labeled glucose added, $^{14}CO_2$ was evolved by bacteria metabolism in quantities adequate for counting in a liquid scintillation detector system. The incubation time required for detectable levels of $^{14}CO_2$ was in the order of 8 to 12 hours. Incubation time was reduced 1 to 2 hours when the liquid media was agitated by means of a shaking incubator. Although the results were satisfactory, the amount of personnel time required was prohibitive for clinical applica-

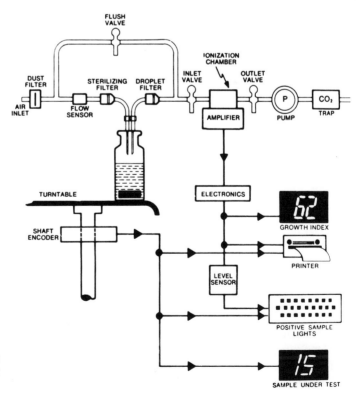

Fig. 26-1. Schematic diagram of the automated detector for radioactive gases.

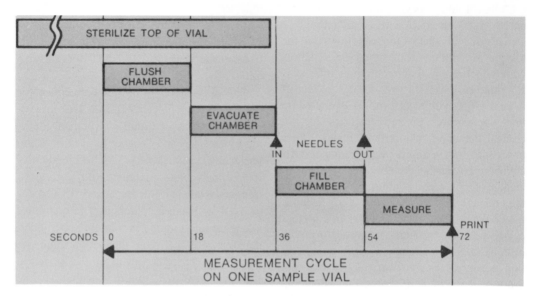

Fig. 26-2. Block diagram of the measurement cycle.

tion, and automation of the system appeared extremely difficult.

An ion chamber was substituted for the liquid scintillation detection system and the incubation vessel was connected by means of plastic tubing with the ion chamber in a closed system which was constantly perfused by a circulating pump. In preliminary trials 500 blood specimens from hospitalized patients were examined for possible bacteremia. Thirty of these specimens were found to be positive as indicated by the release of $^{14}CO_2$ from ^{14}C-U-glucose. By the routine bacteriologic methods, microorganisms were recovered from 26 of these specimens. As a result of this study a completely automated instrument was constructed for the purpose of detecting bacterial metabolism by means of the release of radioactive gaseous compounds from radioactively labeled substrates.

AUTOMATED BACTERIOLOGIC SYSTEM

The culture vessels are standard 50 ml vials with rubber caps. Any labeled substrate can be used in the system if a byproduct of bacteria metabolism is a radio-active volatile gas. In routine work, such as detection of bacteria in blood specimens, trypticase soy broth* or fluid thioglycolate with indicator is used.† Neither of these media contains glucose. To the culture media 1 μc of uniform label, ^{14}C-glucose is added. Each vial contains a bar magnet.

The instrumentation used for measuring the radioactive volatile by-products of bacterial metabolism is completely automated. Figure 26-1 is a diagram of the instrument and Figure 26-2 is a diagram of the cycling.‡ The component parts of the instrument are:

1. A "lazy-susan" tray that holds 25 culture vials and rotates for sequential sampling of the specimens.

2. A dual needle aspirating system, one for air intake and one for air exhaust from the culture vial.

3. Sterilization units for vial and needles.

---

* No. 11774 Trypticase Soy Broth BBL, Cockeysville, Md.

† No. 11724 Fluid Thioglycolate with Indicator, BBL, Cockeysville, Md.

‡ Bac Tec, Johnston Laboratories, Inc., Cockeysville, Md.

4. A circulating pump for purging the vial and instrument.

5. An ion chamber for measuring the amount of volatile radioactive gas released.

6. A rotating magnet system in each vial for agitation of the culture media.

7. An electromechanical system for sequentially sampling each vial.

8. An electronic component for measuring the radioactivity released and translating this to the display system.

Prior to sampling of a vial the first step is to sterilize the rubber stopper by exposing it to an intense ultraviolet light for 70 seconds. This occurs just before the turntable moves the vial into position under the twin needles. While the vial is moving into position, the air lines and ion chamber are flushed with clean room air to remove and trap any residual $^{14}CO_2$ from the previous sample vial. Air is sucked through all 3 valves (flush, inlet and outlet) and is cleansed by dust filters on the inlet port. After 18 seconds the inlet and flush valves close, but the circulating pump continues to run in order to lower the air pressure within the ionization chamber to approximately one-third of an atmosphere. After 36 seconds of the cycle the outlet valve closes and effectively isolates the ionization chamber, and at the same time the turntable advances one step moving the vial beneath the twin needles. The needles are driven down through the rubber stopper of the bottle; the inlet valve then opens causing air to rush through the inlet dust filter and into the culture vial sweeping any $^{14}CO_2$ present within the vial into the chamber. At 54 seconds the chamber pressure has returned to atmospheric, the inlet valve closes again, and the needles are withdrawn from the valve. Radioactivity is measured by the ionization chamber and an additional 18 seconds is allowed for the measurement to stabilize. The ionization chamber current is converted to a digital form and displayed by electronic register and print-out. If the radioactive

level exceeds a preset value, then an appropriate sample light is activated.

The instrument can be operated manually or automatically. In the automatic mode it can be programmed to sample each vial sequentially at 1- to 4-hour intervals. The chamber containing the culture vials is incubated at $37°C$ ($\pm$ 1). The culture media is continuously agitated by means of a bar magnet in each culture vial and a corresponding rotating bar magnet directly beneath each vial. Cross-contamination between vials is prevented by: (a) sterilization of the rubber stopper of the vials by means of an ultraviolet light, and (b) sterilization of the needles by means of a block heater. When the instrument is purged by room air, $^{14}CO_2$ and CO_2 are trapped in a soda lime vessel connected to the output of the circulating pump.

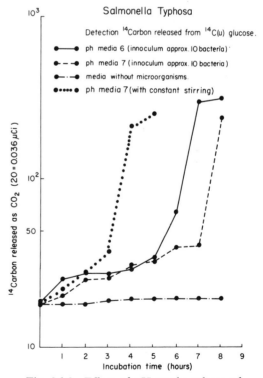

Fig. 26-3. Effect of pH on the release of $^{14}CO_2$ from cultures of *Salmonella typhosa* which contained uniformly labeled carbon-14 glucose.

CHARACTERISTICS OF THE $^{14}CO_2$ DETECTION SYSTEM

The $^{14}CO_2$ detection system depends upon the release of radioactive volatile gases from solution into the atmosphere above the culture media. Most frequently this gas is $^{14}CO_2$. The solubility of carbon dioxide in a solution with a pH of 5 or higher is 100 per cent and at a pH of 3 the solubility is still about 85 per cent. Since the pH culture media is 7.2, release of $^{14}CO_2$ from the liquid media is limited to surface exchange and is closely related to the concentration of carbon dioxide in the media and that in the atmosphere above the media. In order to enhance the exchange or release of carbon dioxide, pH of the culture media can be lowered but at those ranges, which enhance discharge of the CO_2 from the media, growth of bacteria is inactivated. Figure 26-3 illustrates the effect of lowering the pH of the media from 7 to 6. After an original inoculum of approximately 10 bacteria per cu ml, significant release of $^{14}CO_2$ occurs at 6 to 7 hours of incubation in a culture media with a pH of 7. The level of radioactivity at this time is approximately double that of the background (*horizontal curve*). When the pH of the culture media was reduced to 6 (*solid curve*), significant levels of $^{14}CO_2$ were obtained about 1 hour earlier, but the rate of bacterial growth was diminished. When the culture media were constantly agitated (as with the rotating magnetic bars), significant radioactive levels were detected at 3 hours with a culture media of pH 7 (*dotted curve*). Agitation of the media not only promotes a more rapid exchange of the radioactive CO_2 in the media with the non-radioactive CO_2 in the atmosphere above the media but also promotes more rapid bacterial growth.

Uniformly labeled ^{14}C-glucose was selected as the substrate of choice because nearly all bacteria utilize glucose in one or more metabolic pathways.[6] Figure 26-4 is a simplified diagram of glucose metabolic pathways used by bacteria. There are 2 major pathways both of which produce carbon dioxide as released by decarboxylation of the first carbon, and the metabolic product is ribose.

Figure 26-5 illustrates the first pathway release of $^{14}CO_2$ in a culture that contains *Staphylococcus aureus* from glucose molecules labeled in different positions.[7] The time-rate release of $^{14}CO_2$ from ^{14}C-D-glucose labeled in the 1 position only is similar to that released from uniformly labeled ^{14}C-D-glucose. The quantity of activity re-

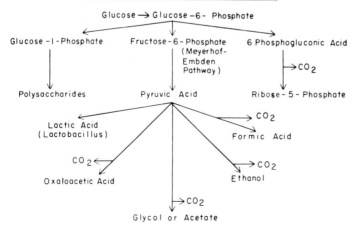

Fig. 26-4. Abbreviated diagram of metabolic pathways of glucose.

Fig. 26-5. The detection of carbon dioxide from cultures of *Staphlococcus aureus* which contained uniformly labeled carbon-14 glucose, or carbon-14 glucose labeled in the first carbon position or the sixth carbon position. (DeLand, F. H., and Cohen, M.: Antimicrob. Agents Chemother., 2:405, 1972)[7]

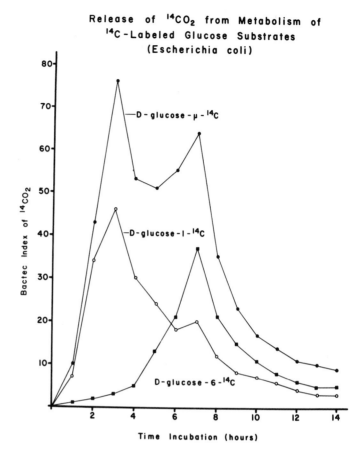

Release of $^{14}CO_2$ from Metabolism of ^{14}C-Labeled Glucose Substrates (Escherichia coli)

leased from each of these 2 substrates was about equal. But when ^{14}C-D-glucose labeled in position 6 only was incubated with *Staphylococcus aureus,* the level of radioactivity did not exceed background. A number of organisms were found to have this characteristic type of metabolic release of $^{14}CO_2$, and the quantity that was released varied between 16 and 18 per cent, indicating that one carbon was metabolized to $^{14}CO_2$.

The second major pathway for metabolism of glucose by bacteria is the Meyerhof-Embden pathway from glucose to pyruvate. Pyruvic acid may decompose through at least 5 major pathways with the release of CO_2 at several states (see Fig. 26-4). Figure 26-6 is an example of both the "pentose-shunt" pathway and the pyruvic-acid path-

way. When a culture media containing D-glucose-μ-^{14}C was inoculated with *Escherichia coli* (10^5 microorganisms per ml), $^{14}CO_2$ was first noted after 1 hour of incubation, peaked at 3 hours, and by 4 hours the level of radioactivity released was decreasing. However, by the fifth hour of incubation, the amount of radioactivity released was increasing again with a secondary peak of activity occurring at 7 hours. When *E. Coli* was inoculated in a culture media that contained D-glucose-1-^{14}C, the release of $^{14}CO_2$ corresponded to the first peak of activity observed with the ^{14}C uniformly labeled glucose. When *E. Coli* was inoculated in a culture media that contained D-glucose-6-^{14}C the release of $^{14}CO_2$ coincided with the secondary peak that was found with uniformly labeled glucose. When

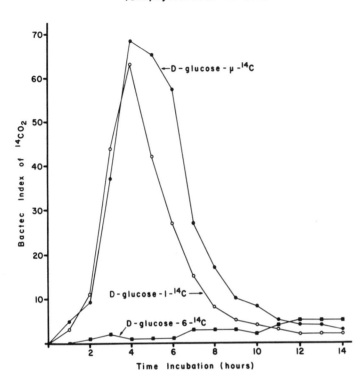

Release of $^{14}CO_2$ from Metabolism of ^{14}C-Labeled Glucose Substrates (Staphylococcus aureus)

Fig. 26-6. The detection of carbon dioxide from cultures of *Escherichia coli* which contained uniformly labeled carbon-14 glucose or carbon-14 glucose labeled in the first carbon position or the sixth carbon position. (DeLand, F. H., and Cohen, M.: Antimicrob. Agents Chemother., 2:405, 1972)[7]

glucose is metabolized by means of the Meyerhof-Embden pathway to pyruvic acid, the carbon-6 chain divides between carbons-3 and -4 into two 3-carbon atoms pyruvic acid. Decarboxylation of the pyruvic acid occurs at the carbon-1 position of one of the molecules and at carbon-6 position of the other half. The secondary peak seen with ^{14}C-labeled glucose at the carbon-6 position is the decarboxylation of carbon-6 which occurs after the split of the glucose molecule into pyruvic acid. Investigations with glucose labeled at either the third or fourth carbon did not reveal evidence of decarboxylation at those points.

The quantity of $^{14}CO_2$ released by bacterial metabolism can be enhanced, particularly for the more fastidious organisms, by adding radioactive-labeled amino acids that are also decarboxylated. Two common amino acids used for this purpose are ^{14}C-glycene and ^{14}C-alinine.

The total production of $^{14}CO_2$- from ^{14}C-labeled substrates is never measured in this automated detector. In order to utilize the system for procedures that require quantitation, such as the measurement of bacterial metabolism, the relative amount of CO_2 which is released to the atmosphere must be determined.

Figure 26-7 illustrates the result of the measurement of the amount of $^{14}CO_2$ that is sampled at each hour for 8 hours.[7] In order to determine the relative amount of $^{14}CO_2$, that is sampled at each period a series of culture vials containing one μc of ^{14}C-U-glucose was inoculated with *Escherichia coli*. The vials were sampled hourly for the re-

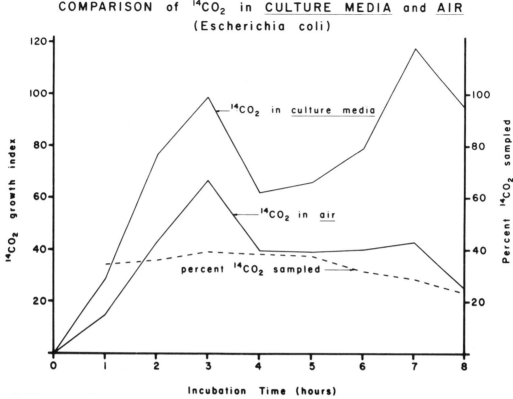

Fig. 26-7. The distribution of $^{14}CO_2$ in the culture media and air above the media from the metabolism of ^{14}C-U-glucose by *Escherichia coli*. (DeLand, F. H., and Cohen, M.: Antimicrob. Agents Chemother., 2:405,1972)[7]

lease of $^{14}CO_2$ and at each hour hydrochloric acid was added to 1 vial, reducing the pH to less than 1 and the solubility of carbon dioxide in the liquid media to nearly 0. This vial was immediately resampled several times in order to obtain the total amount of $^{14}CO_2$ which was in both the liquid media and the atmosphere. The dashed line represents the per cent of total $^{14}CO_2$ obtained from each vial by the first sampling during the first 8 hours of incubation. The relative amount of $^{14}CO_2$ which was detected by the ionization chamber was nearly constant during the first 5 hours of incubation, even though the level of decarboxylation varied markedly during this period. Since the fraction of $^{14}CO_2$ measured was relatively constant, quantitative results could be obtained.

BLOOD CULTURES

The detection of bacteremia by means of current microbiologic methods is usually not possible for 18 to 24 hours. Evaluation of blood cultures depends on visual assessment of turbidity, microscopic examination, and subculturing when the presence of bacteria is suspected. A not infrequent problem encountered in bacterial cultures is the death of fastidious organisms prior to visual evidence of bacterial growth. For example, *Diplococcus pneumoniae* may be lost in culture media before sufficient growth has occurred to produce a detectable turbidity. By the $^{14}CO_2$ method, these organisms were detected prior to visual evidence of growth and were recovered by early subculturing.[8]

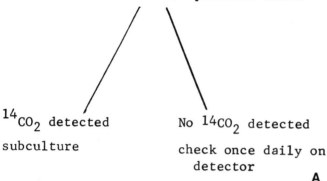

Fig. 26-8. *A*, Radiometric examination of blood cultures. *B*, Routine examination of blood cultures.

DAY 1

Inoculate culture vial with patients blood

$^{14}CO_2$ detected

subculture

No $^{14}CO_2$ detected

check once daily on detector

A

DAY 1

Inoculate culture vessel with patients blood

DAY 2

a. Visually inspect culture for growth
b. Subculture to appropriate solid media
c. Microscopic examination of smear from culture

DAYS 3 through 13

a. Visually inspect culture daily for growth
b. Subculture to appropriate solid media if suspicious
c. Microscopic examination of smear if suspicious

DAY 14

a. Visually inspect culture for growth
b. Subculture to appropriate media   **B**

Figure 26-8 illustrates the comparable efforts expended by the radiometric and routine methods for examining blood cultures.

DeBlanc, *et al.*[9] reported their results on the detection of bacteria in blood cultures. Of 2,967 cultures from 1,280 patients suspected of having bacteremia, they found that 138 cultures from 57 patients were positive by either the radiometric method or by the routine bacteriologic method, or by both. In 48 patients 111 cultures were positive radiometrically and in 50 patients 125 were posi-

tive by routine bacteriologic testing. Table 26-1 lists the organisms detected radiometrically and Table 26-2 lists those detected by the routine method. In 111 cultures from 48 patients that were positive by the radiometric method, bacterial growth was found in all by subcultures from the radiometric medium. Of these, the routine laboratory detected 98 cultures from 40 patients. Of 125 cultures found to be positive by routine laboratory methods, 102 were positive by the radiometric method and 23 were

Table 26-1. Organisms Detected by the Radiometric Method.

Organism	No. of Samples	No. of Patients
Pneumococcus	34	15
Staphylococcus aureus	23	9
Escherichia coli	12	4
Klebsiella	10	6
Beta streptococcus	6	3
Gonococcus	2	1
Pseudomonas	1	1
Hemophilus	1	1
S. epidermidis	2	1
S. aureus and *Klebsiella*	4	2
S. aureus and beta streptococcus	2	1
Proteus and *Streptococcus faecalis*	3	1
Yeast	11	3
Total	111	48

(DeBlanc, H. J., Jr., *et al.*: Appl. Microbiol., *22*:846, 1971)[9]

Table 26-2. Organisms Detected by Routine Techniques.

Organism	No. of Samples	No. of Patients
Pneumococcus	32	14
Staphylococcus aureus	20	7
Escherichia coli	15	5
Klebsiella	11	7
Beta streptococcus	5	2
Gonococcus	3	1
Pseudomonas	1	1
S. epidermidis	2	1
Streptococcus faecalis	1	1
Microaerophilic alpha-streptococcus	8	1
S. aureus and *Klebsiella*	4	2
S. aureus and beta streptococcus	4	2
Proteus and *S. faecalis*	3	1
α-Streptococcus	3	1
γ-Streptococcus	2	1
Yeast	11	3
Total	125	50

(DeBlanc, H. J., Jr., *et al.*: Appl. Microbiol., *22*:846, 1971)[9]

negative. No viable bacteria were found in the subcultures of 11 of the 23 negative cultures, suggesting that the organism may not have been present at the time or that original inoculation was due to sampling errors, since the volume of blood used by the conventional method is 5 to 10 times that used by the radiometric method (1-2 ml). Of the remaining 12 negative cultures by the radiometric method, a microaerophilic alpha streptococcus was subcultured from 8 of the specimens and all cultures were from the same person. In addition a gonococcus, a pneumococcus, and 2 mixed cultures containing *Staphylococcus aureus* and beta-hemolytic streptococcus were negative by the radiometric method. Most of the organisms not detected by the radiometric method are fastidious and require specific atmospheric conditions for growth. As a result of this investigation the culture media were enhanced with ^{14}C-labeled amino acids and a system for programming a specific atmosphere such as carbon dioxide was incorporated into the instrument.

The radiometric technique was found to be faster than conventional techniques for the detection of bacteremia (Fig. 26-9). Of the positive cultures 70 per cent were detected first by the radiometric method and 65 per cent of these were detected on the first day of inoculation; 24 per cent were detected by both methods at approximately the same time, and 6 per cent were detected first by routine bacteriological procedures. Only 4 per cent of the cultures detected by the routine method were positive on the day of inoculation.

In a similar comparative study Randall found that 83 per cent of blood specimens proved by subcultures to contain microorganisms were detected by the radiometric method, 78 per cent by routine bacteriologic examination and 49 per cent by the poor plate method.[10] She also observed that some of the microaerophilic streptococci were not detected, due to the use of room air as the atmosphere above the culture media, rather than to partial carbon dioxide.

lations of culture media were made with 10^1 to 10^9 organisms per ml. The cultures were placed in the automated $^{14}CO_2$ detector and the presence of $^{14}CO_2$ in each was evaluated hourly. For most of these organisms there is a similarity in the rate of metabolism and the original concentration of organisms. The main exception is the genus *Pseudomonas* which has a significantly slower initial metabolism for each of the different species. We studied a series of urine samples submitted to the laboratory for culture and found 281 positive cultures by the radiometric method. The routine and $^{14}CO_2$ culture procedures were initiated within 1 hour of each other.

The determination of the concentration of bacteria in urine by the radiometric method was based on a mean relationship between bacterial concentration and hours of incuba-

tion required for a significant level of $^{14}CO_2$. If significant $^{14}CO_2$ was detected within 2 hours the culture was given a value of 10^7 (10,000,000) concentration of organisms per ml at 3 hours 10^6 concentration, 10^4 at 6 hours, and 10^1 at 10 hours. Pseudomonas species were not included in the primary determination because of its slower metabolism.

Table 26-3 compares the results of colony counts by the routine bacteriologic method with those of the estimated bacterial concentration by the radiometric method. Identical colony counts were obtained by both procedures in 126 of 281 specimens (33%) and agreement within 1 order of magnitude was found in 191 of the procedures (68%).

In Table 26-3 the concentrations of bacteria, determined by the routine and $^{14}CO_2$ methods, that agreed within 1 order of mag-

Table 26-3. Concentration of Bacteria in 281 Urine Cultures.

Colony Counts by $^{14}CO_2$ Examination (bacteria/ml³)	0	10^0	10^1	10^2	10^3	10^4	10^5	$>10^5$
$>10^5$	1			1		12	20	43
10^5	6			1	3	10	8	
10^4	4			7	3	17		1
10^3	13			6	5	4		
10^2	9			5	7	1		
10^1	12			2	3	1		
10^0	13			1		2		1
0	48		2	7	1		1	

Colony Counts by Routine Examination (bacteria/ml³)

Fig. 26-12. The relationship between the release of $^{14}CO_2$ from the metabolism of ^{14}C-U-glucose and bacterial growth.

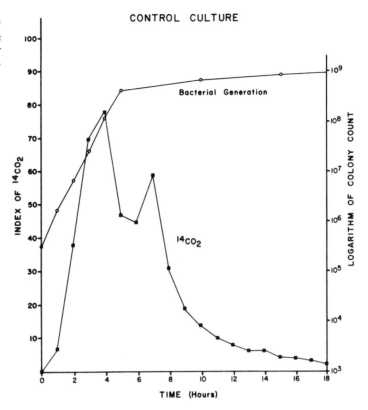

nitude are shown between the atair-step lines. Eleven cultures were found by routine examination to contain bacteria that were not detected by the radiometric procedure; however, in only 1 case (9%) was the concentration of bacteria significant. Surprisingly $^{14}CO_2$ was detected in 58 specimens that were positive by subsequent subculture but bacteria were not recovered by the routine bacteriological procedure. Seven of these cultures, 12 per cent of the 58 cases, produced a significant level of $^{14}CO_2$ not statistically different from the reverse findings (9%).

There are probably several explanations for the large number of positive cultures by $^{14}CO_2$ detection when the routine examination is negative: (a) the greater sensitive by radiometric detection (25 cultures with a concentration of 10^1 or less microorganisms per ml[3]), and (b) lesser incidence of loss of bacteria because of minimal concentration of

fastidious characteristics. It is significant that 11 specimens with 10,000 or greater organisms per ml[3] were detected by means of $^{14}CO_2$ production but were not recovered by routine bacteriologic procedures.

In a series of 156 positive bacterurias, Gaul found agreement between the radiometric method and the routine procedure in 149 of the cultures or 95 per cent. In 4 cases the radiometric gave false-negative results and all of these patients were on antibiotics. In 3 cases the radiometric method gave false-positive results.

MEASUREMENT OF BACTERIAL SENSITIVITY

DeLand and Cohen[7] developed a radiometric method for measuring the bacterial sensitivity to drugs and compared their results to the standard serial broth dilution tests.

Their procedure was based on the degree

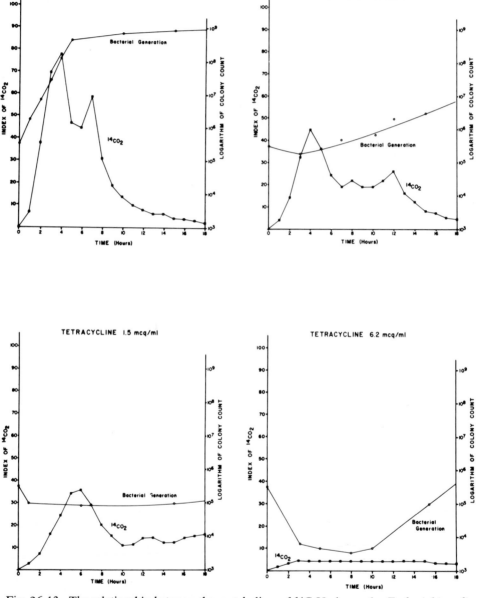

Fig. 26-13. The relationship between the metabolism of ^{14}C-U-glucose by *Escherichia coli* and bacterial growth. (DeLand, F. H., and Cohen, M.: Antimicrob. Agents Chemother., *2*:405, 1971)[7]

of inhibition of glucose metabolism in the presence of serial concentrations of antibiotics. Standard glucose-free media, which contained one μc of ^{14}C-U-glucose, was inoculated with 1 ml of broth culture containing 10^5 microorganisms per ml. To a series of these cultures was added serial dilutions of the antibiotics. The cultures were placed in the bacteriologic detector and sampled at 1-hour intervals for 24 hours. The quantity of ^{14}C-glucose available for bacterial metabolism is very limited (approximately 75 μg glucose). When the peak release of $^{14}CO_2$ from ^{14}C-U-glucose occurs (Fig. 26-12), the maximal rate of metabolism has been achieved for that particular metabolic pathway. This point occurs during the exponential phase of bacterial growth. After the peak $^{14}CO_2$ level is reached the rate of $^{14}CO_2$ production decreases, suggesting that the available glucose is now inadequate for an optimal rate of metabolism.

Since the postpeak period does not accurately reflect metabolic rate, it cannot be used for measuring drug effects on metabolism. Metabolic inhibition is measured only to the peak release of $^{14}CO_2$ and the total amount of gas released during that period is compared to a control. In order to determine the effect of drugs on glucose metabolism, control cultures without antibiotics were run with each investigation and the time of $^{14}CO_2$ peak release was considered as the end-point for optimal metabolism. The amount of $^{14}CO_2$ up to this time released by cultures containing antibiotics was compared to the amount of $^{14}CO_2$ released by the control culture.

Table 26-4 lists the microorganisms and antibiotics investigated. Each bacteria was tested against each of the antibiotics. Figure 26-13 illustrates the relationship between the bacterial generation of *E. coli* and glucose metabolism for several concentrations of tetracyclines. At a concentration of 0.8 μg/ml, bacterial growth was retarded but not

Table 26-4. Microorganisms and Antibiotics Investigated. (Each bacteria was tested against each of the antibiotics.)

Microorganisms	*Antibiotics*
Escherichia coli	Chloramphenicol
Staphylococcus aureus	Erythromycin
Proteus mirabilis	Kanamycin
Enterobacter	Streptomycin
Enterococci	Gentamicin
Pseudomonas	Penicillin G
α-Streptococcus	Ampicillin
β-Streptococcus	Cephalothin
	Colistin
	Tetracycline

inhibited. The amount of $^{14}CO_2$ released in 4 hours of incubation (peak release of $^{14}CO_2$ for control) was less than half that of the control.

These findings indicate that the metabolic systems affected by this group of drugs are particularly sensitive. Of particular significance is the ability of bacteria to escape from the effects of the drug after several hours of incubation, and to commence growth. Thus, for determining drug sensitivity by the serial tube dilution method, which is interpreted after 18 to 24 hours of incubation, tetracycline appears to have little effect on the microorganism. Even with higher concentrations of tetracycline (6.2 μg/ml), *E. coli* escaped the inhibiting effect of the antibiotic after 10 hours of incubation, even though this was preceded by a decrease in the number of viable bacteria. These findings suggest that there is not a direct one-to-one relationship between the radiometric method of determining bacterial sensitivity to drugs by inhibition of metabolism and the minimal inhibitory concentration found by the broth serial tube dilution system.

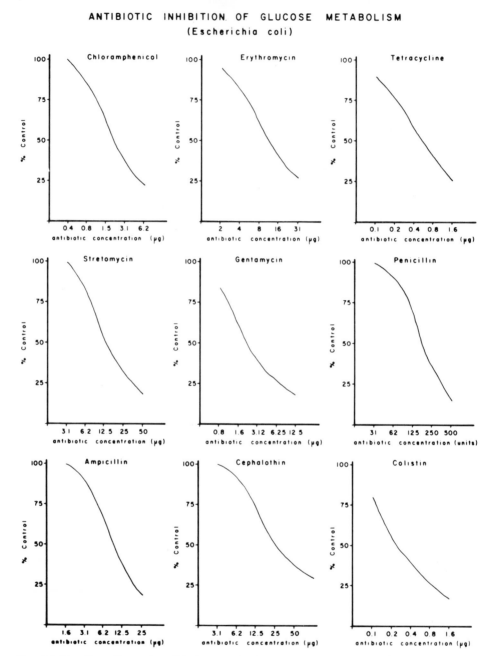

Fig. 26-14. The effect of antibiotics on the bacterial metabolism of ^{14}C-U-glucose by *Escherichia coli*. The response is expressed as a percent of the control culture.

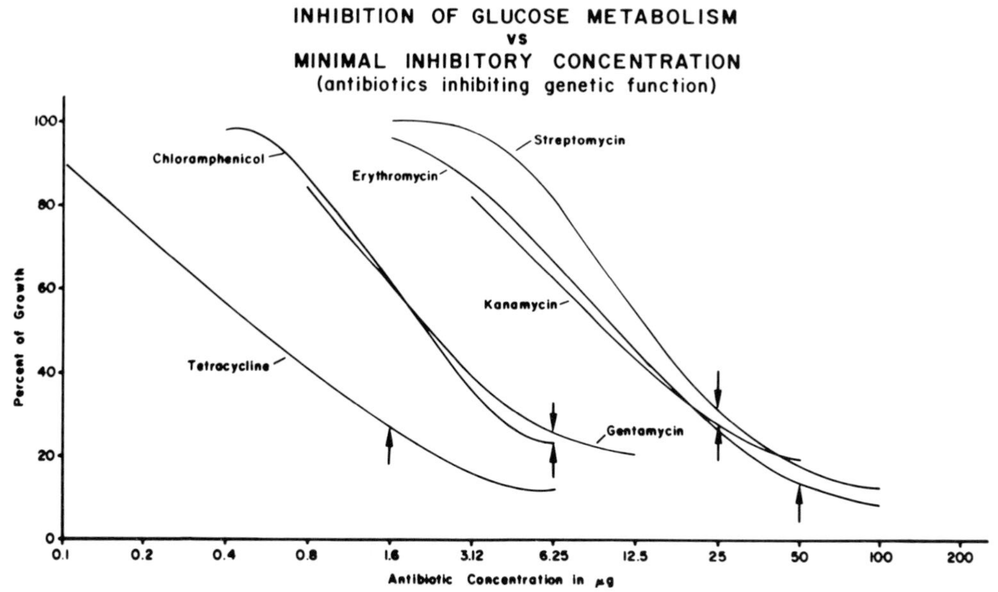

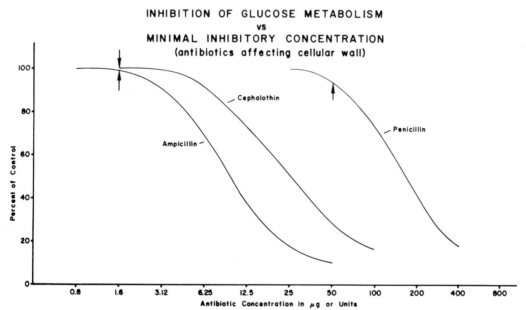

Fig. 26-15. A comparison of the inhibition of glucose metabolism by antibiotics which affect protein synthesis and the minimal inhibitory concentration (mic) by serial tube dilution method. The arrows indicate the mic for each antibiotic. (DeLand, F. H., and Cohen, M.: Antimicrob. Agents Chemother., *2*:405, 1971)[7]

Fig. 26-16. A comparison of the inhibition of glucose metabolism by antibiotics which affect cell walls and the minimal inhibitory concentration (mic) by serial tube dilution method. The arrows indicate the mic for each antibiotic. (DeLand, F. H., and Cohen, M.: Antimicrob. Agents Chemother., *2*:405, 1971)[7]

Figure 26-14 illustrates that the response of bacterial metabolism to different types of antibiotics is quite similar. However, there are differences between the antibiotic concentrations for inhibiting metabolism and those for inhibiting bacterial growth. The effect on glucose metabolism—of *Escherichia coli* by 6 antibiotics classified as those effecting protein synthesis and genetic function—is shown in Figure 26-15. The *arrows* indicate the concentration of each antibiotic required to produce a minimal inhibitory concentration by the serial tube dilution method. For those antibiotics that affect protein synthesis and genetic function, the antibiotic concentration required to inhibit bacterial growth produced marked inhibition of glucose metabolism (approximately 15% to 35% of normal). Whereas for those drugs that affect bacterial cell wall (Fig. 26-16) greater concentrations of antibiotics were required to inhibit glucose metabolism than to produce a minimal inhibitory effect by the serial tube dilution technique. For example, approximately 9 μg ampicillin/ml was required to reduce the release of $^{14}CO_2$ to 50 per cent of the control, whereas the minimal inhibitory concentration was found to be 1.6 μg/ml or about one-sixth the concentration. This indicates that greater concentration of drugs are required to affect glucose metabolism than to affect the cell wall. Table 26-5 compares the concentration of drugs required to produce a minimal inhibitory effect by the serial tube dilution technique with the amount of drug required to reduce glucose metabolism by 50 per cent by the radiometric method.

In the overall evaluation of a new procedure or methodology, cost factors must be considered. There are 2 radiometric instruments designed for use in microbiologic laboratories: (1) the nonautomated—for use in laboratories with a small volume of work and its cost is reasonable for the small institution; (2) the sophisticated automated system—that costs appreciably more but can be justified if the number of specimens is sufficiently large. It has been determined that if a laboratory processes 100 cultures per week,

Table 26-5. Bacterial Susceptibility to Antibiotics by Serial Broth Dilution Versus Inhibition of Glucose Metabolism.*

Antibiotic	*Escherichia Coli* $^{14}CO_2$	MIC	*Enterobacter* $^{14}CO_2$	MIC	*Pseudomonas Morganii* $^{14}CO_2$	MIC	*Staphylococcus Aureus* $^{14}CO_2$	MIC	*Enterococcus* $^{14}CO_2$	MIC	*Proteus Mirabilis* $^{14}CO_2$	MIC	*α-Hemolytic Streptococcus (Viridans)* $^{14}CO_2$	MIC	*Aerobacter Aerogenes* $^{14}CO_2$	MIC
Chloramphenicol	1.5	6.25	1.5	6.25	4	100	1.0	6.25	1.1	3.12	12.5	100	3.12	1.5	3.12	25
Erythromycin	10	50	30	312	30	156	0.03	0.2	0.035	0.4	175	390	0.025	0.025	45	250
Tetracycline	0.4	1.5	1.2	6.25	2.5	12.5	0.04	0.2	1.5	100	7	200	0.8	0.4	1.5	6.25
Streptomycin	12.5	25	3	6.25	12.5	100	1.2	12.5	125	400	4	12.5	50	25	1.6	6.25
Gentamicin	2	6.25	0.6	1.5	0.7	1.5	0.05	1.5	25	100	3.1	3.1	50	6.25	0.7	1.5
Kanamycin	9	25	2	6.25	12.5	100	0.6	6.25	60	200	3.1	25	75	100	3.1	6.25
Penicillin G	150	53	5,500	75,000	250	75,000	0.015	0.03	4.5	3.12	60	500	0.3	0.03	5,000	16,000
Ampicillin	9	1.5	1,200	1,600	40	800	0.015	0.05	0.6	0.8	8	50	0.025	0.025	100	500
Cephalothin	25	1.5	4,000	8,000	625	40,000	0.06	0.1	20	12.5	30	200	0.1	0.1	3,000	2,000
Colistin	0.4	3.12	0.8	3.12	0.5	3.12	75	800	1,600	6,250	1,600	6,250	2,400	730	1.5	12.5

* The minimal inhibitory concentration (MIC) is the lowest concentration of antibiotic (in micrograms) without evidence of bacterial turbidity or sedimentation. Concentration of antibiotic (in milligrams) by the $^{14}CO_2$ method is that concentration (in micrograms) required to attain a 50% reduction in glucose metabolism.

the costs of the automated Bac Tec system (including rental or amortization of the instrument) approximates the costs involved in the standard bacteriologic method. If the work load is 100 specimens per day, the cost of the $^{14}CO_2$ procedure per specimen is decreased by 50 per cent.

The basis for this radiometric methodology is the detection of gaseous by-products from the metabolism of substrates labeled with radionuclides. The possible applications are innumerable. For example, a d-xylose test has been developed to detect intestinal malabsorption and measures the release of $^{14}CO_2$ from ^{14}C-d-xylose excreted in the urine by means of metabolism from the inoculation of the urine with *Escherichia coli*. The advantages of measuring metabolic systems with radioactive-labeled substrates are: specificity, sensitivity, and simplicity.

References

1. Kinney, T. D., and Melville, R. S.: Automation and clinical laboratories. The Proceedings of a Workshop Conference. Lab. Invest., *16*:803, 1967.
2. Levin, G. V., Harrison, V. R., and Hess, W. C.: Preliminary report on a one-hour presumptive test for coliform organisms. Amer. J. Public Health, *46*:11, 1956.
3. Roberts, R. B., *et al.*: Studies of Biosynthesis in *E. coli*. Carnegie Inst. of Washington, Pub. No. 607, Washington, D. C. (Quoted from Levin, G. V., *et al.*, reference No. 2.)
4. Levin, G. V., Harrison, V. R., Hess, W. C., Helm, H. A., and Strauss, V. L.: Rapid bacteriological detection and identification. Second U.N. International Conference on the Peaceful Uses of Atomic Energy, *870*: 291, 1958.
5. DeLand, F. H., and Wagner, H. N., Jr.: Unpublished data.
6. Oginsky, E. L., and Umbreit, W. W.: An Introduction to Bacterial Physiology. ed. 2. San Francisco, W. H. Freeman & Co., 1959.
7. DeLand, F. H., and Cohen, M.: Metabolic inhibition as an index of bacterial susceptibility to drugs. Antimicrob. Agents Chemother., *2*:405, 1972.
8. DeLand, F. H., and Wagner, H. N., Jr.: Automated radiometric detection of bacterial growth in blood cultures. J. Lab. Clin. Med., *75*:529, 1970.
9. DeBlanc, H. J., Jr., DeLand, F. H., and Wagner, H. N., Jr.: Automated radiometric detection of bacteria in 2,967 blood cultures. Appl. Microbiol., *22*:846, 1971.
10. Randall, E. L.: Comparison of a Radiometric Method with Conventional Cultural Methods for Detection of Bacteremia. Presented at the American Society of Microbiology, Philadelphia, 1972.
11. DeBlanc, H. J., Jr., and Wagner, H. J., Jr.: Unpublished data.
12. Gaul, L.: Unpublished data.

27 *Future Pathways*

BENJAMIN ROTHFELD, M.D.

Prognostication in any field of endeavor is difficult at best. This is especially so in the rapidly moving field of Nuclear Medicine. As Will James said, "The present is the interface between the past and the future." From a pragmatic point of view it is essential that some attempt be made to predict the future.

In my opinion the future progress of Nuclear Medicine may be divided into three areas: more widespread use of tests already in use; introduction of new tests or increased sensitivity and specificity of tests already in use; and administrative and logistic problems.

MORE WIDESPREAD USE OF TESTS

There are already tests available to evaluate white cell functions in vitro.[1] By means of these tests both phagocytosis by white cells as well as their bactericidal capabilities may be assessed. Using these tests, persons with chronic granulomatous diseases of childhood may be diagnosed, and those with Chediak-Higashi disease, a disorder in which phagocytosis by white cells is impaired. With more widespread use of these tests, no doubt other diseases caused by disordered white cell function will also be delineated and diagnosed.

Another area in which there is already an assay which is not being widely applied is in the field of allergy. Here the radio-allergo-sorbent test (RAST) is a quantitative and qualitative measure of IgE. This test is done as a competitive protein-binding test and is in use as a research tool. It gives information similar to the Prausnitz-Küstner test in that they are both essentially measures of IgE. However, the Prausnitz-Küstner test has a disadvantage in that it involves injecting foreign serum into test individuals. The RAST test seems to correlate with the drop in the level of IgE during treatment for hay fever. It is specific for IgE for given allergens but is applicable only to a limited number of allergens so far. This test is expensive and time consuming.[2] Currently the NIH is trying to make this test more widely applicable and practical. All in all, it seems to have promise for following the anaphylactoid type of allergic disorder.

As the radioimmunoassay for triiodothyronine becomes simpler it may well become routine in diagnosing hyperthyroidism. There seem to be a significant number of cases of thyrotoxicosis with normal T-4 but elevated T-3 levels. It is essential to keep in mind that the T-3 test referred to here is not the T-3 resin test, but rather a test specific for triiodothyronine. Cases of T-3 thyrotoxicosis are for the most part diagnosed, when suspected, by indirect methods such as thyroid-suppression tests. As use of the T-3 radioimmunoassay becomes more widespread, it will be possible to diagnose these cases more readily. Additionally, as use of the T-4 by radioimmunoassay becomes more widespread, it may well replace the competitive protein-binding technique for assaying T-4 because of the immunoassay's greater inherent sensitivity.

The use of glucagon assay which now seems to have few clinical applications may become more widespread in time and so lead to a better understanding and control of diabetes. Apparently some diabetics do not suppress glucagon normally with rising glucose levels, and this may contribute to glucose intolerance. Reactive hypoglycemia, a somewhat controversial entity, may also become better understood with more widespread use of blood glucagon levels.

Additionally, the gastrointestinal hormones (i.e., gastrin, secretin, pancreozymin-cholecystokinin) apparently have very complex interrelationships. The exact details of the way they influence each other and modulate one another's actions will probably become more apparent as the assays for these various substances become more widely used. Prostaglandin assays may also help to explain the diarrhea which occurs with medullary carcinoma of the thyroid and other disorders.

Although the results using neutron activation analysis have been disappointing so far, possibly with more widespread use of this technique and better realization of the pitfalls inherent in it, new diseases may be discovered and new therapies for old diseases may be worked out. There is also the possibility of mass screening using this technique.

NEW TESTS AND IMPROVED EXISTING TESTS

Although there are in use various methods for measuring the different body compartments by means of radionuclides, they all have their imperfections. Undoubtedly, in time, better and simpler ways of measuring these various body compartments will be developed and they will be a great help in handling surgical and chronically ill patients.

Much the same situation exists regarding platelet and white cell tagging. With better methods of cell tagging, the basic difficulties in various disease entities will be understood much better.

The DU-suppression test, presently a research tool, is the best way for checking for folate deficiency. If this test can be simplified, the possibility of mass screening for folate deficiency in tissues will become possible and the question of the role of folate deficiency in various adult and congenital disorders elucidated.

With more sensitive and specific assays for FSH and LH, there can be better delineation of menstrual and other gonadal abnormalities. More specific urine tests will avoid the errors introduced by rapid fluctuation in blood levels. As assays for Gn-RH become more widely available, the ability to understand the normal physiology and the deviations in gonadal function will improve.

Most current tests for TSH do not have a lower limit of normal. It is of interest to note that in Chapter 15 of this book an assay is presented which represents a major step toward defining the lower limit of normal of TSH. However, 10 percent of normal controls also present with undetectable TSH levels. Use of the TRH-stimulation test is helpful in these cases. The refinements in this test will be helpful for the therapy of thyroid carcinoma and also subtle antithyroid effects of lithium can be picked up.

At this time the existence of the following, among other hypothalamic-releasing hormones, has been either proven or postulated: ACTH-RH, LH-RH, TRF, GH-RF and GH-IF. Assays for some of these substances are available and hopefully in the near future there will be assays for all of them. Once these assays become available numerous questions concerning hypothalamo-pituitary function will be elucidated.

Presently there is work by a number of investigators on tissue receptors using isotopic techniques. When use of these techniques becomes more widespread, we shall have a better understanding of various clinical entities. Receptors are more specific for biologic activity than immunoassay, since the latter often measures only fragments which may or may not have biologic activity. It is evident that assays for receptors will give better correlation with clinical findings than do radioimmunoassays.

Assuming the development of more sensitive assays for various hormones (e.g., thyroid hormones, androgens, estrogens, and cortical steroids) it will be possible to determine their tissue levels. Since tissue levels are the site of action of these substances, we will understand better what is going on both in the normal and abnormal state than we have been able to with only blood levels of these substances. Just as plasma levels of various substances have often given us a much clearer picture of a person's clinical state than urine levels do, so tissue levels will prove to be more accurate. Actually, the transition from urine to plasma to tissue levels of various substances has depended on the sensitivity of the techniques used in measuring these substances.

With better measurements of various hormones involved in pregnancy, it will be possible to improve the monitoring of fetal well-being. At present a single test of HPL is of limited diagnostic value, so that it is necessary to do 2 or more over a period of several days. Further, the understanding of normal and abnormal pregnancies will become clearer.

With the development of more specific antibodies for androgens the necessity for chromatography, extraction and other tedious steps will lessen. Thus, use of assays for specific androgens will become more widespread.

With more specific tests it should become possible to distinguish between ectopic and primary parathyroid overactivity. It will then be possible to avoid expensive and difficult work-ups to rule out extraparathyroid causes of hypercalcemia. It may also become possible with highly specific assays to distinguish between molecules with similar biologic activity but different molecular structure. Thus, a distinction between the hormone produced by a parathyroid adenoma and parathyroid hyperplasia may become possible.

It is also possible that a more sensitive test for calcitonin will be developed which will enable the detection of values in the normal range. Such a test will enable us to understand some abnormalities of bone metabolism better.

The current carcinoembryonic antigen (CEA) test is the most widely used radioimmunoassay for tumor. However, in my opinion this test is but a start in the problem of first picking up tumors and distinguishing them from inflammatory processes. It is hoped that more specific tests will be developed and become available for screening purposes—the dream of clinicians for many years. However, the CEA test does seem to be a step in this direction.

As has been mentioned in various chapters of this book, many of the peptide hormones—gastrin, parathormone, glucagon, growth hormone and ACTH—exist in several forms. It is not certain exactly what the roles of these various forms of given hormones are, but they will undoubtedly be determined. For instance, better understanding of the various forms of gastrin in the body will help us diagnose Zollinger-Ellison syndrome as well as increase our understanding of peptic ulcer.

Additionally, just as the Australia antigen serves as a marker for serum (long incubation) hepatitis, before long we hope to have a similar marker for infectious (short incubation) hepatitis.

Finally, there seem to be definite possibilities for serum drug assays using isotopic techniques, probably by enzymatic methods. Currently, there is some promise of such techniques for assaying gentamycin and kanamycin.[3]

PROBLEMS FACING NUCLEAR MEDICINE LABORATORIES

In our field of In Vitro Nuclear Medicine as in any other field in which there is a large amount of data to be handled, computer processing and filing of results seem inevitable in the near future. These steps seem to be necessary to keep us from being overwhelmed with paperwork.

Another area in which changes seem to be underway is that of certification of products.

More and more laboratories are using kits to meet their needs in the field of radioimmunoassay. Many manufacturers have taken great pains to insure the accuracy, sensitivity and reproducibility of their results. However, there seems to be a real need for a federal role in this area. For most Nuclear Medicine laboratories, evaluation of kits is a matter of great difficulty. At the present time (May, 1974) the Bureau of Biologics, Food and Drug Administration has approved only 2 kits: the Carcino-Embryonic Antigen* (CEA) kit and the HAA† kit. According to this agency, their future plans to approve such kits are contingent upon a submission by manufacturers of adequately documented license applications.[4] There is a definite

---

* Trademark, Hoffman-LaRoche.
† Trademark, Abbott.

possibility that other kits involving hepatitis-associated antigen may be approved in the future. As this field grows, there will probably be more and more efforts by manufacturers to secure FDA approval for their kits and indeed in certain areas this might become mandatory.

References

1. Root, R.: Studies of leukocyte function. Course on In Vitro Nuclear Medicine. Johns Hopkins Hospital, November, 1972.
2. Frick, O. L.: Personal communication.
3. Leitman, P.: Course on In Vitro Nuclear Medicine. Johns Hopkins Hospital, November, 1972.
4. Barker, L. F.: Personal communication with Director, Division of Blood and Blood Products, Bureau of Biologics, Food and Drug Administration.

Index

Page numbers in *italics* indicate illustrations; "t" indicates tabular matter; "n" indicates a footnote.